INFORMATION PROCESSING IN MEDICAL IMAGING

INFORMATION PROCESSING IN MEDICAL IMAGING

Proceedings of the 8th conference, Brussels, 29 August–2 September 1983

edited by

F. DECONINCK, PhD

Department of Nuclear Medicine
Vrije Universiteit Brussel
Brussels, Belgium

1984 **MARTINUS NIJHOFF PUBLISHERS**
a member of the KLUWER ACADEMIC PUBLISHERS GROUP
BOSTON / THE HAGUE / DORDRECHT / LANCASTER

Distributors

for the United States and Canada: Kluwer Academic Publishers, 190 Old Derby Street, Hingham, MA 02043, USA
for the UK and Ireland: Kluwer Academic Publishers, MTP Press Limited, Falcon House, Queen Square, Lancaster LA1 1RN, England
for all other countries: Kluwer Academic Publishers Group, Distribution Center, P.O. Box 322, 3300 AH Dordrecht, The Netherlands

Library of Congress Cataloging in Publication Data

```
Main entry under title:

Information processing in medical imaging.

  "Information Processing in Medical Imaging Conference"
--Foreword.
  Includes bibliographies.
  1. Diagnosis, Radioscopic--Data processing--Congresses.
2. Imaging systems in medicine--Data processing--
Congresses.  I. Deconinck, F.  II. Information
Processing in Medical Imaging Conference (8th : 1983 :
Brussels, Belgium)  [DNLM: 1. Diagnosis, Computer
Assisted--congresses.  2. Nuclear Magnetic Resonance--
congresses.  3. Radiography--congresses.  4. Radionuclide
Imaging--congresses.  5. Technology, Radiologic--
congresses.  WN 200 I43 1983]
RC78.A2I5  1984      616.07'5'02854      84-1121
```

ISBN-13: 978-94-009-6047-3   e-ISBN-13: 978-94-009-6045-9
DOI: 10.1007/ 978-94-009-6045-9

Copyright

FOREWORD

The Information Processing in Medical Imaging Conference is a biennial conference, held alternatively in Europe and in the United States of America. The subject of the conference is the use of computers and mathematics in medical imaging, the evaluation of new imaging techniques, image processing, image analysis, diagnostic decision making and related fields. The conference brings together the top specialists in the field (both scientists and medical doctors) and other participants doing active research on the subject of the conference.

The success of a meeting primarily depends on the enthusiasm of the participants. It also greatly depends on the financial support as well as on the personal efforts of the technical staff and collaborators of the organizers. To all who made this conference a success, the members of the organizing committee want to express their sincere thanks.

In particular, the organizers want to acknowledge the help received from:

De Vice-Voorzitter van de Vlaamse Executieve
De Minister van Onderwijs
Het Nationaal Fonds voor Wetenschappelijk Onderzoek
De Vrije Universiteit Brussel

Adac
Agfa-Gevaert
Bruker Spectrospin
Byk Belga
Elscint
Instituut voor Radioelementen, IRE
Nucleobel
Solco
Sonotron

TABLE OF CONTENTS

Foreword.   V

A. VENOT, J.L. GOLMARD, J.F. LEBRUCHEC, L. PRONZATO, E. WALTER, G. FRIJA and
J.C. ROUCAYROL:
        "Digital Methods for Change Detection in Medical Images".   1

E.A. GEISER, L.H. OLIVER, L.F. ZHANG, K.J. FU, D.D. BUSS, C.R. CONTI:
        "An Approach to Endocardial Boundary Detection from
        Sequential Real Time Two-dimensional Echocardiographic
        Images: Status of the Algorithm and its Validation".   17

K.S. NIJRAN, D.C. BARBER:
        "Analysis of Dynamic Radionuclide Studies Using Factor
        Analysis - a new approach".   30

G. KONSTANTINOW, S.M. PIZER, R.H. JONES:
        "Decontamination of Crosstalk in First-Pass Radionuclide
        Angiocardiography".   46

Y. BIZAIS, R.W. ROWE, I.G. ZUBAL, G.W. BENNETT, A.B. BRILL:
        "Coded Aperture Tomography Revisited".   63

M. DEFRISE, C. DE MOL:
        "Resolution Limits for Full- and Limited-Angle
        Tomography".   94

H.H. BARRETT, H.B. BARBER, P.A. ERVIN, K.J. MYERS, R.G. PAXMAN, W.E. SMITH,
W.J. WILD, J.M. WOOLFENDEN:
        "New Directions in Coded Aperture Imaging".   106

A. TODD-POKROPEK, G. CLARKE, R. MARSH:
        "Preprocessing of SPECT Data as a Precursor for
        Attenuation Correction".   130

M.O. LEACH, W.D. FLATMAN, S. WEBB, M.A. FLOWER, R.J. OTT:
        "The Application of Variable Median Window Filtering
        to Computerised Tomography".   151

B.E. OPPENHEIM, C.R. APPLEDORN:
        "ART vs. Convolution Algorithms for ECT".   169

E. TANAKA, H. TOYAMA:
        "A Generalised Weighted Backprojection
        Algorithm for SPECT".   185

J. DUVERNOY, J.C. CARDOT, M. BAUD, J. VERDENET, XIA YUNG, P. BERTHOUT, R.
FAIVRE, J.P. BASSAND, R. BIDET, J.P. MAURAT:
        "Application of Linear Classifiers to the Recognition of
        the Temporal Behavior of the Heart".   202

A.S. HOUSTON, M.A. MACLEOD:
"A Comparative Review of Methods of Obtaining Ampl./Phase
and Related Images for Gated Cardiac Studies".   223

N.J.G. BROWN, S.R. UNDERWOOD, S. WALTON, P.H. JARRITT, M.A. SEIFALIAN, P.J.
LAMING:
"Rapid Automatic Functional Imaging of the Heart and the
Application of Time Images".   238

D.G. PAVEL, P.A. BRIANDET, R.B. FANG, K. ZOLNIERCZYK, J. SYCHRA:
"The Normal Heart: Patterns for Various Functional Images
Obtained from Radionuclide Gated Equilibrium Studies".   250

S.L. BACHARACH, M.V. GREEN, D. VITALE, G. WHITE, M.A. DOUGLAS, R.O. BONOW,
A.E. JONES, S.M. LARSON:
"Fourier Filtering Cardiac Time Activity Curves:
Sharp Cutoff Filters".   266

R. LUYPAERT, A. BOSSUYT:
"Data Processing in Nuclear Ventriculography: Assessing
Cardiac Function from Noisy Data".   282

M.L. GORIS:
"The Definition of a Single Measure of Regional Wall
Motion Abnormality in Scintigraphic Ventriculography".   299

A. TOET, J.J. KOENDERINK, P. ZUIDEMA, C.N. DE GRAAF:
"Image Analysis - Topological Methods".   306

C.N. DEGRAAF, A. TOET, J.J. KOENDERINK, P. ZUIDEMA, P.P. VANRIJK:
"Some Applications of Hierarchical Image Processing
Algorithms".   343

J.C. SOMER, F.H.M. JONGSMA:
"Acousto-Optic Deconvolution System for Real-Time
Echography".   370

D.A. ORTENDAHL, R.S. HATTNER, E. BOTVINICK, L. KAUFMAN, W. O'CONNELL, D.
FAULKNER, L.T. KIRCOS:
"A Bayesean Algorithm for Resolution Recovery in
Clinical Nuclear Medicine".   392

P. SCHMIDLIN, J.H. CLORIUS:
"Discriminant Analysis of Exercise Renograms".   408

M. GORIS, E. GORDON, D. KIM:
"A Stochastic Interpretation of Thallium
Myocardial Perfusion Scintigraphy".   421

C.E. METZ, P. WANG, H.B. KRONMAN
   "A New Approach for Testing the Significance of
   Differences Between ROC Curves Measured from
   Correlated Data".   432

D.C. BARBER, B.H. BROWN, I.L. FREESTON:
   "Imaging Spatial Distributions of Resistivity Using
   Applied Potential Tomography - APT".   446

S.K. CLAYTON, S. ANGHAIE, A.M. JACOBS:
   "An Uncollimated Compton Profile Method for Determination
   of Osteoporotic Changes in Vertebral Bone Density
   and Composition".   463

D.A. ORTENDAHL, N.M. HYLTON, L. KAUFMAN, L.E. CROOKS:
   "Automated Tissue Characterization with NMR Imaging".   477

T. SANDOR, D.P. HARRINGTON, L. BOXT, W.B. HANLON:
   "Zonal Parametric Imaging".   494

S.M. PIZER, H. FUCHS, E.R. HEINZ, E.V. STAAB, E.L. CHANEY, J.G. ROSENMAN, J.D.
AUSTIN, S.H. BLOOMBERG, E.T. MacHARDY, P.H. MILLS, D.C. STRICKLAND:
   "Interactive 3D Display of Medical Images".   513

B. BAXTER, C. BLACKBURN, R. NORMANN:
   "Can We Predict Visual Performance Using a Model
   of the Human Eye?".   527

R.F. WAGNER, D.G. BROWN:
   "Unified Analysis of Medical Imaging System
   SNR Characteristics".   544

List of addresses.   561

Proceedings of previous IPMI conferences.   580

DIGITAL METHODS FOR CHANGE DETECTION IN MEDICAL IMAGES

A. VENOT, J.L. GOLMARD, J.F. LEBRUCHEC, L. PRONZATO, E. WALTER, G.FRIJ.
and J.C. ROUCAYROL

FR Synthèse et Analyse d'Images Médicales and Service d'Exploration
Fonctionnelle par les Radioisotopes, Hopital Cochin, Paris.
INSERM U194, Pitié-Salpétrière, Paris.
Laboratoire des Signaux et Systèmes, CNRS-ESE, Gif sur Yvette
Service de Radiologie, Hopital Ambroise Paré, Boulogne.

1. INTRODUCTION

The detection and visualisation of the changes between two images is
the basis or the goal of several imaging techniques. Thus, digitized
subtraction angiography consists in visualizing the differences between
two images obtained without and with iodine contrast, intravenously injected. In Nuclear Medicine, the comparison of two scintigraphic images
of the same organ explored under varying conditions (images acquired at
different times, with different tracers, after various physiological or
pharmacological interventions) is a routine problem. The visual comparison of the images is often a difficult task for the following reasons:
The differences can be too low to be visually identified. In certain types
of images, there are normal statistical fluctuations which can mask or
simulate a difference. The gray level intensities can be different in
the images which must be first normalized. Therefore, it seems reasonable
to use the capacities of a computer and the knowledge about the count fluctuations to perform an automated comparison of the images. Better performances than those given by the visual inspection can be expected from such
a procedure. To form this comparison, it is necessary to first register
the images (alignment, normalization, magnification,...) (1,2,3,4,5) and
second detect the changes by analyzing the images point by point (6,7).

In this paper, we propose original methods which are well suited for
the successive registration and statistical comparison of images, with
applications in X and Gamma ray imaging techniques.

2. STUDY OF THE REGISTRATION STEP

2.1. The choice of a similarity measure

The registration step is usually performed by optimizing a similarity measure with respect to the registration parameters. For the registration of similar images, three particular similarity measures are representative of those used in the algorithms of interest (1,3): The correlation coefficient CC, the correlation function CF and the sum of the absolute values of the differences SAVD. These criteria are defined as follows. Consider two images $F_1(i,j)$ and $F_2(i,j)$ of the same object (i,j=1,2,..n are the coordinates of the digitized image) and a window in image $F_2(i,j)$ i and j varying respectively from m to o and p to q. One has the expressions:

$$CC= \frac{N^2 \sum \sum F_1(i,j).F_2(i,j)-\left[\sum \sum F_1(i,j)\right]\left[\sum \sum F_2(i,j)\right]}{\left[N^2 \sum \sum F_1^2(i,j)-(\sum \sum F_1(i,j))^2\right]\left[N^2 \sum \sum F_2^2(i,j)-(\sum \sum F_2(i,j))^2\right]}$$

$$CF=\sum \sum F_1(i,j).F_2(i,j)$$

$$SAVD=\sum \sum |F_1(i,j)-F_2(i,j)| \qquad \text{with } N=(o-m)(q-p)$$

Using these similarity measures for the registration of dissimilar images can lead to a misregistration (10). Therefore we have developed a new class of similarity measures whose optimization with respect to the registration parameters permits robust registration procedures (8,9,10). This new class is derived from non parametric statistical considerations (11,12) sometimes used in the field of mathematical modeling. Two cases must be distinguished a stochastic and a deterministic one. When the noise level in the images is far greater than the digitization precision, the similarity measure called the stochastic sign change criterion (SSC) is defined as the number of sign changes in the sequence of the values of the subtraction image $D(i,j)=F_1(i,j)-F_2(i,j)$ scanned line by line or column by column. The SSC criterion has useful statistical properties. In the case of similar images, the asymptotic SSC criterion density function is normal with a mean and a variance respectively equal to $N/2 - 1$ and $N/4$ (10,12). This distribution permits to derive a 95% interval of confidence for the SCC criterion: $\frac{N}{2} -1 \pm 2. \sqrt{N/4}$. This criterion was succesfully used for the registration of very dissimilar scintigraphic images (8,9,10) when classical methods had led to wrong registration parameter values. The optimized SSC criterion value (in the case of similar images) must be in the range of the interval of confidence. This is useful to determine (i) if the assumptions concerning the noise are valid (additive, zero mean with a symmetric density function), (ii) if the set of transformations proposed for the registration can lead to a correct registration. When the noise level is low (under the precision of the digitization), the SSC criterion value becomes null and therefore cannot be considered as a similarity criterion. Such assumptions are valid for subtraction angiography images where the signal to noise ratio reaches values of 400 which are very high compared with the precision due to an 8 bit depth coding(13). In this deterministic case, we have proposed an other criterion called the deterministic sign change criterion (DSC) which is defined as the number of sign hanges in the sequence of the values of a new subtraction image :

$D(i,j)= F_1(i,j)-F_3(i,j)$ scanned line by line or column by column with:
$F_3(i,j)= F_2(i,j) + q$ if $i + j$ is even
$F_3(i,j)= F_2(i,j) - q$ if $i + j$ is odd
q is a smal real or integer value.

In the case of similar images, if there are N pixels, the DSC criterion value is N-1 (10). This criterion remains maximum for the right registration parameter values even when large disparities exist in the images to compare (the classical methods leading to wrong values of the registration parameters (10)). Therefore we propose to use this method for the registration of subtraction angiography images to correct for patient motions. If such a displacement occurs during the investigation, the images with contrast medium must be registered prior to their subtraction from those without contrast medium.

2.2. Example of application

An application of this new class of similarity measure in controlled conditions is illustrated by Fig. 1 where digitized subtraction angiography images are shown. Fig. 1a is a 512X512 image obtained before the arrival of the contrast medium during a carotid angiography (no displacement of the patient occured during this investigation). The figured zone corresponds to a 128X128 area which was selected for the calculations because it contained much contrast medium at the angiographic times.

4

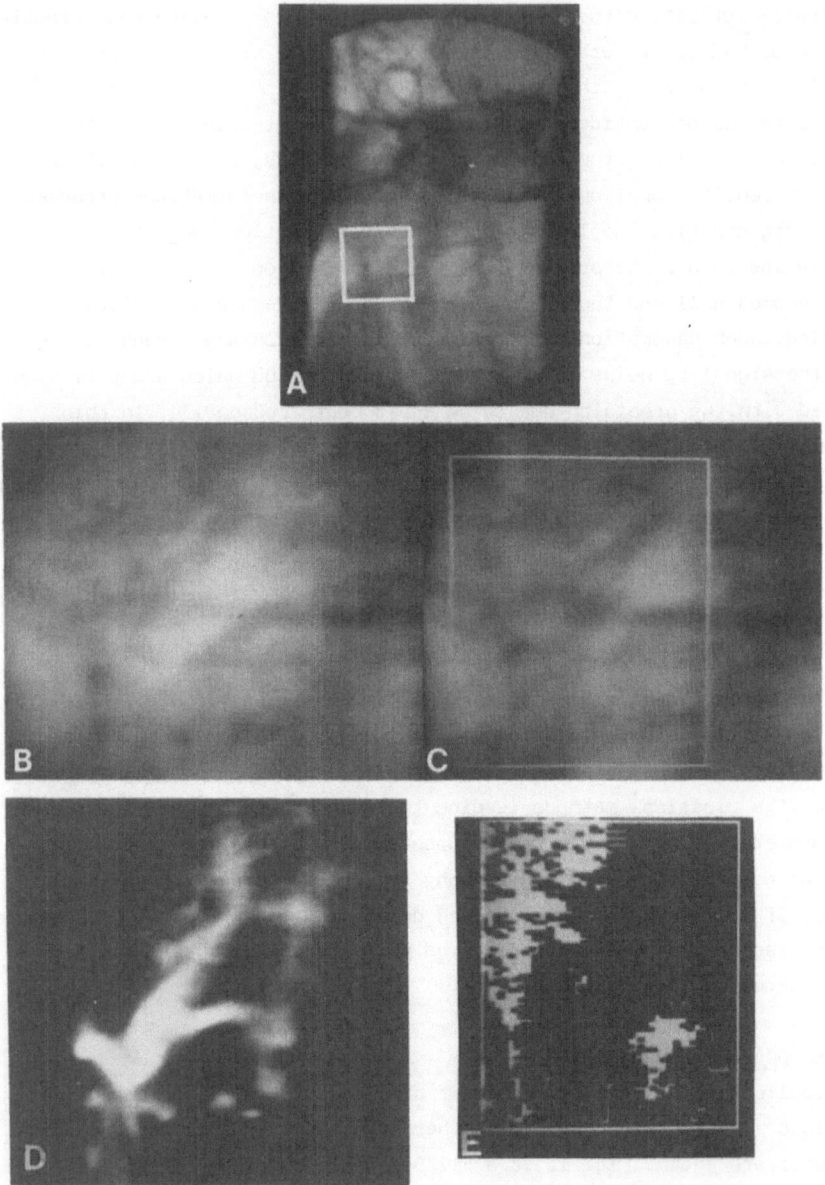

FIGURE 1. a) 512X512 carotid angiography image. b) 128X128 zone of image la without contrast medium. c) Same zone with contrast medium. d) Subtraction image of this zone. e) Sign change image in this zone.

This area is shown without (Fig.1b) and with (Fig.1c) contrast medium.
Fig 1d is the subtraction image corresponding to pure vascular structures.
In Fig. 1c a periodic pattern +1,-1,+1,-1,+1... was added for the calculation of the DSC criterion. In the 6660 pixel area figured in image 1c,
the DSC criterion was found equal to 1529. The repartition of the sign
changes in the subtraction image (see 2-1) is illustrated by Fig. 1e
(white corresponds to a sign change and black to none). This image would
be completely white if the images to compare were similar and the DSC
criterion value would be 6659. When image 1c is translated along the
horizontal axis, the DSC, CC, CF and SAVD criteria were found optimum
for respectively 0, 3, -10 and 1 pixel translations. This illustrates
the robustness of the registration method using the DSC criterion. It is
the only one to provide a correct value of the translationnal shift while
the other criteria are optimum for wrong values of the shift.

2.3. THE AUTOMATED OPTIMIZATION OF THE SIMILARITY MEASURE

2.3.1. The registration parameters. The registration step is performed
by optimizing (maximizing or minimizing) a similarity measure with respect to the registration parameters p. These ones depend on the suspected
transformations which can lead to a correct registration. The most currently used transformations in Radiology and Nuclear Medicine are:

-Normalization: $F_1(i,j)= NF. F_2(i,j)$ NF is the normalization
factor. It takes into account the changes of exposure in Radiology (assuming a linear relationship between the exposure and the gray level value
(13)). In Nuclear Medicine, it permits to correct for the changes in the
injected activity, acquisition time, length of the spectrometric window,
detection efficiency and for the radioactive decay(8).

-Translation: $F_1(i,j)= F_2(i+\Delta i,j+\Delta j)$ where Δi and Δj are the
translational shifts. In subtraction angiography the movement of a patient
which occurs during the arrival of the contrast medium can often be considered as a strict translation. This corresponds in Nuclear Medicine to
the case of scintigraphic studies when the repositioning of the patient is
necessary(5).

-Rotation: $F_1(i,j)=F_2(i',j')$. The location of the pixel i, j
after it has been rotated by an angle ϕ around a point (i_0,j_0) is (i',j')
defined by the two equations: $i'=i_0+(i-i_0).\cos\phi-(j-j_0)\sin\phi$
$$j'=j_0+(i-i_0).\sin\phi+(j-j_0)\cos\phi$$

The details of the calculations are given in (14).

Other transformations can be considered especially in Nuclear Medicine, such as a magnification, when the acquisition of two scintigraphies has been carried out with two different scintillation cameras. Double tracer studies can necessitate the addition of an unknown background for registration. It could be useful to correct for the geometric distorsions and inhomogeneities induced by the different locations of the radioactive organs in the field of the camera.

2.3.2. <u>The choice of an optimization method</u>. The optimization theory had a great developement(15) and a lot of methods are available to minimize a function (the negatived similarity measure) with respect to several parameters (the registration parameters). The choice of a method must be considered in terms of efficiency and speed.

The problem of the minimization of a criterion with respect to only one parameter is easily solved by the use of a unidimensional method such as the Fibonacci or the golden section (if the function to minimize is unimodal in the search interval). In this context, the Fibonacci method (15, 16) was succesfully used (8) to automatically normalize scintigraphic images.

When one wants to minimize a criterion with respect to several parameters, the most commonly used algorithms proceed by iterative global refinements. At each iteration k, they start from a point p^k in the parametric space, associated to a value c^k of the criterion and try to find a point p^{k+1} in the neighborhood of p^k such that $c^{k+1} < c^k$. If the criterion is sufficiently regular, expansion of the criterion in Taylor series around p^k can be used to produce efficient algorithms which converge to a local minimum of the criterion(15). When the criterion is unimodal, this minimum is also a global minimum and such a procedure is satisfactory.

For the minimization problem considered in this paper, the situation is different because (i) the criterion may be multimodal and (ii) the criterion is not differentiable with respect to the parameters. Among the many methods (17) which have been proposed for a global approach of optimization, a good number have to be eliminated because they require an evaluation of the gradient of the criterion with respect to the parameters to be available (17), or because they are so complex that they cannot be used for problems with more than two parameters. We were thus, naturally conducted to a random search approach. The basic idea is as follows. At each iteration k, a vector $\lambda \mu^k$ is generated according to some suitably chosen probability density function and an intermediary parameter value is obtained by: $x^k = p^k + \lambda \mu^k$ (λ is a real value). The next parameter value is:

$$p^{k+1} = x^k \text{ if } C(x^k) < C(p^k) \text{ and}$$
$$p^{k+1} = p^k \text{ if } C(x^k) \geqslant C(p^k) .$$

When $\lambda \mu^k$ is small enough, the parameters converge to the nearest local minimum of the criterion, whereas for higher values of $\lambda \mu^k$ attempts are made to reach the domain of attraction of a better minimum. Therefore, most algorithms combine several values of λ to alternate local and global searches. it can be shown that such a procedure converges in probability to the global minimum of the criterion. This result is valid only when the number of iterations tends to infinity and the speed of convergence highly depends on various choices made during the implementation of the algorithm, so that many of the algorithms proposed in the litterature depend upon the particular tunings selected. We have tried to avoid the necessity of such tunings and our algorithm is only provided with the rules for the calculations of the criterion and with the domain of the parametric space to be explored. Several ideas of the litterature have been combined (18,19) which allow some self tuning of the algorithm. The resulting program has been tested on several test cases of the litterature as well as on realistic problems of control theory. It has proven to be extremely efficient. For the registration of images, the calculations were carried out on a classical Nuclear Medicine data processing system[*] connected with an array processor[**].

The SSC or DSC criteria were calculated by the array processor at each iteration, but the global random search program was written in Fortran and implemented on the minicomputer of the system. This program was successfully tested on practical problems in controlled conditions corresponding to the minimization of the criteria with up to four parameters (the normalization factor, the translations along the vertical and horizontal axis, the addition of a background). Convergence was achieved after approximatively 1000 calculations of the criterion and the total duration of this registration step required approximatively one minute. Lower calculation times were sufficient (20 seconds) when only normalization and

* IMAC 7300, CGR Médecine Nucléaire(French version of ADAC system 1) .
**AP120B,Floating Point System.

translations were considered. It must be emphasized that there is absolutely no limitation to increase the number of the registration parameters
(adding of a rotation,..) in this minimization procedure.

3. THE POINT BY POINT COMPARISON OF THE REGISTERED IMAGES
3.1. The assumptions

When the noise level in the images is very low, subtraction images are
sufficient for a pictorial description of the changes. When important
fluctuations occur, we propose now a processing which takes into account
the knowledge about the statistical properties of the noise to determine
which pixels significantly differ in the images. Afterwards, only the
subtraction images of these significant changes will be generated.

The images are supposed well aligned and the normalization factor NF
has been calculated during the registration step. The fluctuations in the
images are assumed to follow a Poisson law so that this section is specific to scintigraphic images. We present now the construction of statistical
tests of comparison of Poisson variables which take into account the NF
value. These tests will be applied point by point as decision rules to
select the significant differences.

3.2. Construction of the statistical tests

3.2.1. The different approaches. The comparison of two random variables
which have a Poisson density function is not a trivial task. The distribution function of the difference of two Poisson variables is a Bessel
function which does not permit to derive simple statistical tests (20).
Therefore, two different approaches were used, first the maximum likelihood ratio test approach (21), second an adaptation of the UMP test of
comparison of two Poisson parameters (20). The construction of these tests
is presented in section 3.2.2. and 3.2.3. and section 3.3 is devoted to
the comparison of these tests in terms of their respective powers which
are theoretically and numerically appreciated.

3.2.2. The maximum likelihood ratio test. Consider X a random variable
whose density function depends on q parameters $\theta_1,....,\theta_q$. Let θ^1 be the
vector $(\theta_1,...,\theta_k)$ and θ^2 the vector $(\theta_{k+1},..\theta_q)$ and θ the vector $(\theta_1,...$
$..,\theta_q)$. One wants to test the null hypothesis $\theta^1=\theta_o^1$ against the composite
hypothesis $\theta^1 \neq \theta_o^1$. Let define L as :

$$L = \frac{L_{max}(X,(\theta_o^1, \hat{\theta}^2))}{L_{max}(X,(\hat{\theta}, \hat{\theta}))}$$

where $L_{max}(X,(\theta_o^1, \hat{\theta}^2))$ and $L_{max}(X,(\hat{\theta}, \hat{\theta}))$ are the maximum likelihood of the sample X calculated by maximizing these functions with respect to θ^2 and θ. One can demonstrate that without very restrictive conditions, the expression $-2.Log\ L$ has a χ^2 asymptotic distribution law with q-k degrees of freedom (21).

Therefore, we have to calculate the expression $-2.Log\ L$ with the following assumptions. In two corresponding pixels, the number of counts X_1 and X_2 have been measured; they are considered as samples of two Poisson laws with respectively λ_1 and λ_2 parameters. The null hypothesis is H_o: $\lambda_1 = NF.\lambda_2$ (the radioactivity in first pixel is differing from the second one just because of the preceedingly calculated value of the normalization factor). The composite hypothesis is $H_1 : \lambda_1 \neq NF.\lambda_2$. To apply the maximum likelihood ratio test approach, one must first calculate the likelihood of the sample (X_1 and X_2) under H_o and H_1.

a) Maximum likelihood under H_o. The probability of observing X_1 and X_2 values are :

$$\frac{e^{-NF.\lambda_2} . (NF.\lambda_2)^{X_1}}{X_1!} . \frac{e^{-\lambda_2} (\lambda_2)^{X_2}}{X_2!}$$

Hence: $Log\ L(X,(\lambda_2)) = -\lambda_2.(NF+1)+(X_1+X_2).Log\lambda_2+X_1.Log\ NF-Log(X_1!)-Log(X_2!)$

The maximum likelihood estimator of λ_2 is solution of $\frac{d(Log\ L(X,\lambda_2))}{d\lambda_2} = 0$

Hence: $-(NF+1) + \frac{X_1+X_2}{\lambda_2} = 0$ and $\hat{\lambda}_2 = \frac{X_1+X_2}{NF+1}$

The maximum likelihood under H_o is :

$$Log(L_{max}(X,(\hat{\lambda}_2))) = -(X_1+X_2)+(X_1+X_2).Log(\frac{X_1+X_2}{NF+1})+X_1.Log\ NF -Log(X_1!)$$
$$-Log\ (X_2!)$$

b) Maximum likelihood under H_1. The probability of observing X_1 and X_2 is:

$$\frac{e^{-\lambda_1} (\lambda_1)^{X_1}}{X_1!} . \frac{e^{-\lambda_2} (\lambda_2)^{X_2}}{X_2!}$$

Hence: $\text{Log } L(X,(\lambda_1,\lambda_2))=-\lambda_1+X_1.\text{Log}\lambda_1-\text{Log}(X_1!)-\lambda_2+X_2.\text{Log}\lambda_2-\text{Log}(X_2!)$

The best estimation of λ_1 and λ_2 are X_1 and X_2 so that the maximum

likelihood under H_1 is :

$$\text{Log}(L_{max}(X,(\hat{\lambda}_1,\hat{\lambda}_2)))=-X_1+X_1.\text{Log}X_1-X_2+X_2\text{Log}X_2-\text{Log}(X_1!)-\text{Log}(X_2!)$$

c) Final expression of the test . The expression :

$$-2.\text{LogL}=C_1=2(X_1.\text{Log}X_1+X_2.\text{Log}X_2-(X_1+X_2)\text{Log}\frac{(X_1+X_2)}{NF+1} - X_1\text{LogNF}) \text{ must be cal-}$$

calculated pixel by pixel and compared to the x^2 tabulated values with 1

degree of freedom (for example 3.84 for a 0.05 value of the size test)

    3.2.3. <u>Approximation of the UMP test</u>. The null and composite hypothe-
sis are similar. It has been demonstrated (20) that when two independant
random variables X_1 and X_2 follow a Poisson law with parameters λ_1 and λ_2
the conditional distribution law of $(X_1/X_1+X_2=s)$ is a binomial law with
parameters $\lambda_1/\lambda_1+\lambda_2$. Using this conditional law leads to a UMP test.
Nevertheless, the practical utilisation of this UMP test is limited because of the numerical difficulties occured by its implementation. Therefore, the binomial law was approximated by the normal law in order to
derive a more practical test. The approximation of the binomial law $B(n,p)$
is the normal law $N(np,np(1-p))$. This approximation in our problem leads
to the law :

$$\left\{\frac{X_1}{s} /X_1+X_2=s\right\} = N(\frac{s.\lambda_1}{\lambda_1+\lambda_2}, \frac{\lambda_1\cdot\lambda_2}{(\lambda_1+\lambda_2)^2}.s)$$

Under the null hypothesis we have: $\dfrac{\lambda_1}{\lambda_1+\lambda_2} = \dfrac{NF}{NF+1}$

Hence:

$$\left\{\frac{X_1}{s} /X_1+X_2=s\right\} =N(\frac{.NF}{NF+1}, \frac{NF}{s(NF+1)^2})$$

so that the expression:

$$\frac{\dfrac{X_1}{s} - \dfrac{NF}{1+NF}}{NF/s(1+NF)^2} \text{ is distributed according a normal law.}$$

The final expression of the test consists to calculate the expression C_2:

$$C_2 = \frac{(X_1 - NF \cdot X_2)^2}{NF(X_1 + X_2)}$$

C_2 has a χ^2 distribution with one degree of freedom and must be calculated pixel by pixel as C_1 test.

3.3. Study of the power of these tests.

3.3.1. General considerations. When a statistical test is applied, there are always type I and type II errors(21). In our problem, type I error consists in deciding that two pixels are different when they are similar (false detection of a change), type II error consists in deciding that two pixels are similar when they differ (missed detection of a change). The probability of type I and II errors are respectively quantified by α (for ex. $\alpha = 0.05$) which is the size of the test and β. The complementary probability $1-\beta$ is called the power of the test of the null hypothesis against the alternative hypothesis H_1. If for given H_0 and H_1 $\alpha = 0.05$ and $\beta = 0.05$, 95% of the pixels which really differ will be detected and 5% of similar pixels will be declared falsely different. Therefore, when a new test is used, it is necessary to know its power for the different values of the parameters. In our problem, the power of the test is function of four parameters: α, NF_0 and NF_1 the ratios of the parameters of the two Poisson laws under the null and alternative hypothesis and s the sum $X_1 + X_2$ of the counts in the pixels to compare. The numerical calculation of the power C_1 and C_2 tests was carried out for a large number of these parameter sets in order to (i) obtain absolute values of these powers (ii) be able to select the best of these two tests (iii) get indications concerning the best way of performing a point by point comparison of the images.

3.3.2. Calculation of C_1 and C_2 test powers. The power of C_1 and C_2 tests were derived from a numerical simulation according to the following way. First a NF_1 and a s value were selected. A n dimensional sample of the binomial law with parameters s and NF_1/NF_1+1 was numerically generated, giving n values of X_1 and X_2 under the alternative hypothesis. For this set of NF_0, NF_1 and s values, the C_1 and C_2 criterion values were calculated n times; an α value was selected and the corresponding β value was calculated; it was, in this n dimensional sample, the proportion of the pixels declared similar under the null hypothesis. The numerical values selected for the parameters were: NF_1= 0.5, 1., 2., 5. NF_0=0.5, 1., 2., 5., s=10, 30, 100, 200, α=0.2, 0.1, 0.05, 0.01 and n=10000. Thus 256 βvalues were calculated for each test C_1 and C_2. These values were compared to the analytically calculated βvalues of the approximated UMP test.

3.3.3. Results of the calculations.

s	10	30	100	200
$1-\beta_1$	0.31	0.44	0.93	1.00
$1-\beta_2$	0.11	0.44	0.93	1.00

Table 1. Comparative values of C_1 and C_2 test powers ($1-\beta_1$ and $1-\beta_2$) for different values of s (NF_1=2, NF_0=1, α =0.05)

The powers of these tests are very low for s=10, low for s=30; the powers become fairly good when the sum of the counts in the pixels to compare reach a 100 value (Tab.1). For such s values the theoretically and numerically calculated power values are in a good agreement.

The results of these numerical simulations have practical implications. The pixel by pixel comparison will be inefficient in the zones where the sum of the pixel values is under 100. If such a case occur it is necessary to first modify the format of the image in order to increase the number of counts in the pixels. For example a 128X128 image will be transformed in 64X64 or 32X32 image before the application of the tests.

It must be emphasized that when this statistical processing is applied to an entire image with a fixed α value, the β values will differ in the whole image, depending of the various s values in the pixels. This is a simple way of applying the test but an other approach including the use of a fixed β value on the entire image could be more convenient for certain applications where it is important not to fail to detect a change.

3.3.4. Example of application. Fig. 2a and 2b show two low count (30000) scintigraphic images of a liver phantom. In the case of image 2b, a small piece of lucite has been set in front of the left lobe during the acquisition of the image. It is impossible to detect a change from the visual inspection of either the original 128X128 images (2a and 2b) or even the classical image 2c. Test C_1 was applied to images 2a and 2b whose format was first reduced to 32X32 in order to increase the number of counts by pixel. Image 2d is the 32X32 subtraction image (2a-2b) where are only figured the pixels which significantly differ in terms of C_1 test ($\alpha=0.05$) This image permits an excellent identification of the change of image 2b.

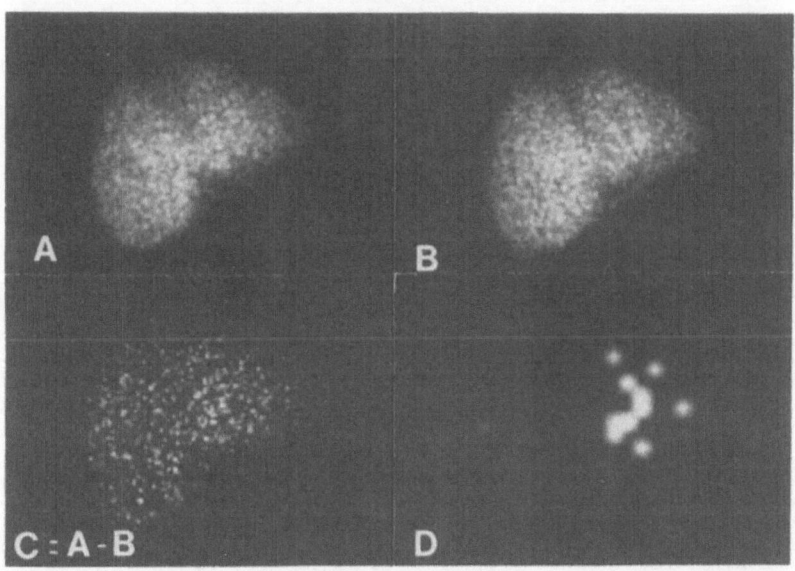

FIGURE 2. a) Scintigraphic 128X128 image of a liver phantom. b) Modified version of image 2a. c) Classical subtraction image. d) Subtraction image of the significant differences.

4. THE SEQUENTIAL APPLICATION OF THESE METHODS

4.1. Description of the software.

We have combined all these methods in a software which permits the successive registration and point by point comparison of two scintigraphic images with very few operator interventions. The first step is the selection of the images, determination of a rectangular window. Afterwards, the images are automatically aligned and the normalization factor is calculated. After the end of the registration step, the sign change image is generated because it permits to visually check the quality of the registration. Test C_1 is then applied pixel by pixel either with the original format or in a more packed form (64X64 or 32X32), using the preceedingly calculated value of the normalization factor. This image processing ends with the generation of images of the positive and negative significant changes for various α values

4.2. Example of application in controlled conditions

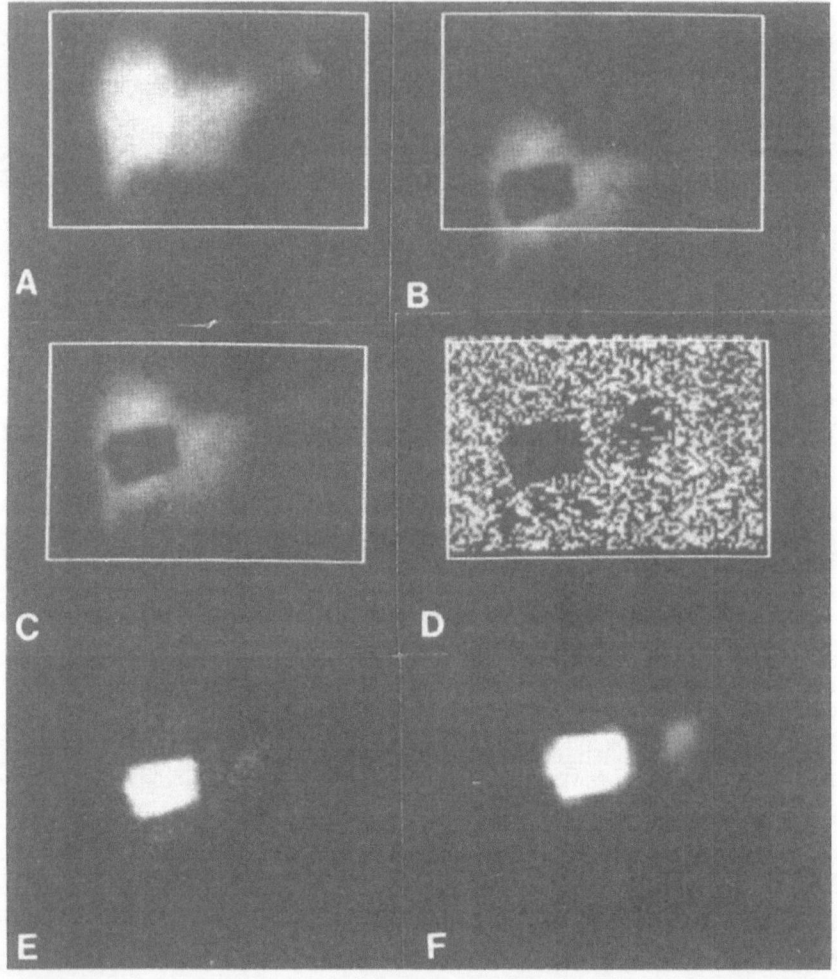

FIGURE 3. Comparison of two scintigraphic images in controlled conditions. a) Anterior liver scan of a patient. b) Translated, unnormalized, modified version of image a. c) Registered image b. d) Sign change image after registration. e) Classical subtraction image. f) Subtraction image of the significant differences.

Fig. 3. shows the automated comparison of two scintigraphic images in controlled conditions. Image 3a (128X128) is the anterior liver scan of a patient; the acquisition time was 30 seconds. Image b is an image of the same liver obtained after having translated the patient under the camera and set absorbant materials in front of his right and left lobe. The acquisition time was 20 seconds. Image c is the aligned version of image b. For the registration step, the SSC criterion was maximized with respect to Δi and Δj the abcissa and ordinate translation parameters and NF the normalization factor. The maximum SSC criterion value (2423) was found for $\Delta i=0$, $\Delta j=-21$ pixels and NF=1.46 (the true NF value is 1.50). Correlation methods (5) gave wrong values of the parameters ($\Delta i=1$, $\Delta j=-19$). Image d is the sign change image after this registration step; in the rectangular window (6003 pixels) used for the calculation of the SSC criterion. It demonstrates the correctness of the registration. Image e is the classical subtraction image A-NF.C. Image f is the image of the significant differences derived from the application of C_1 test. Two modified zones are visualized corresponding to a piece of lead (right lobe) and a piece of lucite (left lobe) set on the patient. The changes in the right lobe are well appreciated from a visual inspection of image a and b but image f is the only one to clearly demonstrate the occurence of a change in the left lobe.

5. CONCLUSION

These digital methods of image comparison have many powerful clinical applications. In the context of the subtraction angiography, the DSC criterion registration method represents an important contribution to the registration of unnoisy but dissimilar images. Its practical implementation would require fraction of pixels translations of the images as it is done for correlation methods of registration. In Nuclear Medicine, we find these methods useful for different investigations: Follow up of patients with liver and lung scintigraphies, interpretation of stress and rest myocardial images, double tracer studies and also for the sequential check of the camera field homogeneity. The registration step would benefit of the adding of new registration parameters but this is only a software and not a basic problem. The point by point comparison actually only concerns the scintigraphic images but new developements concerning the statistical comparison SPECT images are actually under investigation in our laboratory.

REFERENCES

1. Barnea DI, Silverman HF. 1972. A class of algorithms for fast digital image registration. IEEE C21, 353-357.
2. Pratt WK. 1974. Correlation techniques of image registration. IEEE AES10, 353-358.
3. Svedlow M, Mc Gillem CD, Anuta PE. 1978. Image registration: similarity measure and preprocessing method comparisons. IEEE AES14,141-149.
4. Lillestrand RL. 1972. Techniques for change detection. IEEE C21, 654-659.
5. Appledorn CR, Oppenheim BE, Wellman HN. 1980. An automated method for the alignment of image pairs. J. Nucl. Med.,21, 165-167.
6. Eghbali H. 1979. K-S test for detecting changes from Landsat imagery data. IEEE SMC9, 17-23.
7. Barnard ST, Thompson WB. 1980. Disparity analysis of images. IEEE PAMI2, 333-340.
8. Venot A, Lebruchec JF, Golmard JL, Roucayrol JC. 1983. An automated method for the normalization of scintigraphic images. J. Nucl. Med., 24, 529-531.
9. Venot A, Lebruchec JF, Golmard JL, Roucayrol JC. 1983. Digital methods for change detection in scintigraphic images. J. Nucl. Med.,24, p67.
10.Venot A, Lebruchec JF, Roucayrol JC. 1983. A new class of similarity measures for robust image registration. Submitted to Computer vision, graphics and image processing.
11.Draper NB, Smith H. 1966. Applied regression analysis. John Wiley and sons. New York.
12.Gibbons JD. 1971. Non parametric statistical inference. Mc Graw Hill. New York.
13.Cohen G, Wagner LK, Rauschkolb EN. 1982. Evaluation of a digital subtraction angiography unit. Radiology, 144, 613-617.
14.Pavlidis T. 1982. Algorithms for graphics and image processing. Springer Verlag, Berlin.
15.Himmelblau DM. 1972. Applied non linear programming. Mc Graw Hill. New York.
16.Richalet J, Rault A, Pouliquen R. 1971. Identification des processus par la méthode du modèle. Gordon and Breach. Paris.
17.Towards global optimization 1 and 2. 1978. Dixon LCW, Szegö GP Eds. North Holland. Amsterdam.
18.Maszi SF, Bekey GA, Safford FB. 1976. An adaptative random search method for identification of large scale non linear systems. 4th IFAC Symposium on identification and system parameter estimation. Tbilisi.
19.Bekey GA, Ung MT. 1974. A comparative evaluation of two global search algorithms. IEEE SMC4, 112-116.
20.Lehmann EL. 1959. Testing statistical hypothesis. John Wiley and sons, New York.
21.Kendall M, Stuart A. 1979. The advanced theory of statistics 2. Griffin. London.

AN APPROACH TO ENDOCARDIAL BOUNDARY DETECTION FROM SEQUENTIAL
REAL TIME TWO-DIMENSIONAL ECHOCARDIOGRAPHIC IMAGES: STATUS OF
THE ALGORITHM AND ITS VALIDATION.

E.A. Geiser, M.D., L.H. Oliver, Ph.D., L.F. Zhang, K.J. Fu,
D.D. Buss, D.V.M., Ph.D., C.R. Conti, M.D.
From the Division of Cardiology, Department of Medicine and
the Department of Computer and Information Sciences, University
of Florida, Gainesville, Florida, U.S.A.

1. INTRODUCTION

1.1. Two-dimensional echocardiography

Over the last several years numerous papers have been published on the quantitation of 2-dimensional echocardiograms.
This seems to have come about for several reasons. Echocardiography is easy to use and completely non-invasive. The technique is also relatively inexpensive and is portable. These
features mean that it can be used at the patient's bedside
conveniently and even that it is not necessarily hospital
based.

Quantitation has been mainly directed toward analysis of
wall motion during the cardiac cycle, calculation of volume,
both systolic and diastolic, and the calculation of ejection
fraction. Two-dimensional echocardiography is well suited
towards the first of these since it is currently the only convenient real time tomographic imaging technique available.

With the above considerations in mind, it seems that
accurate quantitation of echocardiographic data may well ful-
fill the current void in clinical cardiology for an accurate,
convenient method to serially assess ventricular function in
patients using quantitative techniques. Thus, the basic
hypothesis followed in this research is that accurate data
concerning cardiac structure and motion is present in real
time echocardiographic images.

1.2. Background

In terms of cardiac structure, volume has been the most
frequently studied quantitative measure from real time echo.

Numerous studies have been published in which the volume of
the left ventricular muscle mass or the volume of the left
ventricular chamber has been compared to either angiography or
objective in vitro measurements. In 1980, we predicted on
theorectical grounds that there should be a ±16% variability
of predicted chamber volume in a 3-dimensional reconstruction
(1). Our first experimental work in formalin fixed hearts
substantiated this and found a predictability of approximately
±18%. A similar figure was found using a 4 cross-section
Simpson's Rule calculation by Wyatt et al (2). More recently,
in vivo human studies (3) have again bracketed this range of
predicted chamber volume at ±16% to ±30% in normals. In all of
these studies, a major contribution to this variability seems
to be inter- and intraobserver variability in defining the
endocardial borders from which the volumes are calculated.
With this in mind, we and others have sought to develop a
computer program to extract endocardial borders from the
2-dimensional echocardiographic images. The purpose of develop-
ing such an algorithm is twofold. First of all, it is difficult
and very time-consuming to manually digitize the endocardial
borders from sequences of echocardiographic images. Secondly,
development of a computer algorithm would be aimed at producing
an accurate, objective, and reproducible set of borders. The
objectivity of computer defined borders would hopefully
eliminate, or at least reduce, the inter- and intraobserver
contributions to the predictive error.

1.3. Previous work

Several groups have used image processing techniques to
help define borders. Skorton et al (4), described the use of
computer image processing in static single frames to assist in
edge detection. several other groups have reported experience
with edge detection in sequences of 2-dimensional echocardiograms (5,6,7). We and others have also attempted to use the
temporal redundancy of the data in order to limit the regions
of search and help define borders on sequential frames (8,6).

A basic assumption was made when the development of this

algorithm was started. This assumption was that the best
information in the real time echocardiographic image is present in the motion of the spots in the B-mode display rather
than the grey levels displayed. This assumption is supported
clinically by the observation that the endocardium is readily
identified by most observers in the moving image, but is
difficult to trace from stop-frame images once integrated
motion is lost. The high degree of variability in motion
patterns in clinical 2-dimensional echocardiograms, however,
has made it difficult to develop an algorithm which uses
frame-to-frame change as a primary feature for the selection
of endocardial edges. Instead, the algorithm to date has
developed as a complex integration which now utilizes a plan-
guided windowing technique. The final position of these windows
can be adjusted depending on the position of temporally and
spatially adjacent windows. In addition, the temporal information is also used to modify the border points selected within
these windows.

2. DESCRIPTION OF THE ALGORITHM
2.1. Digitization
The algorithm thus far developed is diagramed in Figure 1.
In order to utilize the motion information during the entire
cycle, all video frames for the cycle are digitized and stored.
Several cycles are digitized from a video input signal at 30
frames per second to form a 256 X 256 matrix of 4 bit pixels.
This data is compressed and passes directly to digital disc.

2.2. Selection of region of interest and rough borders
2.2.1. Operator interaction. The operator next selects,
from the frames on digital disc, the opening end diastolic
frame, the end systolic frame and the closing end diastolic
frame for the cycle to be studied. Next the observer defines
the endocardial edge on these three frames. As will be seen,
these three approximations are used in order to determine the
region of search on the series of images. Since the majority
of echocardiographic images have some translation present

either due to respiratory
motion, motion of the transducer, or patient, we have
found it necessary to digitize both end diastolic frames
in order to define a region
of search which includes this
translation.

2.2.2. Enhancement and
conversion to polar format.
At this point the algorithm
separates and utilizes the
approximate observer defined
borders in two ways. The
maximum X and Y coordinates
of the diastolic borders are
enlarged by three pixels in
the X and Y directions. These
expanded X and Y coordinates
determine a region which has
a high probability of containing the edges for the
entire cycle, but markedly
reduces the region in which
enhancement operators will
be applied. Once an enhancement operator has been
chosen and applied, the geometric center of this maximum diastolic region is
found. Using this center,
the entire region is con-
verted to polar form along
64 radii. Thus, each en-
hanced frame is converted to
a polar image where the rows
represent the 64 radii and

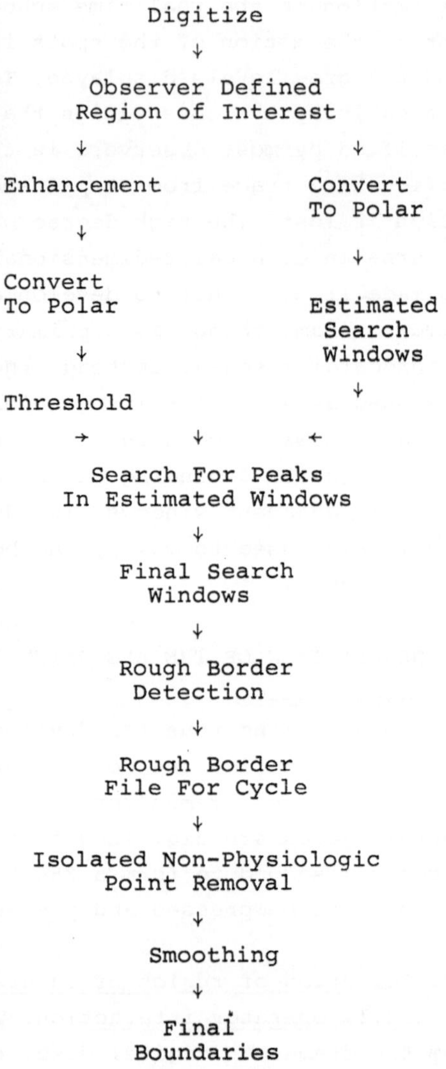

Digitize
↓
Observer Defined
Region of Interest
↓   ↓
Enhancement   Convert
                     To Polar
↓
                              ↓
Convert
To Polar   Estimated
                      Search
↓   Windows
                              ↓
Threshold
→   ↓   ←
Search For Peaks
In Estimated Windows
↓
Final Search
Windows
↓
Rough Border
Detection
↓
Rough Border
File For Cycle
↓
Isolated Non-Physiologic
Point Removal
↓
Smoothing
↓
Final
Boundaries

Figure 1. Flow diagram for full
cycle endocardial boundary
detection algorithm.

the columns represent the grey level at each radial unit
length from the center for the region of interest. The number
of columns i.e. the number of radial units, is set at the
maximum number of radial units in the longest radius of the
interest region.

    2.2.3. <u>Thresholding</u>. In looking at 2-dimensional echo-
cardiographic images, it is obvious that endocardial grey
levels are more intense in the center of the image where the
ultrasound propagation is nearly perpendicular to the position
of the anterior and posterior endocardium. On the other hand,
signals are weak in the lateral portions of the sector. Consequently, regional, rather than global thresholding is more
appropriate. In the polar image files, separate thresholds are
determined for each set of eight rows, thus establishing a
regional threshold for each octant of each image. The threshold
value for each octant is determined either as the average grey
level or as the grey level that maximizes the number of changing pixels in each octant using a temporal co-occurrance
technique (9).

    2.2.4. <u>Estimated search windows</u>. The second way in which
the observer defined boundaries are used is in determining
estimated search windows on each frame of the cycle. In order
to do this, the three observer defined endocardial boundaries
are first converted into polar form using the same center. The
center of the estimated search window is calculated as a linear
interpolation along each radius of each frame between the opening end diastolic and end systolic radius and between the end
systolic and closing end diastolic radius. The estimated
search window has a variable width set between 4 and 7 pixels
from this interpolated center. Once the region of interest
and the center of the estimated windows have been determined,
the observer's borders are discarded.

    2.2.5. <u>Refinement of search windows</u>. These estimated
search windows are then superimposed on the corresponding
polar image file for each frame in the cycle. Since the position of these estimated windows is derived from a linear
interpolation, while cardiac contraction and relaxation is

more sinusoidal, the estimated windows may not be positioned
in the optimal portion of each polar file. Therefore, a re-
adjustment in the position of these windows is performed. This
re-adjustment takes place again within each octant of each
polar image.

Within each octant, the radius length to each peak within
the estimated windows is determined. A peak is defined as a
non-isolated point whose grey level is higher than its neighbors. The mean of these radii is then calculated and forms
the center of the final search window. This window is again of
variable width and extends for 4 to 7 radial positions on each
side of the final center. This final search window should be
optimally positioned over the highest density of peaks within
the thresholded octant. In the case where there is excessive
dropout in one or several frames so that the location of the
final search window cannot be based on the spatial data present,
the position of these final search windows over time can be
analyzed to arrive at a best guess for the position of the
window.

2.2.6. <u>Detection of rough border points</u>. Within each of
these final search windows a rough border point is now selected
along each radius. A border point is defined as the first peak
within the search window along each radius. If no peak is
found, the border point along this radius is left undefined.
Once this process has taken place for all 64 radii on each
image, the missing points are filled using a linear interpolation of the radius length. The number of interpolated points
is displayed on the screen as these rough boundaries are
selected and give the operator feedback regarding the quality
of the image and the confidence he should have in the results.

2.2.7. <u>Spatial and temporal refinement</u>. The radii from
these rough border points selected along all 64 radii in each
frame constitute the rough border file. This file thus contains
all of the points selected as border points over the entire
cardiac cycle. Each row represents the temporal excursion of
the border along a particular radius over the course of the
cycle and each column represents the position of the entire

border at one particular point in time. <u>A priori</u> physiologic
data suggests that this space-time surface should not have any
abrupt discontinuities. Thus, it is very probable that an
isolated point in any column which is more than three pixels
away from <u>both</u> of its neighbors is not a true endocardial edge
point. On the other hand, we know that it is highly improbable
that an individual endocardial point can move more than 3mm in
$1/30^{th}$ of a second. Thus, an isolated point in any row which
is 3 or more radial units from its neighbors can be removed
and replaced with the mean of its neighbors.

2.3. <u>Final borders</u>

Once these "non-physiologic" points have been removed, a
final smoothing of the border matrix is performed using the
weights:

$$\begin{array}{ccc} 1 & 1 & 1 \\ 1 & 0 & 1 \\ 1 & 1 & 1 \end{array}$$

This smoothed matrix is then considered the final border file.
The radial borders are then reconverted to cartesian coordinates and displayed over the original 2-dimensional echo frames
for verification.

3. VALIDATION

3.1. <u>In vitro studies with balloons</u>

3.1.1. <u>Complex motion</u>. Since the beating heart cannot be
cut in cross-section and observed objectively as well as on 2D
echo, the absolute accuracy of this algorithm is difficult to
evaluate. Therefore, the first step in validation has been to
observe pulsating balloons in a test tank. While the balloon
edges are not objectively observed, they are smooth, continuous,
single membranes in which erroneously chosen borders are
quickly identified during superimposition of detected boundaries on the original images. In some of these experiments the
balloon was pulsed in a swinging motion which mimics regions
of dyskinesis and akinesis. The serial borders for both a

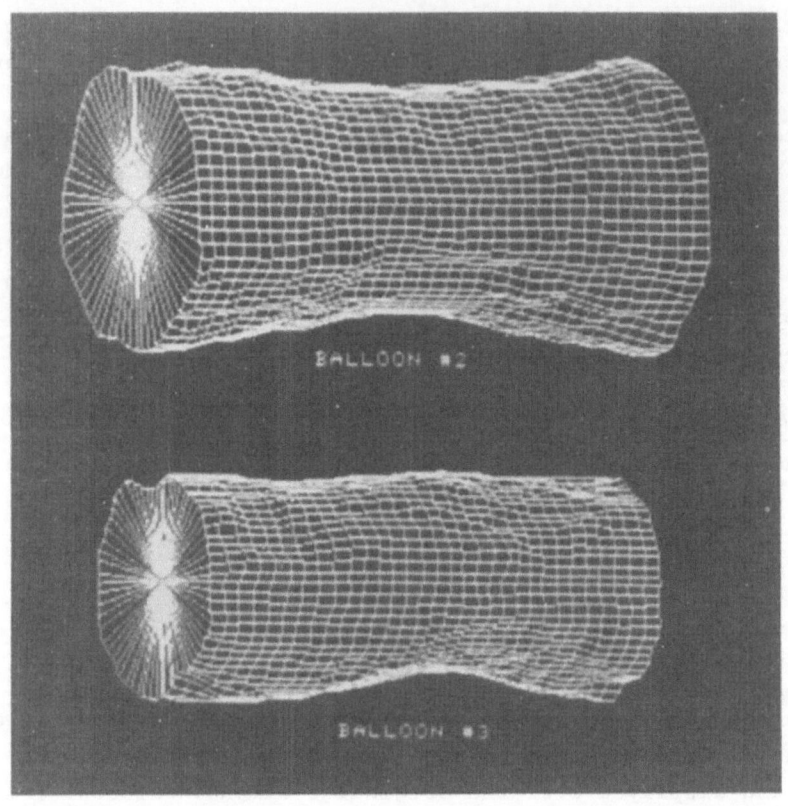

Figure 2. Isometric three-dimensional display of serial
borders defined in two balloon studies. The upper contraction
is concentric while the lower contraction shows motion toward
the transducer during the middle of the cycle.

concentrically contracting and a "dyskinetic" experiment are
shown in Figure 2. Here the borders are displayed consecu-
tively in an isometric projection with an observation angle
of 35°. In the lower panel, the area of apparent dyskinesis
can be seen moving outward towards the observer as the
balloon contracts. Thus, the abnormal wall motion was readily
identified by the algorithm.

3.1.2. <u>Image degradation</u>. In another <u>in</u> <u>vitro</u> experiment, the image was serially degraded while the balloon was kept in as near to a steady state as possible. This experiment was performed in order to test the algorithm over a controlled range of image quality. Image quality was changed by re-adjustment of the damping, reject, and grey scale controls of the rotating head scanner employed for these experiments. Three cycles from each image quality were processed. Table 1 shows the mean areas enclosed by the serial borders for good, inter-mediate, and poor quality images, respectively. Up to 37 of the 64 expected points were interpolated in some of the poor quality images. Columns 4 and 5 in the table show the 2-tailed t-test values between the intermediate and good quality images and the poor and good quality images, respectively. No sig-nificant differences in any of the 36 areas of the intermediate quality images were found with respect to the good. Sixteen out of 36 of the poor images resulted in significant differ-ences at the 0.95 level from the good quality images. Thus, when a large portion of the boundary was not present, there was a tendancy for the algorithm to select other signals that were present in place of the border points. In the case of these balloon studies, the other signals were due to small bubbles either circulating in the water bath or in the fluid being pumped into the balloon.

3.1.3. <u>Calculation of flow</u>. A third method of evaluation was also derived from these balloon experiments. In these studies, 2-dimensional echocardiographic cross-sectional images were obtained at 5 different levels through the balloon. The algorithm was then used to define the sequential borders during one cycle from each of these 5 cross-sectional levels. These borders were used to calculate the volume of the balloon at each 30th of a second during the cycle. From these volumes the rate of change in volume, dV/dt was calculated and this curve compared to the electromagnetic flow signal measured at the inlet to the balloon. Figure 3 shows a comparison between the calculated flow and measured electromagnetic flow in one of these experiments. In the figure, flow out of the balloon

Table 1. Mean sequential areas and t-values for balloon cycles of varying quality.

	Mean Areas			t-values	
				Good VS Excellent	Poor VS Excellent
	Excellent	Good	Poor		
1	19.10	19.03	17.88	0.241	3.118*
2	19.08	18.92	17.90	0.478	2.812*
3	19.02	18.82	17.85	0.600	3.935*
4	18.77	18.59	17.88	0.656	3.133*
5	18.44	18.07	17.53	1.276	2.759
6	18.10	17.68	17.36	1.053	1.711
7	17.57	17.35	16.96	0.463	1.390
8	17.04	16.88	16.53	0.287	0.944
9	16.55	16.31	16.03	0.368	0.866
10	15.94	15.71	15.29	0.543	1.404
11	15.28	15.15	14.84	0.375	1.076
12	14.87	14.49	14.40	0.882	1.012
13	14.24	13.88	13.93	0.779	0.701
14	13.73	13.43	13.47	0.885	0.787
15	13.45	13.00	12.75	1.616	2.133
16	13.07	12.55	12.56	1.370	1.738
17	12.75	12.22	12.32	1.404	2.182
18	12.48	12.08	12.13	0.891	2.461
19	12.35	12.09	11.74	0.709	3.759*
20	12.21	12.18	11.52	0.155	2.489
21	12.16	12.06	11.45	0.501	2.485
22	12.24	12.04	11.62	1.017	2.502
23	12.38	12.17	11.67	1.001	3.139*
24	12.73	12.63	11.72	0.543	4.393*
25	13.01	13.04	11.91	-0.191	3.649*
26	13.35	13.42	12.31	-0.273	4.080*
27	13.64	13.84	12.71	-1.306	7.768*
28	14.19	14.24	13.14	-0.247	5.758*
29	14.73	14.75	13.81	-0.115	5.073*
30	15.23	15.32	14.33	-0.367	4.317*
31	15.81	15.95	14.95	-0.620	3.295*
32	16.43	16.61	15.54	-1.252	3.878*
33	16.81	17.08	16.19	-1.635	3.192*
34	17.22	17.62	16.87	-1.373	1.277
35	17.45	18.07	17.20	-2.290	0.845
36	17.74	18.18	17.28	-1.285	1.176

* Indicates significant difference at the 0.95 level.

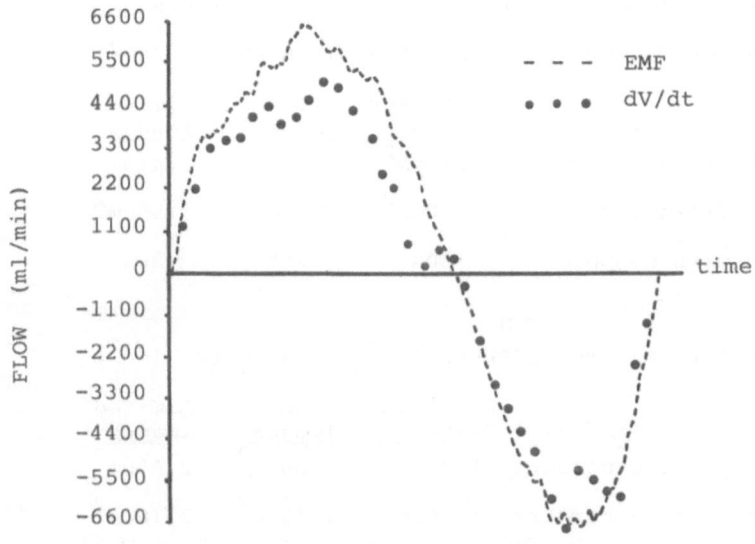

Figure 3. Comparison of the measured electromagnetic flow (EMF) to the calculated rate of change in volume (dV/dt).

is represented as a positive quantity and flow into the balloon is represented as negative. The shape and scale of the computed flow curve correctly follow the measured quantity.

3.2. Human validation studies

Valdiation is also underway comparing observer defined borders from human clinical studies to those derived from the algorithm. The short axis views from six clinical studies were requested from 5 independent clinical laboratories. These six studies were not required to be excellent, but were to cover a spectrum of excellent, good, and poor quality images. One cycle from each of these 30 studies was entered into the computer system in a randomized fashion. Five independent observers from outside of our institution were then asked to grade the images as excellent, good, poor, or inadequate and define the endocardial edges on every other video frame of each cardiac cycle using the joystick. On the second day of the study each observer was asked to define only the opening

Table 2. Intra- and interobserver area differences for manual and computer defined endocardial borders.

MEAN ABSOLUTE INTRAOBSERVER AREA DIFFERENCES (cm^2)

	Excellent Images	Good Images	Limited Images
Manually drawn borders	$1.12cm^2$	$1.23cm^2$	$2.41cm^2$
Computer drawn borders	$0.78cm^2$	$0.92cm^2$	$1.55cm^2$
% change with computer	-30%	-25%	-36%

MEAN ABSOLUTE INTEROBSERVER AREA DIFFERENCES (cm^2)

	Excellent Images	Good Images	Limited Images
Manually drawn borders	$1.71cm^2$	$1.86cm^2$	$2.60cm^2$
Computer drawn borders	$1.06cm^2$	$1.15cm^2$	$2.18cm^2$
% change with computer	-38%	-38%	-16%

diastolic, end systolic, and closing diastolic borders. On both day 1 and day 2 the computer generated all borders in each cardiac cycle. Table 2 shows results compiled from the data of 4 observers processed thus far. These data show reduction in both the inter- and intraobserver variability when the computer is used to define the endocardial borders. In addition, the observers took a mean of 11.4 minutes to draw the borders on every other frame, while the computer took a mean of 3.1 minutes to define borders for the entire cycle.

4. CONCLUSIONS

We have developed an algorithm which has proven effective in extracting endocardial edges from echocardiograms with less variability than trained expert observers and at a substantial saving in time. This algorithm uses both the temporal and spatial continuities of the endocardial borders through the cycle in order to derive these edges. Since the process is initiated by observer defined region of search, the method

itself is not completely objective and has some variability.
It can also be seen that while the algorithm utilizes a combination of image processing methods i.e. predictive windowing,
enhancement, regional thresholding, and a priori knowledge of
cardiovascular structure and motion, it does not use the
motion information as a primary feature in deciding which
points are associated with the endocardial edges.

Thus, work in the future will be directed toward objective
definition of the region of search and better utilization of
the motion or temporal change information as a primary feature.

REFERENCES

1. Geiser EA, Lupkiewicz SM, Christie LG, Ariet M, Conetta DA,
   Conti CR: A framework for three-dimensional time varying
   reconstruction of the human left ventricle: Sources of error
   and estimation of their magnitude. Computers in Biomedical
   Research 13:225-241, 1980.
2. Wyatt HL, Heng MK, Meerbaum S, Gueret P, Hestenes J, Dula E,
   Corday E: Cross-sectional echocardiography. II. Analysis of
   mathematical models for quantifying volume of the formalin
   fixed left ventricle. Circulation 61:1119-1125, 1980.
3. Gordon EP, Schnittger I, Fitzgerald PJ, Popp RL: Reproducibility of left ventricular volume measurement by two-
   dimensional echocardiography. Circulation (suppl)66:II-338,
   1982.
4. Skorton DJ, McNary CA, Child JS, Newton FC, Shah PM: Digital
   image processing of two-dimensional echocardiograms:
   Identification of the endocardium. American Journal of
   Cardiology 48:479-486, 1981.
5. Garcia E, Gueret P, Bennett M, Corday E, Zwehl W, Meerbaum
   S, Corday S, Swan JHC, Berman D: Real time computerization
   of two-dimensional echocardiography. American Heart Journal
   101:783-792, 1981.
6. Delp EJ, Buda AJ, Swastek MR, Smith DN, Jenkins JM, Meyer CR
   and Pitt B: The analysis of two-dimensional echocardiograms
   using a time varying image approach. Computers in Cardiology
   pgs.391-394, October, 1982.
7. Buda AJ, Delp EJ, Meyer CR, Jenkins JM, Smith DN, Bookstein
   FL, Pitt B: Automatic computer processing of digital two-
   dimensional echocardiograms. American Journal of Cardiology
   52:384-389, 1983.
8. Geiser EA, Zhang LF, Buss DD, Franklin BD, Fu KJ, Conetta
   DA, Conti CR: Automated border definition from 2D echocardiograms. Circulation (Suppl)66:II-337, 1982.
9. Zhang LF, Geiser EA: An approach to optimal thresholding
   selection on a sequence of two-dimensional echocardiographic
   images. IEEE Transactions on Biomedical Engineering, BME-29:
   No.8, 577-581, 1982.

ANALYSIS OF DYNAMIC RADIONUCLIDE STUDIES USING FACTOR ANALYSIS
- a new approach

K.S. NIJRAN AND D.C. BARBER

Department of Medical Physics and Clinical Engineering, Royal Hallamshire
Hospital, Sheffield, England

1. INTRODUCTION

In recent years there has been an increasing interest in the use of factor
analysis to analyse dynamic radionuclide studies (Oppenheim, 1978; Schmidlin,
1979; Barber, 1980). Its application has largely centred on providing a means
of compressing large amounts of radionuclide study data, filtering of such
data and for classification of normal and diseased patients. The concept of
physiological factors as introduced by Bazin et al (1979) was a serious
attempt to demonstrate the potential of factor analysis in processing dynamic
studies. This approach was based on the concept that the dynamic structures
imaged by the gamma camera may be decomposed into their fundamental
physiological functions (termed physiological factors). Barber (1980)
presented an iterative method of estimating these fundamental physiological
factors underlying in a study. This method has been adopted by Bazin and his
co-workers (Bazin et al 1982; Aurengo et al, 1982; Cavailloles et al, 1982;
Herry et al, 1982), with some modification and applied to various types of
dynamic studies. This method has produced some interesting results but uses
no a priori knowledge of the underlying physiological model. The consequences
of this is that in certain situations, the assignment of the derived
physiological factors to appropriate anatomical structures in the study is
difficult. Furthermore in some cases it is possible for the unobserved
physiological factor to be contaminated by the other physiological factors
(Barber and Nijran, 1981). In this paper a method is presented which adds a
priori information about the physiology of at least one of the dynamic
structures present in the study, and enable the physiological factor
representing that dynamic structure to be extracted automatically.

The method proposed here is illustrated using kidney function studies.

2. THEORY

A dynamic study consists of a time sequence of digital images or frames, where each frame is sub-divided into small areas or pixel. The time activity curve constructed from the sequence of counts in each frame, in a given pixel is here called a dixel. Vector notation may be used to represent a dixel, where the sequence of numbers associated with a dixel are identified as co-ordinates. If there are N frames in a study, then a dixel is represented as an N-dimensional vector.

It follows from the basic concept of factor analysis that a population of dixels are most efficiently described in terms of orthogonal components of that population. Then any individual dixel in this study is described by the weighted linear sum of the orthogonal components. For the kth dixel

$$\vec{d}_k = \sum_{i=1}^{N} a_{ik} e_i \qquad \cdots\cdots\cdots 2.1$$

in which a_{ik} are the coefficients or weights and $\vec{e}_i$ are the orthogonal components. $\leftarrow$ implies a column vector ($\rightarrow$ row vector). If there are N frames in a study then for a complete reconstruction of any dixel N orthogonal components are required. The N orthogonal components represent a set of N axes. These N axes define an N-dimensional space in which the dixels plot as vectors. If there are P dixels in a study, then these dixels are represented as P vectors in this N-space. There are an infinite number of orthogonal transformations that can be performed on this population of dixels. However, there exists one special type, known as principal components, which maximizes the variance among the dixels such that only a very small number of these principal components, say M (M≪N) are needed to adequately describe any dixel in this study. Then the kth dixel is approximated by the linear combination.

$$\vec{d}_k \sum_{i=1}^{M} c_{ik} \vec{s}_i \qquad \cdots\cdots\cdots 2.2$$

in which c_{ik} are the coefficients or weights and $\vec{s}_i$ are the principal components. The M principal components then represent a new optimal set of axes derived from the distribution of dixels in this study. This means a dixel originally described by N-coefficient in an N-dimensional space can be approximated by M coefficients in an M-dimensional space. The M-principal components define an M dimensional sub-space of the N-space. The N-dimensional vectors drawn from this study will completely be plotted in M space. It must be noted that M-space is unique to this study only. Further properties of this subspace are described in Barber and Nijran (1982). This M-space is called the study space, designated by S.

The variation of activity with time in some dynamic structure underlying in a particular type of study can generally be expressed by the function of the form $f(a_1 \ldots a_i \ldots; t)$, or in vector notation

$$\vec{f} = \vec{f} (a \ldots a_i \ldots) \qquad \ldots\ldots\ldots\ldots 2.3$$

For a particular study, the parameter a_i will take on particular values A_i, and this vector will of necessity plot into S for this study, provided certain conditions of homogenity are satisfied (Barber, 1980). Furthermore if no other structure generates a curve of the form $\vec{f}$ then this is the only curve of this form which plots into S. In Barber and Nijran (1981) an iterative function minimization method was used to find this vector $\vec{f}$ lying in S space by minimizing the difference between the vector $\vec{f}$ and the projection of this vector into S. The curve represented by this vector can be reconstructed using eq.2.2 This curve then represents a physiological factor due to the structure of interest.

In Barber and Nijran (1982) a more efficient and a powerful method of determining the physiological factor was presented. The basic principle underlying this method is as follows. Suppose a population of dixels is generated from eq.2.3 by generating a large sample of vectors f using a realistic range of values of a_i. Then any dixel in this theoretical population of dixels may also be expressed as a weighted sum of the principal components derived for this population and as before only a very small number of principal components, say L, will be needed to adequately reconstruct any theoretical dixel. The L-principal components define an L dimensional subspace of the N-space. This subspace is called the theory space or T space. In general T is not the same as S even if these spaces have the same dimensionality.

There exists at least one vector which lies in both S and T and this vector represents an intersection of these two subspaces

$$T \cap S \qquad . \ldots\ldots\ldots\ldots 2.4$$

If there is only one unique vector which lies in the two subspaces simultaneously then the intersection space, defined by eq2.4 (designated by I) will be one dimensional. A matrix method of determining this one dimensional intersection solution is provided in the appendix and application of this technique to Rose-bengal liver function study was demonstrated in our previous publication (Barber and Nijran, 1982). Now there may be situations where certain types of dynamic structures in a study are described by I space of dimensions greater than one. What this implies is that a structure in the study

is represented by two or more physiological factors although the same
mathematical model describes the physiological processes involved.

2.1 Construction of Renal Theory Space, T

Various models have been proposed by several workers for the renal system
(Oppenheim, 1979; DeGrazin et al, 1974; Lindmo et al, 1974). In general these
models are relatively complex. In this work a primitive three compartment
model is assumed (fig.2.1). It effectively represents the clearance of the
activity by the individual nephrons, where the nephrons in the kidney act only
as transport delays.

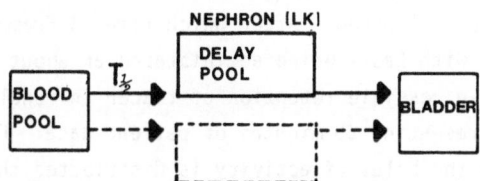

Fig.2.1 A three dompartment model used in this work.

The variation of activity with time in a nephron is given by the function
of the form

$$n(t) = 1 - \exp(-t \cdot 0.693/T_{\frac{1}{2}}) \qquad t \leq td$$
$$= A.\exp(-(t-td).0.693/T_{\frac{1}{2}}) \qquad t \geq td \qquad \cdots\cdots\cdots 2.5$$

where $T_{\frac{1}{2}}$ is the time to half maximum, td is the delay time introduced by the
delay pool, and A is a constant equal to $(1-\exp(-td.0.693/T_{\frac{1}{2}})$. In vector
notation this function may be expressed as

$$\vec{n} = \vec{n}(td, T_{\frac{1}{2}}) \qquad\qquad \cdots\cdots\cdots 2.6$$

The time-activity curve normally obtained over a kidney as a whole is
actually a integral curve resulting from the linear sum of the individual
nephron curves.

A population of 500 theoretical nephron curves was generated by allowing $T_{\frac{1}{2}}$
to take on values ranging from 0.69 minutes to 77 minutes in logarithmic
intervals and td values ranging from 1 minute to 15 minutes in linear steps.
Forty-five data points were calculated for each theoretical curve
corresponding to 45, 20 sec. frames of an actual ^{99m}Tc-DTPA renogram
study. T space was derived for this population and the examination of the
latent roots of the principal components for this space, suggested that at
most the first 5 principal components contained any significant signal i.e.
L = 5 for this T space (for the method of computing principal components the

reader is referred to Barber (1974)). In this T space any total kidney vector
can be plotted which is a weighted sum of the nephron vectors. A vector in
this sub-space is approximately given by the linear combination

$$\bar{n} \sum_{i=1}^{L} b_i \bar{t}_i \qquad \cdots\cdots\cdots 2.7$$

where b_i are the coefficients and $\bar{t}_i$ are the principal components of T space.

3. ONE-DIMENSIONAL INTERSECTION ANALYSIS

Application of one dimensional intersection method to renal function
studies is considered here. Following intravenous injection of Tc-99m DTPA,
20, 2 seconds frames were collected. After which time 73 frames of 20 seconds
duration were recorded, with Lasix being administered at about 15 minutes post
DTPA injection to relieve possible retention of tracer in renal pelvis. A
complete study thus representing 25 minutes of patient data. For approximately
the first half a minute the bolus of activity is distributed throughout the
vascular and extravascular regions and no uptake by kidney tissues takes
place. Therefore, the first 20, 2 second frames were excluded from analysis.
Since the injection of Laxis at around 15 minutes invalidates the renal model
of section 2.1, data processing was restricted to the first, 45, 20 seconds
frames. The representing 15 minutes of recorded data. Figure 3.1 shows a
totalized image of a dynamic renal study. One dimensional intersection
analysis of the right kidney in this study is shown in figure 3.2a, in which
curve R represents the intersection vector in T space and curve S represents
the intersection vector in S space. The intersection of the two spaces occurs
in the least square sense due to noise in the study data. For this study M=3.
To verify the validity of the kidney function obtained, the right kidney was
also processed by the conventional manual region of interest (ROI) method.
Time-activity curves are constructed for a region over the kidney and a second
region identified with blood background activity (i.e. extrarenal activity).
In this work a site superior to the kidney was chosen for background activity
curve, although various other possible areas in the field of view of the
camera have been suggested by other investigators. Background correction
fraction (fraction of background activity component in the composite kidney
curve observed) was evaluated using the procedure outlined in Esser et al
(1973). In figure 3.2b curve T obtained by the manual method and curve S
obtained by the intersection method for the right kidney are superimposed.
Figure 3.3a shows a totalised image of a second dynamic renal study and figure

3.3b shows similar results as figure 3.2b for the left kidney in this study. Curve S is obtained by the intersection method and curve L is obtained by the manual method. Subjective interpretation of these results suggest good agreement between the two methods of analysis. The two examples considered represent two very different renal conditions.

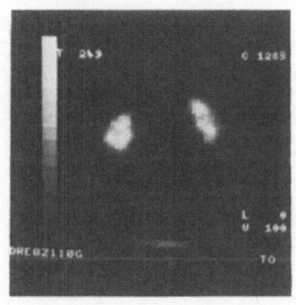

Fig.3.1: A totalized image of
45 frames of a typical
dynamic renal study.

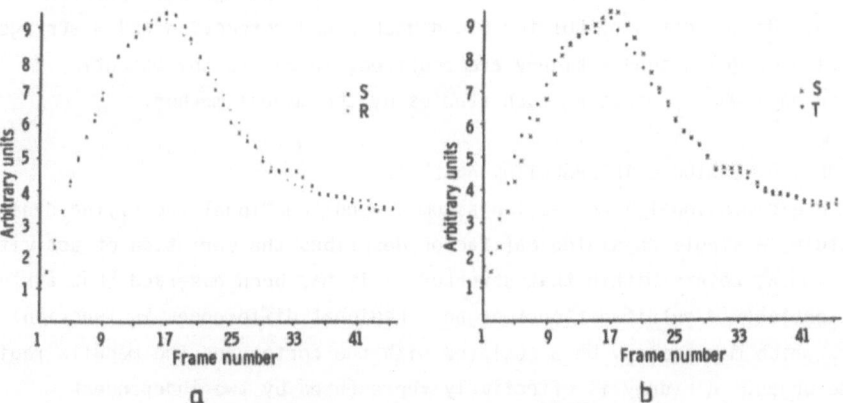

Fig.3.2 (a) Curve R represents the intersection vector in T space and
curve S represents the intersection vector in S space.

(b) Curves S and T correspond to renal function (right kidney
in fig.3.1) determined by the intersection and manual
methods respectively.

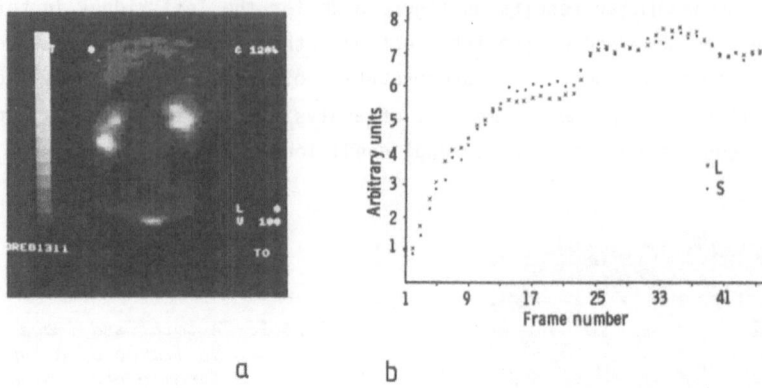

Fig.3.3 *(a)* *A totalized image of a second dynamic renal study.*

(b) *Curves S and L correspond to renal function (left kidney in fig.3.3a) determined by the intersection and manual methods respectively.*

One advantage of the one-dimensional intersection method lies in that the analysis can be performed automatically with little background operator intervention. No selection of ROI for blood background correction and a stringent selection of ROI around a kidney are required, which are the essential requirements when processing such studies by the manual method.

4. MULTI-DIMENSIONAL INTERSECTION ANALYSIS

A one dimensional intersection assumes a unifunctional underlying dynamic structure, a single physiological factor describes the variation of activity with time at points within that structure. It has been observed that a kidney is essentially a multifunctional organ. Regional differences in function occurs which may loosely be associated with the cortex and the medulla region of the organ. A kidney is effectively represented by two independent physiological factors although the same mathematical model describes the underlying physiological processes. The consequences of this observation suggests the solution to equation 2.4 (intersection of S and T) is represented by an intersection space (I) of dimensions greater than one. Nevertheless a one-dimensional intersection solution for the renal case generates an optimal intersection vector which represents renal function of the kidney as a whole. This interpretation has been verified by the results of section 3.0. For dynamic studies in which the structure of interest is unifunctional one-dimensional intersection analysis provides a direct method of computing the true underlying physiological factor attributed to that structure.

A two dimensional intersection solution to equation 2.4 is developed here with respect to the renal problem. Consider the right kidney of figure 3.1 analysed earlier. The study space for this kidney was described by three principal components. It is reasonable to assume that the underlying kidney is best represented by two physiological factors, when considering the quality of data available. Then in this three dimensional S space there must exist a two dimensional space (defining a plane) in which the two renal factors plot completely. This two dimensional space is the renal space. In addition, renal space is represented by the two dimensional intersection of S and T (I space). A simple extenstion of the one dimensional intersection procedure leads to generation of I space as follows.

Intersection of S and T is represented by the linear matrix equation (function A6 in the appendix).

$$Z\overleftrightarrow{x} = 0 \qquad\qquad \ldots\ldots\ldots\ldots 4.1$$

where Z is formed by the L principal components of T and M principal components of S (in the present example M = 3). For a full description of this equation the reader is referred to the appendix. $\overleftrightarrow{x}$ is a vector of coefficients, where the first L elements of $\overleftrightarrow{x}$ represents the coefficients of the intersection vector in T space and the latter M elements represents the coefficients of the intersection vector in S spaces. These two sets of coefficients can be substituted into equations of the forms 2.7 and 2.5 respectively to compute intersection vector in both spaces.

Two dimensional intersection of S and T implies equation 4.1 is satisfied by two solutions for $\overleftrightarrow{x}$ (apart from an arbitrary multiplier). A solution obtained for $\overleftrightarrow{x}$ by the procedure described in the appendix for a kidney defines a vector which plots completely in I space (let this solution for $\overleftrightarrow{x}$ be denoted by $\overleftrightarrow{X}$) this must be so since a vector of this type represents a composite physiological factor of the kidney as a whole. A two dimensional space can be represented by an infinite number of two axes co-ordinate system (orthogonal vectors). Then if the one dimensional intersection vector is taken as the first axis of I the problem reduces to that of determining a second axis (vector) orthogonal to the first such that these two axes form I space. In relation to equation 4.1 a second solution for $\overleftrightarrow{x}$ is required which satisfies the conditions

$$Z\overleftrightarrow{x} = 0 \qquad\qquad \ldots\ldots\ldots\ldots 4.2$$

and $$\vec{x}\overleftarrow{x} = 0 \qquad \cdots\cdots\cdots 4.3$$

i.e. $\overleftarrow{x}$ is orthogonal to $\vec{x}$ and matrix Z. $\overleftarrow{x}$ is evaluated as follows

Premultiply equation 4.1 by the transpose of Z

$$Z^T Z \overleftarrow{x} = Z^T 0 \qquad \cdots\cdots\cdots 4.4$$

$$Z^T Z \overleftarrow{x} = 0 \qquad \cdots\cdots\cdots 4.5$$

$Z^T Z$ forms a square matrix of dimensions (L+M), and let this square matrix be denoted by U.

$$U\overleftarrow{x} = 0 \qquad \cdots\cdots\cdots 4.6$$

The L+M elemental vector $\overleftarrow{x}$ is appended to matrix U as a row rector.

$$\begin{vmatrix} U_{11}\cdots\cdots\cdots U_{1(L+M)} \\[2em] U_{(M+L)1}\cdots\cdots U_{(L+M)(L+M)} \\[2em] X_1 \quad \cdots\cdots\cdots X_{M+L} \end{vmatrix} \overleftarrow{x} = 0 \qquad \cdots\cdots\cdots 4.7$$

or

$$Y\overleftarrow{x} = 0 \qquad \cdots\cdots\cdots 4.8$$

where Y is formed by the left hand matrix of Eq.4.7. The first element of $\overleftarrow{x}$ is set equal to L (fixing the multiplier) and let $\overleftarrow{Y}_1$ be the first column of Y.

$$V\overleftarrow{d} = -\overleftarrow{Y}_1 \qquad \cdots\cdots\cdots 4.9$$

where V is constructed from the matrix Y by deleting the first column (Y_1) and $\overleftarrow{d}$ is formed from $\overleftarrow{x}$ by deleting the first element

$$V^T V\overleftarrow{d} = -V^T \overleftarrow{Y}_1 \qquad \cdots\cdots\cdots 4.10$$

$$\overleftarrow{d} = -(V^T V)^{-1} V^T \overleftarrow{Y}_1 \qquad \cdots\cdots\cdots 4.11$$

The vector $(1, d_1 \cdots d_{L+M-1})$ gives the second solution for $\overleftarrow{x}$, where the first L elements of this vector represents the coefficients of the second vector (second axis) of I in T space, and the latter M elements represents the coefficients of the second vector of I in S space. The two sets of coefficient values are substituted into equations of the form 2.7 and 2.5 respectively to compute the second vector in T and S space. Consider I space in S generated from the two solutions for $\overleftarrow{x}$. Due to the poor quality of study data, an approximate solution for I is obtained. In I space those dixels in the study identified with activity from the renal structures are projected exactly into this space however, in practice no such dixels would be encountered because of contribution of activity due to overlapping extrarenal tissues in the observed dixels. Hence the space represented by I lies outside the distribution of dixels in S. The two vectors describing I do not themselve represent the two renal factors, but only define a subspace in S in which the renal factors plot in their pure form. Further data processing is necessitated to extract the fundamental renal factors.

The three dimensional study space S for the renal example considered here is rotated to a new study space R, by means of a suitable orthogonal transformation procedure such that the first two components of R are represented by the vectors describing I. The new study space R therefore generated is used in extracting the underlying physiological factors by the method of Barber (1980) modified to incorporate additional constraints that the first two factors lie in a space defined by the first two components of R (forming I space). The renal factors obtained in this way have meaning since a priori information of the underlying physiological mechanisms is utilized in extracting the factor model for this study.

Two dimensional intersection analysis developed above was applied to the right kidney in figure 3.1. The left kidney and the bladder were excluded from analysis by means of the ROI procedure. Figure 4.1 shows the three factors extracted for this study and the resulting three factor images. Factors A and B are identified as renal factors and factor C may be attributed to extrarenal activity. Factor images represent total counts contributed by each factor to each dixel in the part of the total study processed. Factor A may be interpreted as representing activity in the cortex region of the kidney and factor B activity in the medulla. Relatively uniform distribution of activity is observed in the kidney region of the background factor image (Figure 4.1d) suggesting effective separation of kidney from background structure. The observed activity in this region may be associated with the vascular pool surrounding the kidney.

In this particular example three physiological factors were found to be adequate for a complete description of the underlying factor model, where a single factor represented extrarenal activity. In general it may be observed that extrarenal activity is best described by several physiological factors. Therefore the appropriate number of factors to extract have to be defined carefully.

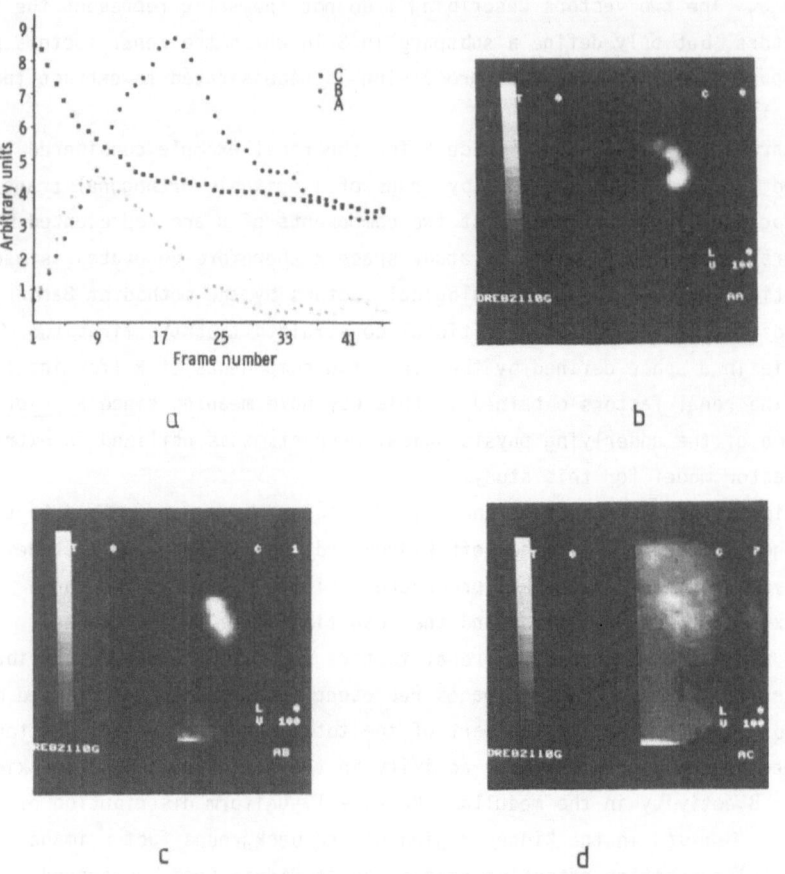

Fig.4.1: (a) The three physiological factor s extracted for the
right kidney in fig.3.1. Curve A is the cortex factor
curve B the medulla factor and curve C is the background factor.

(b) Cortex factor image.

(c) Medulla factor image.

(d) Background factor image.

5. DISCUSSION

The lack of hypothesis of the underlying physiological model in the factorization procedures developed by Barber (1980) and Bazin et al (1979) using factor analysis, introduce uncertainties in the factor solution obtained for a given dynamic study. Some of these uncertainties have been outlined in our previous communication (Barber and Nijran, 1981). In many cases the extracted factors for a particular type of study may not be represented in their pure form but contaminated to some degree by the other unobserved factors since in theory it is not always necessary for the factors to be represented in their pure forms by any of the dixels in the study for the factors to be extractable. In addition, in certain situations it may be difficult to assign computed factors to appropriate anatomical structures underlying in the study.

This paper presents a method of introducing further constraints into the factorization procedure using a mathematical model of at least one of the dynamic structures in a particular study to be analysed. Physiological factors extracted in this way have meaning since a priori information about the physiology of a particular structure is incorporated into the analysis. For a dynamic study in which the structure of interest is unifunctional a direct solution to the true physiological factor representative of that structure is provided by one-dimensional intersection analysis. Such a procedure is useful if this is the only factor required for clinical diagnosis and the extraction of the complete set of factors is not required.

One dimensional intersection analysis of a clinical renal study generates an optimal renal factor which represents the total kidney function, similar to the solution obtained by the manual ROI method of processing. It is necessary to select the appropriate kidney for analysis by marking a region around the kidney of interest. However this procedure can be automated to a certain degree since the only criteria for choosing this region is to ensure the exclusion of the second kidney and the bladder from the data base to be processed. Therefore dynamic renal studies can be performed automatically requiring little operator intervention.

Regional variation of renal function observed suggest a two dimensional intersection of Eq.2.4, which implies a kidney is essentially described by two physiological factors, although the same mathematical model postulates the underlying physiological behaviour. A subspace of S is determined into which the two renal factors plot exactly. Further data processing is necessitated to extract the specific renal factors. In the example given, the two renal factors in figure 4.1a and the factor images obtained suggest the two renal factors may be interpreted as representing activity changes with time in the cortex and the medulla. It appears that one-dimensional intersection solution for a multifunctional structure generates a physiological factor descriptive of the structure as a whole. However, it is necessary to extract the appropriate number of fundamental physiological factors inherent in the structure in order to describe individual dixels associated with this structure and hence to construct factor images.

It has been shown that a primitive physiological model of the kidney is sufficient in generating renal theory space T (section 2.1), although the model itself does not adequately describe the overall kidney function postulated by complex models proposed by other investigators. The model used basically describes activity changes with time in a single nephron and the total kidney function is represented by some weighted sum of the individual nephron functions.

A question remains as to the essential demensionalities of the two sub-spaces T and S. There appears to be no direct method of choosing the appropriate dimensions of these spaces. A procedure found quite satisfactory in this work was to inspect the latent roots of the principal components computed for each space complemented with previous knowledge gained from processing many studies of the same type. Optimal dimensions of T space determined was 5 and 3 for S space.

Two-dimensional intersection analysis has application in sulphur colliod liver function studies where the sulphur collids are removed from the blood stream by both the liver and the spleen but at different rates. The same mathematical model postulates the uptake of activity in the two organs. Therefore if all the dixels constituting this type of study are incorporated into the analysis a two-dimensional intersection solution exists. Hence provides a completely automated method of extracting the physiological factors associated with these organs.

Currently we are evaluating one-dimensional intersection analysis of individual kidney function as an alternative to the conventional manual ROI method of processing such studies and also computer simulated dynamic studies in which the structure is strictly unifunctional. Preliminary results obtained from these studies are very promising. Evaluation of the two-dimensional intersection procedure for regional assessment of kidney function and factor images subsequently generated, is to be undertaken. Results of these studies will be reported in our next communiction.

One-dimensional intersection analysis takes about five minutes on a mini-computer connected to a gamma camera and two-dimensional intersection analysis of a kidney about 10 minutes, where factor image are also generated.

The technique developed in this paper may be extended to other fields of investigation, provided suitable mathematical models can be facilitated to generate T space. Even when such models cannot be given there appears to be no obvious reason why theory space cannot be generated from careful manual processing of many studies of the same kind.

REFERENCES

Aurengo, A., Bazin, J.P., et al. (1982) Factor anlysis as an aid in the interpretation of dynamic scintigrams of transplanted kidney. In: 'Proceeding of the Third World Congress of Nuclear Medicine and Biology', Ed. Raynaud. WFNMB, Paris, 4, 3167-3170

Barber, D.C., Duthie, H.L. et al. (1974) Principal components: A new approach to the analysis of gastric emptying. In: 'Dynamic Studies with Radioisotopes in Medicine'. IAEA, Vienna, 1, 185-196

Barber, D.C. (1980) The use of principal components in a quantitative analysis of gamma camera dynamic studies. Physics Med. Biol., 25, 283-292

Barber, D.C. and Nijran, K.S. (1981) Factor Analysis of Rose Bengal Liver Function Studies. In: 'Information Processing in Medical Images'. Ed. Goris, Stanford, In press

Barber, D.C. and Nijran, K.S. (1982) Factor Analysis of Dynamic Radionuclide Studies. In: 'Proceeding of the Third World Congress of Nuclear Medicine and Biology' Ed. Raynaud. WFNMB, Paris, 1, 31-34

Bazin, J.P., Di Paola, R., et al. (1979) Factor Analysis of Dynamic Scintigraphic data as a Modelling Method. An application to the detection of metastases. In: 'Information processing in Medical Imaging', Eds. Di Paola and Kahn, Inserm Paris, 345-366

Bazin, J.P. and Di Paola, R. (1982) Advances in Factor Analysis Application in Dynamic Function Studies. In: 'Proceeding of the Third World Congress of Nuclear Medicine and Biology' Ed. Raynaud. WFNMB, Paris 1, 35-38

Cavailloles, F., Bazin, J.P., et al (1982) Factor Analysis in Dynamic Cardiac Studies at equilibrium. In: 'Proceeding of the Third World Congress of Nuclear Medicine and Biology'. Ed. Raynaud. WFNMB, Paris, 3, 2361-2364

DeGrazia, P.O., Scheibe, P.E. et al. (1974) Clinical application of a Kinetic Model of Hippurate Distribution and Renal Clearance. J. Nucl. Med., 15, 102-114

Esser, P.D., Bradley-Moore, P.R. et al. (1973) Small computer assisted analysis of camera Renograms. In: 'Proceedings of Third Symposium on Sharing of Computer Programs and Technology in Nuclear Medicine' USAEC Publication, Conf-730627, Miami, Florida, 114-122

Herry, J.Y., Bazin, J.P. et al. (1972) Factor analysis of dynamic scintigraphy structures. Application to kinetics of Hepatobiliary Tracers. In: Proceedings of the Third World Congress of Nuclear Medicine and Biology' Ed. Raynaud WFNMB, Paris, 2, 2240-2243

Lindmo, T., Skretting, A. et al. (1974) An examination of different mathematical model for renal function as measured by ^{131}I-hippuran renography. Medical Physics, 1, No.4, 193-197

Oppenheim, B.E. (1978) Identification of Renograms by Factor Analysis. In: 'Information Processing in Medical Imaging'. Eds. Brill and Price. ORNL/BTIC-2, Springfield, 481-503

Schmidlin, P. (1979) Quantitative evaluation and imaging of functions using pattern recognition methods. Physics Med. Biol., 24, 385-395

APPENDIX

Let T be formed by the L principal components of the theoretical population of dixel generated using a suitable mathematical model of the dynamic structure of interest and let S be formed by the M principal components of the study containing the structure of interest. Then there exists at least one vector, $\overset{\leftarrow}{f}$ which lies in both T and S space simultaneously. This represents an intersection of the two spaces i.e.

$$T \cap S \qquad \ldots\ldots\ldots\ldots A1$$

Let N be the number of frames in the study, then S is a NxM order matrix and T is a NxL order matrix. We have

$$\overset{\leftarrow}{f} = S\overset{\leftarrow}{c} \qquad \ldots\ldots\ldots\ldots A2$$

where $\overset{\leftarrow}{c}$ is the vector of coefficients of the vector $\overset{\leftarrow}{f}$ in study space and

$$\overset{\leftarrow}{f} = T\overset{\leftarrow}{b} \qquad \ldots\ldots\ldots\ldots A3$$

where $\overset{\leftarrow}{b}$ is the vector of coefficients of $\overset{\leftarrow}{f}$ in theory space.
Then

$$T\overset{\leftarrow}{b} - S\overset{\leftarrow}{c} = 0 \qquad \ldots\ldots\ldots\ldots A4$$

Let Z be the matrix formed by concatenating T and -S, i.e.

$$Z = \begin{vmatrix} T_{11}\cdots T_{1L}, & -S_{11}\cdots S_{1M} \\ \\ T_{N1}\cdots T_{NL}, & \cdots -S_{N1}\cdots -S_{NM} \end{vmatrix} \qquad \ldots\ldots\ldots\ldots A5$$

and $\overset{\leftarrow}{x}$ the vector formed by concatenation of $\overset{\leftarrow}{b}$ and $\overset{\leftarrow}{c}$. Then

$$Z\overset{\leftarrow}{x} = 0 \qquad \ldots\ldots\ldots\ldots A6$$

whether or not this has a solution depends on the rank of Z. However, a unique solution of $\overset{\leftarrow}{x}$ is expected (apart from an arbitrary multiplier) from the meaning of the intersection of these two spaces. If the multiplier is fixed by setting $b_1 = 1$ then if T_1 is the first column of Z

$$Y\overset{\leftarrow}{d} = -\overset{\leftarrow}{T}_1 \qquad \ldots\ldots\ldots\ldots A7$$

where Y is formed from the matrix Z by deleting the first column (T_1), and $\overset{\leftarrow}{d}$ is formed from $\overset{\leftarrow}{x}$ by deleting the first element. If Y^T is the transpose of Y.

$$Y^T Y\overset{\leftarrow}{d} = -Y^T \overset{\leftarrow}{T}_1 \qquad \ldots\ldots\ldots\ldots A8$$

and hence

$$\overset{\leftarrow}{d} = -(Y^T Y)^{-1} Y^T \overset{\leftarrow}{T}_1 \qquad \ldots\ldots\ldots\ldots A9$$

The vector $(1, d_1 \ldots d_{L-1})$ represents the coefficients of $\overset{\leftarrow}{f}$ in T and the vector $(d_L \ldots d_{M+L-1})$ represents the coefficients of $\overset{\leftarrow}{f}$ in S. If these vectors (b and c) are substituted back into Eqs. A2 and A3 the two $\overset{\leftarrow}{f}$ vectors generated will not be exactly the same since $\overset{\leftarrow}{d}$ is a solution to Eq.A9 only in a least square sense. $\overset{\leftarrow}{d}$ represents the vector of closest contact of S and T rather than a true intersection.

DECONTAMINATION OF CROSSTALK IN FIRST-PASS RADIONUCLIDE ANGIOCARDIOGRAPHY

George Konstantinow, Ph.D.[*], Stephen M. Pizer, Ph.D.[**], Robert H. Jones, M.D.[*]

[*]Duke University Medical Center, Durham and
[**]University of North Carolina, Chapel Hill, North Carolina

ABSTRACT

Crosstalk is contamination of radionuclide angiocardiographic (RNA) data inherent in the projection of tracer activity within cardiac structures onto the detector of a gamma camera. We describe an algorithm in first-pass RNA for decontaminating crosstalk by modeling tracer activity over time in the isolated chambers of the central circulation. Modeling allows quantification of crosstalk at each individual pixel in the field of view and thus correction of single-pixel time activity curves for this contamination. The resulting decontaminated RNA data are relatively free from crosstalk and from them more accurate and reliable parameters of cardiac function can be evaluated. We present here the decontamination method and discuss its importance in computerized medical image analysis.

INTRODUCTION

First-pass radionuclide angiocardiography (RNA) monitors the passage of a radioactive tracer substance on its first transit with the blood through the central circulation. A problem in first-pass RNA which affects image quality is the distortion of signals in a given region of interest (ROI) due to activity arising from multiple underlying cardiac structures. This distortion, called crosstalk, causes contamination not only of RNA images but also of time activity curves (TAC's) measured at individual picture elements (pixels). Standard methods for dealing with crosstalk in RNA images focus on estimating the distribution of background activity within a given ROI and subtracting this background to correct for the projection of activity from overlapping chambers. Our method focuses rather on the dynamic nature of first-pass data to decontaminate by modeling a characteristic TAC for each isolated chamber of the central circulation. These characteristic curves reflect intrachamber tracer activity relatively free from the contaminating effects of crosstalk; moreover, they allow both the underlying chambers from which a given pixel detects activity and the relative amount detected from each such contributor to be specified for each pixel in the field of view.

When a given single-pixel TAC is decomposed as a linear combination of characteristic curves, the resulting coefficients quantify crosstalk at that pixel. Decontaminated chamber curves can be reconstructed in terms of these pixel-by-pixel decompositions across the entire field of view. These curves lead to new modeled curves, which in turn give a more accurate decomposition of single-pixel TAC's and a better estimation of crosstalk. Iterated in this way, the procedure converges to a final set of characteristic curve estimates reflecting decontaminated activity for each isolated cardiac structure.

The following sections highlight the problem of crosstalk and describe the decontamination procedure. Further details of the algorithm are included in the appendices.

RNA DATA AND CROSSTALK

Data for RNA processing described here are acquired on the BAIRD System-77 multicrystal gamma camera. The detector is a 14x21 array of optically isolated sodium iodide crystals, each of which records counts independently during 25 msec framing intervals. Forty frames per second are stored sequentially in secondary memory. A typical study consisting of 800 frames covers 20 seconds, ample time in most patients for blood to recirculate through the heart. Each frame produces an image for display and within each image the pixels correspond to individual crystals in the detector.

Recorded counts are produced by tracer (Tc^{99m}) injected into the external jugular vein and passing in sequence through the cardiac structures of the central circulation: superior vena cava (VC), right atrium and ventricle (RA and RV), pulmonary arteries (PA), lungs (LL), left atrium and ventricle (LA and LV), and aorta (AO). Counts arising from vasculature in the chest and other organs neighboring the cardiac chambers are referred to as background activity (BK).

Imaging tracer distribution from the anterior view gives the best possible separation of cardiac chambers and vessels overall. Even so, there is considerable overlap between some chambers monitored externally. Consequently, tracer activity projected from areas of overlap contaminates the recorded images - in a given region of interest (ROI) which detects activity from more than one chamber, it may be difficult to determine exactly how much activity comes from each contributing source. The effects of crosstalk are less severe in first-pass RNA than in gated equilibrium studies, since it is possible in the former method to rely on temporal features of the RNA data for chamber separation in ROI's. For example, though the RV and LV overlap significantly in the anterior view, tracer clears the RV for the most part on dispersion through the lungs before it concentrates again in the LV. The TAC from an ROI overlying both ventricles, showing total activity over time from the chambers, has one hump reflecting the increase and decrease of mean tracer concentration in the RV and a second hump reflecting similar concentration changes for the LV. Thus the RV and LV are separated in time by virtue of tracer flow patterns through the catenary system of chambers. Still, crosstalk is evident in the TAC since the actual mean clearance of tracer from the RV (which is approximately exponential) is masked by activity detected from the lungs and appearing early in the LV.

Activity from one chamber may interfere with that recorded from another chamber not only in an entire ROI (comprising many pixels) but also at single pixels. Count rates in first-pass RNA are high enough so that one may determine in most cases the chambers from which a single crystal detects activity according to the low frequency, or mean flow, and oscillatory, or pulsatile, patterns in the TAC for that crystal. It is harder, however, to determine precisely how much activity comes from the individual chambers contributing - to say, for example, that a given crystal detects 30% of its activity from the RV, 60% from the LV, 5% from the lungs, and 5% from other sources. If such information is known locally, it is possible to choose an ROI for any desired chamber and to quantify for the whole ROI the amount of activity arising from the chamber in question (decontaminated activity) and the amount from other regions (crosstalk).

To determine the components of activity at any single pixel it is necessary to have a description of activity over time in each of the cardiac and pulmonary structures without crosstalk. We produce such a description by simulating tracer flow in a catenary model of the central circulation. This model provides a characteristic TAC depicting isolated activity for each chamber in the system. Each single-pixel TAC can then be represented as a linear combination of these "basis" characteristic curves; the coefficients of those combinations quantify the relative amounts of chamber contribution pixel-by-pixel. More important is the ability to reconstruct decontaminated ROI curves as sketched above. Decontaminated curves passed through the catenary model provide a new set of characteristic curves, which in turn provide a more accurate quantification of crosstalk by curve decomposition. When this procedure is iterated, it produces estimates of curves for the ROI's reflecting intrachamber tracer activity relatively free from crosstalk, with coefficients at each point in the field of view corresponding to characteristic curve contributions and thus quantifying crosstalk locally. The algorithm for this procedure is described below.

ALGORITHM FOR DECONTAMINATION

The decontamination program is a three-part iterative procedure:

1) MODEL generates a characteristic curve estimate for each chamber in the catenary sequence as a delayed and spread version of the characteristic curve from the previous chamber.

2) DECOM finds, for each single-pixel TAC, an appropriate linear combination of characteristic curves giving the best least-squares fit to the single-pixel data.

3) RECON produces a new estimate of decontaminated activity for each chamber by a) selecting pixels which detect activity from that chamber, b) summing the TAC's from those pixels, and c) subtracting, from the summed TAC, activity from other chambers.

Single-pixel TAC's $\{f_i(t)\}$ over pixels i and ROI curves $\{F_j(t)\}$ over regions j are functions of time t. The program produces characteristic curve estimates $\{\hat{F}_j(t)\}$ and linear combination coefficients $\{a_{ij}\}$ for each pixel i (j again indexing the chambers).

For initializing program input, each ROI curve F_j is filtered to produce a low frequency component (LFC) reflecting mean flow behavior in chamber j and a high frequency component (HFC) reflecting pulsatile behavior, denoted by L_j and H_j, respectively. Figure 1 presents a typical TAC from the region of RV/LV overlap, showing early appearance of tracer in the RV, subsequent "washout" as tracer passes through the lungs, an increase in activity again as tracer concentrates in the LV, and a final decline as tracer passes to

50

the systemic circulation. The local oscillatory count changes indicate
volume changes as the ventricles alternately contract and relax.
Superimposed on the curve are the LFC and HFC, reflecting the different
aspects of tracer flow being measured. The filters depend on heart rate in
the specific study being processed, as described in Appendix 1. The basic
reason for filtering is to separate the components so that the LFC may be
used in modeling mean flow activity (discussed below). In addition, however,
filtering removes separable, nonphysiologic contributions to the data at
high frequencies (above roughly 6 Hz).

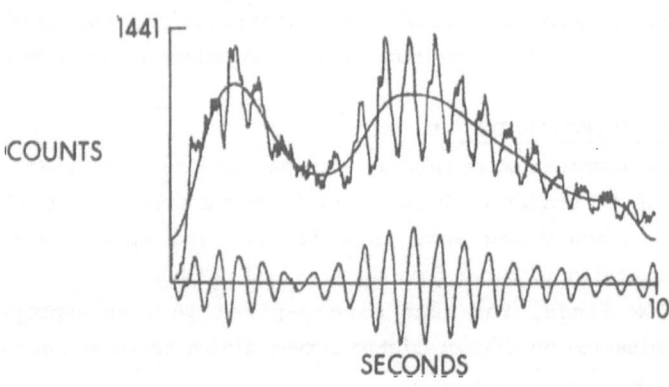

FIGURE 1. Raw data time activity curve with low and high frequency
components.

MODEL

The catenary model produces a low frequency characteristic curve $\hat{L}_j(t)$
by a least-squares fit to the LFC $L_j(t)$ for each chamber j in sequence. Low
frequency behavior for a chamber is modeled as low frequency activity
delayed and spread from the preceding chamber, in accordance with the
principle of mass balance of tracer. Figure 2 is a schematic description of
the modeling process, with a derivation of the accompanying equation given
in Appendix 2. In this figure, the input curve from chamber j-1 is shown
spreading across a volume V_j. Convolution using a factor k_j reflects the

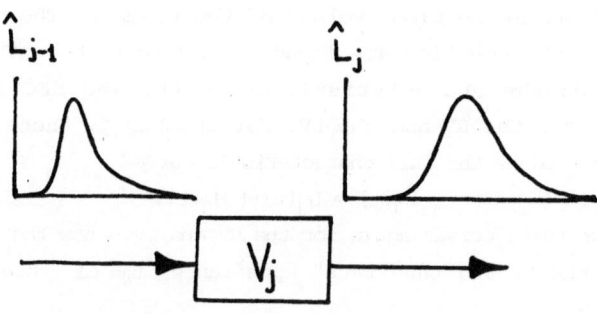

$$\hat{L}_j(t) = m_j \, \hat{L}_{j-1}(t-d_j) * e^{-k_j t}$$

FIGURE 2. Schematic description of modeling. Input from chamber j-1 is delayed and spread across chamber j to produce the low frequency component.

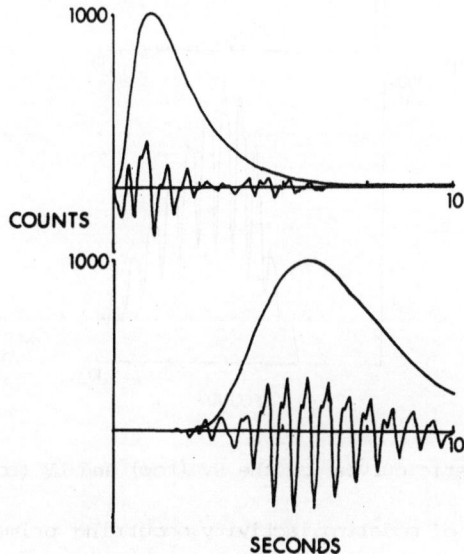

FIGURE 3. Low and high frequency components of the characteristic curves for the RV (top) and LV (bottom).

52

spread of tracer in the bloodstream and a delay d_j reflects the time needed for tracer to mix in the blood volume of the chamber. The values for the parameters in the equation are found by fitting to the LFC for chamber j. Figure 3 shows the characteristic curve LFC and HFC separated and superimposed for the RV and the LV. For chamber j, these components are recombined to produce the full characteristic curve

$$\hat{F}_j(t) = \hat{L}_j(t) + H_j(t).$$

Figure 4 shows these curves again for the RV and LV - now the "true" washout pattern for the RV and the "true" appearance time of tracer in the LV are apparent.

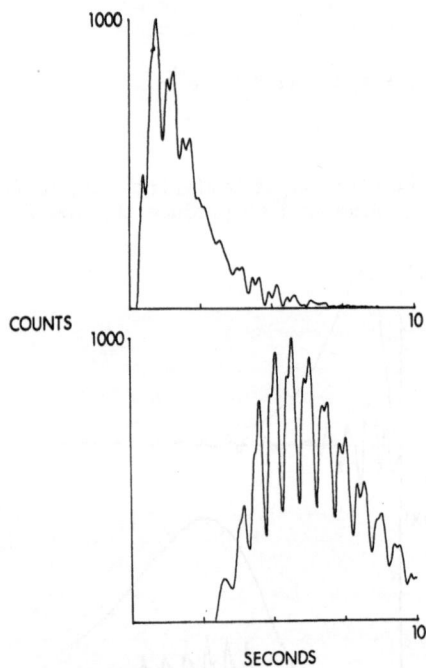

FIGURE 4. Characteristic curves for the RV (top) and LV (bottom).

In the last step of modeling, activity occurring primarily late in the left heart phase, a type of background unaccounted for by activity in any of the regular chambers, is modeled as a combination of counts shifted and spread from the LV and the AO. Appendix 2 describes this formulation of residual flow through the coronary circulation and the lower systemic vasculature. Once all characteristic curve have been computed, they are normalized to maximum counts so that later relative activity detected from contributing chambers may be quantified at each pixel.

DECOM

For each single-pixel curve $f_i(t)$, decomposition produces coefficients $\{a_{ij}\}$ of the linear combination $\sum_j a_{ij} \hat{F}_j(t)$ best approximating $f_i(t)$. Because the characteristic curves are sometimes highly correlated, however, fitting all curves simultaneously at a given pixel can produce negative coefficients and hence meaningless results. To avoid this problem the algorithm is designed instead to search for the triplet of standard characteristic curves (and possibly BK) which offers for pixel i the best nonnegative least-squares fit to f_i among all possible linear combinations of triplets. Appendix 3 discusses the potential fitting problem and describes the algorithm used. Figure 5 shows a single-pixel curve from the region of RV/LV overlap decomposed as a linear combination of the RV, lung, and LV curves (without the background component displayed).

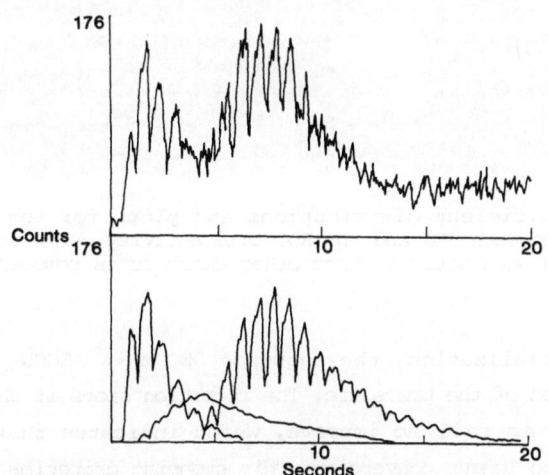

FIGURE 5. Single-pixel curve (top) approximated by activity from the RV, lungs, and LV (bottom).

RECON

The reconstruction step produces a new ROI map for each region j, $R_j = \{i: \text{pixel } i \in \text{ROI } j\}$, from the fitting coefficients computed in DECOM.

The map R_j marks pixels with positive coefficients for the curve $\hat{F}_j$, signaling the appearance of activity for chamber j in the single-pixel TAC's. Figure 6 shows this map along with the decontaminated ROI curve for the RV and the LV to illustrate the procedure. For ROI j the TAC's for pixels in R_j are summed for total activity in the region with crosstalk. The contributions of curves other than $\hat{F}_j$ are then removed from the curve summed over R_j pixel-by-pixel by using the crosstalk coefficients. The resulting decontaminated residual curve becomes part of the next input set to MODEL. Appendix 4 gives the details of the reconstruction algorithm.

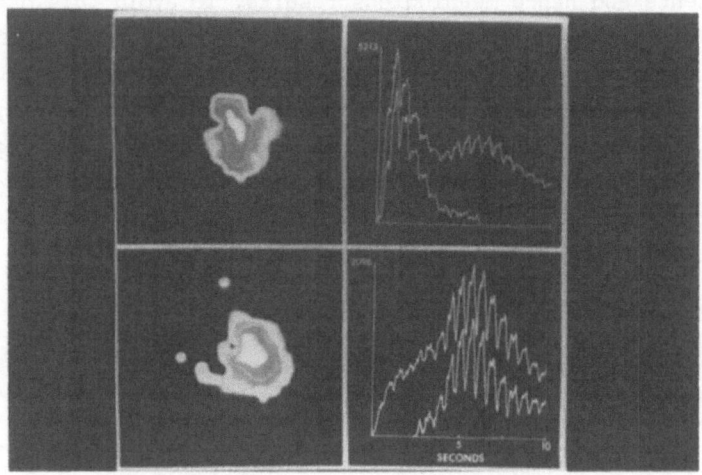

FIGURE 6. Coefficient distributions and plots for the RV (top) and LV (bottom) showing each ROI and the ROI time activity curve with the residual curve resulting when activity from other chambers is removed.

Iteration

After initialization, the sequence DECOM -> RECON -> MODEL forms a single iteration of the procedure. The iteration stops if the characteristic curve estimates fail to improve, which indicates that the successive estimates are no longer converging. This stopping criterion is based on the normalized difference, defined in Appendix 5, between each new characteristic curve from MODEL and its predecessor from the previous iteration. Nonconvergence implies either that the curve estimates are beginning to diverge or that they do not describe underlying characteristic activity in a significantly different way from the previous set.

RESULTS

Figure 7 shows the distribution in the anterior view of the fitting coefficients and indicates their usefulness in ROI selection. The array for each chamber is shown along with an image of the distribution of counts at the time of peak concentration in that chamber. In some cases (for example, the LV and AO here), the coefficient arrays isolate ROI's even though no single raw data image is available for separating adjacent chambers in the field of view. Figure 8 shows similar images in the LAO projection, indicating that the decontamination procedure is not sensitive to the view used for data acquisition (since the dynamic activity within the chambers is independent of the recording position).

Figure 9 shows characteristic curves along with the raw chamber curves for each of the regions. The characteristic curves preserve the correct mean flow and pulsatile patterns of tracer activity in the catenary system of chambers and are relatively free from the effects of crosstalk (unlike the double-humped raw curves or those like the LV curve which reflect activity at times during which no tracer is present in the underlying chamber).

Figure 10 illustrates the capability for detecting chamber overlap locally. Here a single-crystal TAC is shown decomposed as a linear combination of the RA, RV, and AO curves, indicating that crosstalk can be quantified even for pairs of chambers for which the times of peak tracer concentration are not greatly separated.

DISCUSSION

Previously reported results of testing the routine on normal resting studies[1] indicate that the procedure reliably decontaminates TAC's for the central circulatory chambers, verified according to principles of cardiac physiology and indicator dilution theory. Problems sometimes arise on applying the method to data from exercise studies in normal subjects and studies involving various cardiac abnormalities. In exercise studies, especially at high heart rates, it can be difficult at times to generate accurate characteristic curves since flow can be quite brisk and peak concentration times for successive chambers can be hard to separate. In abnormal studies, anomalies of cardiac physiology reflected in the chamber curves can affect the modeling procedure in attempting fits to poor quality data. Research is in progress to document the performance of the procedure

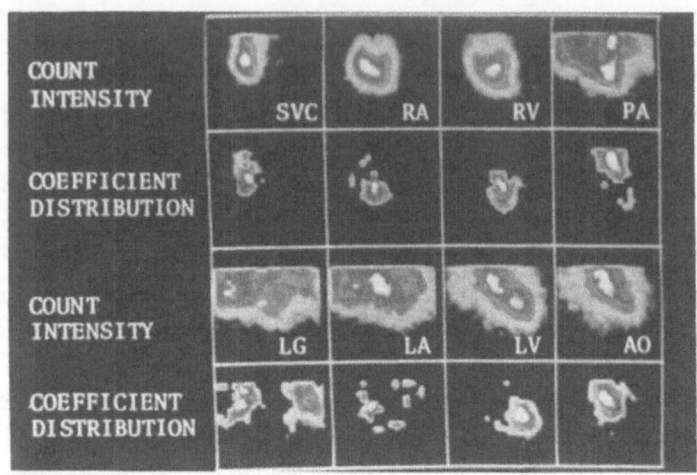

FIGURE 7. Coefficient distributions displayed with raw data frames at a chamber's peak time for the chambers of the central circulation (anterior view). Each image is normalized to its own maximum value.

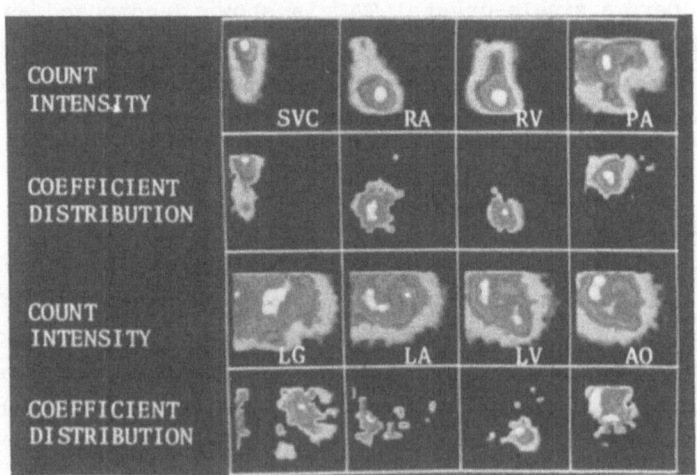

FIGURE 8. Coefficient distributions and images as in figure 7, seen from the LAO projection.

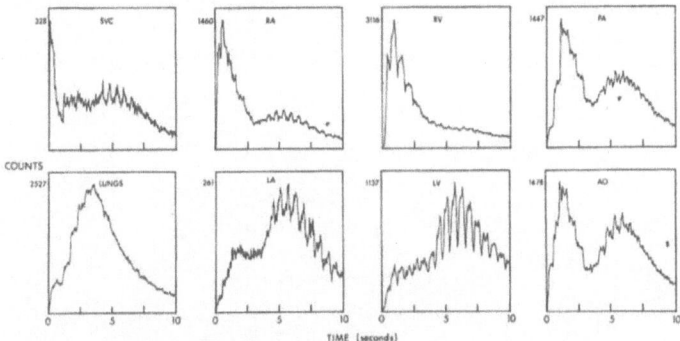

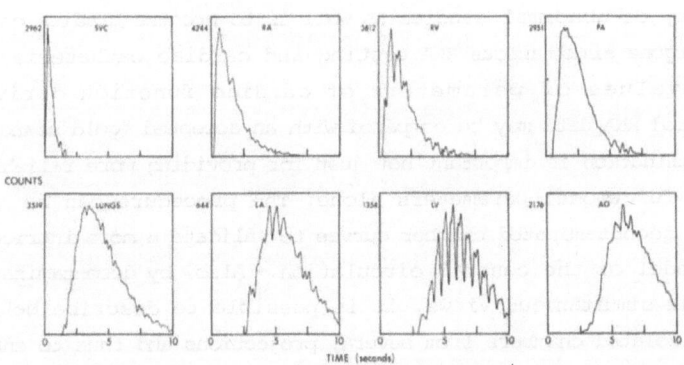

FIGURE 9. Raw data chamber curves (top) and final characteristic curves (bottom) for the chambers of the central circulation.

58

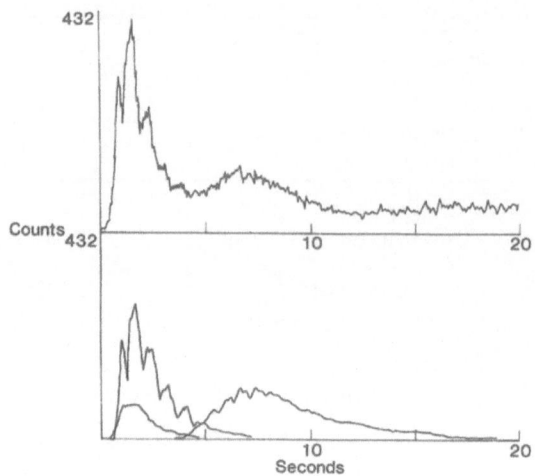

FIGURE 10. Single-pixel curve (top) approximated by activity from the RA, RV, and AO (bottom).

on a variety of abnormal studies as well as to process studies on patients having undergone simultaneous RNA testing and cardiac catheterization (so that the values of parameters of cardiac function derived from decontaminated RNA data may be compared with an accepted "gold standard").

Decontamination is important not just for providing more reliable values of cardiac functional parameters alone. The procedure can be used for simulating decontaminated chamber curves to validate a more intricate state variable model of the central circulation.[2] Also, by decontaminating data from multiple simultaneous views, it is possible to describe behavior of tracer in isolated chambers from several projections and thus to enhance the reconstruction of three-dimensional dynamic images of cardiac structures.

The value of the procedure overall is in its relying on physiologic modeling to describe the dynamic behavior of tracer in the central circulation and on the self-governing iterative construction which controls the quality of the characteristic curve estimates. The successful performance of the method emphasizes the importance of modeling in general for RNA data analysis.

REFERENCES

1. Konstantinow G, Pizer SM, Jones RH: Decontamination of time-activity
    curves in first-pass radionuclide angiocardiography. In Emission
    Computed Tomography, Society of Nuclear Medicine, New York, 1983,
    pp. 251-262.

2. Spencer JL, Regina A, Castellana FS, Friedman MI, Pierson RN:
    Decontamination of region of interest curves using models of the
    central circulation. In Nuclear Cardiology: Selected Computer Aspects,
    Society of Nuclear Medicine, New York, 1978, pp. 181-191.

Appendix 1 - Filtering

The low frequency component (LFC) L_j is produced from the curve F_j by
lowpass filtering in the frequency domain using a multiplicative filter:

$$\frac{3 \{\sin(z)/z\}^4}{1 + 2 \cos(z)^2}$$

with $z = \pi u/h$ at frequency u and cutoff frequency h (corresponding to heart
rate). The high frequency component (HFC) H_j is produced by bandpass
filtering over the range of frequencies from the heart rate to its first
harmonic. Higher "nonphysiologic" frequencies above this range are removed
when the ROI curve F_j is rewritten as the sum

$$F_j(t) = L_j(t) + H_j(t).$$

Typically in RNA studies the frequencies encountered are at the low end of
the frequency spectrum. Heart rates above 240 beats/min (4 Hz) are extremely
rare. Hence one would not expect to find significant information in routine
RNA studies at frequencies higher than the first or second harmonic of that
value.

Appendix 2 - Modeling

The compartmental or catenary model is a sequence of chambers and
vessels through which blood with mixed tracer flows. Let q_j be the flow from
chamber j, c_j the concentration of tracer in the chamber, and v_j the volume

of the chamber. The principle of mass-balance specifies that the change in tracer mass during a given time interval is the amount which flows into the chamber less the amount which flows out:

$$d/dt \{c_j(t) \ v_j(t)\} = q_{j-1}(t) \ c_{j-1}(t) - q_j(t) \ c_j(t)$$

If low frequency behavior is modeled, in which case v_j is fixed ($v_j(t) = V$), $dv/dt = 0$ and

$$d/dt \{c_j(t) \ v_j(t)\} = v_j(t) \ dc/dt + c_j(t) \ dv/dt$$
$$= V \ dc/dt.$$

Furthermore, it may be assumed that flow across the chamber is constant ($q_{j-1} = q_j = Q$):

$$V \ dc/dt = Q \ c_{j-1}(t) - Q \ c_j(t).$$

The Laplace transform gives

$$Vs \ C_j(s) = Q \ C_{j-1}(s) - Q \ C_j(s), \ or$$
$$C_j(s) = [\ Q \ / \ (Q+Vs) \ ] \ C_{j-1}(s).$$

The solution for $c_j(t)$ is the convolution

$$c_j(t) = c_{j-1}(t) * e^{-kt}, \ \ k = V/Q.$$

This convolution is reflected in the form of the low frequency characteristic curve $\hat{L}_j(t)$ for chamber j:

$$\hat{L}_j(t) = m_j \ \hat{L}_{j-1}(t-d_j) * e^{-k_j t},$$

with parameters d_j, k_j and m_j reflecting delay, spread and scaling, respectively, of the input activity $\hat{L}_{j-1}(t)$ to the chamber.

The input to the catenary system is an impulse into the VC. The VC characteristic curve is modeled at the outset by linear inflow and exponential washout of tracer, since the first VC ROI curve used can reflect activity from the PA and AO. This correction is necessary only for initializing the procedure, since the reconstruction step subsequently produces a decontaminated curve for the VC along with the other chambers. Output from the catenary system is background activity modeled as a combination of activity from the LV and the AO:

$$\hat{F}_{bk}(t) = k_1 \ \hat{F}_{1v}(t-t_1) + k_2 \ \hat{F}_{ao}(t-t_2).$$

The constants k_1 and k_2 reflect the fact that roughly 5% of the cardiac output with each beat flows through the coronary circulation and 60% flows through the lower systemic vasculature. The time delays t_1 and t_2 are 1- and 3-beat delays for blood from the LV and AO, respectively, to reach the above-mentioned areas within the field of view.

Appendix 3 - Decomposition

The goal of decomposing a single-pixel TAC f_i is to find a linear combination $\sum_j a_{ij} \hat{F}_j(t)$ best approximating $f_i(t)$. If all curves $\{\hat{F}_j\}$ are used simultaneously, it can happen that two characteristic curves cancel each other (with substantial positive and negative coefficients) to fit to low-count activity in the target single-pixel curve. To avoid this error, the search for a linear combination is constrained so that, for a given f_i,

1) no more than three characteristic curves are used in linear combination except when BK appears as a fourth, and

2) a characteristic curve can give only a positive coefficient of contribution to f_i.

These constraints state that a crystal will rarely record significant activity from more than three chambers and will never record negative activity.

For 8 ROI's there are 56 possible triplets of characteristic curves to check. With the above constraints the triplet

$$\{\hat{F}_{j1}, \hat{F}_{j2}, \hat{F}_{j3}\} \text{ (and possibly background, } \hat{F}_{j4})$$

is found which depends on i and which among all triplets minimizes the difference

$$U_i = \sum_t \{f_i(t) - \sum_j a_{ij} \hat{F}_j(t)\}^2, \quad j=j_1,\ldots,j_4.$$

Algorithm

For each triplet:

1) Fit the triplet plus BK to f_i. If all coefficients are positive, retain the coefficients $\{a_{ij}, j=j_1, j_2, j_3, j_4\}$.

2) If at least one negative coefficient results, fit again without BK (set a_{ij_4} to zero).

3) If in this second fitting attempt a negative coefficient occurs again, discard the triplet (retain no coefficients).

Among all triplets retained, find that linear combination which best fits f_i. The final values $\{a_{ij}\}$ specify the relative contributions to f_i from the underlying chambers indexed.

Appendix 4 - Reconstruction

The goal of reconstruction is to produce new ROI maps
$$R_j = \{i: \text{pixel } i \in \text{ROI } j\}$$
from the decomposition coefficients $\{a_{ij}\}$ across the field of view.

Algorithm

1) Expand the 4-tuple $\{a_{ij}, j=j_1,j_2,j_3,j_4\}$ for each pixel i to a 9-tuple (8 regions plus BK):
$$a_{ij} = 0 \text{ for } j \neq j_1,j_2,j_3,j_4.$$

For each region j:

2) Compute the maximum, $\max_j$, of $COEF_j = \{a_{ij}, i=1,\ldots,n\}$ and a threshold level $A_j = 20\%$ of $\max_j$ to threshold $COEF_j$:
$$\text{for } i=1,..,n: \text{ IF } a_{ij} < A_j \text{ THEN set } a_{ij} = 0.$$

3) Sum the single-crystal TAC's indexed by $R_j = \{i: a_{ij} > 0\}$ and remove activity not related to ROI j:
$$F_j(t) = \sum_i f_i(t) - \sum_k a_{ik} \hat{F}_k(t),$$
$$\text{for } i \in R_j, a_{ik} \in COEF_k, \text{ and } k \neq j.$$

Appendix 5 - Iteration

Convergence is measured according to the "normalized difference" between each new chamber characteristic curve $\hat{F}_j$ and its predecessor $\hat{G}_j$ from the previous iteration. The curves are normalized to the same total counts (area) and their least-squares difference evaluated relative to the common total counts:

$$d_j = \sum_t \{ \hat{F}_j(t)/A_j - \hat{G}_j(t)/B_j \}^2,$$

$$A_j = \sum_t \hat{F}_j(t),$$
$$B_j = \sum_t \hat{G}_j(t).$$

The iteration stops if more than half of the d_j's (for all regions except BK) increase over the corresponding values from the preceding pass.

CODED APERTURE TOMOGRAPHY REVISITED

Y. BIZAIS, R.W. ROWE, I.G. ZUBAL, G.W. BENNETT, A.B. BRILL

1. INTRODUCTION

If the goal of Nuclear Medicine is to quantify the distribution
of a radiolabelled pharmaceutical inside an organ, then the two major
drawbacks of the gamma camera when used with parallel hole collimators (the
most commonly used imaging device in Nuclear Medicine) are low sensitivity
and poor depth resolution of imbedded sources. The former leads to low
statistics (and therefore noisy) images. Improved depth resolution can be
achieved by rotating the camera around the patient (1) (SPECT system) for
imaging stationary distributions.

The gamma-camera inherently is a sensitive instrument (2) for the
energy range used in clincial studies, and the lack of sensitivity arises
from the very poor efficiency of parallel-hole collimators. Besides, this
collimator geometry does not provide any depth information. Consequently,
a great deal of interest has been given to alternative means of collimating
gamma-rays in order to improve efficiency and to code depth information.
Two major approaches have been studied. Multiple pinhole tomography (3),
which can be considered as a degenerate case of coded aperture imaging,
does not exhibit a significantly better sensitivity over parallel hole
collimator imaging, but does provide information on source depth, and
has achieved widespread clinical use. On the other hand, real coded
aperture imaging (4) (e.g. Fresnel Zone Plate, Pseudo-random pinhole
arrays) has a much higher sensitivity, and also provides depth information
but is not used clinically because of severe artifacts induced by the
decoding process.

Actually, depth resolution achieved by both methods is rather limited
and clinically disappointing (5). This arises from the fact that both
collimation techniques sample the 3D distribution within a very limited
angular range. Advent of large diameter dual camera systems make it

64

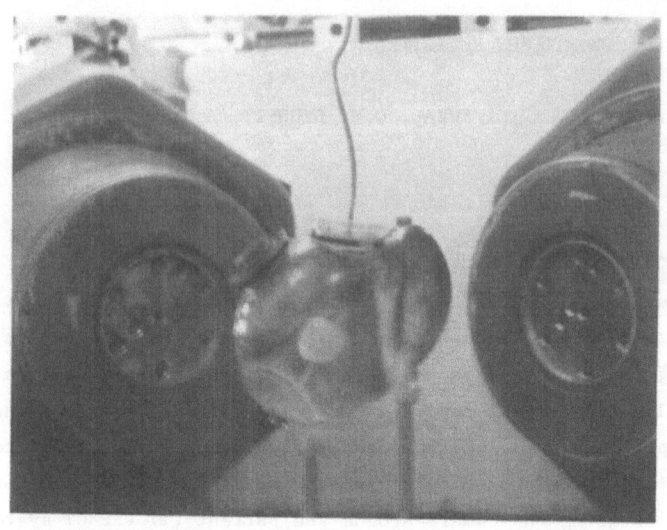

Fig. 1 The UNICON imaging device with detectors
orthogonally oriented and mounted with seven pinhole
collimators.

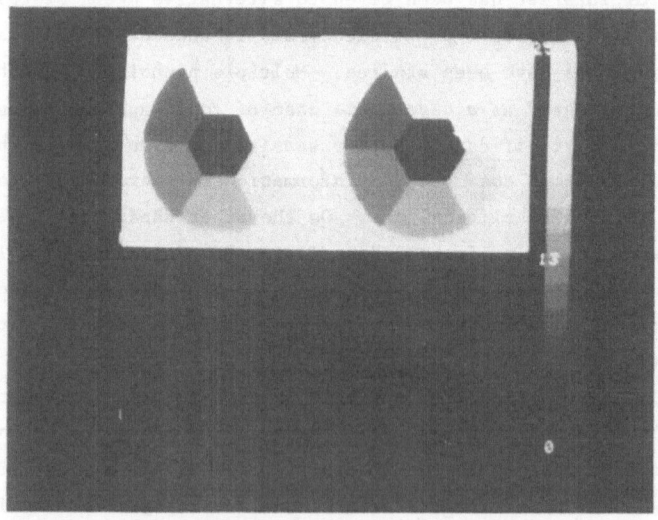

Fig. 4 Projection masks.

possible to increase this angular range to a point where depth resolution
is of the same order of magnitude as lateral resolution. In other words,
a dual static coded aperture imaging system should permit high detection
efficiency and enhanced tomographic ability.

Presented in Section 2 of this paper is the experimental work done in
our laboratory about dual seven pinhole tomography (6). This work is
intended to present and validate the clinical usefulness of dual coded
aperture imaging systems. In Section 3, imaging properties of such a
system are analyzed theoretically and a filtered back projection algorithm
is derived. Section 4 presents a method to build optimal decoding
functions for a given coding aperture. This permits one to analyze the
tomographic ability of a coding-decoding process and to define a coded
aperture imaging device suitable for Nuclear Medicine studies. The paper
concludes with the comparison of multi-pinhole systems and coded aperture
imaging (CAI) systems in the framework of Nuclear Medicine.

2. DUAL SEVEN PINHOLE TOMOGRAPHY

Experimental measurements were made with a dual camera system, the
detectors of which are orthogonally oriented and mounted with seven pinhole
collimators. Seven pinhole collimators were chosen because such
collimators are commercially available, and reference data for single seven
pinhole tomography can be found in the literature. By using such an
imaging system, doubled sensitivity and improved depth resolution are
expected. The latter property can be explained by the fact that the
sampling angular range is increased, or otherwise stated, that the lateral
resolution of one detector corresponds to the depth resolution of the
second one.

2.1. Acquisition hardware and calibration images

Each detector of the dual camera system is a large field-of-view
(LFOV) 40 cm diameter Searle camera mounted with a commercial seven pinhole
collimator (distance collimator - crystal = 5 inches, distance between
adjacent pinholes = 2.5 inches, pinhole diameter = 5.5 mm). The two
detectors are orthogonally oriented but could be angulated differently
according to requirements of specific clinical studies (Fig. 1).

The camera events are digitized and stored in a PDP 11/34 computer
via a special purpose interface, capable of encoding spatial and energy
information of camera events as well as physiological signals. List mode

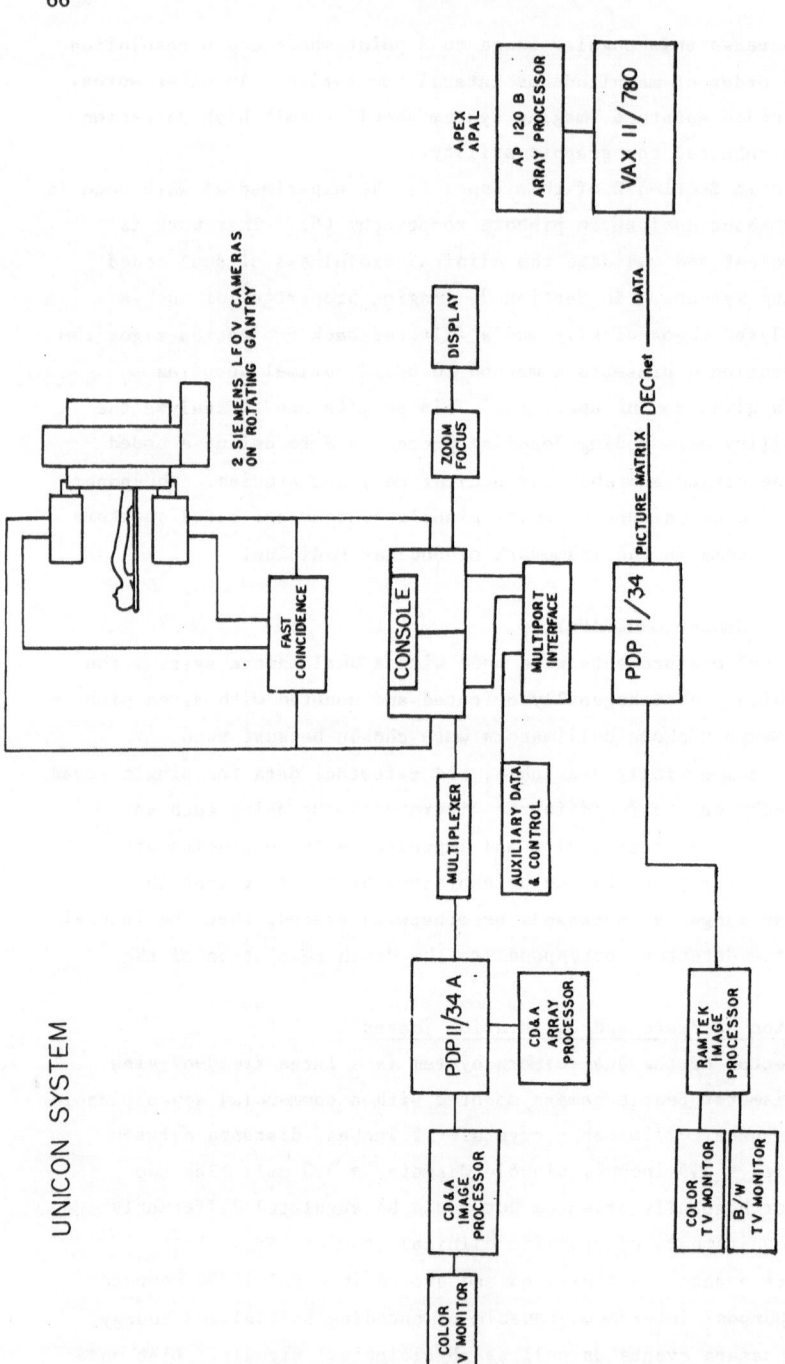

Fig. 2 Block diagram of the computer system used for image acquisition, processing, and display.

files are sent to a VAX 11/780 through a DECNET link where they are
processed to correct for energy and spatial distortions, using an algorithm
described elsewhere (7) (Fig. 2). All images shown in this paper have been
acquired and processed in this way. (For more details about the
acquisition hardware, see (8)).

Parameters describing the system geometry are the following (Fig. 3):
- The system center is defined as the intersection of the two detector
axes. By construction, this point always lies on the axis of rotation of
the system gantry.

- the distances from the system center to the center of each
detector. They do not need to be equal, which makes the system more
versatile for clinical applications.

These parameters are used to calibrate the system using the
projection images of a point source at the system center and of a flood
field parallel to each detector, as explained below. The calibration
procedure is hence very similar to the one used in single seven pinhole
tomography. It must be done every time the system geometry, or the camera
characteristics change appreciably. In other words, only one set of
calibration images is needed for imaging a series of dynamic distributions.
In addition to the calibration images, two images, each containing 7
projections, are acquired for each distribution to be reconstructed.

2.2. Reconstruction volume

The reconstruction volume of single seven pinhole tomography is a
hexagonal section cylinder topped with a hexagonal pyramid (9). Therefore,
the region where two complete sets of 7 projections are available in the
case of dual seven pinhole tomography is the intersection of two such
cylinders. This region is included in a 5 inch wide cube. The true
reconstruction region can be useful only when small organs like the heart
are imaged. Nevertheless, in a wider region (extension of the pyramid),
less than 14 projections are available (usually 2 are missing) and can be
used for reconstruction, because sampling angles are quite different.

In single seven pinhole tomography, plane thickness and pixel size
increase with depth. Despite the fact that this voxellation follows
naturally from sampling considerations (see Section 3), it makes
reconstructed images difficult to interpret. Since dual seven pinhole
tomography cannot use such a voxellation, and because of its drawbacks, the

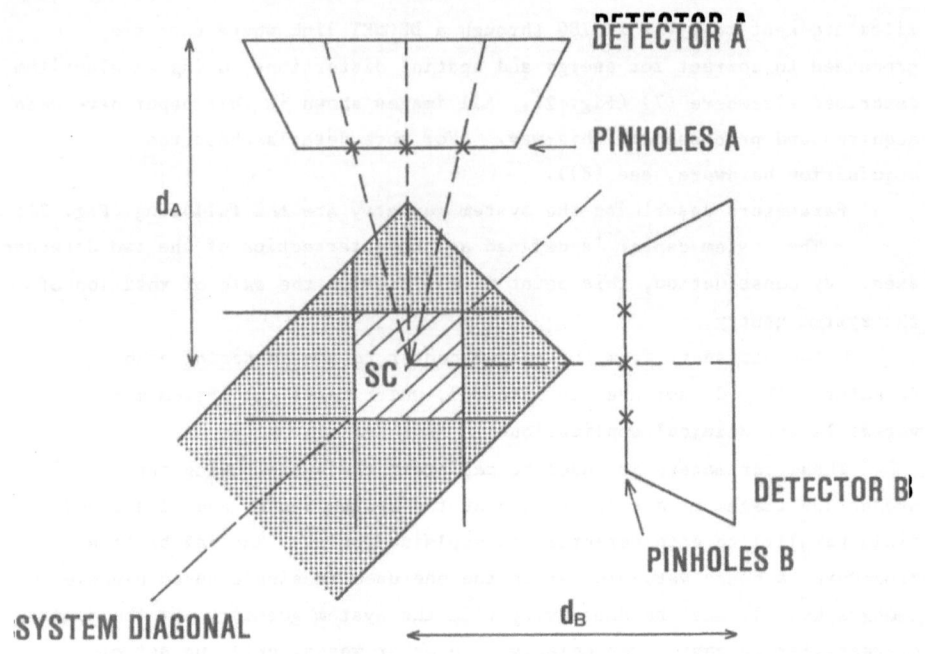

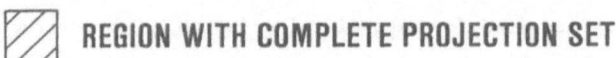

REGION WITH COMPLETE PROJECTION SET

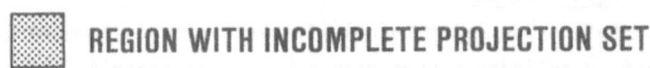

REGION WITH INCOMPLETE PROJECTION SET

Fig. 3 Reconstruction volume.

reconstruction volume is a cube and voxels are of equal size. This choice does not imply that resolution is perfectly uniform throughout the reconstruction volume.

2.3 Reconstruction algorithm

The algorithm is broken into two parts: a projection – independent section in which calibration files are processed and the geometric relationship between projections and reconstruction volume is defined; and a projection – dependent section where tomographic images are actually reconstructed. This scheme allows one to make the algorithm efficient when time-varying distributions are to be reconstructed.

2.3.1. Projection – independent section. Fitting a hexagon to the seven projections of the point source at the system center allows one to estimate the relationship between the reconstruction reference system (defined by the system center, the two camera axes, and the axis orthogonal to the two camera axes) and each digital image system. The algorithm derives offsets, rotation, and an index of residual distortion for each camera (Table 1).

At this point, the center of each projection is known and a mask is built for each camera. This mask contains, in each pixel, a number referring to the pinhole through which the pixel samples the radioactivity distribution. Information from the flood field image is included, such that pixels outside the FOV or under septa are set to eight (code for non sampling pixel) (See Fig. 4).

When masks have been built and reconstruction volume characteristics have been defined, a projection array can be generated. This projection array contains 14 triples (one for each projection) for each voxel of the reconstruction volume. In turn, each triple defines completely one projection: x, y, w, where w is a weight taking into account ray attenuation under a constant attenuation model.

With such a projection array, reconstruction is simply a matter of combining projection values at coordinates given by the projection array after correction for attenuation. This corresponds to a very simple and therefore very fast algorithm.

2.3.2. Projection – dependent section. First of all, the two projection images acquired for each radioactivity distribution are flood-field corrected. The rationale for flood-field correction is not to remove

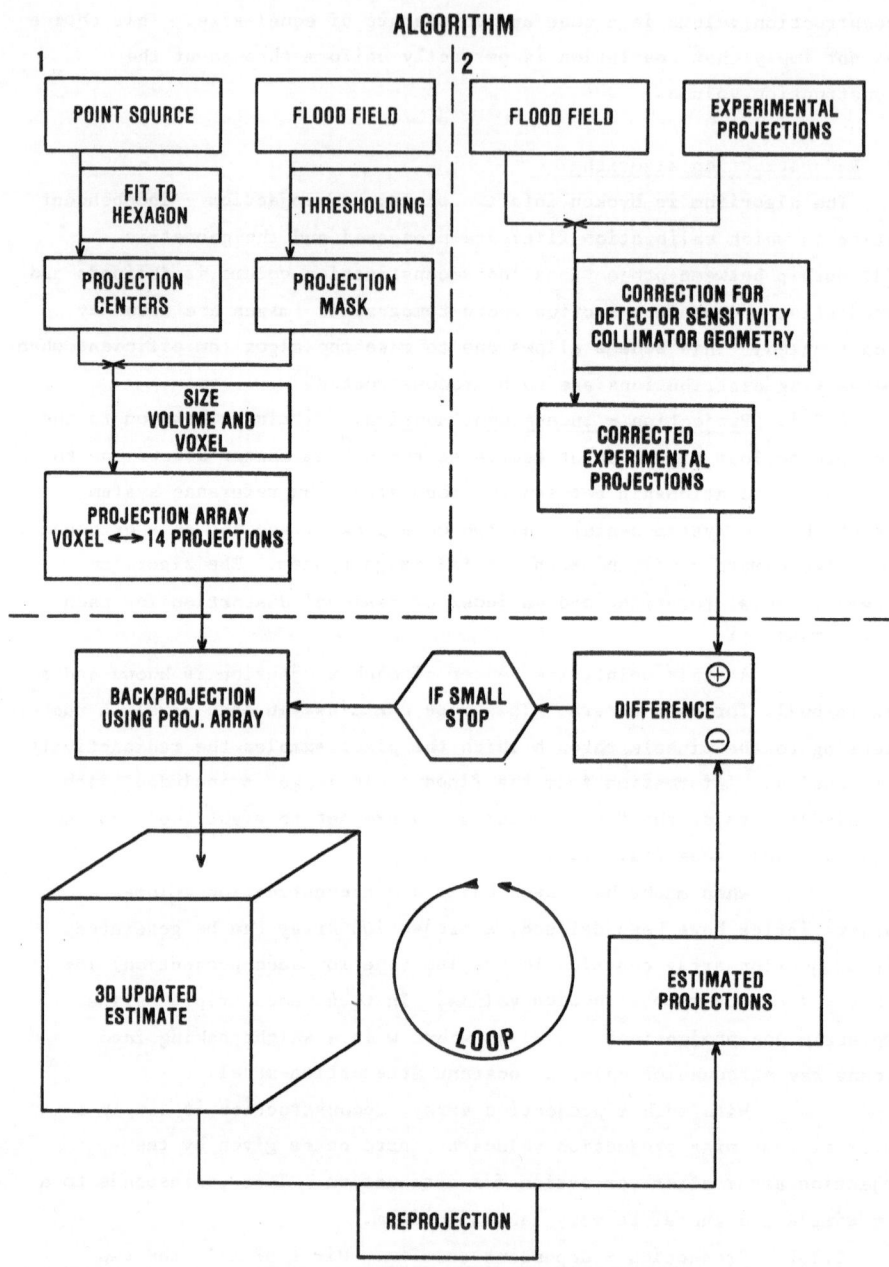

Fig. 5 Diagram of reconstruction algorithm. Top left is projection-independent. Top right corresponds to preprograming of projections. Bottom part sketches iterative reconstruction process.

residual non uniformities as for planar images, but rather to correct for geometric variations of collimator sensitivity. As developed later, collimator sensitivity varies with the cosine of the angle made by the ray and the normal to the collimator. This correction is therefore absolutely necessary to weight every projection pixel in the same way. The reconstructed distribution and its corresponding projections (called later estimated projections or reprojections) are initialized to zero.

The iterative reconstruction can be summarized as follows:

1) a first estimate of the radioactivity distribution is given by the minimum estimator:

$$f_1(k) = \min_{i,j} \left(w_{ij}(k) \cdot p(\ell_{ij}(k)) \right)$$

where k refers to one of the voxels of the reconstruction volume, i refers to a detector (1,2), j refers to a pinhole (1 to 7), ℓ refers to the location of the projection of voxel (k) through pinhole (i, j), and $p(\ell)$ refers to the pixel value at location (ℓ).

Rationale for using such an estimator is that a projection value is a ray sum (integral of a positive function) which is a majorant of any voxel value along that ray. By taking the minimum of all projections a majorant of the pixel value is still obtained. Therefore, this estimator tends to overestimate the distribution at inner points but has proven to be very effective to suppress streaking artifacts.

This first estimate (f_1) is reprojected (p_1) and both are scaled in such a way that the total number of counts in experimental projections (p) and estimated projections are equal.

2) for each subsequent iteration (n = 2,...), distance (d) between experimental projections and estimated projection is formed:

$$d_n = \sum_{\ell} \left(p_n(\ell) - p(\ell) \right)^2 / d_2$$

If d_n is less than a preset value, the iterative process is stopped. Otherwise, the difference between experimental projections and estimated projections is computed:

$$\Delta p_{n-1}(\ell) = p_{n-1}(\ell) - p(\ell)$$

and the estimated distribution is updated, using simple back projection:

$$f_n(k) = f_{n-1}(k) + \lambda \sum_{ij} \left(w_{ij}(k) \cdot \Delta p_{n-1} \left(\ell_{ij}(k) \right) \right)$$

where λ is a damping factor arbitrarily set to 0.25 (9). At each iteration, f_n is reprojected as p_n and both are scaled such that the total number of counts in p_n and p are equal.

Because every complex computation has been performed in the projection-independent section, this algorithm is fast and therefore well-suited to the reconstruction of time-varying distributions. A second important feature of this algorithm is its ability to take into account the two projection sets simultaneously.

2.4. <u>Sensitivity</u>. Point source sensitivity has been evaluated by measuring the count rate obtained with one seven pinhole collimator mounted camera, using a 20% energy window for various locations of a 250 µCi Tc-99m point source. In graphs of Fig. 6, d denotes the distance from the system center to the detector, and r the offset of the point source with respect to the system center. By convention, this offset is negative when the point source is closer to the detector than the system center. Measurements were performed with the point source on the system diagonal (see Fig. 3).

Count rate at each point source location is the sum of count rates detected in every projection. When gamma rays are not stopped by septa, count rate is proportional to the solid angle with which the point source is seen by the corresponding pinhole (10). If θ_j is the angle made by incident γ-rays and the pinhole plane normal, then:

$$N_j = \frac{AS \cos^3 \theta_j}{4\pi Z^2} = A \left(\frac{R}{2Z} \right)^2 \cos^3 \theta_j$$

where A is the point source activity, $S = \pi R^2$ is the pinhole area, and $Z = d+r-s$ is the distance from the point source to the pinhole plate.

Therefore

$$N = A \left(\frac{R}{2Z}\right)^2 \sum_{j=1}^{7} \delta_j \cdot \cos^3\theta_j$$

where $\delta_j = 0$ if γ-rays are stopped by septa and $\delta_j = 1$ if not.

Therefore count rate is 0 when the point source is too close to the detectors on the system diagonal to be seen by any projection and increases to a maximum where the imaged point source enters the complete projection region. Then count rate falls off inversely with the square of the distance from the point source to the detector. When the point source leaves the complete projection region, count rate decreases faster each time that one (or more) projection is lost from the field-of-view.

This model describes experimental data of Fig. 6 quite accurately, and therefore, will be used in the next section. It also agrees well with the data published by Le Free et al (9). Finally, it implies that positioning of the radioactivity distribution is critical: if it is too close to the detector, parts of it are not projected and hence cannot be reconstructed; if it is too far, count statistics will decrease accordingly and the reconstructed distribution will be noisy.

For a typical situation where 5.5 mm diameter pinholes are used, where the source is confined in the complete projection region, and where the distance from the system center to each detector is equal to 280 mm, a count rate of 2 Kcpm is obtained as compared to 0.7 Kcpm which the dual camera system records when LEAP collimators are used. This corresponds to a 3-fold increase in sensitivity.

2.5. Resolution

In order to study variations of resolution with source location, point source projections in air for various distances from the system center to the detectors and for various offsets of the imaged point source with respect to the system center, have been acquired following the procedure described in 2.1. Furthermore, the point source was not always located within the complete projection region.

Point source reconstructions have been carried out using the algorithm described in 2.3 with the reconstruction volume centered at the expected location of the point source and by oversampling the

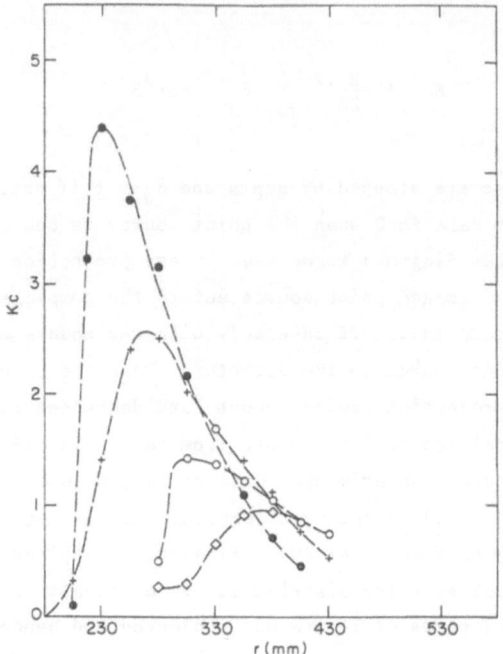

Fig. 6 **Variations of sensitivity with point source location.**

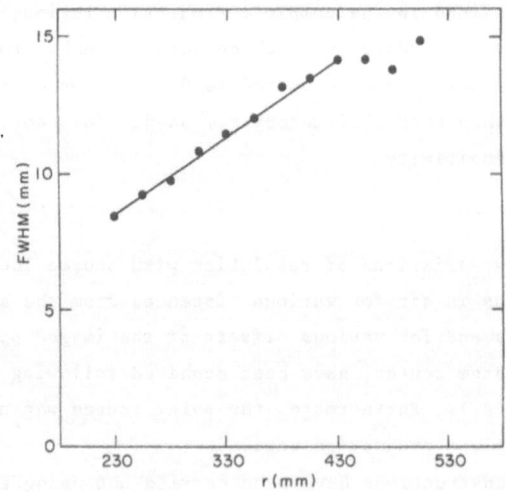

Fig. 8 **Variations of resolution with point source location.**

reconstruction volume with respect to the expected resolution.
Reconstructions have been characterized by measuring FWHM along each axis
and by visual inspection.

Because of the use of the minimum estimator to build the first
estimate, no major streak artifacts are noticed in the reconstruction (see
Fig. 7). LeFree et al. (9) obtained the same type of result using the so
called impedance estimator. For a given point source location, differences
of FWHM along the three axes are considered as negligible (<2 mm). It can
be explained by the fact that angular sampling is nearly isotropic, and
this justifies the even sampling of the reconstruction volume.
Consequently, FWHM along each axis were averaged for each point source
location. Figure 8 shows variations of the average FWHM with point source
location. This graph demonstrates how the use of an orthogonal geometry
improves resolution in the reconstructed distribution and minimizes
resolution variations. Indeed, FWHM is equal to 9 mm for a distance from
the point source to each detector of 230 mm, and to 15 mm for a distance of
480 mm. With a single detector (9), a 8 to 9 mm FWHM is also obtained
close to the detector, but FWHM is approximately equal to 40 mm for a point
source at 430 mm from the detector. Improvements in resolution variations
with source location is still more important than improvement of absolute
resolution, in order to achieve quantitation in emission tomography.

2.6. A realistic example

Resolution measurements using point source in air are required to
evaluate performances of a tomographic system, but do not provide any
information about its ability to generate clinically relevant data. In
order to test the latter point, the following experiment has been
performed. During open chest surgery of a dog, a 1 mm diameter catheter
has been wrapped around the dog pericardium. As shown in Fig. 9, one
extremity of the catheter goes into the dog thorax, loops around the
auriculo-ventricular plane, then follows the interventricular plane towards
the apex, and finally describes a second, smaller loop close to the apex
before going out of the dog thorax. This setting was considered as complex
enough in terms of geometry and attenuation properties, and stable enough
to allow meaningful comparisons between expected distribution and
reconstruction.

76

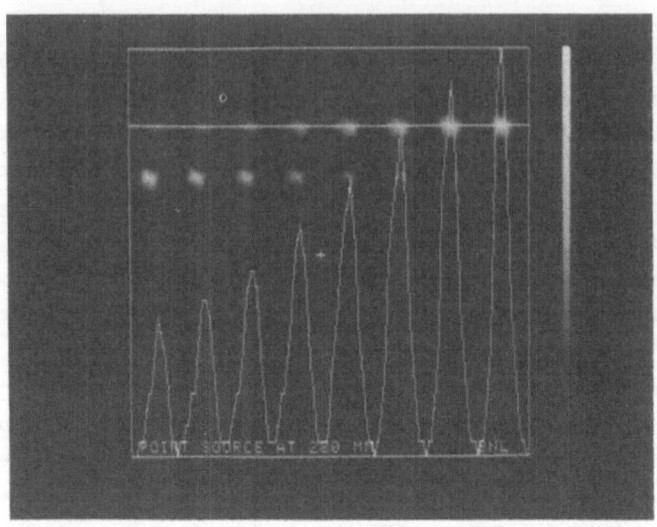

Fig. 7   Point source reconstruction.

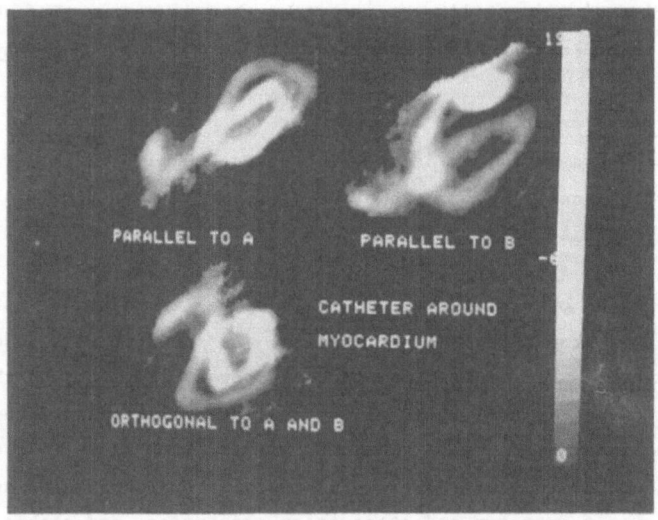

Fig. 10   Pseudo isometric view of catheter loops: (A) seen
from detector A; (B) seen from detector B; (C) reconstructed
planes orthogonal to both detectors.

The catheter was filled with Tc-99m, and two sets of projections were recorded following the techniques described in 2.1, along with calibration files. Reconstruction was performed as detailed in 2.3.

Because loops are not coplanar with planes parallel to either detector, or perpendicular to both detectors, the following visualization method was used to generate Fig. 10. Each 64 x 64 image representing one of 64 planes parallel to one detector (Fig. 10A and 10B) or orthogonal to both detectors (Fig. 10C) was written in a 256 x 256 buffer with the location of the bottom left corner shifted by one along both x and y for each plane. This technique produces a pseudo-isometric representation of the 3-D scene.

The following semi-quantitative conclusions can be drawn from comparison of Fig. 9 and 10:

- Reconstructed images are virtually artifact-free,

- A realistic attenuation geometry does not degrade significantly resolution as measured from point source in air. Resolution is fairly constant over the reconstruction volume.

- Phantom geometry is properly reconstructed, which proves ability of D7PHT to reconstruct complex distributions from projections.

- Constant attenuation within an arbitrary volume can be considered only as a first-order approximation, since intensity should be constant throughout the catheter. Improvements of attenuation correction scheme are important for single photon rotating tomography.

2.7. Conclusion

Experimental validation of dual coded aperture imaging was made possible by the use of a dual camera system and seven pinhole collimators.

The present section of this paper demonstrates that a substantial improvement in sensitivity is obtained by using seven pinhole collimators over LEAP collimators. Results given for resolution of reconstructed point source and the cardiac loop phantoms prove that acceptable resolution and resolution variations can be achieved using this technique. When volume limited distributions are to be reconstructed, dual seven pinhole tomography is a modality comparing well with rotating single photon tomography. Furthermore, the former has the advantage of using a static detector, which potentially allows dynamic tomography.

At this point, two questions are left unanswered:

- Is there any alternative approach to the iterative reconstruction technique, which would be faster and/or better? Theoretical developments, presented in Section 3, lead to a filtered backprojection algorithm which is definitely faster than the iterative method, but for which no experimental data are available yet.

- Can an optimal decoding procedure be developed for dual coded aperture imaging, such that resolution comparable to that obtained by dual seven pinhole tomography can be achieved, along with improved sensitivity? Partial answer to this question is given in Section 4 of this paper.

3. PROPERTIES OF NON OVERLAPPING MULTIPINHOLE PLANAR DETECTORS

In this section, sampling properties of multipinhole detectors are analyzed. This study was motivated by the need to evaluate the theoretical limitations of such tomographic devices, in order to assess their potential for quantitation. It also provides a means to compare seven pinhole tomography with other multipinhole systems in order to define configurations optimal with respect to intrinsic resolution of state-of-the-art gamma cameras and to the size of distributions to be imaged.

The key element of this section is a space transformation which maps the fan beam geometry into a parallel beam geometry. This transformation has been described by Tam et al. (11) but has not yet been fully exploited. It has also been used by Gindi et al. (12) in the case of true coded aperture imaging for which restrictive assumptions are necessary.

In the transformed space, the relationship between pinhole plate geometry and planes sampled in the associated Fourier space is easily derived. This allows one to understand the fundamental limitations of multipinhole systems about depth resolution, and to optimize the pinhole plate parameters for given gamma-camera characteristics.

Because of the parallel beam geometry in the transformed space, a filtered backprojection approach to the reconstruction problem is possible. In particular, a stable realization of the filter is proposed. Such an alternative to the iterative algorithm described in Section 2 is faster and should lead to more reliable results in clinical situations.

Finally, since the transformation can be carried-out only for one planar detector at a time, a scheme to combine independent information from two orthogonal detectors is proposed.

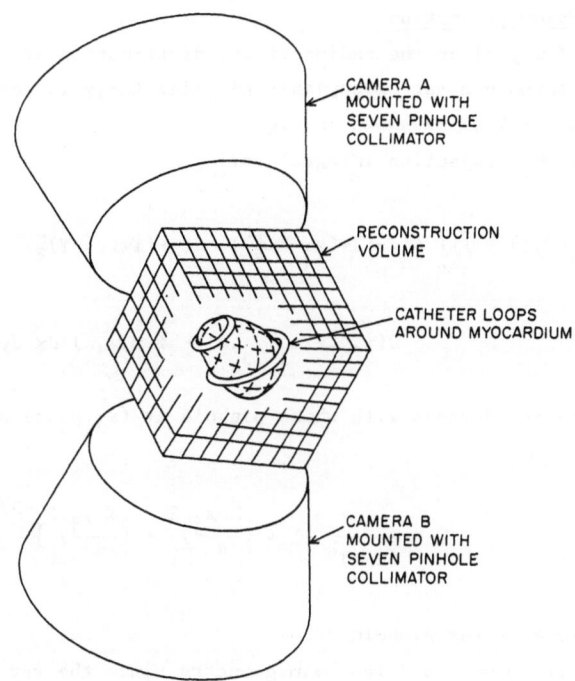

Fig. 9 **Schematic of catheter loops around myocardium.**

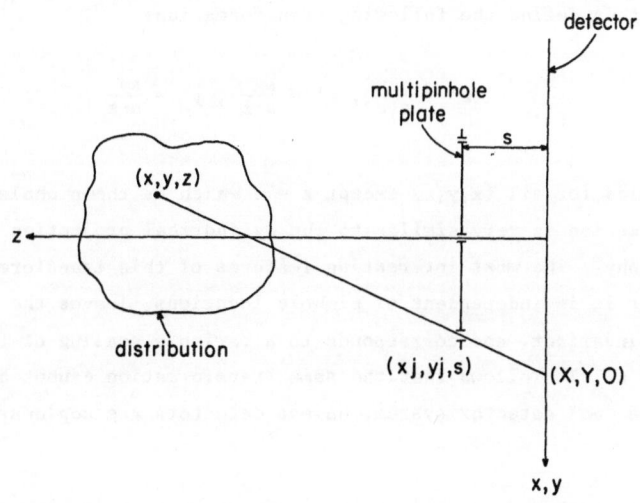

Fig. 11 **Image formation geometry for multipinhole detector system.**

3.1. Fan beam projection

Let $f(x,y,z)$ be the radioactivity distribution of a 3D structure projected through a set of coplanar pinholes (x_j, y_j, s) onto a planar detector at $(X,Y,0)$ as shown in Fig. 11:

Then the projection integral is:

$$P_j(X,Y) = \iiint_{z=s}^{\infty} \delta(x-(X+(x_j-X)\frac{z}{s})) \cdot \delta(y-(Y+(y_j-Y)\frac{z}{s}))$$

(Eq. 1)

$$\cdot \, \Omega(x,y,z,x_j,y_j,s) \cdot f(x,y,z) \, dx \, dy \, dz)$$

Ω being the solid angle with which pinhole at (x_j, y_j, s) sees (x,y,z) i.e. (13):

$$\Omega = \frac{A}{(z-s)^2} \left(1 + (\frac{X-x_j}{s})^2 + (\frac{Y-y_j}{s})^2\right)^{-3/2}$$

(Eq. 2)

where A is the pinhole area.

(Eq. 1) corresponds to a fan beam geometry since the ray slope $((x_j-X)/s, (y_j-Y)/s$ in delta functions) depends on the projection location (X,Y).

3.2. Geometric transformation

Let us define the following transformation:

$$z' = \frac{sz}{s-z} \, , \quad x' = \frac{sx}{s-z} \, , \quad y' = \frac{sy}{s-z}$$

which holds for all (x,y,z) except $z = s$ which is the pinhole plane. This transformation is very similar to the cylindrical projection used in cartography. The most interesting features of this transformation are the fact that it is independent of pinhole locations, leaves the detector plane $(z = 0)$ invariant, and corresponds to a variable scaling of (x,y) according to depth z. It follows that the same transformation cannot be used in the case of a dual detector system, unless detectors are coplanar.

In the resulting space, the projection integral is written:

$$P_j(X,Y) = \int\int\int_{z'=-\infty}^{-s} \delta(x'-(X + \frac{x_j}{s}z')) \cdot \delta(y'-(Y + \frac{y_j}{s} z'))$$

(Eq. 3)

$$\Omega(X,Y,x_j,y_j,s) \cdot f'(x',y',z') (\frac{s}{s+z'})^2 dx'dy'dz'$$

where the last term is the product of the Jacobian with the scaling factors arising from the change of variable in the delta functions.

When Ω is replaced by its value given in (Eq. 2), the following equation is obtained:

$$q_j(X,Y) = \int\int\int_{z'=-\infty}^{-s} \delta(x'-(X + \frac{x_j}{s}z')) \cdot \delta(y'-(Y + \frac{y_j}{s} z'))$$

(Eq.4)

$$f'(x',y',z')dx'dy'dz'$$

where

$$q_j(X,Y) = \frac{s^2}{A} \left[1 + (\frac{X-x_j}{s})^2 + (\frac{Y-y_j}{s})^2 \right]^{3/2} p_j(X,Y) \qquad \text{(Eq. 5)}$$

(Eq. 3) has the following meaning: in the new space, the 3D radioactivity distribution (f') is projected along parallel rays onto the detector, since the slope $((x_j)/s, (y_j)/s)$ of the beam line is independent of the projection point (X,Y), contrary to (Eq.1). However, the projection intensity $(p_j(X,Y))$ must be corrected $(q_j(X,Y))$ for sensitivity variations induced by the beam angulation in order to obtain a truly parallel beam formula. Each projection samples the 3D distribution along parallel rays characterized by the angle $((x_j)/s, (y_j)/s)$. Therefore a J aperture imaging system generates a set of J parallel beam projections in the new space, and the tomographic ability of this device is related to how well the range of projection angles covers the unit hemisphere.

3.3. Fourier representation

Because the above transformation maps a fan beam projection into a parallel beam projection, inferences about the sampling properties of a multipinhole system can be made in the Fourier space associated to the transformed space. For this purpose let $Q_j(\lambda,\mu)$ be the Fourier transform of $q_j(X,Y)$.

By replacing $q_j(X,Y)$ by its value (Eq. 4) and by substituting orders of integration, we obtain

$$Q (\lambda,\mu) = F'(\lambda,\mu, - \frac{x_j\lambda + y_j\mu}{s})$$

(Eq. 6)

where F' is the Fourier transform of f'. Therefore each corrected projection (q_j) corresponds to one plane of the Fourier transform of f'. In other words, a J-pinhole system provides information about J planes of the 3D Fourier transform of the radioactivity distribution.

Each plane sampled in the Fourier space characterized by its normal $v_j(\alpha_j,\beta_j,\gamma_j) =$

$$\alpha_j = \frac{x_j}{s} \left(1 + \frac{x_j^2 + y_j^2}{s^2}\right)^{-1/2}$$

$$\beta_j = \frac{y_j}{s} \left(1 + \frac{x_j^2 + y_j^2}{s^2}\right)^{-1/2}$$

$$\gamma_j = \left(1 + \frac{x_j^2 + y_j^2}{s^2}\right)^{-1/2}$$

The distribution of this set of vectors on a unit sphere defines the tomographic properties of a multiphinhole detector, which are related very simply to the collimator geometry (x_j,y_j,s).

As an example, sampling properties of a seven pinhole collimator, as the one described in Section 2, are given. Central pinhole (index 0) is located at $(x_0 = 0, y_0 = 0)$ while peripheral pinholes (index = 1, 6) are located at

$$x_j = \frac{s}{2} \cos \frac{2j-1}{6} \pi, \ y_j = \frac{s}{2} \cos \frac{2j-1}{6} \pi$$

Therefore the Fourier plane associated to the central pinhole is characterized by vector $v_o(0,0,1)$ and Fourier planes associated to peripheral pinholes are associated with

$$v_j \left(\frac{1}{\sqrt{5}} \cos \frac{2j-1}{6} \pi, \frac{1}{\sqrt{5}} \sin \frac{2j-1}{6} \pi, \frac{2}{\sqrt{5}}\right)$$

Figure 12 is a graphic representation of this set of vectors on a unit sphere where the latter is seen from the north pole (positive ν). In a real implementation, each projection is sampled within a given surface with a given mesh. The latter determines the highest known frequency of the Discrete Fourier Transform. Each sampled plane in the 3D Fourier space is given by a 2D Fourier Transform of a projection, and therefore is known up to the same spatial frequency. If a sampled plane is drawn in plane

$$\left(\lambda \cos \frac{2j-1}{6} \pi + \mu \sin \frac{2j-1}{6} \pi, \nu\right),$$

as shown in Fig. 13 for $j = 0$ and $j = 1$, it becomes evident that:

- plane associated to v_o completely samples plane (λ,μ) but does not contain any information about the ν axis (no depth information).

- planes associated with any peripheral pinhole contain information about the ν axis in a bandwidth $\sqrt{5}$ narrower than along the λ or μ axes.

Therefore resolution along z' can be expected to be coarser than along x' or y', by a factor of $\sqrt{5}$, if projection images are sampled at Nyquist rate or more finely. In other words, even after space transformation where the multipinhole system samples the 3D distribution according to a parallel beam geometry, strong anisotropy in resolution can be expected due to the bandwidth limitation along the Fourier axis corresponding to depth. Furthermore, projection images (p_j) are evenly sampled, which implies that $F'(\lambda,\mu,\nu)$ and $f'(x',y',z')$ are evenly sampled as well. Therefore $f(x,y,z)$ is known at coarser and coarser mesh points with increasing depth. This fact is acknowledged empirically in the way the original single seven pinhole tomography algorithm performs reconstruction, since plane thickness and pixel size increase with depth.

As an attempt to increase depth resolution, one can imagine to decrease (s) in order to increase ratios $(x_j)/s$ and $(y_j)/s$. Unfortunately

it further decreases the complete projection region, which is already quite
limited, and overall resolution in the reconstruction region would not be
improved significantly, because of the combined effects of decreased
magnification and finite intrinsic resolution of the detector. Therefore,
the current design of seven pinhole collimators is well adapted to the
performances of present gamma-cameras, and improved reconstruction can be
sought for only in the use of dual camera systems.

Very qualitatively because the space transformation is by no means
the same for two non coplanar detectors, improvements obtained by using a
dual camera system can be understood from Fig. 12 and Fig. 13. In the case
of an orthogonal geometry, respective roles of axes ν and (λ, μ) are
exchanged. Since the angle made by v_0 and any v_j for one detector is about
30° (26.57° exactly), the angle made by any two vectors normal to planes
sampled by peripheral pinholes of the orthogonal detector pair is also
close to 30°. It follows that an orthogonal geometry samples the 3D
distribution almost evenly along each axis of the Fourier space.
Furthermore, the inverse space transformation being different for each
detector, resolution variations induced by resampling are reduced when
compared to the single detector case.

3.4. Filtered backprojection algorithm

The above space transformation is useful to understand sampling
properties of multipinhole imaging systems, and represents the basis for
deriving a filtered backprojection algorithm.

3.4.1. Impulse response of simple backprojection.

Let a point
source located at (x_0', y_0', z_0') in the transformed space be imaged with a
multipinhole system. It can be derived from (Eq. 4) that for each pinhole
(j), a point source corrected projection (q_j) is obtained:

$$q_j(X,Y) = \delta(X-X_j) \cdot \delta(Y-Y_j)$$

with

$$X_j = x_0' - \frac{x_j}{s} z_0'$$

$$Y_j = y_0' - \frac{y_j}{s} z_0'$$

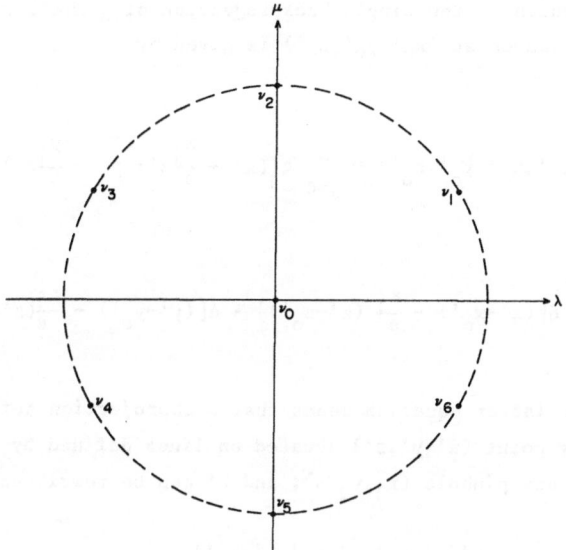

Fig. 12 Distribution of vectors normal to sampled planes in the Fourier space associated to the transformed space.

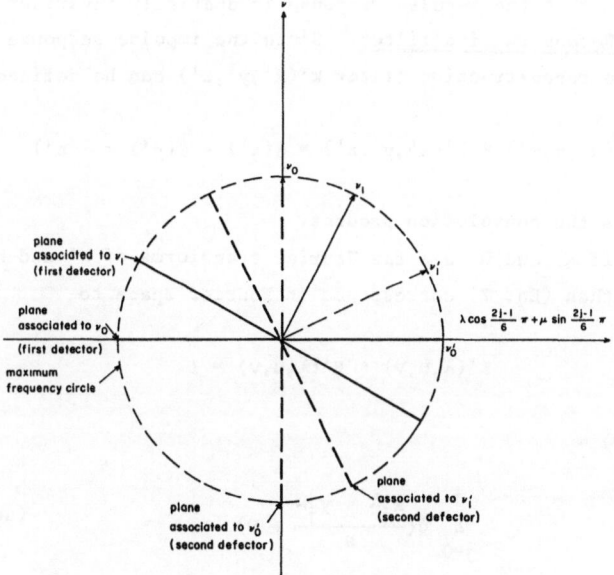

Fig. 13 Angulation of vectors normal to the Fourier plane associated to the central pinhole and to the Fourier plane associated with any peripheral pinhole. Locations of vectors associated with the second detector demonstrate improvements in angular sampling uniformity achieved with an orthogonal geometry.

The function h', which is the simple backprojection of pinhole projections (q_j) of the point source at (x_o',y_o',z_o') is given by:

$$h'(x',y',z',x_o',y_o',z_o') = \sum_{j=0}^{J} q_j(x' - \frac{x_j}{s}z', y' - \frac{y_j}{s}z')$$

$$= \sum_{j=0}^{J} \delta((x'-x_o') - \frac{x_j}{s}(z'-z_o')) \cdot \delta((y'-y_o') - \frac{y_j}{s}(z'-z_o'))$$

Geometrically, the latter equation means that backprojection defines the intensity of every point (x',y',z') located on lines defined by (x_o',y_o',z_o') and any pinhole (x_j,y_j,s); and h' can be rewritten as:

$$h'(x'-x_o',y'-y_o',z'-z_o').$$

This is a direct consequence of parallel beam geometry in the transformed space and means that the impulse response is spatially invariant.

3.4.2. <u>Reconstruction filter</u>. Since the impulse response is stationary, the reconstruction filter $k'(x',y',z')$ can be defined by:

$$k'(x',y,z') * h'(x',y',z') = \delta(x') \cdot \delta(y') \cdot \delta(z') \qquad \text{(Eq. 7)}$$

where * denotes the convolution product.

If K' and H' are the Fourier transforms of k' and h' respectively, then (Eq. 7) corresponds in Fourier space to

$$K'(\lambda,\mu,\nu) \cdot H'(\lambda,\mu,\nu) = 1 \qquad \text{(Eq. 8)}$$

Since $H'(\lambda,\mu,\nu) =$

$$\sum_{j=0}^{j} \delta(\frac{x_j\lambda + y_j\mu}{s} + \nu) \qquad \text{(see Eq. 6)},$$

H' is equal to zero at most points of the Fourier space, and Eq. 8 cannot be inverted for every point due to incomplete sampling. However, a stable approximation of k' can be derived using a regularization technique (14):

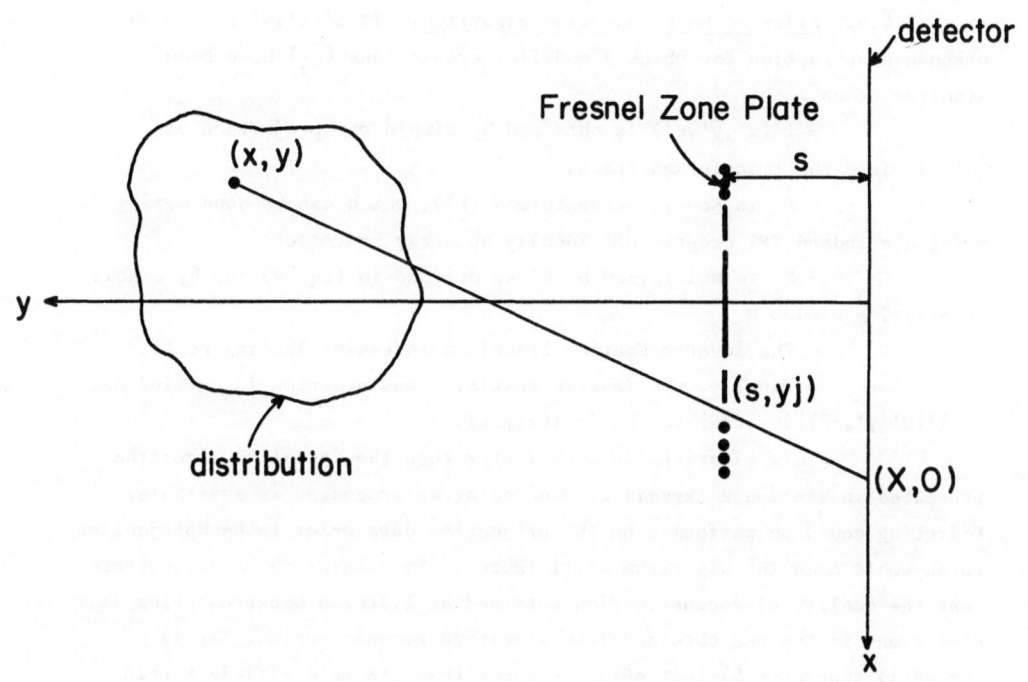

Fig. 14 Image formation geometry for coded aperture imaging system.

$$K'(\lambda,\mu,\nu) = \frac{H^*(\lambda,\mu,\nu)}{||H(\lambda,\mu,\nu)||^2 + C} \qquad\qquad (Eq.\ 9)$$

where C is an appropriate constant.

The reconstruction filter thus obtained formerly corresponds to the ramp filter of single photon tomography and should be multiplied by a window (e.g. Hanning window) to avoid noise amplification.

3.4.3. <u>Filtered backprojection algorithm</u>. If f'(x',y',z') is an unknown distribution for which J modified projections (q_j) have been acquired, then

- f'(x',y',z') is obtained by simple backprojection of $q_j(X,Y)$ into the transformed space,

- f' is Fourier transformed (F'), which can be done easily using a standard FFT program and ideally an array processor.

- F' is multiplied by K' as defined in (Eq. 9) and by a noise suppressing window W.

- The inverse Fourier transform is taken, leading to f',

- finally, the inverse spatial transformation is carried out on f'(x',y',z') in order to obtain f(x,y,z).

This algorithm is much faster than the iterative algorithm presented in Section 2 expecially when an array processor is available. Filtering could be performed on the projection data prior to backprojection which would make the algorithm still faster. It remains to be demonstrated that the quality of reconstruction obtained by filtered backprojection is equivalent to the one obtained from iterative reconstruction. It is currently thought (15) that ART-type algorithms are more efficient than filtered backprojection when a small number of projections is available.

As pointed out already, the same spatial transformation cannot be used for two orthogonal sets of projections. This means that an estimated distribution must be computed for each detector, and then both estimates combined. This can be done fairly simply by performing the above algorithm for both sets of projections independently but the last step, and to use both estimates adequately weighted to perform the resampling step.

3.5. <u>Conclusion</u>

The space transformation described above maps the original fan beam geometry of multipinhole detector systems into a parallel beam geometry.

In the Fourier space associated to the transformed space, sampling properties of such detectors are easily described in terms of the geometric characteristics of the pinhole plate. Poor depth resolution can be explained both by undersampling along the depth axis in the transformed space (limited angular range) and by the inverse space transformation of an evenly sampled reconstruction, such that plane thickness and voxel size increase with depth. Another major result is the fact that use of two orthogonally oriented seven pinhole collimators ensures an almost uniform angular sampling of the distribution. This fact explains why decreased variations in resolution were experimentally demonstrated with such a device.

In the transformed space, a filtered backprojection has been derived, and is much faster than the iterative algorithm of Section 2, especially if filtering is performed prior to backprojection. However, experimental evidence is still needed to demonstrate that this type of reconstruction performs significantly better than an iterative procedure, for incompletely sampled distributions.

4. DISCUSSION

The theoretical developments presented above make clear the relationship between the multipinhole detector geometry and its sampling properties (hence its tomographic ability). In particular, they demonstrate that conventional seven pinhole collimators are a good compromise between efficient use of the crystal area, the size of the reconstruction volume, and depth information. Furthermore, based on theoretical and experimental observations, the use of an orthogonal geometry has been shown to result in improved tomographic resolution.

It remains now to determine whether orthogonal true coded aperture imaging systems can provide the same type of resolution as orthogonal multipinhole detectors, with a much higher collection efficiency. We favor time-invariant coded apertures like Fresnel Zone Plate, over time-varying apertures which prevent the study of fast dynamic 4-dimensional processes (x,y,z,t). This section describes the image formation process when time-invariant coded apertures are used, presents the current state of decoding procedure, and discusses the problems to be solved before coded apertures can be used in clinical situations.

4.1. Image formation process

The image formation process is described in the 2-D case without loss of generality. Let $f(x,z)$ be a radioactive distribution coded by an aperture mask $A(x_j)$ as $p(X)$. From Fig. 14 it is obvious that:

$$p(X) = \int_0 \frac{A(x_j)}{\left(1+(\frac{X-x_j}{s})^2\right)^{3/2}} \iint \frac{f(x,y)\delta(x-(X+(x_j-X)\frac{z}{s})}{z^2}dxdz\ dx_j^2$$

(Eq. 10)

This equation can be seen as a generalization of (Eq. 1), since $A(x_j)$ is a delta function for a pinhole. The correction factor for angulation $\left(1 + (X-x_j)/s^2\right)^{3/2}$ depends both on the projection point (X) and the point of the aperture mask (x_j) through which the distribution is sampled. This fact prevents the correction of projections for geometric variations of efficiency, and therefore the use of space transformation, as was done for multipinhole systems. In practical situations, this angulation factor cannot be neglected as claimed in Gindi et al. (12).

4.2. Reconstruction

It follows that reconstruction should be performed by filtering (decoding) the projection image with a different kernel for each point of the reconstruction volume. As this cannot be done actually, reconstruction is carried out using only one decoding function matching the aperture mask, by analogy to optical methods. This approach is by no means optimal and has led to clinically disappointing results.

A more precise method has been proposed by Steinbach (16) where the decoding function is defined as the product of the usual decoding function by the Fourier expansion of an apodisation function. Optimal coefficients of the expansion are obtained by minimizing the distance between the ideal image of a point source at the center of the reconstruction volume and the actual decoded image. According to results published by Steinbach, improvements provided by such an optimal decoding function are impressive in terms of bias and mean square distance between ideal and reconstructed distributions. Furthermore, when an orthogonal set of coded apertures is used, resolution is improved and comparable to results obtained in Section 2.

Consequently, simulation and phantom studies are in progress in our laboratory to study the effects of the number of coefficients in the development of the apodisation function, and to analyze the variations of the optimal decoding function throughout the reconstruction volume. If the decoding function can be considered as constant, then reconstruction of radioactivity distributions of quality comparable to that of dual seven pinhole tomography could be achieved with a much higher sensitivity.

4.3. Noise and attenuation

Two important issues have to be considered before coded aperture imaging can be used clinically. The optimal decoding function exhibits high frequency components such that it should perform poorly in the case of noisy projections. This is not peculiar to Fresnel zone plates and has been known for long for a variety of coded apertures. This is a more serious problem for parallel hole collimators, since they pass very much lower count rates than can be achieved with coded apertures. The noise power spectrum of the decoded images has to be analyzed and for clinical situations, low pass filtering might be required.

Correction for attenuation represents a more serious problem. Indeed, when parallel hole collimators are used, a first-order correction using a constant attenuation model usually leads to acceptable results. The reason for this is that a one-to-one correspondence exists between a projection point and a line integral. This is not the case for coded aperture systems, since multiple attenuated ray sums project to the same point on the detector. This is easily seen by inspection of Eq. 10 where $f(x,y)$ should be multiplied by an attenuation factor which depends on the source location and the attenuation boundary, but also on the location of the aperture point under consideration. An iterative correction method should lead to a stable solution however, at the expense of a long execution time.

In conclusion, the used of an orthogonal dual coded aperture system can provide high resolution and low noise images when an optimal decoding function is used; but in practical situations, attenuation should degrade results significantly.

5. GENERAL CONCLUSION

For many years, coded apertures have been considered to be an attractive but impractical imaging technique. This paper shows that, with

present technology in nuclear medicine (high spatial resolution, large
field of view gamma-cameras, good distortion correction methods, and good
counting statistics from short-lived radionuclides), one should be able to
image dynamic radioactivity distributions with such static detectors.

We demonstrate experimentally that a dual seven pinhole tomographic
system exhibits a 3-fold increase in sensitivity as compared to a dual
rotating camera SPECT system, leads to reconstructed images of somewhat
improved resolution without major attenuation related artifacts.
Therefore, when limited size distributions are studied, this technique is
an attractive alternative to rotating SPECT.

These results are formally explained by the analysis of sampling
properties of multipinhole detectors in a transformed space. Limitations
to tomographic ability (poor depth resolution) results from limited angular
sampling of such devices, and seven pinhole collimators are shown to
realize an optimal compromise for relevant clinical situations in terms of
efficient use of crystal area, size of reconstruction volume and depth
resolution. More uniform angular sampling obtained with dual seven pinhole
systems improves spatial resolution and decreases variations in resolution
within the reconstruction volume.

Finally, when a true dual coded aperture system and an optimal
decoding procedure are used, high resolution low noise reconstructed images
can be obtained if the attenuation correction problem is solved.
Consequently, true 3D imaging of fast time-varying structures is feasible
with such high sensitivity, static devices. The key role played by the
analysis of temporal behavior in the understanding of physiological systems
should stimulate the development of such detectors as an adjunct to the
more conventional rotating SPECT.

Medical Department, Brookhaven National Laboratory, Upton, New York U.S.A.
This work has been performed under Contract No. DE-AC02-76CH00016 with the
United States Department of Energy.

REFERENCES

1. Emission computerized tomography: the single photon approach, 1981.
   P. Paras and E.A. Eikman eds. U.S Dept. of Health and Human Services.
   Pub. FDA 81-8177.
2. Hine G.J., Erickson J.J. 1974. Advances in scintigraphic
   instruments. P. 34 in Instrumentation in Nuclear Medicine. Hine
   G.J. and Sorenson eds. Academic Press.
3. Vogel R.A., Kirch D., LeFree M., Steele P. 1978. A new method of
   multiplanar emission tomography using a seven pinhole collimator and
   an Anger scintillation camera. J. Nucl. Med. 19: 648-654.
4. Barrett H.H. 1972. Fresnel Zone Plate imaging in nuclear medicine.
   J. Nucl. Med. 13: 382-395.
5. Williams D.L., Ritchie J.L., Harp G.D., Caldwell J.H., Hamilton G.W.
   1980. In vivo simulation of Thallium-201 myocardial scintigraphy by
   seven pinhole emission tomography. J. Nucl. Med. 21: 821-828.
6. Bizais Y., Zubal I.G., Rowe R.W., Bennett G.W., Brill A.B. 1983 Dual
   seven pinhole tomography. IEEE Trans. Nucl. Sci. NS-30: 703-706.
7. Bizais Y., Rowe R.W., Zubal I.G., Bennett G.W., Brill A.B. 1983. A
   comprehensive method for fast quantitative analysis of gamma camera
   distortions and their corrections. J. Nucl. Med. 24: P67 (abst.).
8. Bennett G.W., Brill A.B., Zubal I.G., Rowe R.W., Bizais Y., Dobert
   R.S. 1982. Unicon - a single instrument for PET, SPECT, and routine
   clinical gamma ray imaging. P21.08 in Proc. of the World Congress on
   medical Physics and Biomedical Engineering. W. Bleifeld ed. MPBE.
9. LeFree M.T., Vogel R.A., Kirch D.L., Steele P.P. 1981. Seven pinhole
   tomography - A technical description. J. Nucl. Med. 22: 48-54.
10. Mallard J.R., Myers M.J. 1963. The performance of a gamma camera for
    the visualization of radioisotopes in vivo. Phys. Med. Biol. 8:
    165-182.
11. Tam K.C., Perez-Mendez V., MacDonald B. 1979. 3D object
    reconstruction in emission and transmission tomography with limited
    angular input. IEEE Trans. Nucl. Sci. NS-26: 2797-2805.
12. Gindi G.R., Arendt J., Barrett H.H., Chiu M.Y., Ervin A., Gilles C.L.,
    Kujoory M.A., Miller E.L., Simpson R.G. 1982. Imaging with rotating
    slit apertures and rotating collimators. Med. Phys. 9: 324-339.
13. Viergever M.A., Vreugdenhil E., Ying-Lie O. 1982. A modelling
    approach to seven pinhole tomography. P. 499 in Proc. of the Third World
    Congress of Nuclear Medicine and Biology. Raynaud C. ed. Pergamon.
14. Phillips D.L. 1964. A technique for the numerical solution of
    certain integral equations of the first kind. J. Ass. Comp. Mach. 9:
    84-97.
15. Steinbach A., Macovski A. 1979. Improved depth resolution with one
    dimensional coded aperture imaging. J. Phys. D: Appl. Phys. 12:
    2079-2099.

RESOLUTION LIMITS IN FULL- AND LIMITED-ANGLE TOMOGRAPHY.

M. Defrise   Theoretische Natuurkunde, Vrije Universiteit Brussel,
             1050 Brussels, Belgium
C. De Mol   Département de Mathématique, Université Libre de Bruxelles,
             1050 Brussels, Belgium

Abstract. We apply regularization methods to the inversion of the Radon transform. Stability with respect to noise is restored by restricting the class of admissible solutions using prior knowledge. In the full-angle case, we derive upper bounds for the global L^2 reconstruction error, and also for local error estimates. In the limited-angle case, we analyse an iterative reconstruction algorithm, and demonstrate its instability in the presence of noise. We explain how this algorithm can be regularized in order to converge to stable solutions.

1. THE FULL-ANGLE CASE.

The problem of inverting the full-angle Radon transform has been extensively studied and many efficient reconstruction algorithms can be found in the literature [1,2,3]. It is well known that exact inversion formulae lead to unstable solutions in the presence of noise. These instability problems are often overcome by means of empirical methods, so that error estimates cannot easily be derived. In regularization methods [4,5,6], however, stability is restored by means of explicit prescriptions on the class of solutions, and furthermore, precise error bounds can be obtained, as will be shown below.

Let us first recall some basic formulae relative to the Radon transform [1]. We will only consider the two-dimensional case, although many results generalize to the three-dimensional case. When solving the tomography problem, we are faced with the following mathematical problem : find the object function $f : R^2 \to R$ from the following set of projections

$$g(s,\theta) = \int_{-\infty}^{\infty} du \; f(s \cos\theta - u \sin\theta, s \sin\theta + u \cos\theta) \tag{1}$$

In the full-angle case, the angle θ giving the direction of projection varies in the interval $(-\pi/2, +\pi/2)$. We will denote by R the operator mapping the solution f onto the data g = Rf. Let us assume, as physically reasonable in most cases, that both the solution and the data are square integrable on their respective domain of definition, so that R can be considered as a linear operator from $L^2(R^2)$ into $L^2(R \times (-\pi/2, +\pi/2))$, the norm in this latter space being

$$\| g \|^2 = \int_{-\pi/2}^{\pi/2} d\theta \int_{-\infty}^{\infty} ds \ |g(s,\theta)|^2 \tag{2}$$

The back-projection operator, which we denote by R^* since it is formally the adjoint of R, is defined as follows :

$$(R^* g)(x,y) = \int_{-\pi/2}^{\pi/2} d\theta \ g(x \cos\theta + y \sin\theta, \theta) \tag{3}$$

The back-projected data $R^* g$ is sometimes considered as a first but very rough estimate of the object function since $R^* Rf$ is easily seen to be the convolution of $f(x,y)$ by the function $r^{-1} = (x^2 + y^2)^{-1/2}$, so that in Fourier space we have :

$$\mathcal{F}_2 (R^* Rf)(\underline{\nu}) = \frac{1}{|\underline{\nu}|} \mathcal{F}_2 f(\underline{\nu}) \tag{4}$$

This formula provides a way for recovering uniquely the object function f from the back-projected data $R^* g$, the so-called "rho-filtered layergram" reconstruction procedure [7], expressed as follows :

$$f = \mathcal{F}_2^{-1} \cdot |\underline{\nu}| \cdot \mathcal{F}_2 R^* g \tag{5}$$

Let us remark that $R^* R$ and R are unbounded operators respectively in $L^2(R^2)$ and from $L^2(R^2)$ into $L^2(R \times (-\pi/2, +\pi/2))$ [8] , as easily seen from (4); they are nevertheless densely defined.

The problem of finding the object f from the projections g has a unique solution, in other words, the operators R^{-1} and $(R^* R)^{-1}$ exist. However, in a L^2 setting, these operators are unbounded and consequently the inversion of the Radon transform is an ill-posed problem : the solution f will not depend continuously on the data g. A practical manifestation of this lack of continuity is the dramatic amplification in the solution of very small errors in the data. In fact, when the data are noisy, the measured function $g(s,\theta)$ need no longer be in the range of the operator R, that is, the equation Rf = g is not necessarily solvable in the usual sense. One can look, however, for any object function f compatible with the data g within a prescribed accuracy, i.e. a function f such that :

$$\|Rf - g\| \leq \varepsilon \tag{6}$$

where ε represents an upper bound for the global error on the data, measured with the norm (2). However, for an ill-posed problem, when R^{-1} is not bounded, the inequality (6) defines in the solution space $L^2(R^2)$ an unbounded set. Arbitrarily close data can correspond to solutions arbitrarily far from each other in the distance generated by the L^2 norm.

According to standard results in regularization theory [4,5,6] , ill-posedness can be cured by restricting the class of admissible solutions with the help of constraints expressing some prior knowledge about the searched-for solutions (upper bounds, smoothness requirements,...). We will thus assume that all admissible solutions satisfy not only the compatibility condition (6) but also an a priori bound of the form :

$$\|Bf\| \leq E \tag{7}$$

where the so-called constraint operator B is a linear operator in $L^2(R^2)$ having a bounded inverse, and E is a prescribed constant. In our case, it is particularly convenient to chose an operator B which is diagonal in Fourier space, and, more precisely [*]:

$$\mathcal{F}_2 \, (Bf)(\underline{v}) = (1 + |\underline{v}|^2)^{\alpha/2} \, \mathcal{F}_2 \, f(\underline{v}) \tag{8}$$

with $\alpha > 0$, so that :

$$\|Bf\| = \{ \int d^2\underline{v} \, (1 + |\underline{v}|^2)^{\alpha} \, |\mathcal{F}_2 f(\underline{v})|^2 \}^{1/2} \tag{9}$$

When α is a positive integer, the constraint (7) involves bounds on the norm of the α first derivatives of f (mathematically speaking, it amounts to requiring that f belongs to a Sobolev space of order α). For $\alpha=0$, $\|Bf\|$ simply reduces to the L^2 norm of f.

The problem of constructing explicitly an approximate solution in the packet K of functions satisfying both constraints (6) and (7) can be solved as follows. In absence of further information, it seems natural to take a central point of K. However, since K has no centre of symmetry, it is easier to consider the following sets sandwiching K :

$$K \supset K_0 = \{ f \mid \phi(f) \leq \varepsilon^2 \} \tag{10}$$

---

[*] A unit of length (e.g. of the same order of magnitude as the diameter of the reconstruction region) is implicitly introduced in eq. (8).

$$K \subset K_1 = \{ f \mid \Phi(f) \leqslant 2\varepsilon^2 \}$$

where the functional Φ is defined by :

$$\Phi(f) = \|Rf - g\|^2 + (\tfrac{\varepsilon}{E})^2 \| Bf\|^2 \tag{11}$$

The sets K_0 and K_1, defined by positive definite quadratic forms, are infinite dimensional "ellipsoids"; their common centre of symmetry $\tilde{f}$ minimizes the functional $\Phi(f)$. As easily seen by a variational argument, $\tilde{f}$ is given by :

$$\tilde{f} = C^{-1} R^* g \tag{12}$$

where C is the following positive-definite operator

$$C = R^* R + (\tfrac{\varepsilon}{E})^2 B^* B \tag{13}$$

Since B is assumed to have a bounded inverse, C^{-1} is a bounded operator substituting for the unbounded one $(R^* R)^{-1}$.

If the sets K, K_0 and K_1 shrink into a point when the error ε on the data tends to zero, then $\tilde{f}$ gets closer and closer to the exact solution and the problem is said to be regularized. The approximate solution $\tilde{f}$ depends continuously on the data and is called a regularized solution of the ill-posed problem. Using Fourier transforms, and equations (4) and (9), the solution (12) can be written as :

$$\tilde{f} = \mathcal{F}_2^{-1} \left(\frac{1}{\frac{1}{|\underline{\nu}|} + (\tfrac{\varepsilon}{E})^2 (1 + |\underline{\nu}|^2)^\alpha} \right) \mathcal{F}_2 R^* g \tag{14}$$

which should be compared to the unregularized solution (5).

An upper bound for the reconstruction error we commit by taking $\tilde{f}$ as approximate solution is then given by half the maximum diameter of the set K_1. It is shown [6] that this diameter is always bounded by the quantity $\sqrt{2}\ \varepsilon \|C^{-1}\|^{1/2}$, so that the following majoration holds for any data g :

$$\|\tilde{f} - f\| \leqslant \sqrt{2}\ \varepsilon\ \|C^{-1}\|^{1/2} \tag{15}$$

In the present case :

$$\|C^{-1}\| = \sup_{\underline{\nu}}\ (\tfrac{1}{|\underline{\nu}|} + (\tfrac{\varepsilon}{E})^2(1 + |\underline{\nu}|^2)^\alpha)^{-1} \leqslant \sup_{\underline{\nu}}\ (\tfrac{1}{|\underline{\nu}|} + (\tfrac{\varepsilon}{E})^2|\underline{\nu}|^{2\alpha})^{-1}$$

$$= (2\alpha)^{-\frac{1}{2\alpha+1}}\ (1 + \tfrac{1}{2\alpha})^{-1}\ (\tfrac{E}{\varepsilon})^{\frac{2}{2\alpha+1}} \tag{16}$$

We then get a result similar to the one obtained by Natterer [8]:

$$\| \tilde{f} - f \| \leqslant (\alpha + \tfrac{1}{2})^{-1/2} \, (2\alpha)^{\frac{\alpha}{2\alpha+1}} \; \varepsilon^{\frac{2\alpha}{2\alpha+1}} \; E^{\frac{1}{2\alpha+1}} \tag{17}$$

Notice that this error estimate contains no unknown constant, and could therefore be explicitly evaluated, for a given α, in function of ε and E, although the values of these parameters could be difficult to assess in practice.

We also see from (17) that the inversion procedure is regularized for any positive α , i.e. :

$$\lim_{\varepsilon \to 0} \| \tilde{f} - f \| = 0 \qquad \alpha > 0 \tag{18}$$

When the only prior knowledge available is $\| f \| < E$ (i.e. $\alpha = 0$) the problem is not regularized strongly, in the sense of equation (18), but it will be shown below that such a constraint is sufficient to ensure regularization in a weaker sense.

The error bound (17) also reflects the fact -which is already evident in view of the great practical efficiency of scanners- that the inversion of the full-angle Radon transform is only mildly ill-posed : the convergence in (17) goes like a power of ε (Hölder continuity), which means that the number of significant digits in the reconstructed image is a fixed percentage of the number of significant digits in the data.

Let us observe that the global error estimate obtained hereabove holds for continuous data only; discretization clearly introduces a supplementary contribution to the reconstruction error [8]. One could of course consider a discrete Radon operator from $L^2(R^2)$ into R^M, where M is the total number of data points. The error estimate for this problem could no longer be evaluated analytically; one should, instead, numerically evaluate the norm of C^{-1}.

On the other hand, it has been pointed by several authors (e.g. [1]) that global error estimates, like (17), are not always sufficient to estimate the ability of a given reconstruction procedure to clearly reproduce the structures needed for clinical diagnosis. In particular, one should be able to estimate the reconstruction error at a given point, or in a small voisinage around a point, in order to answer the question : which resolution do we achieve, i.e. with which accuracy can we reproduce details of a given size? Here too, a possible solution is to completely discretize the Radon transform and to view it as an operator from R^P into R^M, where P is the total number of pixels in the reconstructed image. One could then compute

numerically the error estimate (15), and study its dependence on the number
of pixels.

The approach we follow in this paper is somewhat different and has the
merit of maintaining some analytical simplicity; it consists in studying
the reconstruction of a blurred object :

$$f_w = f * w. \tag{19}$$

where $*$ stands for two-dimensional convolution, and $w(\underline{x})$ is a fixed function
sometimes called a mollifier, peaked in $\underline{x} = \underline{0}$ and satisfying

$$\int d^2\underline{x} \ w(\underline{x}) = 1 \tag{20}$$

The variance σ^2 of w is related to the resolution achieved in such a blurred
reconstruction. Indeed, $f_w(\underline{x})$ is essentially the mean value of $f(\underline{x})$ in a
region of size σ around $\underline{x}$. This approach roughly modelizes a discretized
("pixelized") reconstruction. A possible choice for w is a gaussian :

$$w(\underline{x}) = \frac{1}{2\pi\sigma^2} \ \exp \{ \ -|\underline{x}|^2/2\sigma^2 \ \} \tag{21}$$

Assuming again a constraint of the type (9), we obtain for the
regularized blurred reconstruction :

$$\tilde{f}_w = \mathcal{F}_2^{-1} \{ \frac{\mathcal{F}_2 \ w(\underline{v})}{\frac{1}{|\underline{v}|} + (\frac{\epsilon}{E})^2 (1 + |\underline{v}|^2)^\alpha} \} \mathcal{F}_2 \ R^* g \tag{22}$$

This result is not surprising : working with a finite resolution amounts
to a supplementary filtering.

Let us now study a stability estimate for a local error, defined by :

$$\delta(\epsilon,E,g,w) = \sup_{f \in K_1} |\tilde{f}_w(\underline{0}) - f_w(\underline{0})| \tag{23}$$

where the set K_1 is defined in (10). An upper bound for $\delta(\epsilon,E,g,w)$ can be
derived, which is independent of the data g [6].

$$\delta(\epsilon,E,g,w) \leqslant \delta(\epsilon,E,w) = \sqrt{2} \ \epsilon (C^{-1}w,w)^{1/2} \tag{24}$$

Similarly, the following bound holds for the relative local error [6] :

$$\delta_{rel}(\epsilon,E,g,w) \leqslant \delta_{rel}(\epsilon,E,w) = \frac{\epsilon}{E} \ \frac{(C^{-1}w,w)^{1/2}}{((B^*B)^{-1}w,w)^{1/2}} \tag{25}$$

In the case of the Radon transform, using a constraint of the type (9),
one gets :

$$\delta^2_{rel}(\epsilon,E,w) = \frac{\epsilon^2}{E^2} \; \frac{\int d^2\underline{\nu} \; \frac{|\mathcal{F}_2 w(\underline{\nu})|^2}{\frac{1}{|\underline{\nu}|} + (\frac{\epsilon}{E})^2 \; (1 + |\underline{\nu}|^2)^\alpha}}{\int d^2\underline{\nu} \; \frac{|\mathcal{F}_2 w(\underline{\nu})|^2}{(1 + |\underline{\nu}|^2)^\alpha}} \tag{26}$$

Notice that this expression only depends on the modulus of $\mathcal{F}_2 w(\underline{\nu})$, and is therefore invariant with respect to translations.

The following results can then be proved straightforwardly :

1. For any fixed resolution length $\sigma = \sqrt{\int d^2\underline{x} \; |\underline{x}|^2 \; w(\underline{x})}$, and for any non-negative value of α, the blurred reconstruction is regularized, i.e. :

$$\lim_{\epsilon \to 0} \; \delta_{rel}(\epsilon,E,w) = 0 \tag{27}$$

The stability is therefore restored even when $\alpha=0$, i.e. when the constraint operator is the identity. The convergence is faster than in the unblurred case : for any $w(\underline{x})$ satisfying a constraint of the type (9) with $\alpha > 1/2$, one has $\delta_{rel} \propto \epsilon/E$.

2. For $\alpha > 1$ and for non-negative $w(\underline{x})$, one has :

$$\delta^2_{rel}(\epsilon,E,w) \leqslant \frac{2\pi \; (\frac{\epsilon^2}{E^2})^{\frac{2\alpha-2}{2\alpha+1}} \; (\frac{1}{2\alpha-2} + \frac{1}{3})}{\int d^2\underline{\nu} \; \frac{|\mathcal{F}_2 w(\underline{\nu})|^2}{(1 + |\underline{\nu}|^2)^\alpha}} \tag{28}$$

Notice that the integral at the denominator is independent of ϵ and remains finite even when σ tends to zero. Therefore, when the constraint on the solution is sufficiently strong, the regularized reconstructed object converges locally to the true object, however sharp the mollifier w is. Notice that the rate of convergence for this local error is slower than for the global error estimate (17).

3. For $\alpha < 1$ (i.e., in particular, for classes of objects defined by (7) with $\alpha < 1/2$, classes which include objects with sharp contrasts), one has for any value of ϵ :

$$\lim_{\sigma \to 0} \; \delta_{rel}(\epsilon,E,w) = 1 \tag{29}$$

Therefore, for any fixed signal-to-noise ratio, the error becomes unacceptably large if one tries to resolve a finer structure, i.e. to reconstruct details having a size smaller,than some critical resolution length. Such a phenomenon is typical for ill-posed problems.

Let us now study in more details the relationship between reconstruction error, signal-to-noise ratio, and resolution length, in the case $\alpha=0$. We take as mollifier a gaussian with standard deviation σ . Then :

$$\delta^2_{rel}(\varepsilon,E,w) = 2 \int_0^\infty \frac{x \ dx \ exp(-x^2)}{(1 + \frac{2\pi\sigma E^2}{x \ \varepsilon^2})} \tag{30}$$

Figure 1 shows the relative error δ_{rel} versus the dimensionless factor $\beta = 2\pi\sigma \ E^2/\varepsilon^2$. In order to interprete this, notice that ε^2/E^2 has the dimension of a length. If the reconstruction region has a diameter L, the link between ε^2/E^2 and the dimensionless signal-to-noise ratio η^{-1} is expressed by the following proportionality :

$$\frac{\varepsilon^2}{E^2} \propto \eta^2 L \tag{31}$$

In the limit $2\pi\sigma E^2/\varepsilon^2 \gg 1$, equation (30) becomes

$$\delta^2_{rel}(\varepsilon,E,w) = \frac{\sqrt{\pi}}{2} \ \frac{\varepsilon^2}{2\pi\sigma E^2} \ (1 + \ 0 \ (\frac{\varepsilon^2}{2\pi\sigma E^2}) \ ) \ \propto \ \eta^2 \ \frac{L}{\sigma} \tag{32}$$

the same dependence on σ , in this limit, was derived by Natterer [9], using a different approach.

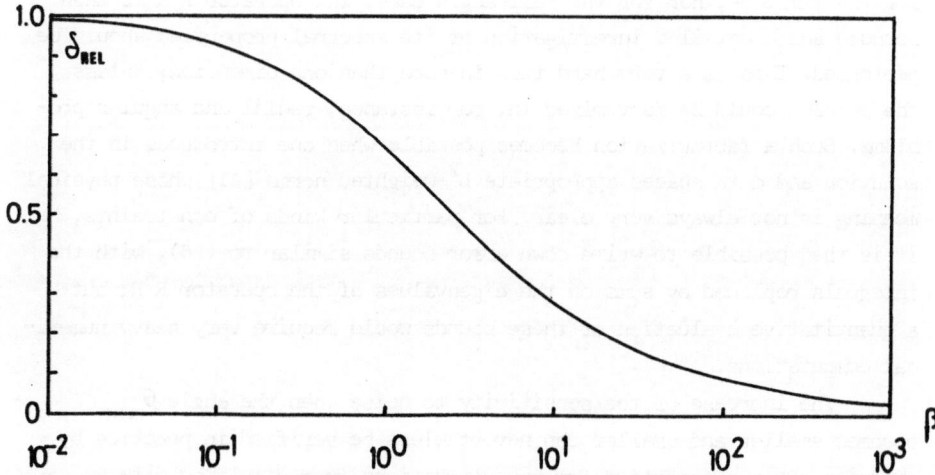

Figure 1. The upper bound for the relative reconstruction error versus $\beta = 2\pi\sigma E^2/\varepsilon^2$.

2. THE LIMITED-ANGLE PROBLEM.

In this case, the projections $g(s,\theta)$ defined by (1) are given only for $-\theta_{max} < \theta < +\theta_{max}$. With the following back-projection operator

$$(R^* g)(x,y) = \int_{-\theta_{max}}^{+\theta_{max}} d\theta \ g(x \cos\theta + y \sin\theta, \theta) \tag{33}$$

equation (4) is replaced by :

$$(R^* R f)(\underline{v}) = \chi_\Omega \frac{1}{|\underline{v}|} (\mathcal{F}_2 f)(\underline{v}) \tag{34}$$

where χ_Ω takes the value 1 in the angular sector Ω defined by $|\tan\theta| < \tan\theta_{max}$ and 0 in the complementary sector, which is called the "missing cone". It is clear that the values of $\mathcal{F}_2 f$ in the missing cone cannot in general be uniquely retrieved from the back-projected data $R^* g$. However, when it is known a priori that the object function $f(x)$ vanishes outside a finite support D, $\mathcal{F}_2 f$ is an entire function and its values in the missing cone are uniquely determined by analytic continuation. Of course, the ill-posedness of analytic continuation is then superimposed to the ill-posedness of full-angle inverse Radon transform [10,11] , we therefore expect significantly greater reconstruction error as well as worse achievable resolution. To demonstrate this assertion, one should incorporate explicitly into the formalism the knowledge of the finite support D of f. This is no longer possible in a simple Fourier-space analysis, neither for the limited-, nor for the full-angle case. The operator $R^* R$ is then bounded and a detailed investigation of its spectral properties should be performed. This is a very hard task in more than one dimension, unless the problem could be factorized in, for instance, radial and angular problems. Such a factorization becomes possible when one introduces in the solution and data spaces appropriate L^2-weighted norms [11] whose physical meaning is not always very clear. For particular kinds of constraints, it is then possible to write down error bounds similar to (26), with the integrals replaced by sums on the eigenvalues of the operator $R^* R$; but a quantitative evaluation of these bounds would require very heavy numerical computations.

The increase of the sensitivity to noise when the angle θ_{max} becomes smaller and smaller can nevertheless be verified in practice by studying error propagation for reconstructions from simulated data by

means of an iterative algorithm which allows the analytic extrapolation
to the missing cone. This algorithm was developed by Gerchberg [12] ,
De Santis and Gori [13] and Papoulis [14] for extrapolating band-limited
signals in one dimension, and its application to limited-angle tomography
has been discussed by several authors [10,15,16,17] . Let us briefly recall
the principle of this method. We see from (34) that the Fourier components
of the object function in the sector Ω can be retrieved by multiplying the
Fourier transform of the back-projected data by $|\underline{y}|$, the modulus of the
two-dimensional frequency (this first step should of course be regularized
in the same way as for the full-angle case, see eq. (14)). Then, the Fourier
components obtained so are set to zero outside the cone Ω, as they should
be if the data were noiseless; the resulting spectrum is the first estimate
of the function $\mathcal{F}_2$ f. The Gerchberg algorithm then proceeds by repeated
back and forth Fast Fourier Transform between object and frequency space,
the available information about the solution being incorporated at each
iteration step into the current object estimate : this means setting the
n^{th} iterate $f_n(\underline{x})$ to zero outside the known support D and replacing
$\mathcal{F}_2 f_n(\underline{y})$ by its known values inside the cone Ω.

The Gerchberg algorithm has been shown to converge to the unique
solution of the inversion problem, when starting from noise-free data.
However, as could be expected from the ill-posedness of analytic continua-
tion problems, one cannot ensure convergence of the Gerchberg algorithm
to a meaningful solution whenever the data are corrupted by noise. The
reconstruction error will then grow out of control when the number of
iteration increases beyond some limit. We have demonstrated this phenomenon
by means of numerical simulations, an example of which is given below.
It is clear, therefore, that the constraint that f should have bounded
support is not sufficient to guarantee the stability of the solution in
the presence of noise. Notice that this observation is by no means restricted
to the Gerchberg method : any algorithm leading exactly to the solution of
the noise-free equation, such as a Gerchberg algorithm with relaxation
parameter [18] , or the conjugate-gradient method [19] , will be subject to
the same instability. As a matter of fact, noise propagation will be all
the more dramatic as the convergence of the algorithm is faster in the
noise-free case.

As in the full-angle case, stability can be restored by incorporating supplementary prior knowledge into the algorithm, e.g. of the type considered previously (eq. (7)-(9)). This amounts to replacing the original equation by a quadratic optimization problem, the solution of which can then be obtained iteratively, e.g. by implementing the usual Jacobi method by means of successive back and forth Fast Fourier Transform, much in the same way as for the original Gerchberg method.

The regularized algorithm thus obtained is described in details in a previous paper, for a constraint of the type $\alpha=0$ [20]. Its efficiency has been demonstrated by numerical simulations. Figure 2 shows, for instance, the evolution of the relative reconstruction error with the number of iterations n, for a particular model object reconstructed on a 64 x 64 lattice, and for a signal-to-noise ratio of 10. Curves 3 and 6 clearly demonstrate the instability of the Gerchberg algorithm in the presence of noise, and also show how this instability worsens when θ_{max} gets smaller. On the other hand, the regularized algorithm is seen to lead to a stable solution after a few tenths of iterations. We have also checked that imposing a positivity constraint at each iteration, although it significantly improves the reconstructions, is not sufficient by itself to fully restore stability [20]. Further work is in progress in order to obtain more general results on resolutions limits in function of θ_{max}.

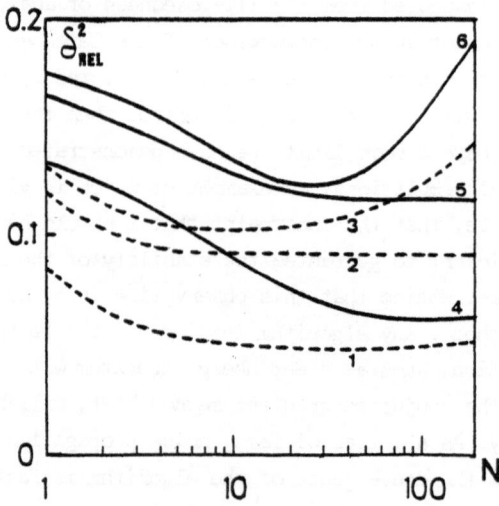

Figure 2. Relative reconstruction error versus the number of iteration N. Dotted lines : θmax = 1.4 rad, full lines : θmax = 1.2 rad. Curves 1,4 : noise-free; curves 3,6 :η=0.1,unregularized; curves 2,5 :η=0.1,regularized.

ACKNOWLEDGEMENTS.

M. Defrise is in receipt of a fellowship from the Inter University Institute for Nuclear Sciences (Belgium). C. De Mol is Research Associate with the National Fund for Scientific Research (Belgium).

REFERENCES.

1. Herman, G. T. 1980, Image reconstruction from projections. London, New-York, Academic Press.
2. Lewitt R.M. 1983, Proceedings of the IEEE, 71, n°3, 390,408.
3. Censor Y. 1983, Proceedings of the IEEE, 71, n°3, 409,419.
4. Tikhonov A. N. and Arsenin V. Y. 1977, Solutions of ill-posed problems. Washington D.C., W.H. Winston & Sons.
5. Miller K. 1970, SIAM J. Math. Anal. 1, 52,74.
6. Bertero M., De Mol C., Viano G.A. 1980,in Inverse scattering problems in optics (H.P. Baltes, ed), Topics in Current Physics, 20, Berlin, Heidelberg, New-York, Springer-Verlag, 161, 214.
7. Bates R.H.T. and Peters T.M. 1971, New Zealand J. Sci., 14, 883,896.
8. Louis A.K. and Natterer F. 1983, Proceedings of the IEEE, 71, n°3, 379, 389.
9. Natterer F. 1978, Numer. Math., 30, 81, 91.
10. Grünbaum F.A. 1980, Numer. Funct. Anal. Optimiz., 2, 31.
11. Davison M.E. 1980, SIAM J. Appl. Math. 43, 428, 448.

12. Gerchberg 1974, Optica Acta, 21, 709, 720.
13. De Santis P. and Gori F. 1975, Optica Acta, 22, 691, 695.
14. Papoulis A. 1975, IEEE Trans. Circuits Syst., CAS-22, 735,742.
15. Sato T. et al. 1981, Appl. Optics, 20, 395, 399.
16. Tam K.C. and Perez-Mendez V. 1981, J. Opt. Soc. Amer., 71, 582, 592.
17. Baba N. and Murata K. 1982, Optik, 60, 327,332.
18. Lent A. and Tuy H. 1981, J. Math. Anal. and Applic., 83, 554, 565.
19. Maitre H. 1981, Optica Acta, 28, 973, 980.
20. Defrise M. and De Mol C. 1983, Optica Acta, 30, 403, 408.

NEW DIRECTIONS IN CODED-APERTURE IMAGING

H.H. BARRETT, H.B. BARBER, P.A. ERVIN, K.J. MYERS, R.G. PAXMAN, W.E. SMITH
W.J. WILD, J.M. WOOLFENDEN

1. INTRODUCTION

It has now been over a decade since the idea of coded apertures as an alternative to conventional pinholes and collimators was first proposed in the nuclear medicine literature. During this period, many different codes and decoding algorithms have been studied. Several workers have carried out extensive experimental and theoretical investigations, and a few clinical trials have been performed. For a review, see Barrett and Swindell (1981) or Simpson and Barrett (1980). However, in spite of these efforts, coded-aperture imaging has not yet blossomed into a routine clinical tool. The method has been perhaps a scientific success, yielding new insights into the physics and mathematics of radiological imaging, but so far it has been a practical failure.

Several reasons can be suggested for this failure. The hoped-for advantages in dose or signal-to-noise ratio have proven to be modest or in some cases nonexistent. The kind of longitudinal tomography usually offered by coded apertures is complicated, subject to artifacts, and distinctly inferior to emission computed tomography (ECT). Also, there is still no detector available that is really well suited to use with coded apertures. Finally, and perhaps most importantly, there is no clinical application where the peculiar characteristics of coded apertures are of proven value.

Is it, then, perhaps time to give up the quest, to abandon this once-promising idea? It is the central thesis of this paper that to do so would be a mistake. We believe that the past decade has been a period of steady if unspectacular progress in our understanding of coded imaging systems, and that we can now envision radically new approaches to scintigraphic imaging based on the coding principle.

2. THE TOMOGRAPHY PROBLEM

The original application of coded apertures was in x-ray astronomy, where the object is at an infinite distance from the aperture and can thus be treated as a single plane. When the coding concept was carried over into nuclear medicine, it was natural to think of a three-dimensional (3D) distribution of radioactivity as composed of discrete planes. The goal of the early research in this area was therefore to devise coded imaging systems that would give good reconstructions of planar objects. The first apertures investigated, the Fresnel zone plate and the random-pinhole array, were found to be deficient for even this limited task, but other apertures, including the annulus, rotating slit, and uniformly redundant array, were soon demonstrated to yield high-quality images of planar objects. Much of the subsequent research was devoted to deciding whether the statistical accuracy of reconstructions from coded images was superior to that of conventional images of these mythical planar objects; this debate continues today and is discussed briefly in a later section.

It was, of course, apparent from the outset that coded apertures offered a kind of tomographic imaging capability. Each point in a 3D object casts a shadow of the aperture onto the detector, and depth information is encoded in the scale of the shadow. The simplest method of decoding is correlation of the coded image with a scaled version of the aperture code function. This method is equivalent to matched filtering for a particular object plane; object points in that plane are imaged as sharp points, while points in other planes are blurred in some manner.

Coded-aperture tomography may be classified as longitudinal, limited-angle, multiplexed tomography. "Longitudinal" means that the focal planes are parallel to the aperture plane and hence usually parallel to the long axis of the patient's body. The detector is most commonly a stationary scintillation camera, which means that the projection data set is necessarily limited in angle. (See Fig. 1). Furthermore, even the projections that are recorded are scrambled together or "multiplexed". That is, the radiation reaching one detector element is not a measure of a line integral of the activity distribution as in ECT, but rather represents a linear combination of line integrals.

These two problems, the limited angular range and the multiplexing, make the reconstruction problem very ill-posed. A unique solution does not, in general, exist. One way to see this is to think in digital terms,

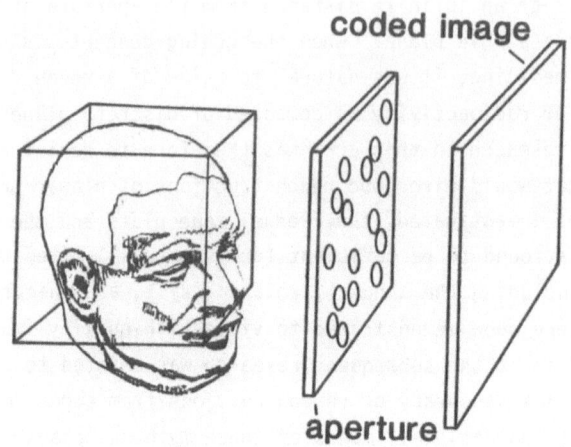

Figure 1. Coded-aperture imaging geometry: one view.

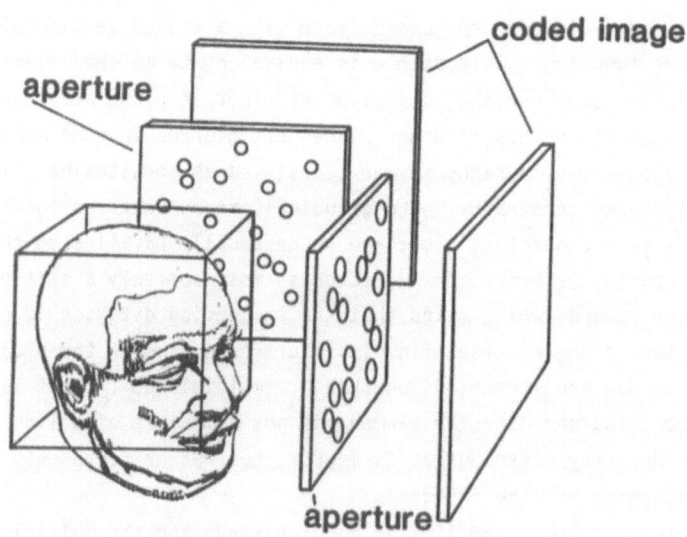

Figure 2. Coded-aperture imaging geometry: two orthogonal views.

where the coded image is divided into N^2 picture elements or pixels, while the 3D object is divided into N^3 volume elements or voxels. A true reconstruction would be equivalent to solving N^2 equations in N^3 unknowns, clearly an impossible task. Note that this ill-posedness is not specific to coded-aperture tomography; it occurs also in other forms of limited-angle tomography, such as seven-pinhole systems and rotating slant-hole collimators. Indeed, we shall demonstrate below that the limited angular range is a much more serious problem than the multiplexing.

Several attempts have been made in the past to circumvent these deficiencies in coded-aperture imaging. The multiplexing can be avoided by using multiple apertures, as in the so-called stochastic aperture at the University of Michigan (May et al., 1974) or the Fourier aperture at the University of Toronto (Renaud et al., 1979). To understand how this works, consider a coded aperture consisting of M pinholes. Then each point on the detector receives radiation that originates along M distinct lines passing through the object. In other words, M separate line integrals of the activity distribution are multiplexed together. If M different apertures are used, and the code functions are properly chosen, it is possible to undo the multiplexing (Chiu et al., 1979); the resulting data set is then equivalent to the one that would have been obtained if the pinholes had been opened sequentially instead of simultaneously. The Michigan and Toronto workers succeed in carrying out this demultiplexing, but they are still left with an incomplete data set because of the limited angular range.

A few workers have considered coded-aperture systems with more than one detector in an attempt to fill in the missing projection angles. Tipton (1978) and Steinbach and Macovski (1979) proposed the use of two orthogonal coded apertures, and Lefkopoulos et al. (1982) have recently successfully implemented this approach in clinical practice. (See Fig. 2). In this case, the data set is multiplexed but it covers a wide angular range. By using both multiple code functions and multiple aperture planes, it would be possible in principle to obtain a complete data set that would allow accurate tomographic reconstruction. Such a system does not seem to have been considered in the literature, and its practicality is open to question. Furthermore, it is our contention, supported below, that it is not necessary to have unmultiplexed data in order to get useful

reconstructions; a wide angular range, on the other hand, is definitely
necessary.

3. TWO DECODING ALGORITHMS

Given a coded data set, the goal of the decoding algorithm is to
find an object distribution that could have produced the data and that
satisfies any known prior constraints on the object. The most useful
constraints are that the object is positive and contained in a finite
volume. It is important to note that the algorithm can do nothing more
than find <u>an</u> image that is consistent with the data and constraints. This
image may or may not be an accurate reconstruction of the original object.
If it is not, then no modification of the algorithm will help; instead,
the data-collection system must be modified.

We have investigated in detail two specific reconstruction algorithms.
The first of these is an iterative algorithm known in the literature on
numerical analysis as the Jacobi method and in the optics literature as
the van Cittert method. It is closely related to the familiar ART and
SIRT algorithms from computed tomography.

An operator notation is a convenient way to describe the iterative
steps in the van Cittert algorithm. Let the original object be defined
by a function f in a two- or three-dimensional space as appropriate, and
let g be the measured data set. Note that f is the quantity that is to
be <u>found</u> and g is the <u>given</u> data. The data function g is related to the
object f by a linear operator P, so that

$$g = Pf \quad .$$

The operator P is a generalized projection operator. In the case of a
multiple-pinhole coded aperture, P corresponds to projecting each object
point through each of the pinholes to the detector plane. The coded image
g thus consists of many overlapping pinhole images of f.

Another useful operator is the generalized back-projection operator
B. For the multiple-pinhole aperture, B corresponds to back-projecting
each point in the coded image through each pinhole to the object space.
Of course, B is not the mathematical inverse of P, and Bg is not equal to
f. Indeed, the exact inverse of P does not in general exist.

We can now use these operators to define the van Cittert iteration scheme. An initial estimate of f, denoted f_i, is obtained by back-projecting the data, i.e., $f_i = Bg$. After n iterations, a corrected estimate f_n is formed in accordance with the recursion relation,

$$f_{n+1} = f_n + \alpha(f_i - BPf_n) \quad .$$

Here, α is an acceleration parameter that affects the rate of convergence of the algorithm. One important feature of this algorithm is that it is very easy to impose constraints on the reconstruction. For example, if at any stage a portion of the estimated object becomes negative, that portion can simply be set back to zero. We know of no general proof that this algorithm will always converge, but in practice it seems to do so and to always produce a reconstruction consistent with the data and the constraints. Results are presented in the next section.

In addition to the iterative algorithm, we are also studying another approach to the problem of obtaining true tomographic reconstructions from coded images (Smith et al., 1983). This approach, called simulated annealing, is based on some recent I.B.M. work on optimal design of integrated circuits (Kirkpatrick et al., 1983). In this problem, the goal is to place a large number of gates on a chip in such a way that the manufacturing cost of the chip is minimized. It is thus a problem in constrained optimization, the constraint being that the final circuit must perform its intended function. Since the number of conceivable designs is enormous, it is impractical to compute the cost of each of them. Instead, the I.B.M. workers start with a trial configuration and then systematically perturb it by changing the location of a single gate. If this perturbation lowers the cost of the chip, then it is accepted and a new trial configuration is formed. However, in order to avoid getting stuck in a local minimum in the optimization space, it is also necessary to accept some perturbations that increase the cost of the chip. If we denote the cost by E and its change due to moving one gate by ΔE, then negative values of ΔE are always accepted, and positive values are accepted with a probability

$$\text{Probability} = \exp(-\Delta E/kT) \quad .$$

Since this expression has the same form as the Boltzmann probability
from thermodynamics, the parameter kT is naturally interpreted as a
"thermal energy", while T itself may be thought of as a "temperature".
At high temperature, positive values of E are accepted with high probability and the chip design can randomly take on a wide variety of
configurations. As the temperature is systematically lowered, changes
that increase the cost become increasingly unlikely, and an optimum
configuration is "frozen in".

Simulated annealing gets its name from an analogy with crystal
growth. If a melt is quickly quenched, the result is an amorphous solid
or, at best, a highly imperfect crystal. Even though a perfect single
crystal would have lower energy, the system does not have the opportunity
to reach this optimum state. If the temperature is lowered gradually,
on the other hand, the imperfections are annealed out and a good crystal
is produced.

To carry this idea over into coded-aperture imaging, we define the
energy E to be the root-mean-square difference between the actual,
measured coded image and our current estimate of it. As mentioned above,
the goal of the algorithm is to make the estimated coded image agree with
the measured one or, in other words, to make E tend to zero. Thus we
start with some initial estimate of the object, calculate its coded image,
and compare it to the measured one, thereby determining E. Then the
object estimate is perturbed by adding a small increment of brightness,
called a "grain", to it and the change in energy ΔE is computed. As in
the I.B.M. work, negative values of ΔE are always accepted, and positive
values are accepted according to the Boltzmann law. The temperature
parameter T is slowly lowered, and an accurate reconstruction of the
object gradually evolves. Results obtained by this method are shown
below.

4.   SIMULATION RESULTS

The coded imaging system of primary interest in this study uses two
orthogonal aperture planes as shown in fig. 2. Digital simulation of
this system is, however, very time-consuming because of the large number
of object voxels. We have therefore chosen to reduce the dimensionality
in most of the simulations by considering the simpler problem of reconstructing a two-dimensional object from two orthogonal one-dimensional

coded images. (See Fig. 3). We have also performed a few simulations of the actual problem of reconstructing a three-dimensional object from a pair of two-dimensional coded images, with qualitatively similar results.

The first test of the simulated annealing algorithm used a binary object in the form of a letter E. The aperture in this case was a uniformly redundant, one-dimensional array of eight pinholes in each of the two "planes" (now collapsed to lines). The two coded images were each digitized to 256 pixels, and the object was represented as a 64 by 64 array. Thus there were at most 512 measured data values but 4096 unknown object values. Nevertheless, good reconstructions were obtained, as shown in Fig. 4. The only constraint used in this case was that the object was positive.

It could be argued that the quality of the reconstruction in Fig. 4 was because the object was binary (black and white), consisted only of straight lines, or filled a small part of the reconstruction space. Therefore, we also studied a more realistic object as shown in Fig. 5. The same imaging geometry was used and, once again, very good reconstructions were obtained (Fig. 5). In addition to the positivity constraint, a smoothness constraint was added in this case. The images were found to be quite insensitive to noise in the data and to be quantitatively accurate. As a general rule, more accurate results were obtained with more pinholes in the code, but computer memory requirements restricted us to a total of sixteen (eight in each aperture).

Similiar results were obtained with the iterative algorithm, as shown in Fig. 6. There are, of course, artifacts and imperfections in the reconstructions with both algorithms, but they have a qualitatively different appearance. The iterative algorithm gives streak artifacts while simulated annealing leads to a grainy or blobby appearance. Both of these problems appear to be related to computer limitations; if more pinholes could be used, along with more grains in the simulated annealing case, still better reconstructions would likely result. The two algorithms are, however, about equally effective in producing object estimates that are consistent with the constraints and the data; the remaining differences between the two reconstructions or between either reconstruction and the actual object reflect a fundamental indeterminacy inherent in the data set.

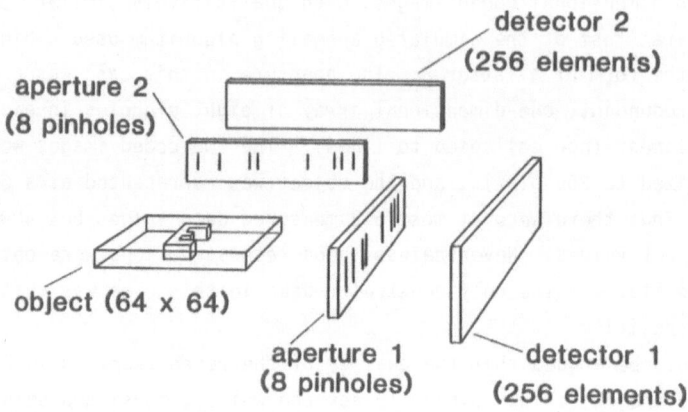

Figure 3. The collapsed geometry: tomographic imaging of a two-dimensional object with two orthogonal one-dimensional coded apertures.

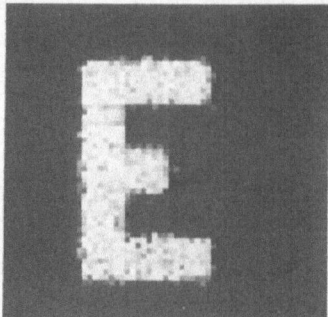

Figure 4. The reconstruction of a binary "E" using simulated annealing. Only a positivity constraint has been applied.

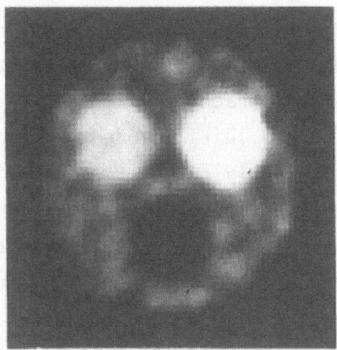

Figure 5. The reconstruction of a circular phantom with four grey
levels using simulated annealing. Positivity and smoothing
constraints have been applied.

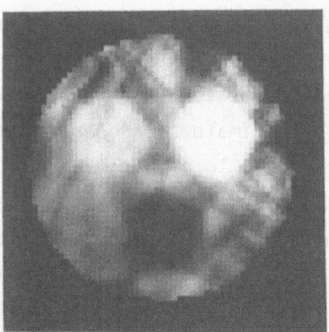

Figure 6. The reconstruction of the circular phantom, using the
iterative algorithm. Positivity and lateral limit
constraints have been applied.

5. COMPARISON OF LIMITED-ANGLE AND MULTIPLEXED IMAGING

To assess the relative importance of limited-angle viewing and multiplexing, we carried out the simulation shown in Fig. 7. To "turn off"
the multiplexing, we simply kept track of which pinhole a given object
ray passed through in forming the initial coded image. This is equivalent
to opening the pinholes sequentially rather than simultaneously, thereby
obtaining nonoverlapping pinhole images of the object.

Quite surprisingly, this made almost no difference in the reconstructed images with either algorithm (see Fig. 7). On the other hand,
the second aperture plane made an enormous difference; if it was not
present, very poor images were obtained.

Although Fig. 7 is just one anecdotal example, it strongly suggests
that multiplexing is, in general, a far less serious deficiency than a
limited view angle. Theoretical support for this contention may be found
in some recent work by Davison (1983), who showed that the limited-angle
tomography problem is horribly ill-conditioned. The corresponding
calculation for the multiplexed case has not been performed, but our
results suggest that this problem is not so badly behaved. Further
theoretical investigation is clearly needed.

6. COMPARISON OF SPECT SYSTEMS

Coded-aperture imaging is a form of single-photon emission computed
tomography (SPECT). In this section, we examine its relationship to
other forms of SPECT, including rotating Anger cameras, seven-pinhole
systems, rotating slant-hole collimators, and tomographic scanners. What
is the niche for coded apertures? To answer this question, we first
discuss some of the limitations of the competing systems.

The rotating Anger camera is clearly the most successful approach to
SPECT to date. Modern systems give good, artifact-free images with
moderate resolution. The linear resolution is typically 1.5-2.0 cm, but
a better way to specify resolution for tomographic systems is by the
volume of the resolution cell. A linear resolution of 2 cm corresponds
to a resolution volume of some 8 cm^3. To appreciate the significance of
this number, suppose that a 1 cm^3 tumor is to be imaged. Since the tumor
fills just 1/8 of the resolution cell, its apparent contrast is reduced a
factor of 8, greatly reducing the probability of detection. Thus, even
modest improvements in resolution would have great clinical significance.

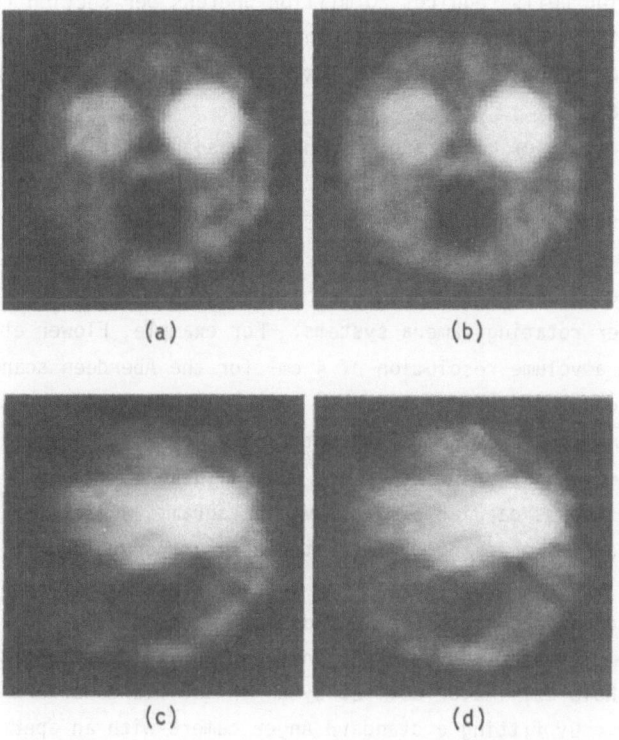

Figure 7.   Reconstruction of the circular phantom with simulated
            annealing:
            (a)   same as Fig. 5; 2 views, multiplexing
            (b)   2 views, no multiplexing
            (c)   1 view, multiplexing
            (d)   1 view, no multiplexing.

Unfortunately, it is not likely that these improvements in rotating-camera systems will be forthcoming. The resolution limitation arises mainly from the collimator, and any improvement in this area must come at the expense of photon collection efficiency. Such a trade-off is unacceptable because the images are already photon-starved. For example, an image of just 30×30 resolution cells requires 20 million photons per section for an RMS uncertainty of 5% (Budinger, 1980). In practice, far fewer photons can be recorded in an acceptable time, and lower resolution or greater uncertainty must be tolerated.

A wide variety of tomographic scanners has appeared, including the Mark IV brain scanner (Kuhl et al., 1976), the Aberdeen section scanner and the Tomogscanner (Bowley et al., 1973), the Cleon brain imager (Stoddart and Stoddart, 1979), and the Anger tomographic scanner or Pho/Con. Some of these instruments achieve a slight improvement in resolution over rotating-camera systems. For example, Flower et al. (1981) report a volume resolution of 4 cm^3 for the Aberdeen scanner and 2 cm^3 for Cleon.

Since tomographic scanners and rotating cameras require mechanical motion of a heavy instrument, they are not suitable for rapid dynamic studies. First-pass cardiac studies, venacavagrams, and cerebral blood-flow studies are examples of dynamic studies that cannot now be performed tomographically. There is thus a need for a tomographic system that will give good reconstructions without any detector motion.

One attempt at filling this gap in tomographic instrumentation was the seven-pinhole collimator devised by Kirch and his coworkers (Vogel et al., 1978). By fitting a standard Anger camera with an aperture plate having seven pinhole apertures, they were able to obtain simultaneously seven nonoverlapping (unmultiplexed) pinhole projections of small objects. With an ingenious reconstruction algorithm, they were able to get very respectable reconstructions of the myocardium. Unfortunately, it soon became apparent that the method was applicable only to the heart, and that, even there, severe artifacts resulted if the camera was slightly tilted with respect to the axis of the heart.

The basic difficulty with the seven-pinhole approach is the paucity of data it collects. Only seven projections are available, compared to typically 72 in rotating-camera SPECT. But, more importantly, the angular field of view is very limited; no projection data at all are recorded over a wide range of angles. Finally, the spatial resolution is very poor. Each pinhole image occupies about 10% of the available area of the Anger camera and must, of necessity, consist of a very small number of resolvable elements if overlap of the images is to be avoided.

The rotating slant-hole collimator is in some respects an improvement on the seven-pinhole collimator. It has better resolution in each projection and collects a larger data set. However, it is still a limited-angle system and cannot, in our view, ever be expected to give quantitatively accurate reconstructions. Moreover, it requires mechanical motion and is therefore unsuited for dynamic studies.

The niche for coded apertures can now be seen. They form the basis for a wide-angle, high-resolution tomographic system without detector motion. To get the necessary wide viewing angle, at least two orthogonal detector planes are required. We are currently building a system of modular scintillation cameras for this purpose (Milster et al., 1983). In addition, the goal of high spatial resolution dictates the use of a multiplexed aperture so that each projection can be recorded with the full space-bandwidth product of the detectors.

7. STATISTICAL CONSIDERATIONS

Of course, high resolution must not be bought at the expense of a large degradation in statistical accuracy, and here again coded apertures might prove advantageous. For planar objects, there is a large literature on the statistical properties of coded imaging systems. If one specifies the statistical quality of a reconstruction by the pixel signal-to-noise ratio (SNR), which is defined as the ratio of the ensemble average of the image at a particular pixel to its standard deviation, then it is straightforward to show that coded apertures are superior to conventional imaging systems of similar resolution for very small objects and inferior for very large objects. Rogers has put it succinctly by saying that coded apertures are a way of effectively utilizing the available detector area. If the image already fills the detector, coded apertures are of little or no use. This statement is, however, subject to criticism on two grounds. First, pixel SNR may not be a good measure of image quality, and second, the statistical considerations for tomographic reconstruction may be very different from those for planar imaging. We shall discuss each of these points in turn.

Although pixel SNR is a traditional measure of image quality, recent work of Burgess et al. (1981) indicates that its applicability is limited. Building on an earlier suggestion of Harris (1964), they propose instead to frame the image quality question in terms of an ideal observer who is trying to make a decision or test an hypothesis on the basis of the given image data. If the hypothesis is binary, an appropriate test statistic is the likelihood ratio (van Trees, 1968), and the SNR associated with this statistic is another possible measure of image quality. Burgess et al. found a reasonable correlation between this ideal-observer SNR and the SNR demonstrated by a human observer in psychophysical experiments. More recently, however, Voss et al. (1983) have found situations in which the ideal-observer SNR is a very poor predictor of human performance.

Wagner et al. (1981) have approached the coded-aperture problem from the ideal-observer viewpoint. They compared a URA coded aperture to a large open aperture for the task of deciding whether a planar object consisted of one Gaussian blob or two. By calculating the ideal-observer SNR for the two apertures, they concluded that the large open aperture was almost always superior to the URA. They claimed, therefore, that the large aperture had better "resolution" for this task than the URA. It must be emphasized that this usage of the word resolution is rather unconventional; it does not correspond, for example, to the usage else- where in this paper, where resolution refers to the width of the point spread function of the system. By this traditional usage of the term, the URA in Wagner's comparison had some twenty times <u>better</u> resolution than the large open aperture.

Wagner et al. did not consider the question of the optimum size of the large open aperture. Rather, they chose arbitrarily to set the area of the open aperture equal to the open area of the URA. Specifically, the URA was 29×31 elements, 50% of which were open, and the open aperture was 21×21 elements (all open, of course). In other words, in this comparison the coded aperture did not have any advantage at all in collection efficiency. Previous workers have chosen, equally arbitrarily, to compare coded apertures to pinholes with the same resolution (in the traditional sense). The appropriate comparison in this viewpoint would be between the 29×31 URA and a 1×1 aperture or pinhole. Wagner et al. did not carry out this comparison, but they indicated that they expected the coded aperture to be superior to this small pinhole.

The Wagner study also did not address the question of human performance with these apertures. In fact, no decoding operation was performed on the coded data, so it was left in a form that was not useful to a human observer. Several open questions thus remain: (1) How would the human observer perform with the large open aperture? (2) How would the ideal and human observers perform with a small pinhole? (3) Does the simple binary decision problem have any predictive value for the immensely more complicated tasks encountered in the clinic?

To summarize, the objective statistical properties of coded-aperture imaging of planar objects are well understood. There is no difficulty in calculating the pixel SNR or any other proposed measure of statistical accuracy. The far more difficult question of assessing image quality requires more study. In particular, the relative performance of human and ideal observers must be determined, and the role of spatial resolution, as traditionally defined, must be clarified.

On the other hand, even the objective statistical properties of coded apertures need further attention when true tomographic reconstruction is considered. This question has not been addressed until now because it was not clear that such a reconstruction was possible. With limited-angle geometries, there are such huge inaccuracies due to the incomplete data that it makes little sense to consider the residual statistical effects. With the orthogonal-view geometry, on the other hand, we get good reconstructions with noise-free data, and the statistical limitations must now be studied.

Unfortunately, it is very difficult to treat the statistics analytically because the reconstruction algorithms are nonlinear. We must resort to digital simulation to compare coded and non-coded systems. An example of such a simulation is shown in Fig. 8, which shows essentially the same comparison of coded and non-coded imaging as in Fig. 7, but with noise added. The imaging system consisted of two orthogonal aperture planes, with eight pinhole apertures in each plane. In the coded case, all pinholes were open simultaneously, while in the non-coded case they were open sequentially. The overall imaging time was held constant in this comparison, so that the coded data set contains eight times as many photons as the non-coded set. Subjectively, the reconstruction from the coded data seems to be substantially better. It should be noted that the object fills a substantial portion of the field in this comparison; if the same

122

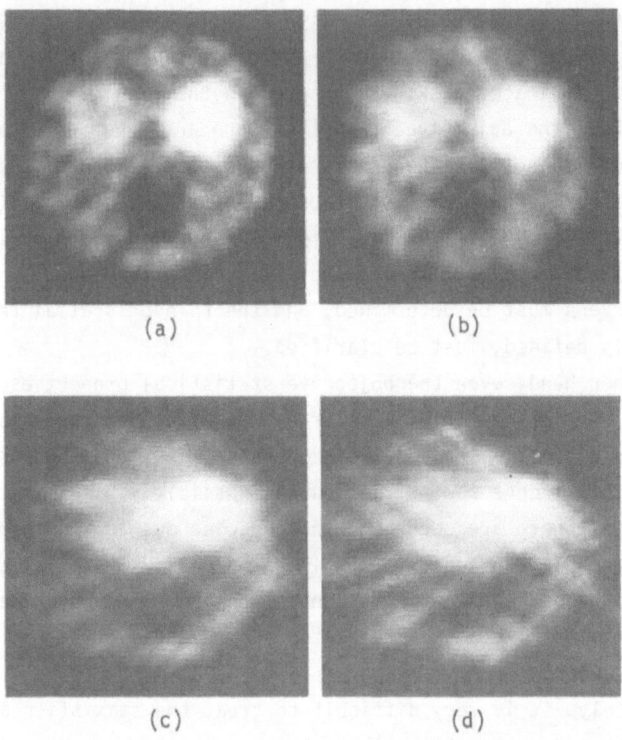

(a) (b)

(c) (d)

Figure 8. Simulated-annealing reconstruction of the circular phantom
with Poisson noise in the projection data.
(a) two views, with multiplexing (pinholes open
simultaneously)
(b) two views, no multiplexing (pinholes open sequentially,
each for 1/8 of the total exposure time.)
(c) one view, with multiplexing
(d) one view, no multiplexing

considerations as in the case of coded imaging of planar objects were valid here, little or no advantage would be expected from coding.

8. ENDOSCOPIC IMAGING

Traditionally, nuclear medicine has involved the use of a large scintillation camera outside the patient's body. A severe limitation to this method is that the camera must be rather far from the object of interest, resulting in loss of resolution and poor contrast because of attenuation and scatter. In clinical terms, this makes it very difficult to detect lesions less than two or three centimeters in diameter.

A few investigators have sought to circumvent these problems by using an endoscopic detector. For example, we have had considerable success in detecting lung tumors with a miniature scintillation detector capable of passing through the biopsy channel of a bronchoscope. The detector had no imaging capability, and tumors were detected merely by proximity. Nevertheless, nonvisible submucosal and extraluminal tumors as small as 6 mm were detected (Barber et al., 1979).

A problem with this kind of endoscopic probe is that it is sometimes difficult to distinguish small tumor foci from nonuniform distributions of background activity. An imaging endoscopic probe, on the other hand, could potentially give high spatial resolution and contrast, resulting in improved sensitivity and specificity for detection of small tumors.

There are a great many possible designs for an imaging endoscopic probe. The detector itself could have a two-dimensional imaging capability, analogous to a miniature Anger camera, or it could be a one-dimensional array of individual detectors or even a single nonimaging detector. We shall refer to these three options as, respectively, 2D, 1D, and 0D detectors. In all cases, however, the goal is to produce a 2D image. Therefore, with a 0D or 1D detector, some kind of scanning motion must be used. With each of these generic detectors, many different imaging apertures can be used. With the 2D detector, for example, we could use a pinhole, a collimator, or some form of coded aperture, just as with external imaging.

A numerical example will illustrate the feasibility of this approach. Consider a 2D detector array consisting of 400 semiconductor detectors, each 0.5 mm square. The overall array is thus 1 cm square. A miniature parallel-hole collimator, perhaps made of gold, could have a bore diameter

of 0.25 mm, a septal thickness of 0.25 mm, and a bore length of 4 mm.
This system would have a spatial resolution of 0.5 mm for objects close to
the collimator face, and it would have a geometric collection efficiency
of about 2.5×10^{-4}, comparable to conventional collimators for external
imaging. The important point is that efficiency need not be sacrificed
for resolution if <u>all</u> dimensions, including the distance from the detector
to the object, are scaled in proportion.

There is, however, one dimension that cannot be scaled, and that is
the attenuation length of the gamma rays in the collimator and shielding
material. The collimator described above would be suitable for cobalt-57,
with a gamma-ray energy of 122 keV, and marginally useful for technetium-99m
(140 keV), but septal penetration would be a severe problem for higher
energies. Coded apertures offer one way to alleviate this problem. Since
they allow a larger geometric collection efficiency in the first place,
penetration through the shielding and apertur- material is less important.
An endoscopic probe based on coded apertures will, therefore, be lighter
and more compact than one based on collimators.

9. A PROTOTYPE IMAGING PROBE

To demonstrate the concept of endoscopic imaging, we have constructed
a prototype probe based on a simple OD (non-imaging) detector. As shown
in Fig. 9, the aperture consists of a lead cylinder, 2 cm in diameter,
with azimuthally coded slits. The code function is a uniformly redundant
array (URA) with either 15 or 31 elements. This code cylinder may be
rotated around its axis by means of a drive cable. The detector is a NaI
scintillation crystal attached via a fiber-optic light guide to a
photomultiplier. Parallel lead discs provide axial collimation.

To understand the operation of this system, a cylindrical coordinate
system (r, θ, z) is useful. The z axis coincides with the axis of the lead
cylinder, and the transmission of the cylinder as a function of θ is the
URA code function. An angular coded image, a function of θ, is formed
during one rotation of the cylinder. Decoding is carried out by correlating
the coded image with a bipolar version of the code function. This decoding
operation has the effect of converting the code function into a sharply
peaked point spread function. The 1D decoded image has an angular
resolution of 2π divided by the number of elements in the URA. The disc
collimator provides resolution in the z direction, and image information

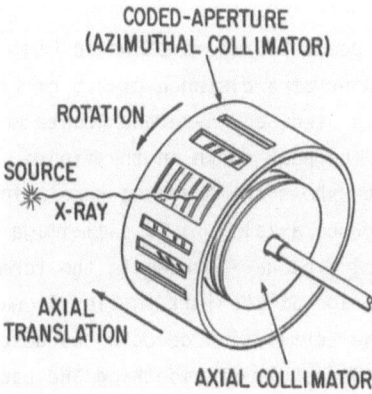

Figure 9. Schematic of an endoscopic imaging probe using a rotating coded aperture

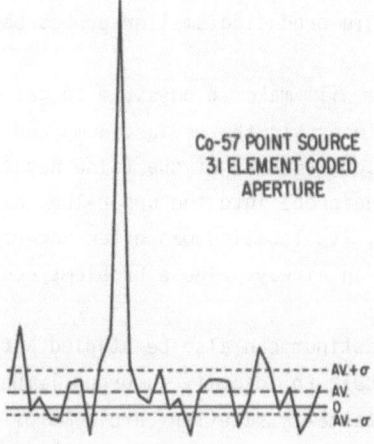

Figure 10. Reconstructed image of a point source using the probe of Fig. 9.

in this direction is obtained by scanning the probe axially. The final image is thus a function of θ and z; no information about the r direction is obtained.

A decoded image of a point source is shown in Fig. 10. The source was a 1.5 mCi cobalt-57 point at a distance of 2.5 cm from the probe. The 31-element aperture was used, and 5-second counts were taken at each of 31 angular positions. The peak shown in the figure, which is the decoded image of the point, shows the expected resolution.

By translating this probe axially, a 2D(θ-z) image can be formed. To illustrate this feature, a planar phantom in the form of a letter E, 13×15 cm, was used. The image at the left in Fig. 11 was acquired with the 31-element aperture and correlation decoding as described above. The image at the right shows the result of smoothing and background suppression.

10.   OUTLOOK FOR ENDOSCOPIC IMAGING

The primary uses of an endoscopic probe would be in the esophagus and colon. The prototype probe described above is somewhat too large for the esophagus, where a diameter of 10-12 mm appears to be a practical limit, but it might be useful in the colon. However, there does not seem to be any fundamental problem in producing smaller probes based on OD, 1D, or even 2D detectors.

An esophageal probe will make it possible to get close to tumors in the upper lobes of the lungs, in the mediastinum, and in the hilar regions. In our bronchoscopic study, several of the false negatives resulted from inability to maneuver the probe into the upper-lobe airways. And even when we detected a tumor, its location was often uncertain if it wasn't immediately adjacent to an airway. These problems could be circumvented with esophageal imaging.

Tumors in the mediastinum can also be studied with an esophageal probe. It is now difficult to identify tumorous lymph nodes in the mediastinum, a major metastatic site for carcinoma of the lung.

The use of radiolabelled monoclonal antibodies in conjunction with an esophageal imaging probe for lesions in the mediastinum is also attractive. Heavy smokers, the high-risk group for lung cancer, frequently have inflammatory airway changes, and tumor-seeking tracers such as cobalt-57 bleomycin are taken up to some extent at sites of inflammation. Similarly, inflammatory diseases involving mediastinal lymph nodes may show a pattern

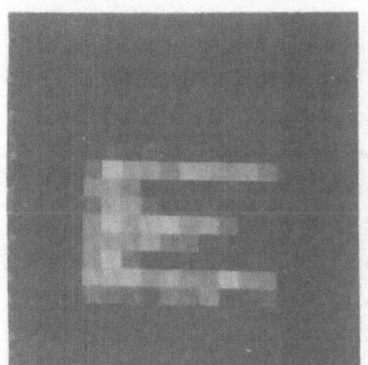

left   right

Figure 11.   Reconstructed image of an E-shaped radioactive source.
             Left - unsmoothed.
             Right - smoothed.

of bleomycin uptake similar to that in metastatic disease. Monoclonal antibodies would not be expected to concentrate in these sites of inflammation.

Radiolabelled antibodies and an imaging probe should be equally applicable in detecting and localizing colon cancer. In addition, a colon probe could provide information about antibody deposition in adjacent structures such as retroperitoneal lymph nodes.

11. SUMMARY AND CONCLUSIONS

Two new approaches to coded-aperture imaging have been suggested in this paper. The first of these, external imaging with two orthogonal apertures, has been shown by digital simulation to yield high-quality tomographic reconstructions in spite of the multiplexing of the data. Two different algorithms, the van Cittert iterative method and simulated annealing, were shown to be effective reconstruction techniques. Orthogonal-view coded-aperture imaging makes it possible to get high-resolution, quantitatively accurate tomographic images without any detector motion.

The second new approach, endoscopic imaging, is in a very early stage, but the principle has been demonstrated with a prototype probe 2 cm in diameter, and smaller probes are certainly possible.

ACKNOWLEDGMENTS

Helpful discussions with Dennis Patton, George Seeley, Mark Borgstrom, Mark Stempski, Ellen Cargill, Tom Milster, and Lars Selberg are gratefully acknowledged. This work was supported by the National Cancer Institute under grant no. P01 23417.

REFERENCES

Barber, H.B., Donahue, D.J., Woolfenden, J.M., and Silverstein, M.E. 1979. "Miniature Radiation Detectors for Surgical Tumor Staging." Proceedings of the 32nd Annual Conference on Engineering in Medicine and Biology, Denver, Colorado. Paper 16.8, p. 142.

Barrett, H.H., and Swindell, W. 1981. "Radiological Imaging: Theory of Image Formation, Detection, and Processing." Academic Press, New York.

Bowley, A.R., Taylor, C.G., Causer, D.A., Barber, D.C., Keyes, W.L., Undrill, P.E., Corfield, J.R., and Mallard, J.R. 1973. Br. J. Radiology $\underline{46}$, pp. 262-271.

Budinger, T.F. 1980. "Physical Attributes of Single-Photon Tomography." J. Nucl. Med. $\underline{21}$, pp. 579-592.

Burgess, A.E., Wagner, R.D., Kenning, R.J., and Barlow, H.B. 1981. "Efficiency of Human Visual Signal Discrimination." Science $\underline{214}$, pp. 93-94.

Chiu, M.-Y., Barrett, H.H., Simpson, R.G., Chou, C., Arendt, J.W., and
    Gindi, G.R. 1979. "Three-dimensional Radiographic Imaging with A
    Restricted View Angle." J. Opt. Soc. Am. 69, p. 1323.
Davison, M.E. 1983. "The Ill-conditioned Nature of the Limited Angle Tomogra-
    phy Problem." SIAM J. Appl. Math. 43, pp. 428-448.
Flower, M.A., Rowe, R.W., Webb, S., and Keyes, W.I. 1981. "A Comparison of
    Three Systems for Performing Single-Photon Emission Tomography." Phy.s
    Med. Biol. 26, pp. 671-691.
Harris, J.L. 1964. "Resolving Power and Decision Theory." J. Opt. Soc. Am.
    54, pp. 606-611.
Kirkpatrick, S., Gelatt Jr., C.D., and Vecci, M.P. 1983. "Optimization by
    Simulated Annealing." Science 220, pp. 671-680.
Kuhl, D.E., Edwards, R.Q., Ricci, A.R., Yacob, R.J., Mich, T.J., and Alavi, A.
    1976. "The Mark IV System for Radionuclide Computed Tomography of the
    Brain." Radiology 121, pp. 405-413.
Lefkopoulos, D., Fonroget, J., Devaux, J.Y., Guilhem, J.B., Roucayrol, J.C.,
    and Gu.raud, R. 1982. "Quantitative 3D Imaging with Coded Apertures by
    Using SVD Decomposition of the Transmission Matrix." World Federation
    of Nuclear Medicine and Biology. Paris.
May, R.S., Akcasu, Z., and Knoll, G.F. 1974. "Gamma-Ray Imaging with
    Stochastic Apertures." Appl. Opt. 13, p. 2589.
Milster, T.D., Selberg, L.A., Easton, R.L., Barrett, H.H., and Rossi, G.R.
    1983. "A Modular Imaging System in Nuclear Medicine." 30th Annual
    Meeting of the Society of Nuclear Medicine, St. Louis.
Renaud, L., Joy, M.L.G., and Gilday, D.L. 1979. "Fourier Multiaperture
    Emission Tomography. J. Nucl. Med. 20, p. 986.
Simpson, R.G., and Barrett, H.H. 1980. "Coded-Aperture Imaging." Imaging
    in Diagnostic Medicine (S. Nudelman, ed.), Plenum, New York,
    pp. 217-311.
Smith, W.E., Barrett, H.H., and Paxman, R.G. 1983. "Reconstruction of
    Objects from Coded Images by Simulated Annealing." Opt. Lett. 8,
    p. 199.
Steinbach, A., and Macovski, A. 1979. "Improved Depth Resolution with One-
    dimensional Coded Aperture Imaging." J. Phys. D: Appl. Phys. 12,
    pp. 2079-2099.
Stoddart, H.F. and Stoddart, H.A. 1979. IEEE Trans. Nucl. Sci.:NS-26,
    pp. 2710-2712.
Tipton, M.D. 1978. "The Odcat: One Dimensional Coded Aperture Tomography."
    Rec. Fut. Devel. Med. Imaging SPIE 152.
Van Trees, H.L. 1968. "Detection, Estimation, and Modulation Theory,
    Part I." John Wiley and Sons, New York.
Vogel, R.A., Kirch, D., LeFree, M., and Steele, P. 1978. "A New Method of
    Multiplanar Emission Tomography Using a Seven Pinhole Collimator and
    an Anger Scintillation Camera." J. Nucl. Med. 19, p. 648.
Voss, K.J., Varrett, H.H., Borgstrom, M.C., Patton, D.D., and Seeley, G.
    W. 1983. "Effect of Texture on Detectability of Abnormalities in
    Medical Imaging." J. Nucl. Med. 24, 66.
Wagner, R.F., Brown, D.G., and Metz, C.E. 1981. "On the Multiplex
    Advantage of Coded Source/Aperture Photon Imaging." SPIE 314,
    pp. 72-76.

PREPROCESSING OF SPECT DATA AS A PRECURSOR FOR ATTENUATION CORRECTION

A. TODD-POKROPEK, G. CLARKE and R. MARSH

University College London U.K.

1. INTRODUCTION

Almost all systems available for performing single photon emission computed tomography (SPECT) reconstruct images by filtered backprojection, and perform some kind of attenuation correction. These systems give qualitatively reasonable images. However, for the purposes of quantitation, the results are far from satisfactory. Specifically, it may be observed that, often, when procedures designed to perform attenuation correct are tested and evaluated, usually simulated data is employed (as in [1] for example). The attenuation at the centre of such simulated objects is much greater than that observed in reality (see Fig 16). Alternatively, the results of correcting for attenuation in a real uniform phantom are studied [2]. Such tests are inadequate since a variety of physical effects such as the presence of scatter, and the effect of the collimator response function, have been ignored. It may also be observed that, firstly, such procedures do not work if the known linear attenuation coefficient μ for the photon energy of the isotope used (e.g 0.15cm^{-1} for 140Kev for Tc99M) is employed, and, secondly, tend to over- or under-correct depending on the form of the activity distribution. These problems occur both when a distribution of values of μ , or when a single value based on the attenuation of water, is used. The purpose of this paper is to present a series of preprocessing techniques such that an attenuation correction may be applied which is, to a reasonable approximation, object

independent. A secondary problem is that errors in the data
are amplified by such correction, and methods of reducing
the importance of such errors are given.

Some results are presented for the following
preprocessing techniques:

1. Uniformity correction
2. Artefact filtering
3. The use of non-circular orbits
4. Noise reducing filters
5. Collimator response function correction
6. Scatter correction

These preprocessing techniques have all been applied to the
data in the form of sinograms, where each sinogram
corresponds to one tomographic 'slice'. A sinogram is a
matrix where each row of the data corresponds to a
projection (every position on the detector, for one given
angle), and each column to one position on the detector for
every angle.

2. UNIFORMITY CORRECTION

It is well known [3,4] that the presence of
non-uniformity can introduce artefacts in tomographic
reconstructions. This applies in particular to systems with
circular symmetry such as rotating gamma camera SPECT
systems. As shown in Fig 1, the effect of variation in
sensitivity in the detector may be considerably amplified in
the tomographic image, dependent on (the inverse of the
square root of) the distance of the error from the
perpendicular through the axis of rotation. In addition, the
error introduced is an increasing function of spatial
frequency. Thus, for example, stripes caused by the
differential non-linearity of ADCs may cause artefacts.

While, in general, it is highly desirable that the
detectors used be as uniform as possible by using
appropriate correction for spatial distortion etc [5], post
acquisition correction procedures may also be employed. The
simplest and most common technique used is that of a

pointwise matrix division of the projection data by that from a uniform source, i.e. a flood field correction. However, ignoring the problem of variations in sensitivity as a function of rotational angle, a problem that has been solved by manufacturers by the use of appropriate shielding, it may be observed that apparent uniformity also varies as a function of the form of the uniform source used, and in particular, the amount of scatter. It should also be noted that the physical distortion of a flood field (bowing), contrary to what has been suggested elsewhere [6] is of little importance since it is a low frequency effect, and does not cause artefacts. However, pixelation and the statistical error on a point in the correction matrix, being of high frequency, can cause severe artefacts [7]. Although it has been suggested that very high numbers of counts be collected for such correction matrix (e.g. >100M counts), it has been found that conventional image processing and interpolation performed so as to reduce any spurious high frequency content of the image at frequencies greater than about 3 times the spacing of the photomultipliers is a powerful preprocessing technique which may be applied to such correction matrices.

An experiment was performed using a uniform source with various amounts of scatter in order to evaluate the potential error in the estimate of planar uniformity. The results are summarised in Table 1, for one particular (Siemens ZLC) camera.

Thus it is clear that, as a function of the amount of scatter, and in particular, as a function of the energy window, the apparent uniformity changes. This is particularly true as the energy window is offset towards higher energies. Thus while it is desirable to attempt to achieve uniformity which is of the order of say better that 2%, in practice, for an object with a variable amount of scatter, this cannot be achieved. In fact, it is unreasonable to expect better than 4% uniformity, even with a perfect flood field correction, with current systems.

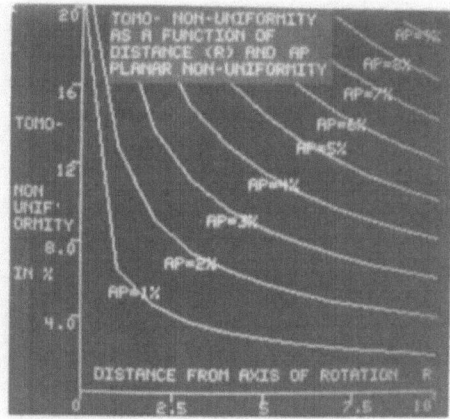

Fig 1. A plot of tomographic uniformity against distance from the axis of rotation for various amounts of planar uniformity (AP) from 1% to 9%. Note that the amplification on the axis of rotation is by about a factor of 20.

Fig 2. A map of 's' the sinogram uniformity map, for a circular orbit. Note that non-uniformity takes the form of vertical stripes.

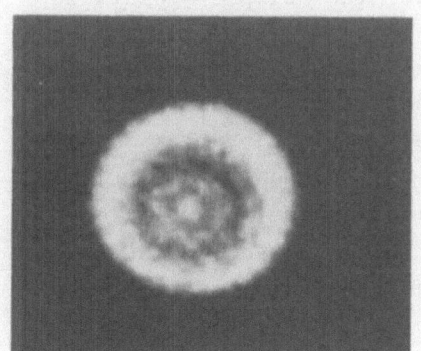

Fig 3. A uniform phantom showing a classic (severe) uniformity artefact.

Since this implies a maximum error in the tomogram of the order of 80%, it is clear that other techniques must be used.

Table 1. Error in uniformity for various types of flood sources and energies, expressed as the maximum error between the given image and a reference image.

Type of Source	Window Kev	Maximum error in Central field of view
Tc99m flood, 2cm thick	130–150	Reference image
Co57 disk	115–125	17%
Tc99m flood +5cm of scattering medium	130–150	4.5%
Tc99m flood +5cm of scattering medium	135–155	9.5%
Tc99m flood +5cm of scattering medium	125–145	7.5%
Tc99m flood +5cm of scattering medium	110–135	6%

3. ARTEFACT FILTERING

The observed value in a sinogram $p_o(x, theta)$ is related to the incident number of photons $p(x, theta)$ is terms of the sensitivity of the camera $s(x,y,theta)$ at the point x, for the given slice y, at an angle theta by:

$$p_o(x, theta) = p(x, theta) \cdot s(x,y,theta)$$

Thus the observed sinogram is the simple pointwise multiplication of the 'incident' sinogram, and a mapping function s. However, in most current systems s is independent of theta. For conventional circular orbits, s is only a function of x, as illustrated in Fig 2. Variations in uniformity may be observed in this image as vertical stripes, which after reconstruction, become the well known circular artefacts, as illustrated in Fig 3. Removal of such stripes is a simple problem in image processing. If a 2-D Fourier transformation is made of s, the vertical stripes tend to have a high spatial frequency in x, and low angular frequency. A filter may be designed such that power

Fig 4. Left, the artefact filter (with the Nyquist frequency in the centre, and the fundamental top left), and right, the filtered 2-D Fourier transform of a sinogram.

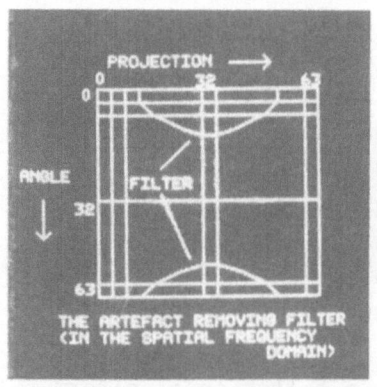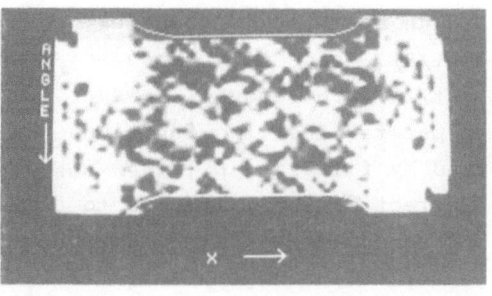

Fig 5. The result of filtering a uniform phantom, showing left, the image before filtering, and, right, the image after filtering

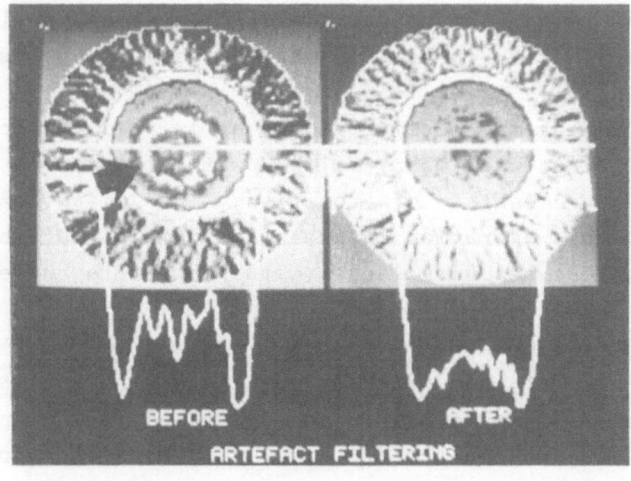

associated with such vertical stripes is removed, as shown in Fig 4. Note that fundamental is at (0,0) and that the central point corresponds to the Nyquist frequency. This filter has in fact been used previously in X-ray CT [8]. Thus high spatial frequencies in x (greater than about Nyquist/8), and low frequencies in theta (less than about Nyquist/10) are removed. However, since it is not possible to separate the two functions s and p, the filter must be applied by filtering p_o, the observed projection. Thus a side affect of the filter is to eliminate such components in the true projection data. Fortunately, such components in p (e.g. vertical stripes) are rare, but nevertheless, the filter must be used with some caution.

An example of the use of such a filter on a uniform phantom is shown in Fig 5. In clinical practice, circular artefacts are difficult to recognise as such, since they are typically incomplete circles. Fig 6 shows the result of the use of the filter on a clinical lung scan. The filter has also been tested to check the loss of resolution, which is slight, and the quantitative distortion of the data, which is minimal with the exception of data with circular form such scalp activity in brains, where the effect is still reasonably small.

The filter may be improved by applying it in the space domain, as a non-stationary filter, with increasing weight towards the centre of rotation. The disadvantage of performing this operation in the space domain is that the filter then becomes very large (with respect to angle).

4. NON-CIRCULAR ORBITS

The use of non-circular orbits may be analysed in a simple manner. Essentially, as described in a previous paper [9] any non-circular orbit may be reconstructed by shifting the data from such an orbit to the corresponding circular orbit. Fig 7 shows the observed centre of gravity for a point source as a function of angle, for a circular, and for a non-circular orbit (without of course moving the

Fig 6. The result of filtering a clinical lung scan. This shows: 1) the original reconstruction, 2) the artefact filtered reconstruction, 3) the difference between the sinograms before and after filtering, and 4) the difference between the reconstructions before and after filtering.

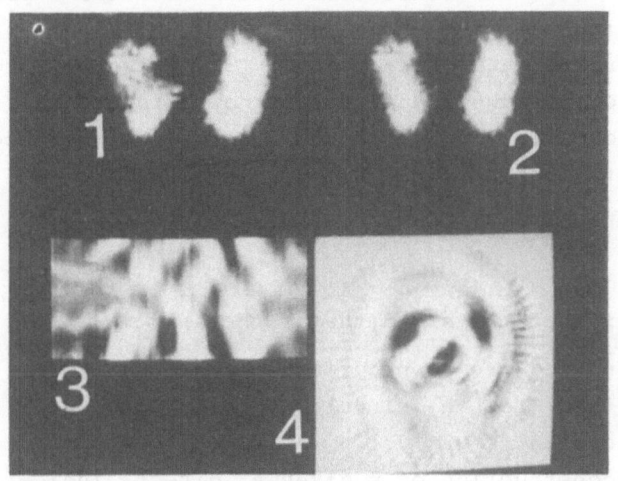

Fig 7. The centre of gravity of a point source plotted as a function of angle, for a circular orbit and for an elliptic orbit. The difference between the two is the correction factor.

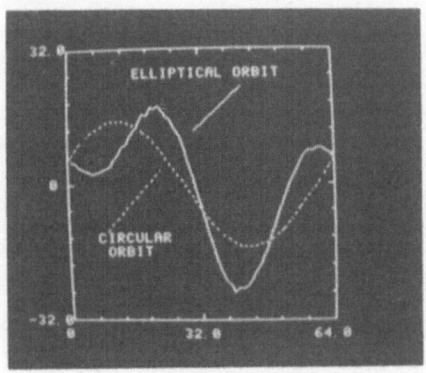

point source). Thus the differences between these functions
gives a vector of shift values as a function of angle. These
values are used to shift $p_o(x,theta)$. Thus the observed
shifted p_o may be considered to be the pointwise
multiplication of the true unshifted $p(x,theta)$ for a
circular orbit, and the shifted $s(x,y,theta)$. For an
elliptical orbit, the function s is now a function of theta,
but not normally of y. Such an orbit is generated by a
displacement d(theta) given by:

$$d(theta) = c1. cos(2.theta + c2)$$

and thus:

$$s'(x,theta) = s(x+d(theta),theta)$$

where c1, and c2 are appropriate constants, s() is the
uniformity map for a circular orbit, and s'() for the
elliptical orbit.

The reconstruction of s gives a direct indication of
the amplitude of the tomographic non-uniformity. The shape
of the artefacts, as has been demonstrated by Gullberg [10]
is that of the hypocyloid with four cusps. The amplitude of
such artefacts is not a simple function. In general, the
overall amplitude of the artefact reduces as a function of
increasing values of c1.

An alternative type of artefact reduction may be
achieved by altering the slice plane, e.g. moving the
patient in the y direction. The function s is now in
addition a function of y, as illustrated in Fig 8. The
effect of oscillations in y, plus displacements in x may be
combined.

While the overall effect of the reduction of artefacts
by such methods cannot be determined analytically, a simple
simulation using measured uniformity maps can be performed.
Fig 9 shows the amplitude of the resulting artefacts for a
circular orbit, an elliptical orbit, an oscillation in y,
and a combined elliptical orbit plus oscillation in y. It
may be observed that the overall amplitude of the artefacts
is considerably reduced, by, in general a factor of at least

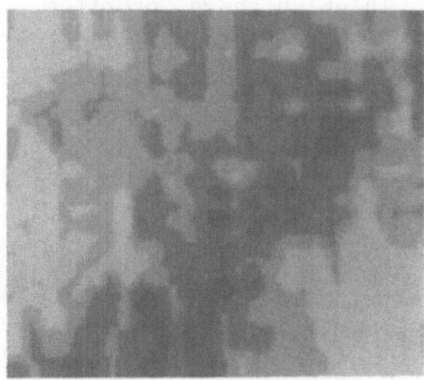

Fig 8. The sinogram uniformity map 's', for an oscillating y. Notice that the stripes are now not continuous.

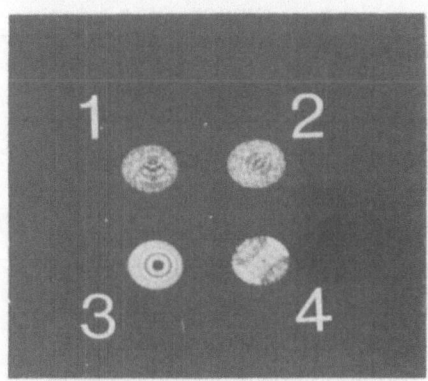

Fig 9. An intercomparison of different types of orbits, based on a simulated uniform object, and a measured uniformity map (using a GE 400AT). The results shown are for:
1) a sinusoidally oscillating value in y,
2) an elliptical orbit (e.g. translation in x) and a sinusoidally varying y,
3) a conventional circular orbit and
4) a conventional elliptical orbit

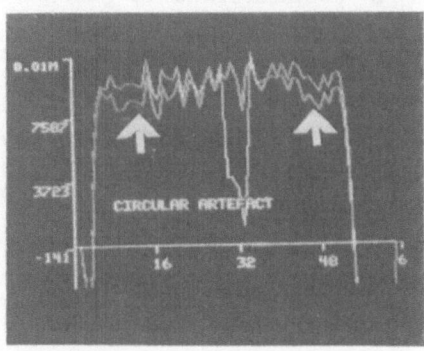

Fig 10. Two profiles though a uniform source after reconstruction: from a circular orbit showing a large central artefact, and from an elliptical orbit with the corresponding artefacts arrowed.

2. A second example is shown in Fig 10 which shows profiles through a uniform source for a circular and an elliptical orbit. It should be stressed that the power associated with the artefact is not eliminated, it is merely distributed differently and does not tend to 'concentrate'.

5. NOISE REDUCING FILTERS

Data in SPECT is very photon limited, and therefore any attempt to improve the signal to noise ratio is important. Several techniques have been compared being:

1. Median filtering
2. Homomorphic filtering
3. Minimum mean square error (MMSE) filtering after the Anscombe transform [11]
4. The use of conventional window functions e.g. the Butterworth window.

Space does not permit a full analysis of these results. In summary, median filtering was found to be rather disappointing. The MMSE filter, after the Anscombe (square root) transform, gave the best results, better than Homomorphic filtering, and were not found to be equivalent to an appropriate choice of an equivalent window functions. An example comparing the MMSE and the Butterworth filters is shown in Fig 11. Preprocessing of data in the form of sinograms, which is normally a 1-D filtering operation, has considerable potential. It is also computationally much cheaper than filtering 2-D reconstructions.

6. CORRECTION FOR THE COLLIMATOR RESPONSE FUNCTION

The importance of a correction for the collimator response function may be estimated from Fig 12. The difference between the observed activity at the two points indicated on the edge of the phantom is due entirely to the effect of the variation in the collimator response function as a function of distance. However, for a given radius of rotation, this function is known, and indeed may be modeled by an exponentially weighted Gaussian [12]. Thus, if the

Fig 11. Two profiles through a reconstruction of a Phelps phantom with, on the left, the result using the MMSE filter after an Anscombe transform, and, on the right, using a Butterworth filter of order 10 with a cutoff frequency of 0.5*Nyquist. Note the differences in the cold lesion, arrowed.

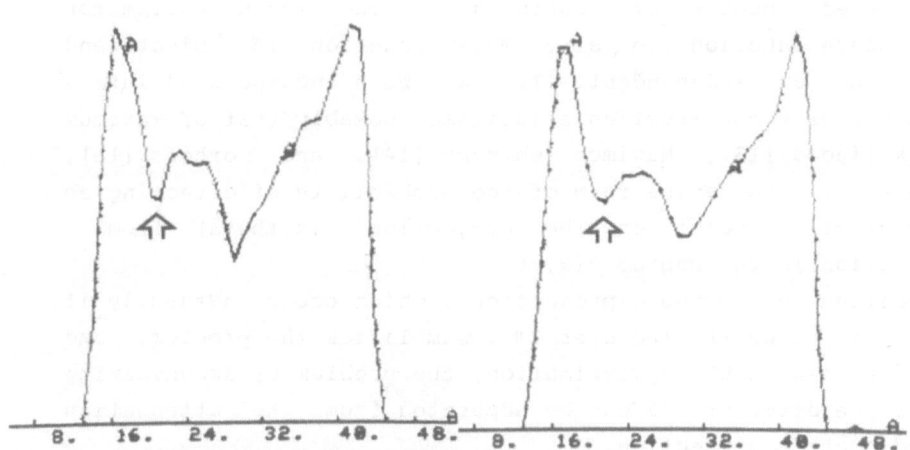

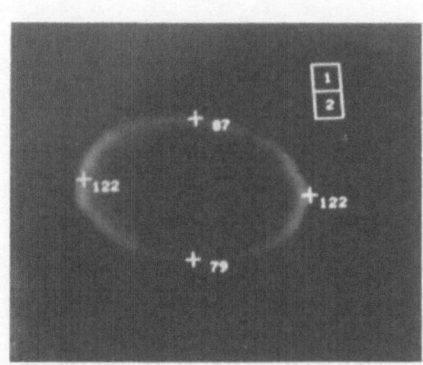

Fig 12. A uniform elliptical phantom, reconstructed without attenuation correction. The values indicated on the edges show variations resulting only from the collimator response function, e.g. a factor of about 50%.

effects of scatter, attenuation and collimator response function are _separable,_ which they are not in general, a simple correction function c(r,theta) can be defined. This is essentially a circularly symmetrical function being the ratio between the observed counts at a point r,theta and the expected number of counts given the known collimator response function in air. This function is object and attenuation independent. It has been incorporated into a number of reconstruction algorithms, notably that of Maximum likelihood [13], Maximum entropy [14], and others [15], where it takes the form of the probability of detecting an event at a point on the projection p(x,theta) from a position in the source f(x,y).

Addition of opposed projections, which occurs naturally if data is reconstructed over 2π , simplifies the problem, and as a reasonable approximation, the problem of deconvolving for the detector PSF can be separated from the attenuation and scatter correction.

7. SCATTER CORRECTION

The central theme of this paper is that applying attenuation correction directly to SPECT data is invalid. Fig 13 shows a profile though a uniform object of a size 19cms in diameter, for the photopeak. An estimate of the scatter contribution is also given. Fig 14 shows a similar profile through an attenuating phantom of the same size, but containing instead a series of uniformly spaced point sources. An estimate of the scatter contribution is also included. The point source at the centre has an amplitude of 24% the edge value, corresponding to the attenuation expected from the physical value of μ for Tc99m. The value at the centre of a uniform distribution, for this system, was measured to be 57%, or 240% greater than expected, whereas all other physical parameters have been kept constant, i.e. radius of rotation, energy window, collimator response function etc. Thus attenuation is _object dependent_ and any attenuation correction procedure which does not take

143

Fig 13. A profile though a Phelps phantom showing, in the
centre, part of the central lesion. The higher curve is for
the photopeak, and the lower curve, is an estimate of the
scatter fraction.

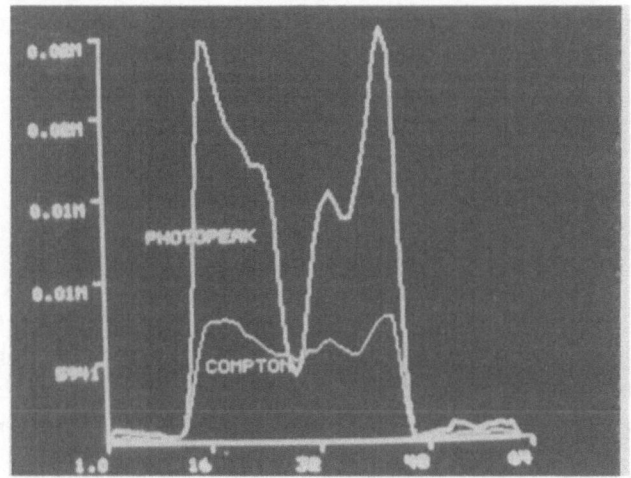

Fig 14. A similar pair of profiles though a uniform
attenuating phantom containing a series of equally spaced
point sources of approximately equal activity. The lower
curve is again an estimate of the scatter fraction.

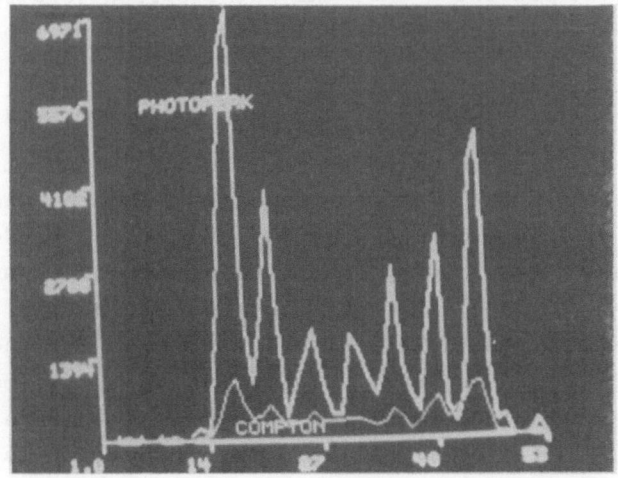

this into account will be in error by up to a factor of two.

In order to correct for this effect, a scatter correction procedure was implemented. The following data collection procedure was used. A series of acquisitions were performed such that sinograms were obtained for various phantoms at the following energies:

1. Normal photopeak   130-150Kev
2. Compton   110-130Kev
3. Low Compton   90-110Kev
4. High photopeak   140-160Kev
5. Low photopeak   120-140Kev

A number of patient acquisitions were also performed but using energy windows 1 and 2 only, a convenient operation with a double headed system.

In addition, a Monte Carlo simulation (using software written by, and in collaboration with, O Ying Lie [12]) was performed. Here a point source in the centre of a circularly symmetrical attenuating medium was simulated, and projections obtained for various energy windows, sizes of scattering medium, and collimator aperture functions. From this data it was found that the point spread function (PSF) of the system could be modelled as the sum of two Gaussian functions:

$$PSF(x) = C1. \exp(-C2. x^2) + C3. \exp(-C4. x^2)$$

where C1 to C4 are constants which are dependent on the energy window, collimator response function, and may be activity distribution and attenuation medium dependent.

It was also observed that there was a considerable difference between the PSF obtained for single scattered events, and for multiple scattered events. In the latter case, the PSF was very flat, and a simple background subtraction should suffice as a correction technique. In particular, the PSF for the photopeak energy was found to have a 'narrow' component where C1 and C2 were object independent, and a 'broad' component where C3 and C4 were object dependent. This suggested the use of a subtraction technique for the data from multiple energy windows. This was applied to the raw projection (sinogram) data where the effects of scatter are essentially a linear summation of unscattered events (object independent, but attenuated), and scattered events (object dependent, and also attenuated).

The complete analytical form of the inverse problem including scatter, attenuation, and spatially variable response function is highly unwieldy. However, the following simplification has been adopted. Let the point spread functions at energies i be called PSF_i, such that at the photopeak (energy window 1) we may observe PSF_1, and at the Compton window we may observe PSF_2. It is thus possible to define a general subtraction operation as:

$$p'(x, theta) = P_1(x, theta) - \sum_j p_j(x, theta) * FILT_j$$

where $p_j(x, theta)$ is the projection data acquired at the jth window, and $FILT_j$ is a corresponding filter function.

The values of $FILT_j$ were chosen such that PSF' is object independent. This does not necessary imply that form of a complex object in terms of scatter and attenuation is now object independent, since the approximation of stationarity is not really valid. Effectively, the aim of the scatter correction described here is to reduce the amount of scatter in the image as far as possible, such that, to a reasonable approximation, the attenuation that is observed in the object is object independent, by testing the operation for a range of different types of object.

Since the PSFs for the various energy windows can be established both from the model, and from experimental measurements (which were also made), then a starting point for the filters that was used was to estimate $FILT_j$ as:

$$FILT_j = F^{-1}\{ F\{ PSF_1(x) \} / F\{ PSF_j(x) \} \}$$

where $F\{\}$ and $F^{-1}\{\}$ represent the Fourier and inverse Fourier transforms. In this case, what is desired for the function PSF_1 is the point spread function of the

Fig 15. The PSFs associated with the Photopeak window, left, and the Compton window, right.

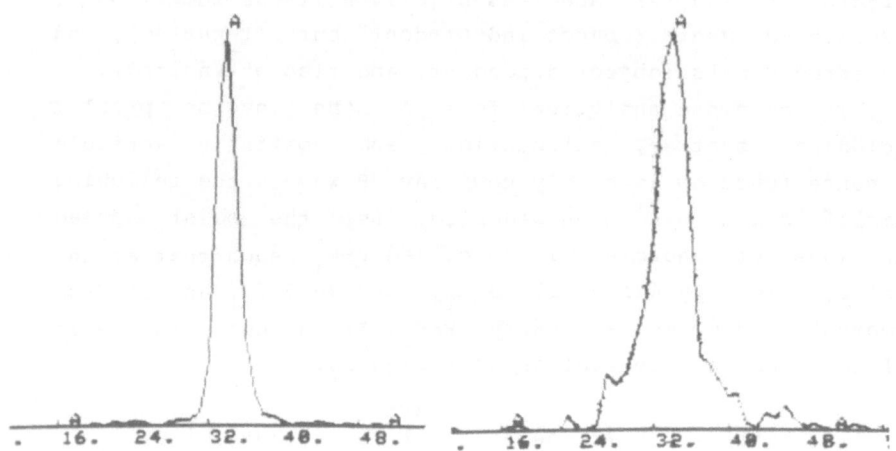

Fig 16. Profiles drawn though the uniform elliptical phantom, on the left, with no attenuation or scatter correction, and on the right, after a scatter correction. Note the difference in amplitude between the edge and the centre in the two cases.

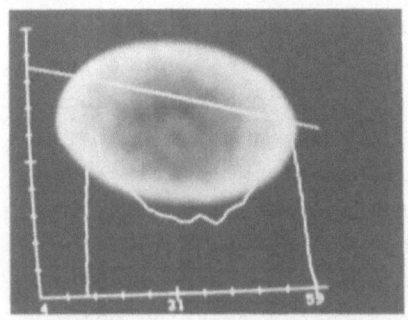
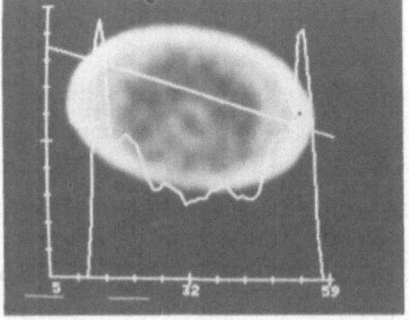

unscattered events alone, a function which can only be estimated from the model. The following procedure was used. Using information from the model, an estimate of a suitable form for PSF_1 was made and equivalent filters derived for the other energy windows using the observed (measured) PSF functions. Fig 15 shows the observed PSFs for the photopeak and Compton windows.

The next problem was to estimate a suitable overall weighting function (i.e. integral of the filter). It should be noted that the scattered events undergo greater attenuation than the unscattered events. It was found that a value for $\int FILT_2$ of the order of 0.9 for the Compton window gave good quantitative results. This value was higher than predicated from the model.

8. RESULTS

Fig 16 shows an example of a phantom study performed with a uniform elliptical phantom, without attenuation correction, but with and without scatter correction. The ratio of centre to edge for the uncorrected image is 41%, and for the corrected image is 28%. The same phantom was also used where three hot lesions were inserted. Here, the images have been attenuation corrected, and a correction for the collimator response function applied. Fig 17 compares the results with, and without a scatter correction. Here only the Compton window was used to estimate scatter. It may be noted that the signal to noise ratio has been degraded, as might be expected since a subtraction has been performed. However, the contrast of the various lesions has been increased significantly. This experiment has been repeated for other phantoms, and distributions of lesions, both hot and cold. In all cases, contrast is significantly improved. In comparison, the use of the high photopeak window alone does not increase contrast. A residual problem was that, for the system used (a double headed Siemens Rota SPECT system), there were still uniformity artefacts present in the Compton window, which have not been removed. Using a

Fig 17. Profiles though the uniform elliptical phantom containing three hot lesions, along the lines indicated, on the left, after attenuation and collimator response function correction, and on the right, after a scatter correction performed in addition. Note the considerable increase in contrast.

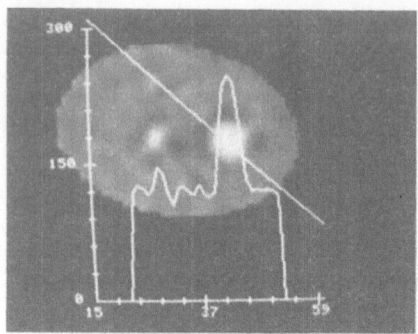 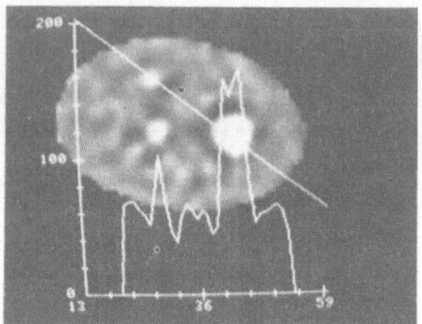

Fig 18. The photopeak sinogram (marked Ph) for the Phelps phantom, plus the scatter correction sinogram (marked Co). The sinogram after scatter correction (marked Sub) is shown below, plus the corresponding reconstruction. Note the increase in constrast in the arrowed regions.

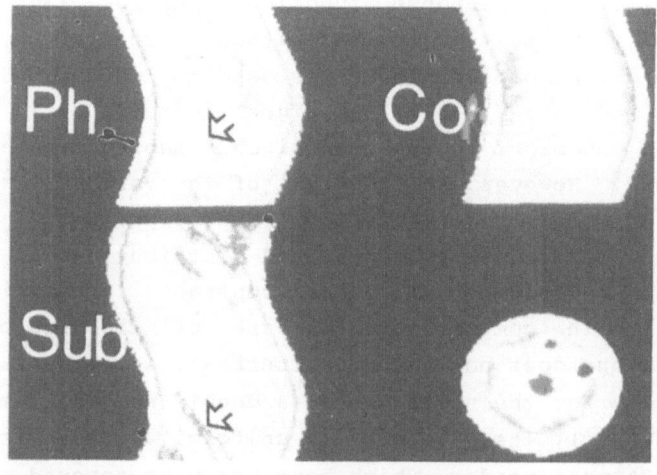

different phantom, Fig 18 shows results from the Phelps cold
lesion phantom, before and after scatter correction, which
also demonstrates the increase in contrast, and the increase
in apparent attenuation. It has been estimated that between
50 and 80% of all the scattered events have been eliminated.
It was also found that, to perform an attenuation
correction, a value for μ of 0.14cm^{-1} gave reasonable
results, still below the theoretical value, reflecting the
fact that not all scattered events have been removed.

9. SUMMARY

In order to quantitate in Single photon emission
computerised tomography (SPECT), four preliminary stages of
data processing are required; to remove artefacts, to
correct for scatter and the collimator response function,
and to perform attenuation correction. To remove artefacts,
firstly, a suitable uniformity correction must be performed
in equivalent scattering conditions to those used for the
real (patient) data. Secondly, an artefact filter may be
used which removes vertical stripes in sinograms. Thirdly, a
non-circular orbit has been found to be helpful. A scatter
correction has been developed, based partly on the use of a
Monte-Carlo model. Using multiple energy windows, an
estimate of the scattered events in the photopeak window is
derived, and subtracted from the projection data. This
results in a considerable gain in contrast. After a
correction for the collimator response function, the
observed attenuation is, to a reasonable approximation,
object independent. If either the scatter correction or the
collimator response function correction are ignored, errors
of a factor of two can occur.

The results of using the scatter correction described
here appear to be very encouraging and suggest that it may
be possible in the near future to extract quantitative data
from SPECT data.

REFERENCES

1. Budinger TF, Gullberg GT, Huesman RH. 1970. Emission computed tomography. In Ed. Herman CT, Image reconstruction from projections. Vol 32 Topics in applied physics, Berlin, Springer-Verlag, pp147-245.
2. Jaszczak RJ, Coleman RE, Whitehead FR. 1981. Physical factors affecting quantitative measurements using camera-based single photon emission computed tomography (SPECT) IEEE Trans. Nucl. Sci. NS-28, pp69-81.
3. Todd-Pokropek AE, Soussaline F, Zurowski S. 1981. Artefact creation and non-uniformity in tomography. In Emission computed tomography: The single photon approach. Washington DC, BRH, pp302-310.
4. Shepp LA, Stein JA. 1977. Simulated reconstruction artefacts in computerized x-ray tomography. In Eds Ter Pogossian MM, Phelps ME, Brownell GL, et al Reconstruction tomography in diagnostic radiology and nuclear medicine. Baltimore MD, University Park Press, pp33-48.
5. Knoll GF, Shrader ME. 1982. Computer corrections of camera nonidealities in gamma ray imaging. IEEE Trans. Nucl. Sci. NS-29, pp1272-1279.
6. Keyes JW, Rogers Wl, Clinthorne NH, et al. 1982. An image quality maintenance program for rotating camera SPECT. In Eds Hofer R, Bergmann H. Radioaktive isotope in Klinik und Forschung, 15 Band. Vienna,Verlag H. Egermann, 2 pp529-537.
7. Gullberg GT, Nowak DJ, Eisner RL, Malko JA, Woronowicz EM. 1982. A theoretical investigation of non-uniformity errors in rotating gamma camera tomography. J. Nucl. Med. 23, P53.
8. Benchimol C. 1981. Personal communication.
9. Todd-Pokropek AE, 1983. Non-circular orbits for the reduction of uniformity artefacts. Phys. Med. Biol. 28, pp309-313.
10. Uniformity artifact reduction with noncircular tomographic detector motion. J. Nucl. Med. 24, P104
11. Appeldorn CR. 1983. Personal communication.
12. O Ying-Lie. 1983. The mathematics and physics of emission computerised tomography. Report to the University of Utrecht.
13. Shepp LA, Vardi Y. 1982. Maximum likelihood reconstruction for emission tomography. IEEE Trans. Medical Imaging MI-1, pp113-121
14. Kemp MC. 1981. Maximum entropy reconstructions in emission tomography. In Medical radionuclide imaging. Vienna, IAEA, 1 pp313-324.
15. O Ying-Lie. 1983. An ECAT reconstruction method which corrects for attenuation and detector response. IEEE Trans. Nucl. Sci. NS-30, pp 632-635.

THE APPLICATION OF VARIABLE MEDIAN WINDOW FILTERING TO COMPUTERISED TOMOGRAPHY

M O LEACH, W D FLATMAN*, S WEBB, M A FLOWER, AND R J OTT.
Physics Department, Royal Marsden Hospital and Institute of Cancer Research,
Downs Road, Sutton, Surrey, SM2 5PT, England.
*Present address: Department of Nuclear Medicine, St. Bartholomew's Hospital,
West Smithfield, London EC1.

INTRODUCTION

The accuracy obtained in reconstructing images from projections is highly dependent upon the degree of noise present in those projections. Although this limitation affects all modes of computerised tomography (CT) where dose to a patient is a consideration, it is a particular limitation in single photon emission CT (SPECT) and in relatively simple transmission CT scanners designed to provide information for radiotherapy treatment planning. Median window filtering provides a method of reducing the noise content of projections, whilst minimising the degradation of resolution which accompanies smoothing with a moving average filter. This paper considers the application of median window filtering to emission and transmission computerised tomography.

In SPECT, the problems of relatively low contrast in projections, with respect to the noise levels arising from low photon statistics, are compounded by the low uptake, in terms of absolute activity, of some of the novel tumour localising agents currently being developed. One of the major objectives of these agents is to indentify the presence of metastatic secondary deposits to a known primary tumour. This then enables appropriate therapy and staging to be carried out, and the efficacy of this therapy to be monitored. In the case of imaging using labelled monoclonal antibodies for instance, the low rate at which the agents are delivered to the secondaries (a function of the proportion of cardiac output delivered to the site) and the limited number of binding sites for highly specific antibodies can limit the absolute uptake of activity at a site. Thus although high up-take in terms of tumour to normal tissue may be achieved, the absolute uptake in tumour sites may be low. Reductions in the noise content of images can enable areas of high uptake to be more accurately delineated, and in sequential studies of changes in radiopharmaceutical uptake, can allow the region of interest to be more precisely localised.

In CT scanners designed for radiotherapy planning purposes (1, 2),

economies have often been made in detector design, leading to relatively inefficient detector systems, which for a given dose, necessarily give rise to
fewer detected photons and a lower signal to noise ratio, than do diagnostic
CT scanners. The former scanners show increased sensitivity to background
radiation and to electronic noise, giving rise to occasional bad data points,
which are not readily removed by moving average smoothing methods. Median
window filtering is particularly suited to removing these bad data points,
as well as to reducing the general noise levels in projections, permitting
tissue interfaces to be more accurately delineated.

The use of a median window filter (MWF) to suppress noise in one dimension
was proposed by Tukey (3). Median window filtering is a process in which the
central value of a string of data of length M is replaced by the median of the
M values. The value of M can be varied to give an increased or decreased
degree of smoothing. The advantages of the method are that the filter tends
to preserve edges and information, of length greater than $(M + 1)/2$, rather
than smoothing edges by the averaging of adjacent pixels. Further the filter
is stable, in that it does not produce oscillations in the data in the way
that a weighted average filter with a sharp well-defined central-peak and
negative lobes can. Frieden (4,5) utilised this property in an edge restoration filter, where the MWF was combined with an edge enhancement filter to
improve edge contrast, on the basis of information derived from the point
spread function of the system.

We have further modified the MWF (6,7) to permit the length of the
filter to be reduced dynamically depending on the nature of the data. This
process is shown in Fig. 1.

5	7	3	4	20	6	4	8	2	RAW DATA
									Filtering central value of data with variable median window filter
	3	4	4	6	7	8	20		E = 10 D = 14
		3	4	4	6	20			D = 16
			4	6	20				D = 14
				20					
									Results of filtering central three points
			5	4	4				W = 5
			5	6	4				W = 3
			5	20	4				W = 1

Figure 1.   The result of applying a median window filter of maximum
length 7 to data containing one large data value.

The top line shows a string of nine data points to be filtered. Below this is shown the initial filter window of length 7, filtering the central value of the string. The data within the window have been ordered in magnitude, thus the central value is the median and is the filtered data point. This is compared with the original unfiltered value. If the modulus of the difference (D) between the original and the smoothed value is greater than the preset constant (E), the length of the median window is reduced by two pixels and the point is refiltered as shown by the next line. The test is then repeated and the process continues until either the constant (E) is not exceeded or until the window is reduced to a preset minimum length (W). This variable MWF permits greater edge retention than is available with the fixed length MWF, and also provides increased control over the acceptance or rejection of information contained in single data points or small regions of data. The bottom three lines of the figure shows the effect of applying a filter of maximum length 7 pixels to the data, which contains one high value, using different minimum filter lengths W, of 5, 3 and 1 pixels length. The high data point is only retained if a value of W equal to 1 is used.

Figure 2 shows the effect of applying the variable MWF to a one dimensional string of data containing edge information of different sizes in the presence of noise. If a MWF of fixed length 7 is applied, detail smaller than 4 pixels in length is lost, but edges or detail of greater length are retained.

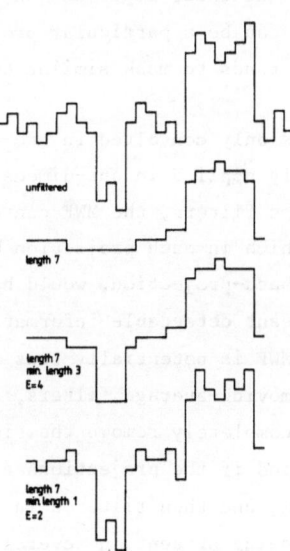

If a variable median window filter with W = 3 and E = 4 is used, detail of length greater than 2 pixels is retained, with little reduction in smoothness. A filter with W = 1 and E = 2 retains most of the detail, but provides limited smoothing.

In some results presented in this paper, a further modification has been added, to permit the filter to respond to changing levels of noise in an image. In projections obtained by either transmission or emission imaging, the standard deviation of each projection pixel can be expressed as $\sqrt{N}$, where N is the number of events recorded in that pixel. In regions of the projection where few events are recorded, the noise is relatively high compared with

Figure 2.

regions recording many events, and for the filter to respond uniformly, a variable factor V is required to accommodate changes in N. Where indicated in the text therefore, the value V will represent the multiple of the preset value E, and the standard deviation of the filtered projection value $\sqrt{a_{MED}}$, at each point in the projections, $V = E\sqrt{a_{MED}}$. That is, if the unfiltered value is N, the filtered value is a_{MED}, the difference $D = N-a_{MED}$. If $|D|$ is greater than V, the length of the filter will be decreased.

METHOD OF APPLICATION OF THE FILTER TO CT SCANS

The use of a non-linear filter such as the MWF, instead of, or together with, a window in the reconstruction process, offers the potential advantage of retaining more high frequency information than may be possible with weighted moving average filters, (which are often equivalent to the window functions, $W(f)$, which are multiplied, in frequency (f) space, with the $|f|$ ramp in the reconstruction process) whilst still offering some reduction in image noise. Filtering the projection data prior to reconstruction can permit the use of a rectangular window in the reconstruction.

A second potential advantage is that the spatial distribution of noise in the reconstructed image can be altered. Reconstruction of noisy projection data will produce mottled images, with the distribution and size of the mottle dependent on the shape of the frequency window, and their amplitude on the noise level in the projection data. This noise can be a particular problem in nuclear medicine applications, where the mottle tends to mask similar hot or cold lesions, particularly in liver tomograms.

The window in the reconstruction process is only convolved in one-dimension with each projection. The MWF is also often only applied in one-dimension to real-space data, but compared with moving-average filters, the MWF can completely remove very low contrast information, which in each projection has a similar amplitude to noise, but when summed by back-projection, would have been spatially coordinated and produced significant detectable information in the reconstructed image. In this respect, the MWF is potentially less sensitive to small projection signals than weighted moving-average filters, as they average a small signal over pixels rather than completely remove the signal. However, this problem can potentially be minimised if the projections are placed in a two-dimensional array, as a sinogram, and then filtered in two dimensions to take advantage of a small signal being present in several projections, providing co-ordinated information in adjacent projections. In multislice transmission CT and in SPECT using rotating gamma cameras, a further dimension of information is present, in that two-dimensional planar images are available and can be filtered. This can permit a degree of three-dimensional filtering, although the results will be dependent upon the order of filtering in the three planes. A sequence independent method would be to map all of the two-dimesional planar images into a three-dimensional array, and then filter each point using three orthogonal intersecting filters. This method has not yet been used due to the long processing time if a large computer memory is not available. In principle, the two-dimensional information present in sinograms and in SPECT planar views can be filtered using a two-dimensional filter shape, such as those discussed by Tyan (8) and Deconinck (9). However, as reported by Deconinck, the use of separate, orthogonal one-dimensional filters provides greater retention of spatial information, and has therefore been used in this study. Two-dimensional (or three-dimensional) filter shapes are likely to be of value where there are strong non-orthogonal components in the filtered data.

For the results from transmission CT scans reported below, only single-slice data have been obtained, and the projection data have only been filtered along the projections. In SPECT, planar gamma-camera views have been filtered in two directions, and for some sets of data, the sinograms have also been filtered, to give a degree of three-dimensional filtering.

Thus the filters used are :-

MWFA   In transmission CT projection data the one-dimensional projections are filtered prior to reconstruction, using the filter with E = constant.

MWFB   In SPECT, the two-dimensional planar views are filtered in the two orthogonal directions, using the filter with E = constant.

MWFC   In SPECT, as for MWFB but with variable $V = E.\sqrt{a_{MED}}$.

MWFD   In SPECT, the sinograms are filtered orthogonally to the projection direction (i.e. across the projections) using the filter with variable $V = E.\sqrt{a_{MED}}$. This may be used prior to MWFC.

NOISE SUPPRESSION IN MEDIAN WINDOW FILTERING

For a normal distribution, Hojo (10) has derived values for the standard error of the median, σ_M for a given sample, in terms of the standard deviation of the sample, σ_N, and the sample size M,

$$\sigma_M = k_M \frac{\sigma_N}{\sqrt{M}}$$

(1)

where values of k_M for small samples are given by Hojo. For large samples, and M odd, Pearson(11) has shown that k_M tends to 1.253. Values of k_M for M = 1, 3, 5, 7 and 9 are 1.000, 1.160, 1.198, 1.214 and 1.223 respectively. Equation 1 can be used to compare the noise to be expected in data filtered with a MWF of fixed length, with the noise if the data were filtered with a moving average filter of the same length. Justusson (12) considered the effect that median window filtering has on the statistical properties of planar images.

The effect that the use of a MWF of fixed length will have on reconstructed image noise can be derived from the formulae of Gore and Tofts (13).

In transmission CT, the projection data, $g = \ln \frac{N_o}{N}$ where N_o and N are respectively the number of photons incident on, and transmitted by, the object, per sampling interval.

Thus the standard deviation in N, $\sigma_N = \sqrt{N}$ \hfill (2)

and the standard deviation of the projection noise

$$\sigma_g = \left|\frac{dg}{dN}\right| \cdot \sigma_N = \frac{\sigma_N}{N} = \frac{1}{\sqrt{N}} \quad \text{if } N \gg 1$$

With no filtering, Gore and Tofts show that the standard deviation at the centre of the reconstructed image

$$\sigma_\mu(0) = \alpha \sigma_g(0) \quad \text{where} \quad \alpha = \frac{\pi}{p\sqrt{12R}}$$

where p is the projection sampling interval, R the number of projections and N(0) the number of photons per projection transmitted through the centre of the object.

If the projection data, prior to taking the logarithm of the projections, were filtered by taking the arithmetic mean of the data within the filter window, the noise in the filtered projections would be characterised by σ_s, the standard error of the mean. If the mean value in the window is $\bar{a}$, and the window length is M, for Poisson statistics

$$\sigma_s = \sqrt{\frac{M\bar{a}}{M}} = \sqrt{\frac{\bar{a}}{M}}$$

hence the standard deviation of the logged projection data after moving average filtering

$$\sigma_{g_A} = \frac{\sigma_s}{\bar{a}} = \frac{1}{\sqrt{M\bar{a}}}$$

thus $\quad\quad\quad \sigma_{\mu_A}(0) = \alpha \sigma_{g_A}$

If the MWF is used instead of the arithmetic mean filter, from formulae 1

$$\sigma_M = k_M \frac{\sigma_N}{\sqrt{M}} \quad \text{where} \quad \sigma_N \cong \sqrt{\bar{a}}$$

and the standard deviation of the logged projection data after median window filtering,

$$\sigma_{g_{MWF}} = \frac{\sigma_M}{a_{MED}} = \frac{k_M \sigma_N}{\sqrt{M} \, a_{MED}}$$

where a_{MED} are the filtered values replacing the unfiltered values N in the projection

hence

$$\sigma_{g_{MWF}} = \frac{k_M \sigma_a}{a_{MED}\sqrt{M}}$$

and

$$\sigma_{\mu_{MWF}}(0) = \alpha \sigma_{g_{MWF}}$$

Thus

$$\frac{\sigma_{\mu_{MWF}}(0)}{\sigma_{\mu_A}(0)} = \frac{\sigma_{g_{MWF}}(0)}{\sigma_{g_A}(0)}$$

$$= \frac{\bar{a}(0)}{a_{MED}(0)} \cdot \frac{k_M \sigma_N(0)}{\sqrt{M} \, \sigma_s(0)} \cong \frac{k_M \bar{a}(0)}{a_{MED}(0)}$$

Thus after median window filtering, both the projection and the reconstructed image noise will be greater, by a factor of $\frac{k_M \bar{a}}{a_{MED}}$ than the noise with a moving average filter.

For emission CT,

the projection data $\qquad g = N$

thus $\qquad \sigma_g = \sigma_N = \sqrt{N}$

and therefore σ_g and $\sigma_\mu(0)$ are both a factor of N greater than is the case for transmission CT. The proportional noise reduction, with a moving average filter and with a median window filter, however, remains the same.

In this derivation, the expression derived by Hojo and by Pearson were for normally distributed data. For Poisson distributed data, the relationship will only be accurate for large N and $\bar{a}$.

RESULTS OBTAINED WITH THE MEDIAN WINDOW FILTER APPLIED TO:

(a) Simulation Studies

Figure 3 shows the results obtained in using the MWF on data simulating the behaviour of a rotate-translate CT scanner. A detector sampling interval and reconstructed pixel size of 1.3 mm was used to produce a 249x249 pixel reconstructed image from 65 views. Figure 3(a) shows the "test" object , prior to imaging. The object diameter is 25 cm, with an attenuation

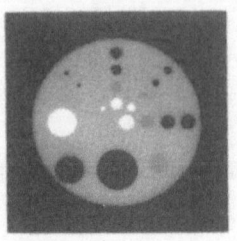

FIGURE 3(a)

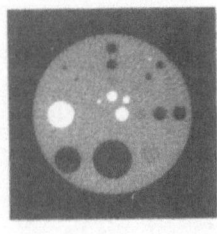

FIGURE 3(b)

FIGURE 3(c)

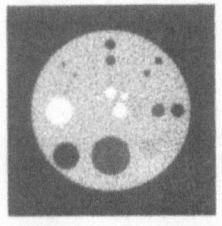

FIGURE 3(d)

FIGURE 3(e)

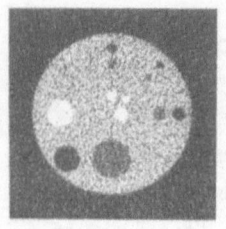

FIGURE 3(f)

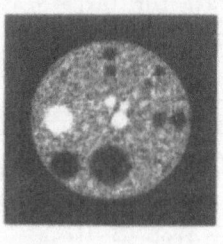

FIGURE 3(g)

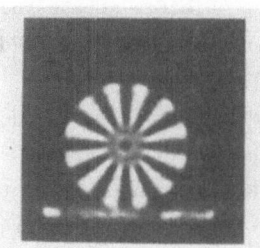

FIGURE 4(a)

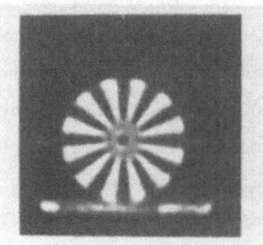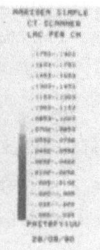

FIGURE 4(b)

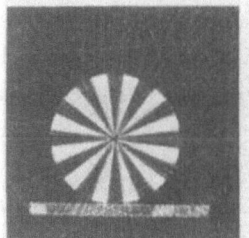

FIGURE 4(c)

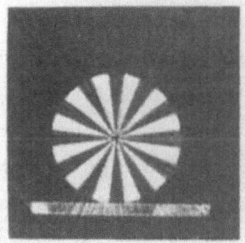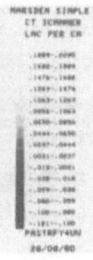

FIGURE 4(d)

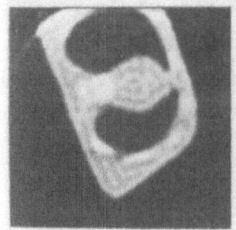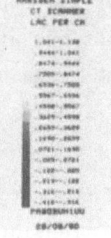

FIGURE 4(e)

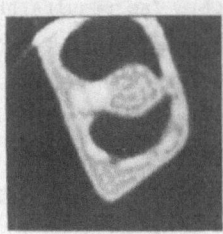

FIGURE 4(f)

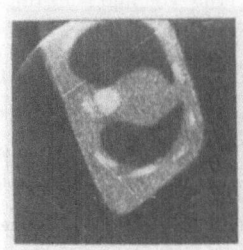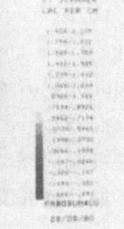

FIGURE 4(g)

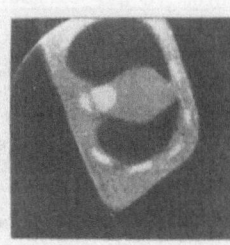

FIGURE 4(h)

coefficient typical of muscle and with holes of varying object-contrast and sizes, the four smallest diameters being 0.5 cm, 1 cm, 1.5 cm and 2 cm. For each of the four small sizes, there are four values of object-contrast, $C_O = \dfrac{D_H}{D_M}$ x 100, where D_H is the density of the hole material and D_M is the density of muscle. The values of C_O are 0.5%, 44%, 95% and 184%. Figure 3(b) shows the result of reconstructing noise-free data, and figure 3(c) shows the effect of using three cycles of MWFA with M = 7, W = 3, and E = 0.007 where $\dfrac{N_O}{N}$ is the function filtered. Figures 3(d) and (e) show results with and without filtering, for noise equivalent to 7000 photons incident on the object per sampling interval, with E = 0.01; and figures 3(f) and (g) show similar results but with a noise level equivalent to 500 incident photons and E = 0.02. In the noise-free filtered data, contrast is lost a little on filtering, but information from the 5 mm diameter hole, with C_O = 95% of the muscle contrast, is primarily lost during reconstruction. With the addition of photon noise, some further loss of contrast in the reconstructed image occurs, making it progressively more difficult to see the 5 mm hole at C_O = 44% in figure 3(e) and finally in figure 3(g) at C_O = 0.5% and 184%. The 1 cm diameter hole at 44% contrast continues to be resolved, albeit at reduced image contrast. Table 1 shows the results obtained by placing regions of interest on different areas of the object. The results show that for the three different levels of photon noise considered, the MWF produced reductions of some 10%, 45% and 76% in order of increasing noise levels, in the image noise, with very little shift in the mean pixel value, the maximum shift being 4% when filtering data with an image standard deviation of 119%.

(b) A simple rotate-translate transmission CT scanner

A number of images obtained from a rotate-translate CT scanner employing a ^{137}Cs source of γ-rays (1) were filtered with MWFA with M = 7, W = 3 and E = 0.01, where the function filtered is $\dfrac{N_O}{N}$. Figures 4(a) and (b) show a Perspex star phantom in air without and with filtering. The reconstruction window used with these data was a pure ramp with a frequency cut-off at f_c = 1.12 cm^{-1}, the value usually used for data from this scanner. Figure 4(c) shows the results of using a high cut-off frequency of $4f_c$ = 4.50 cm^{-1}, close to the Nyquist frequency, with no filtering, and Figure 4(d) shows the effect of using MWFA. It can be seen from the figure that the MWF greatly reduces the number of artefacts from bad data-points, and reduces the noise. Figures 4(e), (f), (g) and (h), show the results of treating an image of a body cross-section phantom in the same way.

Table 1.   Regions of interest in the simulated object.

Region.	Input Photons.	Is MWF applied to data.	Object density. x 10^{-2}.	Image mean pixel density. x 10^{-2}.	% Difference of image mean density from object density.	Pixel % Stand. Devn.	% Difference between filtered and unfiltered values of Stan. Devn.
1.	Object		3.14				
	∞	No		3.14	0	4.29	
		Yes		3.14	0	3.91	8.9
	7000	No		3.15	0.3	12.3	
		Yes		3.16	0.6	7.39	40.0
	500	No		3.18	1.3	45.1	
		Yes		3.18	1.3	10.1	77.6
2.	Object		1.32				
	∞	No		1.23	0.8	13.4	
		Yes		1.34	1.5	12.1	9.7
	7000	No		1.33	0.8	34.2	
		Yes		1.37	3.8	17.7	48.3
	500	No		1.34	1.5	119.1	
		Yes		1.37	3.8	29.8	75.0
3.	Object		2.99				
	∞	No		2.99	0	5.64	
		Yes		2.99	0	4.89	13.8
	7000	No		2.97	−0.7	16.3	
		Yes		3.00	0.3	7.36	54.9
	500	No		2.91	−2.7	56.2	
		Yes		2.97	−0.7	13.1	76.7
4.	Object		5.77				
	∞	No		5.77	0	2.53	
		Yes		5.74	−0.5	2.34	7.5
	7000	No		5.74	−0.5	8.54	
		Yes		5.68	−1.6	4.48	47.5
	500	No		5.68	−1.6	30.7	
		Yes		5.61	−2.8	7.38	76.0

Table 2 shows the percentage standard deviation in regions of interest in the body cross-section phantom, for the same images. The results indicate how a reconstruction filter which passes higher spatial frequencies can be used whilst restricting the increase in image noise to an acceptable level.

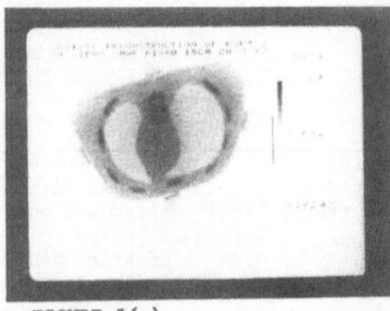

FIGURE 5(a)

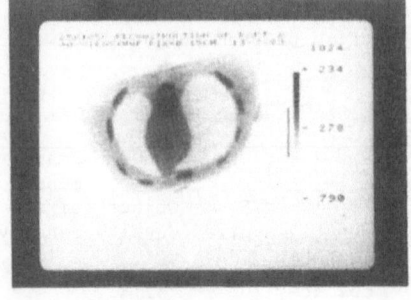

FIGURE 5(b)

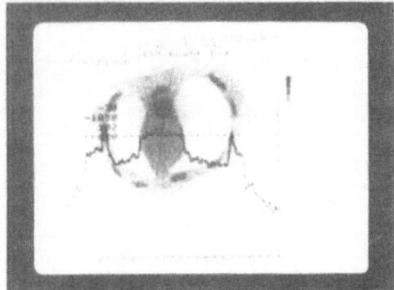

FIGURE 5(c)

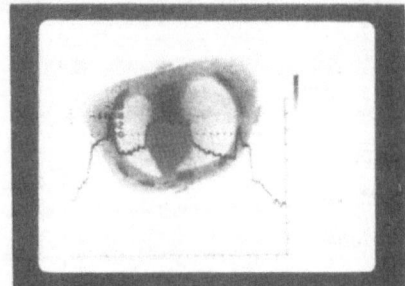

FIGURE 5(d)

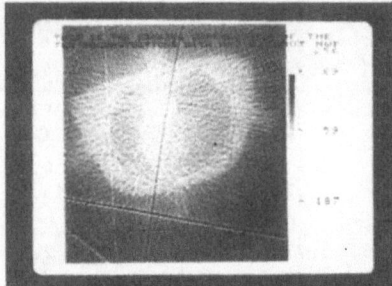

FIGURE 5(e)

Table 2. Region of interest in body cross-section phantom with ^{137}Cs Scanner.

Filter	Cut-off cm^{-1}	% Standard Deviation in Image Muscle	Lung
Unfiltered	1.12	2.9	16.1
Filtered	1.12	2.6	18.8
Unfiltered	4.50	12.8	53.9
Filtered	4.50	5.5	24.9

(c) A transmission CT scanner based on a radiotherapy simulator

A CT scanner based on a radiotherapy simulator and designed to produce images for radiotherapy treatment planning purposes, is currently being developed (2). Figure 5(a) shows the unfiltered image of a body cross-sectional phantom, reconstructed from 90 projections obtained by rotating the phantom in the field of view of the scanner. Figure 5(b) shows the same results using MWFA with M = 7, E = 20, and W = 3 where N is the value filtered. Figures 5(c) and (d) show the same images with profiles through the centering of the image. Figure 5(e) shows a difference image between the two images. The images were obtained using a Siemens Evaluskop CT viewing system. Regions of interest show a slight reduction in image noise which is also evident from the profiles, the removal of streaks arising from bad data-points, and no loss of edge information. The difference image shows the bad data-points removed by filtering. The apparent removal of part of the image information is an artefact of the subtraction procedure, where both images were normalised to their maximum and minimum values.

(d) Emission CT using a rotating gamma-camera system

The MWF has been implemented on the IGE STAR computer system attached to an IGE 400A rotating gamma camera system. Figures 6(a) - (d) show a reconstruction of a cylinder filled with uniform activity, and containing a large rectangular cold area, to provide a measure of the edge response function. Two different frequency windows have been used in the reconstruction; a rectangular window with no high frequency roll-off, to permit maximum use of the available spatial information, and a highly smoothing Hanning window, which is used routinely for many of our clinical studies. Figures 6(e) and (f) show these two window functions multiplied by the $|f|$ ramp in frequency space. Figures 6(a) and (b) show the results of applying these two windows respectively

164

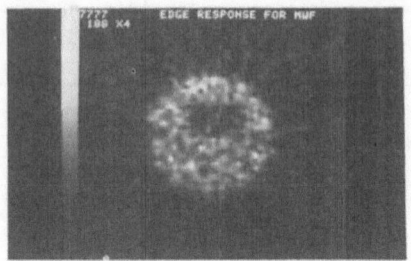

FIGURE 6(a)

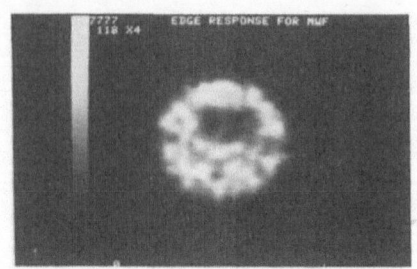

FIGURE 6(b)

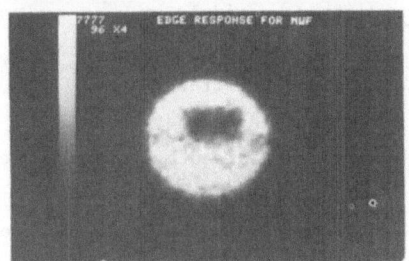

FIGURE 6(c)

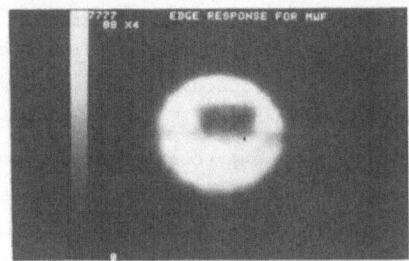

FIGURE 6(d)

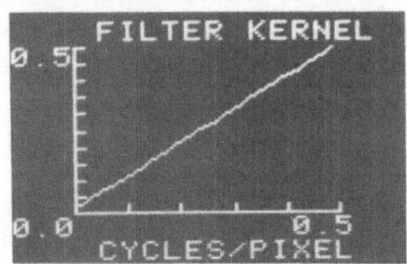

FIGURE 6(e)

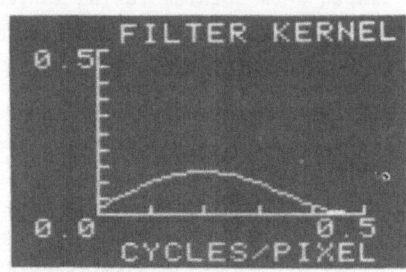

FIGURE 6(f)

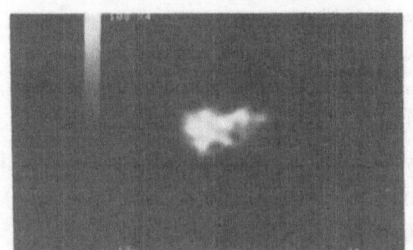

FIGURE 6(g)

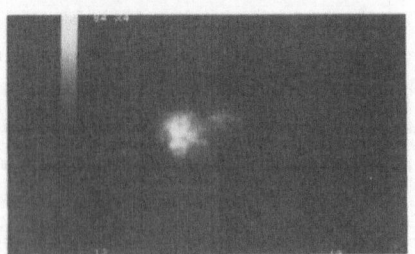

FIGURE 6(h)

during reconstruction from unfiltered projections and figures 6(c) and (d)
show the results with MWFB with W = 3, E = 4 where N is the function filtered,
showing, in particular, the changed distribution of the image noise, the MWF
giving a much smoother image.

Table 3a. Regions of interest and resolution with $|f|$ ramp

Filter	Mean	Stand. Dev.	Resln (cm)
RAW	77.0	30.9	1.46
W = 1, E = 4	79.6	17.9	2.96
W = 1, E = 8	78.0	8.6	1.30
W = 3, E = 2	77.7	24.6	1.22
W = 3, E = 4	78.8	10.1	1.78
W = 3, E = 8	78.4	6.3	2.03

Table 3a gives the mean and standard deviation of the measured activity,
together with a measure of the resolution, derived from the edge response
function, for images filtered with a MWF with different values of W and E, and
the $|f|$ ramp.

Table 3b. Regions of interest and resolution with ramp-Hanning reconstruction
window

Filter	Mean	Stand. Dev.	Resln (cm)
RAW	76.8	15.9	1.86
W = 1, E = 4	79.4	8.0	3.16
W = 1, E = 8	78.2	3.7	2.39
W = 3, E = 2	78.0	12.7	2.09
W = 3, E = 4	78.7	4.9	2.92
W = 3, E = 8	78.0	3.0	3.65

Table 3b gives similar results using the ramp-Hanning window. As these
were low activity images the measure of resolution is not very precise, but
indicates the trend. The results show that increased noise suppression is
obtained at the expense of resolution, but that with the $|f|$ ramp filter, a
smaller image standard deviation than that measured with the normal ramp-
Hanning reconstruction can be obtained, without a major deterioration in
resolution (eg W = 1, E = 8). Figures 6(g) and (h) show a transaxial slice
through the base of the lungs, showing metastatic uptake of a ^{111}In labelled
monoclonal antibody to human milk fat globulin. Figure 6(g) is unfiltered data
reconstructed with a ramp-Hanning window and Figure 6(h) is filtered with
MWFB W = 3, E = 4 and reconstructed with a $|f|$ ramp. The filtered image is

166

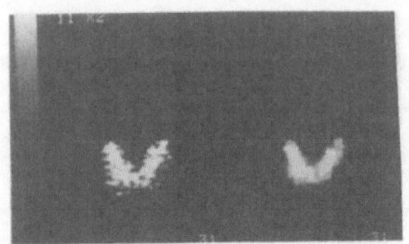

FIGURE 7(a)

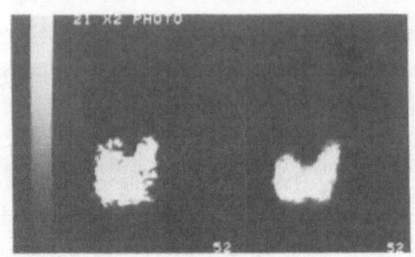

FIGURE 7(b)

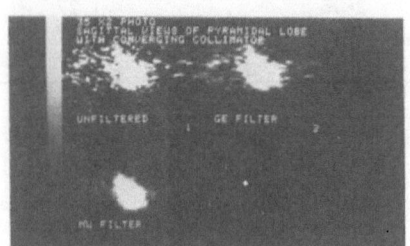

FIGURE 7(c)

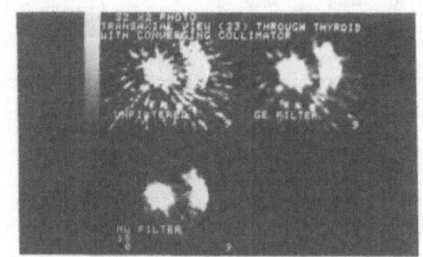

FIGURE 7(d)

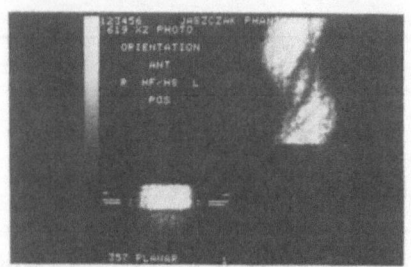

FIGURE 7(e)

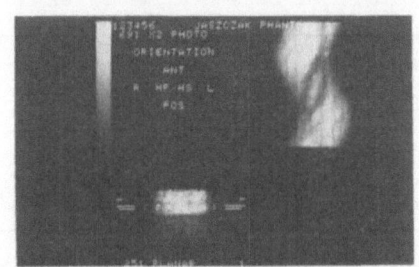

FIGURE 7(f)

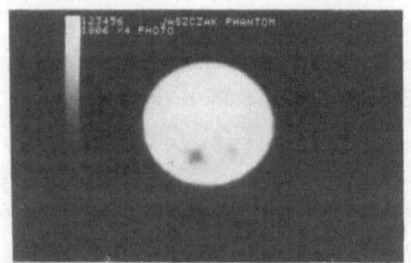

FIGURE 7(g)

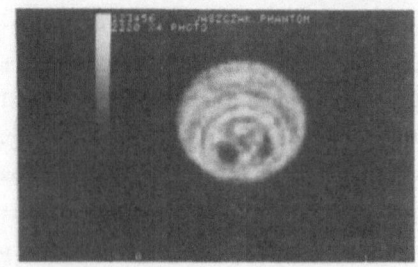

FIGURE 7(h)

markedly less mottled and the uptake is more sharply defined.

Results obtained before and after filtering with an image of a thyroid in a patient with a pyramidal lobe are shown in figure 7. The filter MWFC was used with W = 3 and E = 2. Figure 7(a) shows a planar view while figure 7(b) shows a sagittal plane through the pyramidal lobe. Some data were also obtained from the same patient using a converging/parallel collimator and divergent reconstruction algorithm (14) and figure 7(c) shows similar sagittal plane results obtained with this collimator, and 7(d) shows a reconstructed transaxial view. These two latter figures also show the results of post-processing the non-filtered data with a weighted average smoothing filter supplied by IGE on the STAR system. The MWF appears to give the best results of the two filters, and is substantially better than the unfiltered data. The convergent/parallel collimator data are well suited to median window filtering, as the image is magnified at the camera face, so less high frequency data is lost in applying the filter. This effect also applies to the high resolution parallel collimator thyroid images in figures 7(a) and (b) where a hardware zoom was used during acquisition.

Figures 7(e) and 7(f) show respectively sinograms from unfiltered projections of a Jaszczak phantom, and from MWFD filtered projections, using W = 3 E = 1. As can be seen, the filter appears to retain most of the edge information, but will tend to favour data close to the centre of rotation.

Figures 7(g) and 7(h) show the results of reconstructing after using filters MWFC and MWFD respectively on the data obtained by imaging the Jaszczak phantom with a LEGP collimator. In both cases W = 3 and E = 1. It is evident that this form of sinogram filtering produces some circular artefacts, as a result of the directionality of the filter. It may be that in the case of sinogram filtering, a two dimensional filter would be desirable to allow for the fact that correlated data in different projections will not be orientated orthogonally to the projections.

CONCLUSION

The median window filter has been shown to reduce image noise, permitting higher frequency information to be passed during image reconstruction, and minimising the spatial information lost during smoothing. The filter provides the best results if a minimum filter length of 3 is used, implying that detail of extent less than 2 pixels length will be lost, and therefore for maximum performance, the projections must be sampled more frequently than the highest resolution required in the final image. This is often not the case in emission

CT, and thus some resolution is often lost, although substantial improvements in image quality can be achieved. In SPECT, the MWF performs best when a small acquisition pixel is used, in our case by means of a hardware zoom. In transmission CT, the results have produced significant improvements in image quality.

REFERENCES

1. LEACH M O, WEBB S and BENTLEY R E. A rotate-translate CT scanner providing cross-sectional data suitable for planning the dosimetry of radiotherapy treatment. Med. Phys. 9 269-275, 1982.
2. LEACH M O and WEBB S. A dedicated CT scanner using a position sensitive detector for radiotherapy treatment planning. Paper 20-19 World Congress on Medical Physics and Biomedical Engineering, Hamburg 1982.
3. TUKEY J W. Exploratory data analysis, Addison-Wesley, Reading, Mass. 1971.
4. FRIEDEN B R. Image restoration by discrete convolution of minimal length. J. Opt. Soc. Am. 64, 682-686, 1974.
5. FRIEDEN B R. A new restoring algorithm for the preferential enhancement of edge gradients. J. Opt. Soc. Am. 66, 280-283, 1976.
6. FLATMAN W D. The application of an edge enhancement and smoothing filter to CT data from a simple transmission scanner at The Royal Marsden Hospital, Sutton. M.Sc. Thesis, University of Surrey, 1980.
7. FLATMAN W D, LEACH M O and WEBB S. The use of a median window filter with a simple CT scanner. Paper 20-12. World Congress on Medical Physics and Biomedical Engineering, Hamburg, 1982.
8. TYAN S G. Median Filtering: Deterministic properties in two-dimensional digital signal processing II ed. T S Huang, Springer Verlag, Berlin, 1981.
9. DECONINCK F and LUYPAERT R. Design and evaluation of median filters for scintigraphic image filtering. Proc. ISMIII'82, pp.20-23, IEEE New York, 1982.
10. HOJO T. Distribution of the median, quartiles and interquartile distance in samples from a normal population. Biometrika 23,315-60, 1933.
11. PEARSON K. On the probable errors of frequency constants, III Biometrika 13, 113-132, 1920.
12. JUSTUSSON B I. Median Filtering: Statistical properties in two-dimensional digital signal processing II ed. T S Huang, Springer Verlag, Berlin, 1981.
13. GORE J C and TOFTS P S. Statistical limitations in computed tomography. Phys. Med. Biol. 23, 1176-1182, 1978.
14. WEBB S. A modified convolution reconstruction technique for divergent beams. Phys. Med. Biol. 27, 419-423. 1982.

ART vs. CONVOLUTION ALGORITHMS FOR ECT

B.E. OPPENHEIM AND C.R. APPLEDORN

1. INTRODUCTION

Iterative algorithms were popular in the early days of computed tomography, but fell out of favor because they were considerably slower than convolution algorithms, especially when implemented with the Fast Fourier Transform (FFT). Some of the early work appeared to indicate, however, that iterative methods have better noise handling capabilities than convolution methods (1). In an excellent overview of the iterative reconstruction algorithms Herman and Lent (2) noted that the ART-type were more accurate than the convolution algorithms when the reconstruction problem was underdetermined (too few measurements for the number of unknowns), the picture had high contrast, and there was a large amount of noise in the data. The latter two points describe the usual situation in nuclear medicine tomography, and the first point (an underdetermined problem) would hold if we desired, or were forced, to limit the number of angles at which data were collected.

The low photon detection rate in nuclear medicine forces us to settle for images with rather poor spatial resolution. This is especially true for the new and very promising brain imaging agents, iodoamphetamine and HIPDM. Here the noise handling capability of the reconstruction algorithm may determine the clinical usefulness of the study. A new look at the iterative algorithms appears, therefore, to be appropriate.

We have concentrated on one iterative algorithm, ART (Algebraic Reconstruction Technique), since it is reasonably fast and has been found to give good results. Numerous implementations of ART have been described (2,3). The form we have employed is closely related, but not identical, to Herman's ART2 (4).

In this paper we will compare the ART and convolution algorithms with regard to their effects on image noise and spatial resolution. The relative merits of these algorithms in handling other important problems in nuclear medicine tomography, such as attenuation and distance-dependent spatial resolution, will not be discussed.

2. ALGORITHMS

2.1. ART2 algorithm

The image plane is considered to be subdivided into n pixels, with x_i representing the quantity of tracer in the i-th pixel. The observed data consist of m projection values, each representing the quantity of tracer contained in a strip or ray across the image plane, with the j-th value given by

$$y_j = \sum_i w_{ij} x_i$$

where w_{ij} represents the fraction of the i-th pixel contained within the j-th strip. The reconstruction problem is to determine the x_i given the y_j and the w_{ij}. Let x be a vector representing the true distribution of tracer. In the iterative methods sequential estimates are made, each hopefully closer to x than the preceding estimate. Let x^p be the p-th estimate consisting of n values x_i^p. Corresponding to any observed projection value y_j we can form a forward projection value y_j^p of x_p given by

$$y_j^p = \sum_i w_{ij} x_i^p$$

In ART2 we generate a sequence of unconstrained estimates along with a sequence constrained to be non-negative. Let $\bar{x}^p$ and x^p be the p-th unconstrained and constrained estimates respectively. Choose an angle θ at which some of the y_j were observed, and form the forward projection values y_j^p by the above equation. Then back projection is carried out, using those projection values, by

$$\bar{x}_i^{p+1} = \bar{x}_i^p + \sum_{j \varepsilon \theta} (y_j - y_j^p) w_{ij} / N_j$$

and

$$x_i^{p+1} = \max[0, \tilde{x}_i^{p+1}]$$

where $N_j = \sum_i w_{ij}$ is the area of the j-th strip. We equate the initial estimates $\tilde{x}^0$ and x^0 to the null vector. Note that in ART2 forward projection is carried out on the constrained vector x^p while back projection is carried out on the unconstrained vector $\tilde{x}^p$. ART2 is implemented here on a projection by projection basis, unlike Herman's ART2 which is implemented on a ray by ray basis (4).

Two "tricks" are used to achieve rapid reconstruction. First, it is necessary to evaluate the w_{ij} during execution, or else store them in a very large table. Evaluation becomes very simple and rapid if we first resample the projection data. If the original sampling interval is 1, we resample a projection using linear interpolation with a sampling interval $a_\theta = \max(|\sin\theta|, |\cos\theta|)$ where θ is the angle of the projection. This causes all pixels in a row of the reconstruction array to have the same weight w_{ij}.

Second, convergence is much faster if we utilize projection data in a random or pseudorandom order rather than in the order that they were acquired. We choose each successive projection by incrementing by an integer which is relatively prime to the total number of projections and roughly 40% of that total (e.g., for 18 total projections we choose every seventh).

We call each passage through the entire set of projections a cycle of iterations. It has often been noted with ART that when the projection data are noisy and inconsistent, as is the case with real data, then reconstructions improve for a number of cycles of iterations but then become progressively worse, so one must choose an appropriate stopping point.

The implementation of ART described here is reasonably fast. Excluding the time required for resampling and reordering the projection data, we found that one cycle of iterations of ART executed about 15% faster than convolution-back projection with linear interpolation when convolution was performed in real space, but about 10% slower when convolution was performed using the FFT.

2.2. Convolution algorithm

We investigated three convolution kernels, the Ramachandran, the Shepp, and the modified Shepp formed by convolution of the Shepp kernel with an 0.3,0.4,0.3 weighting function. (4,5). Convolution was carried out either in real space or by use of the FFT, which gave identical results. Since the interpolating function is an integral part of the filter, we investigated three methods of interpolation: nearest neighbor, linear, and modified cubic spline (4). To facilitate comparison of algorithms the resampled projection data that were used for the ART algorithm were also used for the convolution algorithm.

2.3. Implementation

Accurate projections of computer-generated phantoms were made at various angles over 180° onto a projection line 64 pixels wide. Poisson noise was then added to the projection data. When smoothing of the projections was performed it was carried out through one or more convolutions of the projections with an 0.25,0.5,0.25 filter. Resampling as described above was performed using a linear interpolating function. The phantoms were then reconstructed from the projections as a 64 x 64 array by means of the various algorithms.

ART reconstructions were carried out with three cycles of iterations, and convolution reconstructions were carried out using linear interpolation, unless otherwise indicated.

3. METHODS FOR EVALUATION

3.1. Distance measure

The intercomparison of algorithms is usually carried out by generating several representative phantoms with the computer, forming the projection data for each phantom, adding statistical noise, reconstructing the phantoms using the various algorithms, and comparing the reconstructed phantoms with the true phantoms by means of a distance measure such as

$$\delta = [\sum_i (x_i^R - x_i)^2 / \sum_i (\bar{x} - x_i)^2]^{1/2}$$

where x_i and x_i^R are the true and reconstructed values for the i-th pixel and $\bar{x}$ is the average value of the x_i. The smaller the values of δ, the more accurate the reconstruction. The drawbacks of a distance measure are that the value is highly dependent on the phantom chosen, that the results provide little insight regarding why one algorithm works better than another, and the most serious, that the distance measure favors accurate reconstruction of large structures over small structures, although the diagnostic information in the image is mainly dependent on how faithfully the smaller, higher frequency structures are reconstructed. For these reasons we turned to a figure-of-merit approach for evaluating algorithms.

3.2. Figure-of-merit approach

3.2.1. Derivation. Following the leads of Beck (6) and Metz (7), we generated an expression for the probability of detection of an object as a function of the object contrast, the imaging time, and the manner in which the imaging sytem handles contrast and noise. The test object chosen is a circularly symmetric Gaussian spot of peak amplitude A_o and standard deviation σ_o. We let σ_s represent the standard deviation of the imaging system's point spread function (psf), which is assumed constant and independent of the object-detector distance. The perfect reconstruction of a point source in the object plane would be a Gaussian spot whose standard deviation is also σ_s. We define σ_r as the standard deviation of the effective psf of the reconstruction algorithm. Then the standard deviation of the realized reconstruction of a point source is $(\sigma_s^2 + \sigma_r^2)^{1/2}$ and the standard deviation of the reconstruction of the test object is $(\sigma_o^2 + \sigma_s^2 + \sigma_r^2)^{1/2}$. Following the derivation of Metz (7, pp.301-306) it can be shown that the test object, after imaging and reconstruction, has a peak amplitude of $A_o \sigma_o^2 / (\sigma_o^2 + \sigma_s^2 + \sigma_r^2)$. This is the net signal to be detected.

The background upon which the test object is superimposed is a large disk with a uniform amplitude of A_b. Imaging introduces Poisson noise which is dependent on the number of events detected. We define FSDM as the expected fractional standard deviation of reconstructed pixel values for a reconstruction of the disk from projections containing a total of one million detected events. For these many events the noise in the reconstruction is given by $A_b \cdot \text{FSDM}$. Shepp has shown for the convolution algorithm (5,Eq. 20) that the variance of a reconstructed pixel is proportional to the variance of a projection value for a statistically stationary imaging process. It is easy to show from his derivation that for a Poisson process the variance of a reconstructed pixel is proportional to the total number of detected events. The mean value of a reconstructed pixel is, of course, also proportional to the total number of detected events. Then if τ is the actual imaging time and τ_m is the time to image one million events, it follows that the noise in the reconstruction is given by $A_b \cdot \text{FSDM} \cdot (\tau_m / \tau)^{1/2}$. While this relationship has been demonstrated only for the convolution algorithm, it is reasonable to expect that it is at least approximately true for ART. We have carried out computer simulations that confirm this supposition.

The signal-to-noise ratio is thus given by

$$ \text{SNR} \;=\; \frac{A_o}{A_b} \cdot \left[\frac{\tau}{\tau_m} \right]^{1/2} \cdot \frac{\sigma_o^2}{\sigma_o^2 + \sigma_s^2 + \sigma_r^2} \cdot \frac{1}{\text{FSDM}} $$

This is a measure of the probability of detection of the Gaussian spot test object. The four terms in the expression are related, respectively, to the object contrast, the imaging time, the reduction in contrast produced by imaging and reconstruction, and the image noise. Only the third and fourth terms are dependent on the imaging system and the reconstruction algorithm. We therefore define the figure-of-merit as

$$ \text{FOM} \;=\; \frac{\sigma_o^2}{\sigma_o^2 + \sigma_s^2 + \sigma_r^2} \cdot \frac{1}{\text{FSDM}} $$

We will refer to the first term in this expression as the contrast factor (CF) and the second term as the smoothness factor (SF).

3.2.2. <u>Measurement of contrast factor</u>. We assigned a value of two pixels to σ_s, the standard deviation of the imaging system psf, in order to ensure adequate sampling. If a row of the gamma camera image, which spans about 40 cm, is digitized into 128 pixels, then a σ_s of 2 pixels corresponds to a full width at half maximum of about 15 mm, which is typical for the resolution of the gamma camera at distances corresponding to large objects. The term $\sigma_s^2 + \sigma_r^2$ was evaluated through computer simulation: Six psf's with width of σ_s were distributed across a 64 x 64 image array (this array size was used for speed, and may be considered to be the central "zoomed" region of a 128 x 128 array). Exact noiseless projections were obtained at various angles over 180°, and from these projections the psf's were reconstructed on the 64 x 64 array by the different algorithms. The long and short axis of each resulting psf was determined, and the product of the standard deviations along the two axes was computed. Then $\sigma_s^2 + \sigma_r^2$ was equated to the average value of these products for the six psf's.*

The choice of σ_o, which describes the width of the test object, is arbitrary. We chose it to be the same as σ_s, to correspond to one of the smallest objects that we would expect to detect.

3.2.3. <u>Measurement of smoothness factor</u>. A uniform concentric disk with a radius of 26 pixels was generated on a 64 x 64 array. An exact projection was made, which was smoothed slightly to eliminate the Gibbs phenomenon in the subsequent reconstructions. Copies of this projection were made for various angles over 180°, and Poisson noise corresponding to one million total events was added to form a set of noisy projections. The disk was reconstructed by the various algorithms, and the RMS variation and the mean of pixel values within 16 pixels of the center of the disk

---

*We should have actually used the average of the squared standard deviations along each axis. This error has led us to overestimate the contrast factor for 4 projections by about 15% and for 6 projections by about 5%, but for 9 or more projections the error is negligible because the eccentricity of the psf's is so small.

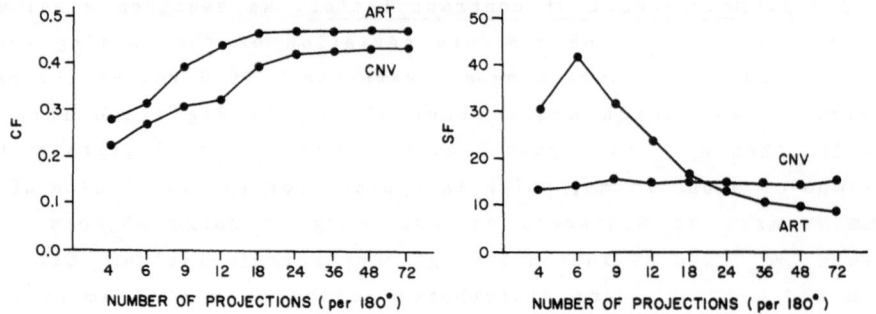

FIGURE 1. Number of projections vs. contrast factor for reconstructions using ART2 and convolution.

FIGURE 2. Number of projections vs. smoothness factor for reconstructions using ART2 and convolution.

were determined. The ratio of these two quantities is the FSDM,
or fractional standard deviation for one million detected events.
Its reciprocal is the smoothness factor. We generally computed
this value from the average of three or four trials.

3.3. Images of phantoms

One is hesitant to accept measured values as indicators of the
goodness of reconstruction unless the results are borne out by
reconstructed images. In parallel with the various figure-of-
merit computations we generated noisy projection data and reconstructed images of the 6-spot phantom superimposed on a noisy
disk, using the same reconstruction algorithms.

4. RESULTS

4.1. Number of projections vs. figure-of-merit

We first investigated the effect of the number of projections
on the reconstruction. Results given here are for ART2 with the
projection data smoothed once, and for convolution using the
modified Shepp kernel, but similar results were obtained with
other implementations of the ART and convolution algorithms.

The contrast factor behaved very similarly for ART and
convolution (Fig. 1). It was found to increase with increasing
number of projections, although little effect was noted beyond 24
projections. The smoothness factor, on the other hand, showed a

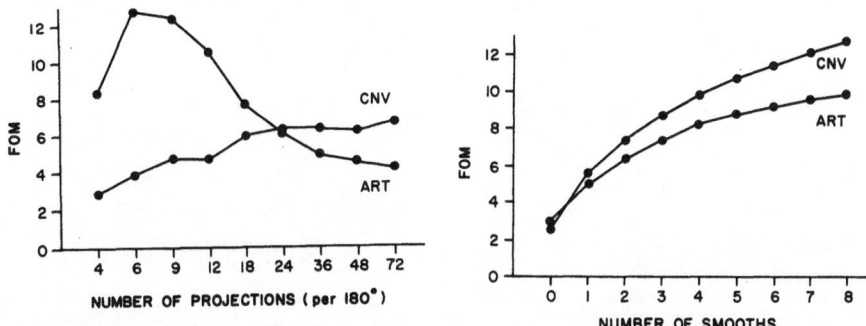

FIGURE 3. Number of projections vs. figure-of-merit for reconstruction using ART2 and convolution.

FIGURE 4. Number of smooths vs. figure-of-merit for reconstructions using ART2 and convolution. For each smooth the projection data are convolved with a 0.25, 0.5, 0.25 filter.

slight increase with increasing number of projections when the convolution algorithm was used, but with ART it was very high for 4 or 6 projections and then decreased rapidly as the number of projections was increased (Fig. 2). The figure-of-merit, which is the product of these two factors, increased steadily with convolution, but with ART it had high values for few projections and decreased rapidly as the number of projections was increased (Fig. 3). The implication here is that with convolution the more projections, the better, while with ART a relatively small number of projections (12 or fewer per 180°) is best. This is supported by reconstructed images (Fig. 5).

4.2. Smoothing vs. figure-of-merit

Early in our investigation we discovered that a small amount of smoothing improved the figure-of-merit. We now attempted to determine how much smoothing was optimal. We applied ART2 and convolution with the Ramachandran filter to 36 projections which had been smoothed 0 to 8 times. We found that the figure-of-merit increased steadily with increasing number of projections (Fig. 4). Images of the 6 spot phantom revealed that the smoothing suppressed noise but the cold spots were preserved (Fig. 6). The implication here is that the more smoothing, the better. This is

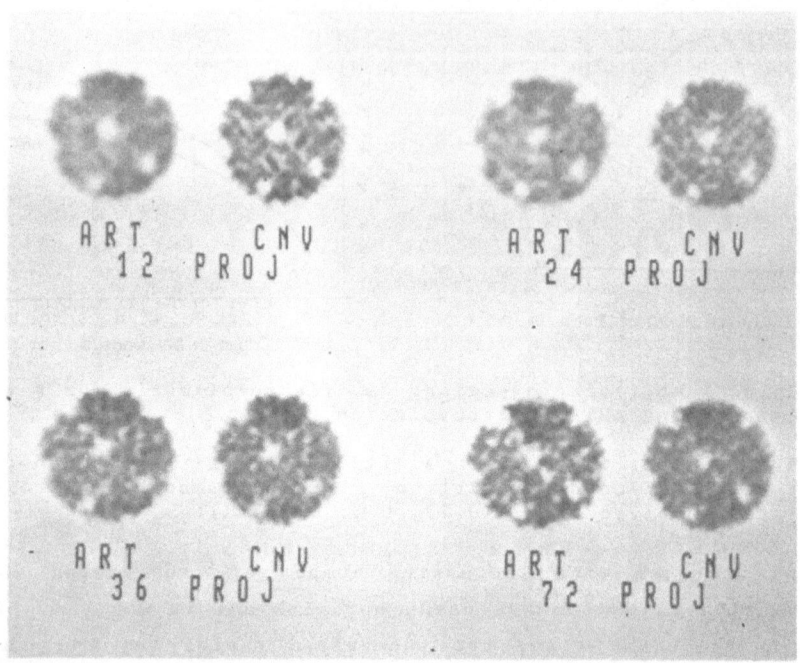

FIGURE 5. Reconstructions of the 6-spot phantom from various
numbers of projections. Each projection set contains one million
total counts. ART reconstructions employ one smooth. Convolution
reconstructions use the modified Shepp kernel with no smoothing.

unrealistic, so we turned elsewhere in our investigation of the
trade-off between noise and resolution.

4.3. CF vs. SF plots

One would expect that one algorithm would be better than
another if it had either greater smoothness (less noise) for the
same spatial resolution, or better spatial resolution for the same
smoothness. We therefore generated plots of the contrast factor
CF (which increases with improving spatial resolution) versus the
smoothness factor SF (which increases with decreasing image
noise)(Figs. 7 through 10). For a particular algorithm the CF vs.
SF plot generated by repeated smoothing of the projection data is
a curve that represents the trade-off between noise and
resolution, analogous to the trade-off between sensitivity and

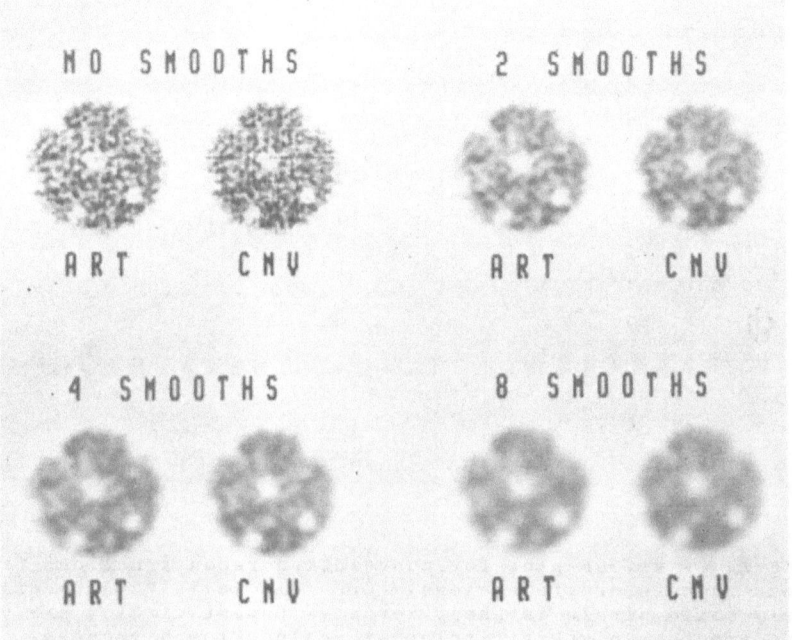

FIGURE 6. Reconstructions of the 6-spot phantom from 36 projections with various numbers of smooths. Convolution reconstructions use the Ramachandran kernel.

specificity that is represented by the well known ROC curve. In the CF vs. SF plot the best values are those closest to the upper right corner. Also in all curves the lowest point corresponds to unsmoothed projection data, and the highest point corresponds to 8 smooths (7 for Fig. 9).

4.3.1. <u>Number of projections</u>. The plots for the convolution algorithm, using the Ramachandran and the Shepp kernels as applied to various numbers of projections, are shown in Fig. 7. This confirms the earlier implications that for the convolution algorithm the more projections the better, although there is very little difference between 36, 48 and 72 projections per 180°.

The plots for ART2 are shown in Fig. 8, with the position of the convolution plot for 72 projections indicated by a dashed line. For a given number of smooths, as the number of projections

180

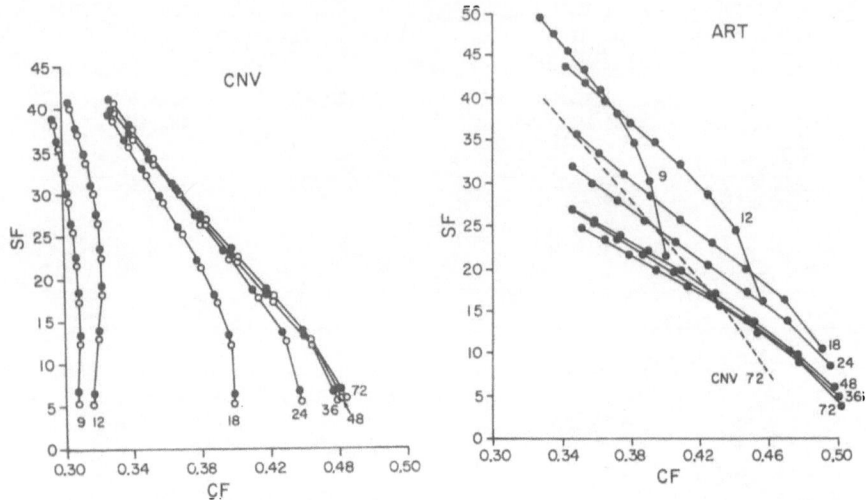

FIGURE 7. CF vs. SF plot for convolution reconstructions from various numbers of projections. Open circle is Ramachandran kernel, solid circle is Shepp kernel. Lowest circles are values for no smooths, highest circles are values for 8 smooths.

FIGURE 8. CF vs. SF plot for ART2 reconstructions from various numbers of projections. Dashed line is plot for convolution from 72 projections.

increases CF generally increases and SF generally decreases. Either 12 or 18 projections is best depending on the desired point of trade-off between noise and resolution. Either curve is noted to be much better than the best convolution curve.

    4.3.2. <u>Alternate implementations of algorithms</u>. Figure 9 gives the plots for convolution reconstructions from 24 projections using nearest neighbor, linear and cubic spline interpolation. Figure 10 gives the plots for 1, 2, 3, and 16 cycles of iterations of ART2 applied to 18 projections. The plots for 4 through 15 cycles were intermediate to those for 3 and 16 cycles.

5. DISCUSSION

    Our principal finding, demonstrated by Fig. 8, is that the trade-off between noise and resolution was much more favorable for reconstructions from 12 or 18 projections per 180° using ART

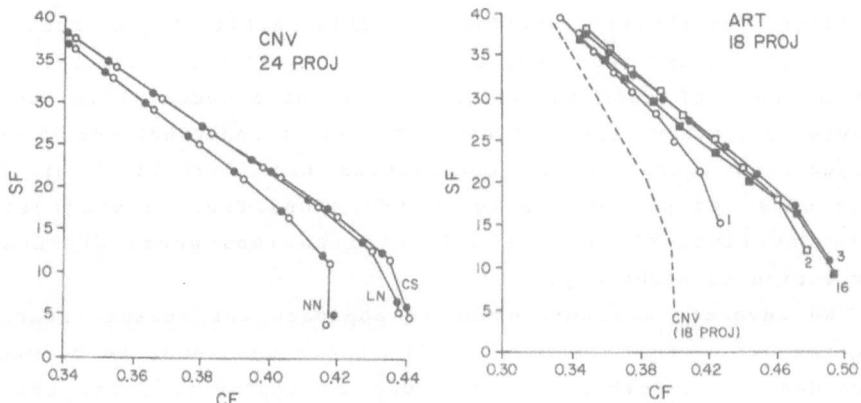

FIGURE 9. CF vs. SF plot for convolution reconstructions from 24 projections using nearest neighbor (NN), linear (LN), and modified cubic spline (CS) interpolation.

FIGURE 10. CF vs. SF plot for ART2 reconstructions from 18 projections for 1, 2, 3, and 16 cycles of iterations. Plots for 4 through 15 cycles were intermediate to those for 3 and 16 cycles. Dashed line is plot for convolution from 18 projections.

than from any number of projections using convolution. This implies that for the noisy, high contrast, low resolution situation encountered in nuclear medicine, ART should be superior to convolution, especially if it were necessary or convenient to image from relatively few angles. One situation which might be especially likely to benefit from this approach is gated cardiac emission tomography (9), since the number of acquisition angles is restricted by the large amount of data that must be acquired at each angle. It must be emphasized, however, that since this investigation is based on computer simulations, our findings require confirmation through clinical studies and observer performance studies.

The penalty for sampling at fewer angles is reduced angular resolution. Simulations that we have carried out suggest that 10° and even 15° angular sampling may be adequate for nuclear medicine since the high noise and low spatial resolution encountered does not permit very good angular resolution. With the convolution algorithm reduced angular sampling carries another penalty, the familiar "starburst" artifact. This artifact is much less noticeable in ART reconstructions. Also, although attenuation was not a topic of this investigation, we have observed in computer simulations that attenuation-corrected reconstructions from 18 projections using ART or convolution had "streaking" artifacts that were not present in reconstructions from 72 projections. This may limit the use of ART in situations where attenuation correction is necessary.

We advocate a figure-of-merit approach for reasons stated in Section 3.1. The figure-of-merit itself was found to be heavily dependent on smoothness. This may be appropriate for the pure detection problem, for which this measure was designed, but it is not appropriate for images that are to be interpreted by human observers who tolerate considerable image noise but require fairly high image contrast. By plotting the two components of the figure-of-merit against each other we were able to generate curves that demonstrate the trade-off between noise and resolution. We cannot tell what location on each curve corresponds to the image that best demonstrates diagnostic information (we would guess that the SF value is between 10 and 20) but we expect that if one curve lies above and to the right of another then the corresponding algorithms should be capable of producing better images. What appealed to us about the CF vs. SF plot is that it became quite linear after two or three smooths. We are unable to explain this phenomenon at this time.

In measuring the contrast factor we have made the simplifying assumption that the reconstructed psf is Gaussian. It is, in fact, decidedly un-Gaussian, especially in convolution reconstructions that demonstrate the "starburst" artifact. The standard deviation of the psf is heavily influenced by spurious "blobs" in its vicinity that are actually reconstruction artifacts. By inspecting reconstructed images we have found that a low contrast factor indicates the presence of these artifacts rather than a loss in amplitude of the psf (which actually changes very little). We feel that it is appropriate, nevertheless, to consider the contrast factor to be a measure of resolution because it is based on the dispersion of the psf that results from reconstruction (as determined by a second moment measure), and because the artifacts that it detects would be expected to interfere with image resolution, however that may be defined.

We estimated CF from six psf´s distributed across the image array in a somewhat random fashion. It would have been preferable, but time-consuming, to have based estimates on multiple trials with varying positions of the six psf´s. Our estimates probably contain a moderate statistical error which we believe accounts for the "bump" in the CNV curve in Fig. 1. Likewise, statistical error in SF probably accounts for the fact that the 48 projection curve lies above the 36 projection curve in Fig. 8.

The CF vs. SF plots help determine which implementations of the algorithms are to be preferred. Figure 9 demonstrates that with convolution the choice of kernel changes the position along the curve, whereas the method of interpolation changes the curve itself with cubic spline being slightly better than linear (and probably not worth the additional computation time) but nearest neighbor being clearly inferior to the others.

Figure 10 demonstrates that with ART three cycles of iterations are better than one or two, but beyond this there is little further improvement. Reconstruction from 18 projections per 180° using three cycles of ART should take roughly 50% longer than reconstructions from 36 projections per 180° using convolution, according to our timings. Thus one should be able to achieve clinically acceptable reconstruction times with ART.

6. CONCLUSION

The CF vs. SF plots appear to be a good means for intercomparing algorithms, since they demonstrate the manner in which each algorithm handles the trade-off between resolution and noise. For the nuclear medicine imaging situation simulated in this study they suggest that reconstructions from 12 or 18 projections using ART should be preferable to reconstructions from any number of projections using convolution. Whether or not this result actually applies to real imaging situations can only be determined through clinical studies and observer performance studies.

184

REFERENCES

1. Herman GT, Rowland SW. 1973. Three methods for reconstructing objects from x-rays: a comparative study. Comput. Graphics & Image Process. 2, 151-178.
2. Herman GT, Lent A. 1976. Iterative reconstruction algorithms. Comput. Biol. Med. 6, 273-294.
3. Gordon R. 1974. A tutorial on ART. IEEE Trans. Nucl. Sci. NS-21, 78-93.
4. Oppenheim BE. 1976. Three-dimensional reconstruction from incomplete projections. In Information Processing in Medical Imaging, C. Raynaud and A. Todd-Pokropek, eds. Orsay, Commissariat a l'Energie Atomique, pp 288-324.
5. Shepp LA, Logan BF. 1974. The Fourier reconstruction of a head section. IEEE Trans. Nucl. Sci. NS-21, 21-43.
6. Beck RN, Harper PV. 1968. Criteria for evaluating radioisotope imaging systems. In Fundamental Problems in Scanning, A. Gottschalk and RN Beck, eds. Springfield, Illinois, Charles C. Thomas, pp 348-382.
7. Metz CE. 1969. A mathematical investigation of radioisotope scan image processing. Ann Arbor, University Microfilms International.

A GENERALIZED WEIGHTED BACKPROJECTION ALGORITHM FOR SINGLE PHOTON EMISSION COMPUTED TOMOGRAPHY

Eiichi TANAKA and Hinako TOYAMA *

National Institute of Radiological Sciences, Anagawa, Chiba-shi, Japan
* Tokyo Metropolitan Geriatric Hospital,Sakae-cho,Itabashi-ku,Tokyo,Japan

1. INTRODUCTION

With expanding use of single photon emission computed tomography (SPECT), development of a more quantitative image reconstruction algorithm is desired. A fundumental problem in the quantitative image reconstruction is to compensate for the effect of photon attenuation in objects. Another important problem is to minimize the propagation of statistical noise in the reconstruction process because the number of accumulated events is usually limited.

In general, iterative reconstruction techniques[1] may provide accurate compensation even for non-uniform attenuation in the objects, but these techniques have not been widely used due to the significant computation capability being required in the implementation. Instead, simpler and faster methods based on filtered backprojection have been developed for practical applications. Most of these methods start from the geometric or arithmetic means of conjugate(antipodal) projections. An earlier method is the "pre-correction method"[2,3], in which simple attenuation correction is applied to the averaged projections prior to the back-projection. Another more widely used method is the "post-correction method"[4.5], in which an image reconstructed with the conventional filtered backprojection is corrected by a correction matrix representing average attenuation at each pixel of the image. In general, however, these simple procedures do not provide adequate correction for objects having large attenuation. Chang[4,5] described a two-step procedure of the post-correction method followed by an iterative method.

Tretiak and Delaney[6] and others[7,8] developed an analytical method

involving exponential backprojection.   In this method, the weight placed
on a projection increases exponentially with the depth in the object, and
this results in appreciable increase in statistical noise at the opposite
peripheral area.   Bellini, et al.[9] described another analytical method
starting from the arithmetic means of conjugate projections.

In SPECT, however, a projection contains more information on source
distribution in a close area from the detector than in a distant area due
to photon attenuation, and the averaging of conjugate projections is not
adequate for reducing the statistical noise.   An off-center area should
be reconstructed with larger weights on the front views than on the rear
views.   The weighted backprojection algorithm described here has been
developed from such point of view.   The point source sensitivity is kept
constant throughout the image, and the relative weights placed on the
conjugate projections are controlled by a reconstruction parameter.   The
details of the mathematical basis are described in reference[10].

2. RECONSTRUCTION ALGORITHM

Consider an object having a constant attenuation coefficent, μ, as
shown in Fig. 1, in which a fixed and a rotated coordinate system are
represented by (X, Y) and (x, y), respectively. The weighted backprojection
algorithm consists of three steps.   The first step is to generate a
set of "normalized projections", $p_n(x)$, from observed projections, $p_o(x)$,
by

$$p_n(x) = p_o(x) \exp(\mu L), \qquad\qquad (1)$$

where $L=L(x)$ is the y-coordinate of the object edge.   We assume here that
the attenuation coefficient is constant throughout the object, but the
following discussion can be extended to an object having non-uniform
attenuation if the source distribution is localized in a convex region
of uniform attenuation, because the non-uniform attenuation of the surrounding medium can be taken into account by incorporating an additional
correction in Eq.(1).   The normalized projections are independent of the
object boundary and of the surrounding attenuation medium.

The second step is a modified convolution.   A set of filtered
projections, $p_f(x)$, is obtained from the normalized projections by

$$p_f(x) = [p_n(x)F(x) * g(x)]/F(x), \qquad (2)$$

where the asterisk denotes the convolution operation, and g(x) is a convolution filter. The function F(x) is introduced to correct the density distortion due to the weighted backprojection. The functions F(x) and g(x) will be given in the next section.

The third step is the weighted backprojection. This step is expressed by

$$I(X, Y) = \sum_{\theta}^{2\pi} p_f(x)W(y), \qquad (3)$$

where I(X, Y) is the image density at a point (X, Y). W(y) is a weighting function defined by

$$W(y) = \exp(k\mu y)/\cosh[(k+1)\mu y], \qquad (4)$$

where k is an arbitrary constant called "reconstruction index". The weighting function is defined so as to provide a constant reconstruction sensitivity for a point source throughout the object. W(y) is plotted in fig. 2.

The reconstruction index determines the relative weights being imposed on two conjugate projections. When k=0, W(y) is equal to W(-y) and images are reconstructed from the arithmetic means of conjugate projections.

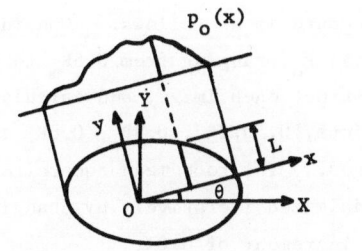

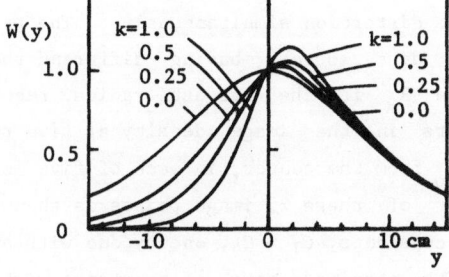

FIGURE 1. Illustration of a fixed coordinate system (X, Y) and a rotated coordinate system (x, y). $p_o(x)$ is an observed projection.

FIGURE 2. Plots of the weighting function defined by Eq.(4). k is the reconstruction index. Attenuation coefficient is 0.15 cm^{-1}.

When k > 0, an off-center area of an image is reconstructed with larger weights on the front views than on the rear views. If a uniform disc source is reconstructed with the coordinate origin at its center, the variance of the statistical noise at an off-center point depends upon the k-value, and it is known that the variance is minimal at k=1. However, the minimum is very broad, and k > 0.2 is a reasonable choice from the view point of noise reduction. We consider the k-value in a range from 0 to 1 in the following discussions.

3. CORRECTION FUNCTION AND CONVOLUTION FILTER

The modified convolution expressed by Eq.(2) involves an approximate correction for image distortion due to the varying weight in the backprojection. In the previous paper[10], the correction function, $F(x)$, and the convolution filter, $g(x)$, were given, which contained one constant each. After further study, it was found that the following functions provide better results for a wide range of photon attenuation.

$$F(x) = \exp[C_1(\mu x)^2] - C_2 \qquad (5)$$

$$g(x) = g_0(x)[1 + C_3(\mu x)^2]/[1 + C_4(\mu x)^4], \qquad (6)$$

where $C_1 \sim C_4$ are constants, and $g_0(x)$ is a conventional convolution filter. A typical filter, $g_0(x)$, is the Shepp-Logan filter[11].

The constants were determined by a computer iteration program so that uniform disc sources having various diameters were reconstructed with the least distortion simultaneously. The procedure is as follows. Consider five disc sources having different radii, R_o, ranging from $0.5R_m$ to R_m where R_m is the largest radius, reconstruct each image, and calculate errors in the image density at five points, 0, $0.2R_o$, $0.4R_o$, $0.6R_o$ and $0.8R_o$ from the center, in each of five images. The root mean square(rms) error of these 25 image points is then minimized iteratively by changing the constants, $C_1 \sim C_4$, one by one with an increment of 0.01.

The obtained sets of constants with $\mu R_m = 2.5$ and $\mu R_m = 3.0$ are shown in Table 1 as #A and #B, respectively. Figure 3 shows the central profiles through the disc images reconstructed with the optimized constants. Since the above computer program works to minimize the error for

Table 1. Optimized constants in the correction function and the convolution filter given by Eqs. (5) and (6), respectively.

	k	c_1	c_2	c_3	c_4	RMS % *
# A	0.00	0.34	−0.16	0.21	0.19	2.50
	0.25	0.38	0.05	0.11	0.21	2.25
	0.50	0.40	0.21	0.01	0.20	2.00
$\mu R_m = 2.5$	0.75	0.42	0.29	−0.06	0.19	2.14
	1.00	0.43	0.34	−0.12	0.16	2.51
# B	0.00	0.28	−0.13	0.27	0.20	4.29
	0.25	0.30	0.11	0.19	0.22	4.05
	0.50	0.33	0.23	0.09	0.21	3.83
$\mu R_m = 3.0$	0.75	0.36	0.32	0.00	0.20	3.49
	1.00	0.38	0.39	−0.09	0.16	2.98

*RMS % is the root mean square error of image densities at 25 points (5 points x 5 images).

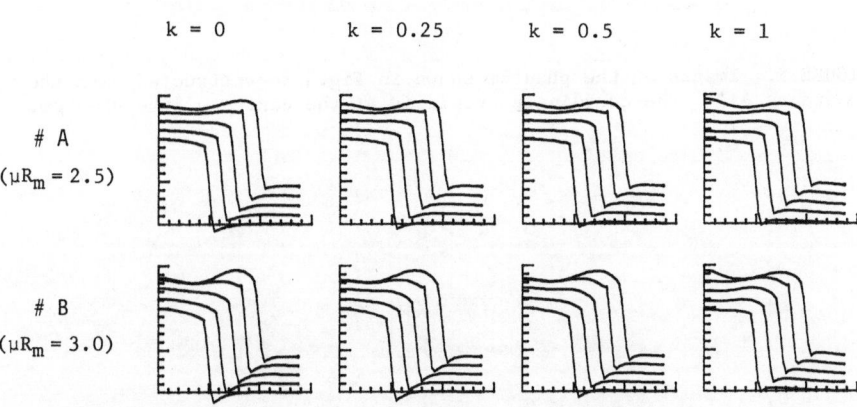

FIGURE 3. Profiles through the images of uniform disc phantoms reconstructed with the optimized constants given in Table 1. The five curves in each figure are the profiles of the disc images having radii, $0.5R_m \sim R_m$ in five steps. The abscissas are the distance from the center. The ordinates are shifted for each curve.

190

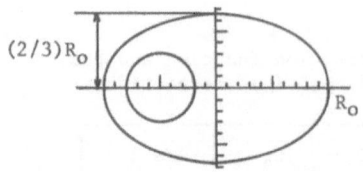

FIGURE 4. The mathematical phantom used for the simulation studies shown in Figs. 5 and 6. The relative activities of the hot area to the body is 2:1.

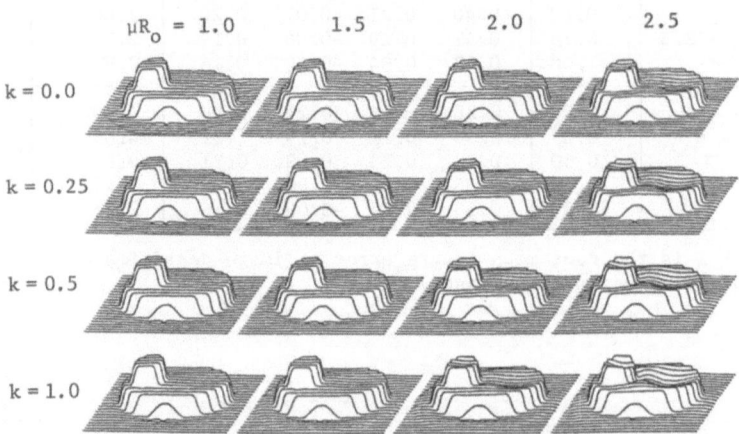

FIGURE 5. Images of the phantom shown in Fig.4 reconstructed with the constants #A. The coordinate origin is at the center of the phantom.

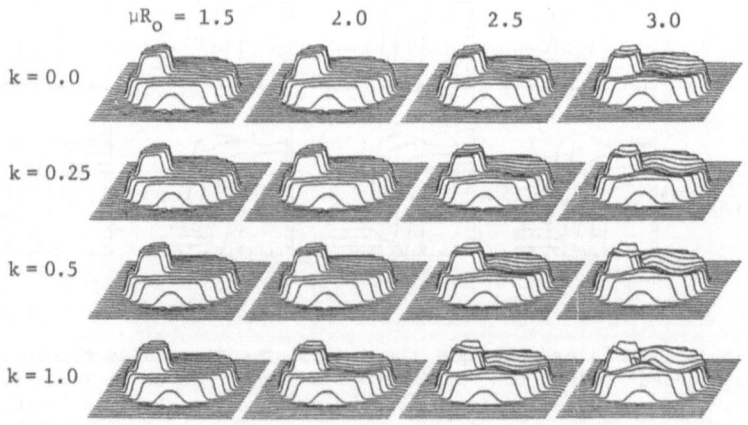

FIGURE 6. Images of the phantom shown in Fig.4 reconstructed with the constants #B. The coordinate origin is at the center of the phantom.

circularly symmetric objects, the tests for non-symmetric mathematical phantoms were performed.

Figures 5 and 6 show the images of the elliptic phantom having a hot area shown in Fig. 4. It is seen that the attenuation compensation is quite satisfactory, but density distortion increases gradually with the increase of μR_o and k-value. It appears that the distortion occurs in tangential direction with respect to the coordinate origin.

The constants #A provide satisfactory images for smaller attenuation ($\mu R_o < 2.0$) with $0 \le k \le 1$ or for medium attenuation ($2.0 < \mu R_o < 2.5$) with k=0 or k=0.25. The constants #B show similar characteristics, but they can handle a little wider range of attenuation (up to $\mu R_o \simeq 3$ with k=0 or 0.25) than #A, allowing for a little increase in distortion for smaller attenuating objects.

4. PROPAGATION OF STATISTICAL NOISE

The quantitative and qualitative usefulness of SPECT depends on the magnitude of statistical noise in the reconstructed images. Assuming that observed projections, $p_o(x)$, obey Poisson statistics, it is shown[10] that the variance, V(X, Y), of the statistical noise of a reconstructed image can be estimated, in a good accuracy, by

$$V(X, Y) = K \sum_{\theta}^{2\pi} [W^2(y)\exp(2\mu L)p_o(x)], \qquad (7)$$

where (X, Y) is the coordinates of a point of interest, (x, y) the rotated coordinates of the point (X, Y) (see Fig.1), and K a constant. The term of the summation represents the variance of image obtained by simple weighted backprojection (skipping the modified convolution process), and the constant K is a factor of noise propagation in the convolution process. The value of K depends on the convolution filter, $g_0(x)$, in Eq.(6) and on the method of interpolation in the backprojection[12]. With the Shepp-Logan filter, $K=0.5/d^3$ for nearest neighbor interpolation and $K=0.25/d^3$ for linear interpolation, where d is the linear sampling interval. If the reconstructed images are smoothed so that the point spread function is Gaussian, $K=0.461/d_F^3$ where d_F is the full-width at half-maximum(FWHM) of the point spread function.

Equation (7) is fairly accurate although it does not include the effect of modification in the convolution expressed by Eq.(2). The reason for this is that the modification affects the low frequency ($\leq \mu$) component of images while most of the noise has much higher spatial frequencies. Equation (7) implies that a given set of observed projections yields various images having different statistical accuracy depending upon the k-value and the position of the coordinate origin.

If a uniform disc image is reconstructed with the coordinate origin at its center, the noise is the largest at the center, and the magnitude of the center noise is independent of k. Figure 7 shows the total number of events required to obtain 10% rms accuracy at the center. The point spread function is assumed to be Gaussian. The rms noise at off-center is dependent upon k. The relative rms noise is plotted in Fig.8 for k=0 (solid curves) and for k=0.5 (dashed curves). The disc radius is 10 cm.

The above analysis was confirmed by simulation. The reconstrucated images of a 20 cm diameter uniform disc with k=0 and k=0.5 are shown in Fig.9(A). The total number of events is 5 x 10^6, and $\mu = 0.2$ cm^{-1}. The detector resolution is assumed to be 6 mm FWHM, and pixel size, d, is 5 mm. The nearest neighbor interpolation was used. Figure 9(B) shows the rms noise at various distances from the center obtained by the simulation (dots and circles) and that obtained by the calculation with K=0.5/d^3 (solid and dashed curves). The two results show a reasonable agreement.

The effect of off-centering of the coordinate origin on the noise is demonstrated in Fig.10. Figure 10(A) is the calculated variance along the X-axis of a uniform disc phantom, and Fig.10(B) is that of a disc phantom having a localized source distribution (see insets). The solid curves are obtained with the centered origin and the dashed curves are with the off-centered origin (off-centered by +3 cm in A and by +2 cm in B). The disc radii are 10 cm and $\mu = 0.225$ cm^{-1}. The images reconstructed by simulation for the localized source phantom (Fig.10(B)) are shown in Fig.11. The total number of events is 10^6. The images well reflect the calculated noise magnitude shown in Fig.10(B).

These results indicate that, for a uniform source distribution, the off-centering generally increases the noise magnitude, but for a localized source distribution, a proper setting of the origin is effective in reducing the noise. It is shown in Appendix that the best result is obtained when the coordinate origin is located at the noisiest point in the image.

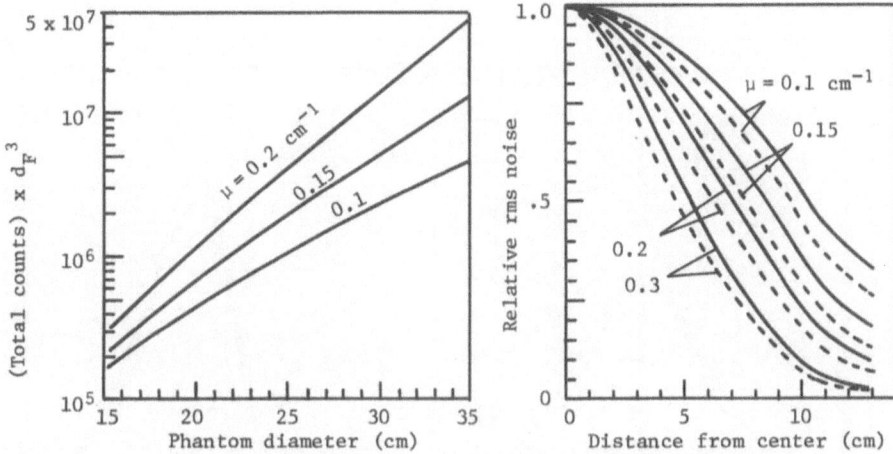

FIGURE 7. Total number of events required to obtain 10% accuracy at the center of a uniform disc image. d_F(cm) is the FWHM of the Gaussian point spread function.

FIGURE 8. Relative rms noise at off-center of a uniform disc image. The disc radius is 10 cm.
Solid curves : k = 0
Dashed curves : k = 0.5

FIGURE 9. (A) Reconstructed images of a uniform disc phantom with statistical noise, and (B) the root mean square noise as a fuction of the distance from the center. The disc radius is 10 cm and $\mu = 0.2$ cm^{-1}. The coordinate origin is the center of the disc. The total number of events is 5 x 10^6.

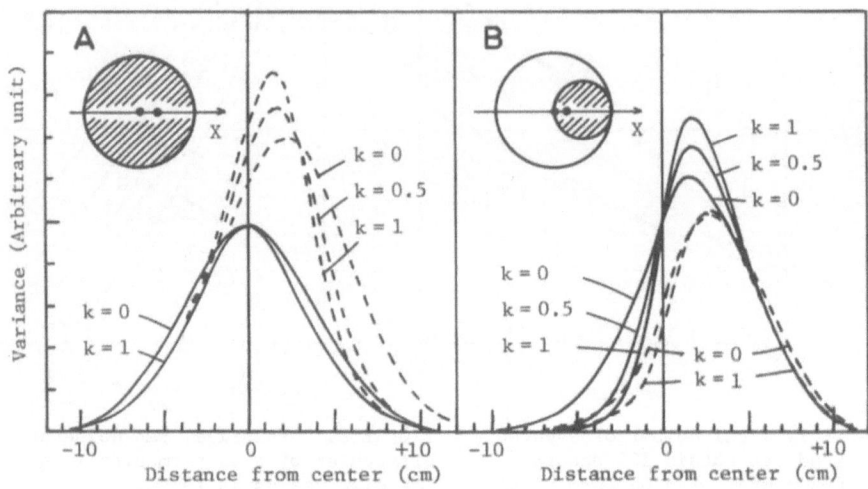

FIGURE 10. Effect of off-centering of the coordinate origin on the magnitude of statistical noise. Variance along the X-axis is plotted. The disc radii are 10 cm and $\mu = 0.225$ cm^{-1}.
  Solid curves : Origin is centered.
  Dashed curves: Origin is off-centered by 3 cm in A and 2 cm in B.

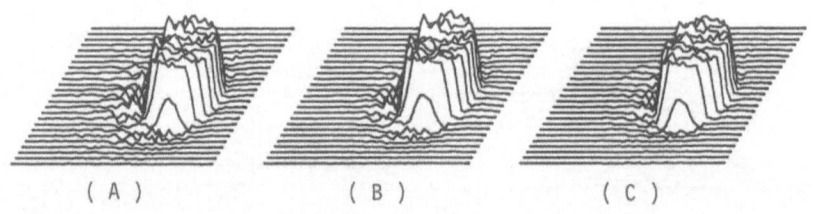

FIGURE 11. Reconstructed images of a disc having localized source distribution (inset of Fig. 10B) with statistical noise. The total number of events is 10^6. The disc radius is 10 cm and $\mu = 0.225$ cm^{-1}.
  (A) Centered origin with k = 0
  (B) Centered origin with k = 0.5
  (C) 2 cm off-centered origin with k = 0.5

5. STARLIKE ARTEFACTS

A sharp hot spot in source distribution may produce starlike artefacts in the image when the number of projections is small. In the conventional filtered backprojection method or in the present method with k=0, the minimum number of projecations, N_m, required to avoid such artefacts at a distance, R, from the hot spot is approximately given by

$$N_m = 2 \pi R/d_o, \tag{8}$$

where d_o is the overall resolution width of the imaging system.

For example, if there is a hot spot near the edge of an object, the value of R in Eq.(8) should be equal to the diameter of the object in order to avoid artefacts at the opposite periphery. On the other hand, in the weighted backprojection method with a positive k-value, a projection gives little effect on the opposite area of the image, and R in Eq.(8) may be reduced to about 70% ∿ 80% of the diameter. This implies that the required number of projections can be reduced by 20% ∿ 30% as compared with the case of k=0 or with the conventional pre- or post-correction method.

Figure 12 demonstrates the comparison of the artefacts for k=0 and k=0.5 generated by a small hot spot (7.5 mm dia.) located at 9 cm from the center. The object diameter is 30 cm and the attenuation coefficient is 0.15 cm^{-1}. The detector resolution is assumed to be 15 mm in FWHM, and the reconstructed images are smoothed with 9–point weighted smoothing (7.5 mm pixel).

6. RECONSTRUCTION FROM LIMITED ANGLE DATA

When a positive k-value is used in the present algorithm, the off-center area of an image is reconstructed mainly by front views, and the contribution of rear views to the image is small. This fact suggests that the off-center area can be imaged adequately with a limited angle scan of less than 360°. Figure 13 shows the images of a disc phantom having two hot areas reconstructed from various scan angles. The scan angles are centered in the direction shown by the arrows in the figure. The reconstruction was made using the constants #B, k=0.5.

It is shown that the right hot area is reconstructed almost completely by a 180° ∿225° scan, while the left hot area does not appear by these

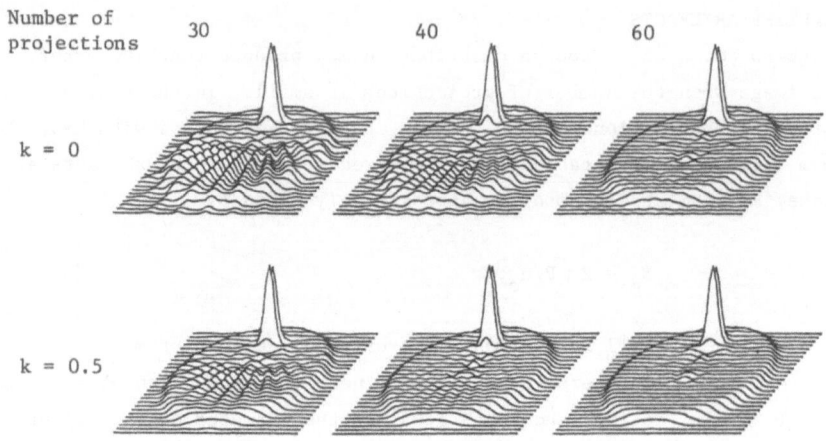

FIUGURE 12.   Effect of k-value on the starlike artefacts due to a hot spot.   The hot spot is located at 9 cm from the center of a 30 cm diameter disc phantom.   The detector resolution is assumed to be 7.5 mm FWHM.   Attenuatin coefficient is 0.15 cm^{-1}.

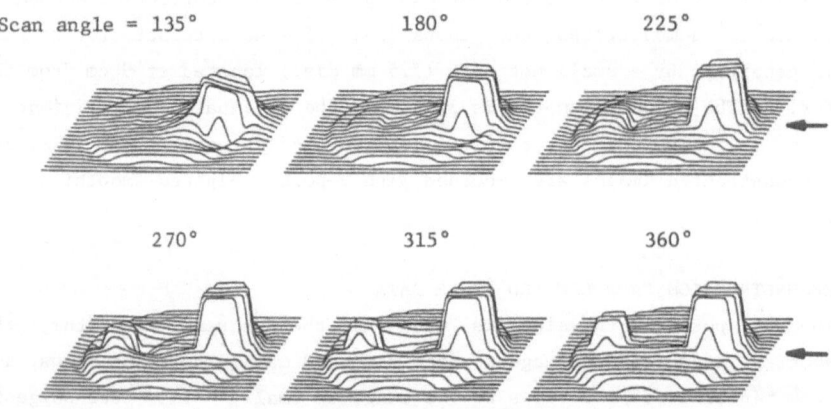

FIGURE 13.   Images of a disc phantom having two hot areas reconstructed with various scan angles.   The center of the scan angles are shown by arrows.   The phantom diameter is 30 cm.   The circular hot areas, having 6 cm and 4 cm diameter each, are located at +6 cm and -6 cm on the X-axis, respectively.   The relative activities of the two hot areas and the body background is 10:6:2. Attenuation coefficient is 0.15 cm^{-1}. The reconstruction was made with the constants #B, k=0.5.

scan angles. On the other hand, the uniform body activity appears almost uniformly by a 180° scan, but its density is half of that of the 360° scan. This result indicates that a small organ such as the heart is adequately reconstructed by a limited angle scan with an angular range of 180° ∿ 360°.

7. EXPERIMENTAL STUDY

The algorithm was tested for experimental data obtained with various phantoms filled with Tc-99m solution. The imaging device was a rotating gamma camera system (GE Maxi Camera 400) provided with a parallel multi-hole collimator(Low-energy general purpose). The energy window was centered on the photo-peak with 20% window width. The pixel size was 6.25 mm, and the number of views was 64 in 360°. The reconstruction was made with the constants #A, k=0.5, assuming μ=0.15 cm^{-1}. The obtained images were smoothed with 9-point weighted smoothing.

Figure 14 shows the reconstructed images of three uniform cylindrical phantoms having diameters of 20, 25 and 30 cm. The total counts are 1.1 x 10^6, 1.9 x 10^6 and 2.4 x 10^6, respectively. The profiles through the X- and Y-axis are also plotted. It seems that the 20 cm diameter image is somewhat convex, while the 30 cm image is concave, as compared with the simulation study. The difference may be due to the effect of scattered photons. The scattered photons tend to increase the image density and to make the image convex for a small object. For a large object, however, photons scattered at the central region of the object will give smaller effect on the image density because the scattered photons attenuate more strongly than the primary photons.

In order to test the effect of scattered photons, a three compartment phantom (see Fig.15) was imaged with different energy windows. Figure 16 shows the projection images (viewed from the direction shown in Fig.15) and the reconstructed images at two slice levels. The energy window was centered (-10% ∿ +10%) on the photo-peak in Fig.16(A), while the window was off-centered (-20% ∿ 0%) in Fig.16(B). It seems that the image density due to the scattered photons at the center of the image of slice 2 is about 20% of that of the active region for the on-peak energy window, and is about 30% for the off-peak window.

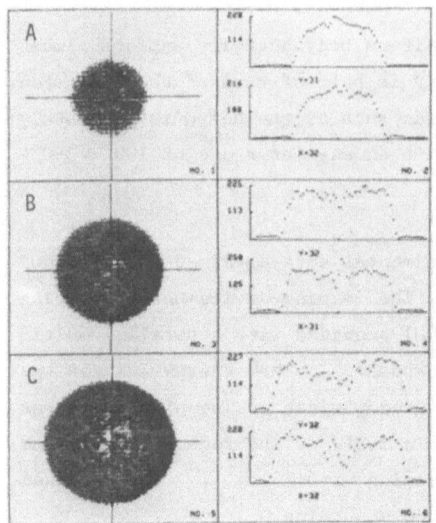

FIGURE 14.   Images of a cylindrical phantoms filled with Tc-99m solution and the profiles.   The diameters are (A):20 cm, (B):25 cm, (C):30 cm.

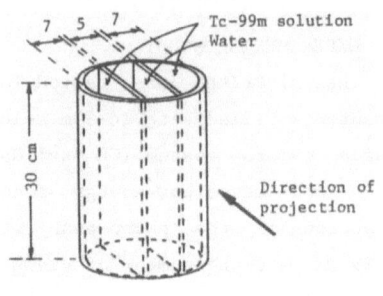

FIGURE 15.   Three compartment phantom used for experiments shown in Fig.16. The diameter of the phantom is 20 cm, and the thickness of the wall and septa is 5 mm.

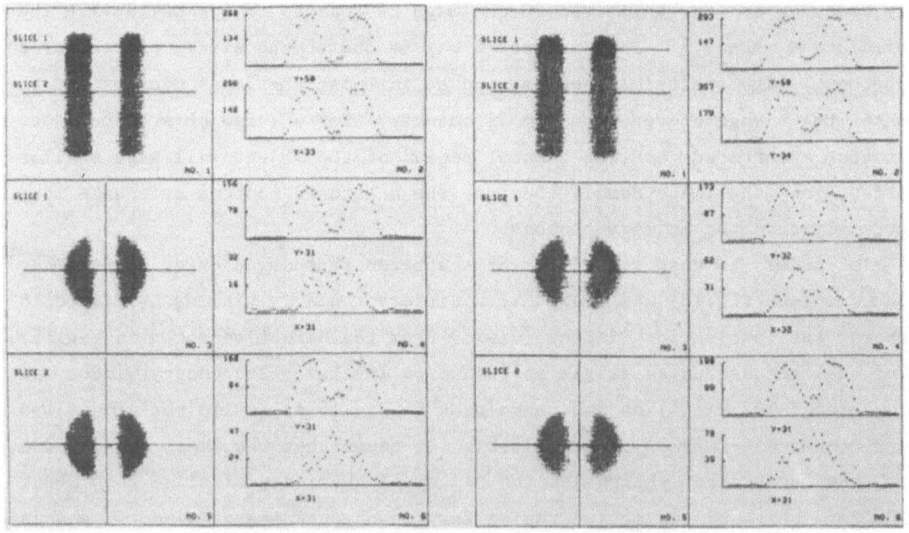

FIGURE 16.   Projection images(Top) and reconstructed images(Middle and Bottom) of the phantom shown in Fig.15 at two slice levels.
(A) Left : Energy window is -10% ∿ +10% of the photo-peak.
(B) Right: Energy window is -20% ∿ 0% of the photo-peak.

8. SUMMARY

A new reconstruction algorithm and its imaging performance have been described. The algorithm consists of normalization of projections, modified convolution and weighted backprojection. The weight in the back-projection is determined so as to provide perfect attenuation compensation for a constant attenuation medium, although non-uniform attenuation in the surrounding medium is properly corrected if the activity in that medium is negligibly small. Image density distortion due to the varying weight is corrected by introducing a correction function in the modified convolution. The optimum correction functions and the convolution filters were determined by an iterative computer program. The relative weights placed on two conjugate projections are controlled by the "reconstruction index", k.

Propagation of statistical noise in the reconstruction was evaluated by a simple formula for various reconstruction indices, and the results were confirmed by computer simulation. A proper positioning of the coordinate origin is important for reducing the largest noise in the reconstructed image, and the use of a positive reconstruction index, k, is effective for reducing the noise in areas apart from the origin (see Appendix).

The use of a positive reconstruction index is also effective to reduce starlike artefacts due to the limited number of views. A small hot organ located at a certain distance from the coordinate origin is adequately imaged with a limited scan angle of $180° \sim 360°$.

Preliminary phantom experiments were performed with a rotating gamma camera system. Somewhat convex and concave images were obtained for small(20 cm in dia.) and large(25 and 30 cm in dia.) objects, respectively. The difference between the results of experiment and the simulation may be due to the effect of scattered photons, but further study is needed to obtain a quantitative conclusion on the effect of scattered photons.

ACKNOWLEDGEMENTS

This work was supported in part by a Grant-in-Aid for Cancer Research (58-42) from the Ministry of Health and Welfare, Japan. The authors would like to thank N. Nohara, T. Tomitani, M. Yamamoto and H. Murayama for their helpful discussions.

Appendix.   COORDINATE ORIGIN FOR THE LEAST STATISTICAL NOISE

The statistical noise of a reconstructed image is not uniformly distributed in the image plane, and the variance has the largest value at a certain point.   A problem is to find the "optimum coordinate origin" which minimizes "the largest variance in the image".

First, we consider the problem in a one-dimensional model.   In Fig.17(A), p_1 and p_2 denote a pair of conjugate projections, and $O(L_1,L_2)$ is a coordinate origin.   The variance at a point, P, is given by the one-dimensional version of Eq.(7):

$$V_1(X) = K[p_1W^2(X)\exp(2\mu L_1) + p_2W^2(-X)\exp(2\mu L_2)]. \qquad (9)$$

The variance, $V_1(0)$, at the origin depends on the position of the origin.   We can determine the origin, $O(\hat{L}_1,\hat{L}_2)$, which yields the smallest $V_1(0)$-value, by solving $dV_1(0)/dL_1=0$ with $L_1+L_2=$constant.   The condition for $\hat{L}_1$ and $\hat{L}_2$ is given by

$$p_1\exp(2\mu\hat{L}_1) = p_2\exp(2\mu\hat{L}_2). \qquad (10)$$

Under this condition, Eq.(9) becomes

$$V_1(X) = Kp_1\exp(2\mu\hat{L}_1)[W^2(X) + W^2(-X)]. \qquad (11)$$

The term in the brackets has a maximum at X=0 for $k \geq 0$.   Therefore, it is apparent that the origin, $O(\hat{L}_1,\hat{L}_2)$, is the optimum coordinate origin.

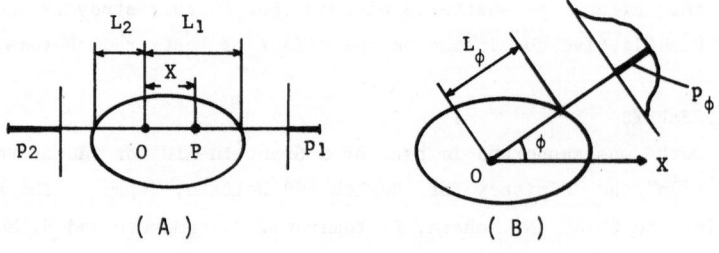

FIGURE 17.   One-dimensional(A) and two-dimensional(B) models for optimizing the position of coordinate origin.

We shall extend the same argument to a two dimensional image without proof. For an arbitrary coordinate origin (see Fig.17(B)), the variance at the origin is given by, from Eq.(7),

$$V(0, \ 0) = K \sum_{\phi}^{2\pi} p_{\phi} \exp(2\mu L_{\phi}).$$ (12)

The origin yielding a minimum $V(0,0)$-value will be the optimum coordinate origin, and the noise magnitude is the largest at the origin.

For example, a calculation shows that the optimum origin in the case of the phantom shown in Fig.10(B) is at X=2.5 cm.

REFERENCES

1. Budinger TF, Gullberg GT: Transverse section reconstruction of gamma-ray emitting radionuclides in patients. In: Reconstruction Tomography in Diagnostic Radiology and Nuclear Medicine. Ed. by MM Ter-Pogossian, et al., Baltimore, University Park Press, 1977, pp 315-42
2. Sorenson JA: Quantitative measurement of radioactivity in vivo by whole-body counting. In: Instrumentation in Nuclear Medicine, Vol.2. Ed. by GJ Hine and JA Sorenson, New York, Academic Press, 1974, pp 311-48
3. Keyes WI: A practical approach to transverse-section gamma-ray imaging. Br J Radiol 49:62-70, 1976
4. Chang LT: A method for attenuation correction in radionuclide computed tomography. IEEE Trans Nucl Sci NS-25:638-43, 1978
5. Chang LT: Attenuation correction and incomplete projection in single photon emission computed tomography. IEEE Trans Nucl Sci NS-26:2780-9, 1978
6. Tretiak OJ, Delaney P: The exponential convolution algorithm for emission computed axial tomography. In: Review of Information Processing in Medical Imaging. Ed. by AB Brill and RR Price, Oak Ridge National Laboratory Report ORNL/BCTIC-2, 1978, pp 266-78
7. Tretiak O, Metz C: The exponential Radon transform. SIAMJ Appl Math 39:341-54, 1980
8. Gullberg GT, Budinger TF: The use of filtering methods to compensate for constant attenuation in single-photon emission computed tomography. IEEE Trans Bio Eng BME-28:142-57, 1981
9. Bellini S, Piacentini M, Cafforio C, Rocca F: Compensation of tissue absorption in emission tomography. IEEE Trans Acoustics, Speech and Signal Processing ASSP-27:213-18, 1979
10. Tanaka E: Quantitative image reconstruction with weighted backprojection for single photon emission computed tomography. J Comput Assist Tomogr. 7:692-700, 1983
11. Shepp LA and Logan BF: The Fourier reconstruction of a head section. IEEE Trans Nucl Sci NS-21:21-43, 1974
12. Tanaka E, Murayama H: Properties of statistical noise in positron emission tomography. In: Proceedings of International Workshop on Physics and Engineering in Medical Imaging (Pacific Grove, 1982), IEEE Comput Soc 82CH1751-7, 1982, pp 158-64

APPLICATION OF LINEAR CLASSIFIERS TO THE RECOGNITION OF THE TEMPORAL
BEHAVIOUR OF THE HEART

J. DUVERNOY, J.C CARDOT, M. BAUD, J. VERDENET, XIA YUNG, P. BERTHOUT,
R. FAIVRE, J.P. BASSAND, R. BIDET, J.P. MAURAT

This paper presents some results obtained by a team of specialists from
different fields who wanted to bring to the disposal of clinicians high-
rated as well as efficient methods of data processing. The emphasis is put
on the evaluation of the techniques that undergo the burden of clinical
routine, and have to meet the capacity of the digital systems already in
place in hospitals.

1. MOTIVATION

We do not intend to present a survey of the methods of data processing
(in the field), which otherwise are widely known and available in the specialized litterature. The organization of this paper will rather give you
an image of the way we followed the information carried by the sequences
of scintigraphic images recorded in heart studies. We did not consider the
problem as a pure exercise of digital image processing, but rather as a
matter of locating and recognizing different temporal behaviours at work
in the data sequence. Each pixel is taken as a vector the components of
which are the measured values of its activity in the successive images of
the sequence. Therefore we have been interested since the very beginning
in the difficulties arising from the handling of sets of vectors, especially
that of a high dimensionality, or that of clustering the temporal behaviours
in spatially disjoined classes. Finally we have been particularly careful
not to propose any technique without the corresponding clinical validation
performed upon a significant number of representative cases by a group of
cardiologists.

2. METHODOLOGY

Without any definite policy in data processing, it is very difficult to
overcome the classical debate about the best method one should have used,

among the well known dilemnas :

- deterministic versus statistical description ;
- linear versus nonlinear transforms ;
- supervised versus nonsupervised training.

Our first goal is to build an image of the heart where at each point we
can tell the respective parts of the temporal behaviours that can be pointed
out. At this stage we do not have any preference for any method ; we just
propose three points :

- going from the 16 images of a scintigraphic sequence to the image which
displays the temporal behaviours, a procedure of information compression
must be applied ;

- identifying the actual temporal behaviours can be achieved either by
a non supervised technique that clusters the points of the image sharing a
given similarity. But it is not said that they are clustered. The other way
of identifying the behaviours consists of using a supervised technique where
a processor is trained to recognize registred temporal behaviours in specified zones of interest ;

- recognizing the temporal behaviours in an image offers the opportunity
of dealing with some questions of interest, such as : what is the signal-
to-noise ratio at each point ? Are there any singular points (e.g. akinetic)
within homogeneous regions ? What is the relative magnitude of each registred
temporal behaviour in the overlapping regions of the projected images of
atrium and ventricle.

These remarks point out that the key of an efficient processing of the
scintigraphic sequences does not lie in an automatic application of a unique
technique, but rather in the definition of efficient features (see Fig. 1.1).
The underlaying philosophy of any feature selection mechanism (1) should be
the optimal retention of a minimum number of dimensions or variables, while
maintaining and maximizing the probability of correct classification. The
latter criterion being difficult to evaluate, other criteria can be used,
which provide sub-optimal but analytically tractable feature selection. In
this way we started from the assumption of maximal ignorance, and we began
our study with the implementation of a statistical transform aimed at compressing the information. The by-product of this transform is a reduction
of dimensionality by means of a set of a few vectors which play the role of
statistical features. These vectors cannot be assimilated to physiological
factors. Moreover their clinical significance may vary from one patient to

another. On the other hand, the nice thing with statistical features is
that they point out temporal behaviours as whole entities. For instance,
akinetic points or other wall motion abnormalities benefit from the same
representation as that of overall behaviours of atria and ventricles. Nevertheless the expected result from such a non-supervised learning is just the
description of the number of clusters the unclassified data fall into. When
it comes to the identification of these classes, supervised techniques become meaningful. This led us to an attempt to specify the statistical features by introducing an additional training. This method was applied to the
problem of discriminating the content of the overlapping areas. At this
stage the differences become very narrow between the statistical features
matched to the principal temporal behaviours and those obtained by a deterministic classifier -such as the perceptron- trained on characteristic regions of interest (ROI's). That is the reason why we recently tried to compare the relative efficacy of the statistical features to that of some classical, and somehow simpler, linear classifiers. It is known indeed that if
N classes are linearly separable, then a feature space of N dimensions will
be sufficient for classification. In such a case the necessary features can
reduce to the set of N normals to the hyperplanes separating each pair of
classes.

Required are representative prototypes of the temporal behaviours one
wishes to recognize. We payed special attention to the choice of such prototypes by designing statistical estimators, recursive or not, that extract
useful informations from registred ROI's (e.g. atrium, ventricle, and background noise). Our ambition has not been to write any consumer report on
linear classifiers : therefore we will present as a conclusion what we think
to be optimal from the view point of routine processing, depending on each
specific application, and with a special reference to clinical usefulness.

Finally we tried to illustrate the efficiency of the investigated techniques by making up the error-image which makes visible the limitations of
the techniques. Such an image is defined by the difference between the original data and their reconstruction by means of the selected features.

FIGURE 1.1

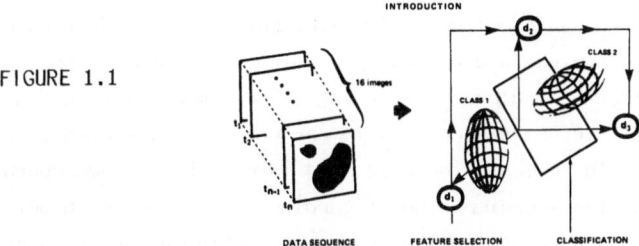

3. FURTHER PROBLEMS

Obviously the question of processing the scintigraphic sequences will remain an ill-posed problem as long as it is taken as a matter of digital processing of a set of fixed images. In fact, when looking at a given pixel, what is being observed is not the temporal evolution of a fixed point of the organ under study. It is rather the travelling of different parts of the three-dimensional organ ; at different stages of their evolution, through the window made up by the pixel. The goal of analyzing the temporal behaviour of what is going on in the pixel is still justified when looking at a region of the organ where all points have almost the same behaviour. The job becomes difficult when dealing with areas of superimposition, or border-line regions. Our next research project includes the study of the heart as that of the motion of a three-dimensional object. We intend to reconstruct the trajectory of a given number of elements of this volume, according to a limited number of reasonable assumptions on the local motion of this organ.

4. MATERIAL

The study group consisted of 21 patients (pts) suffering from chronic ischemic heart disease, hospitalized in the Cardiac Unit. All patients were in normal sinus rhythm and presented no interventricular conduction abnormalities. All underwent cardiac catherization with biplane angiography (RAO 30° - LAO 60°). As established by contrast angiography analysis 3 pts out of 21 had normal left ventricular wall motion and 18 out of 21 had wall motion abnormalities depicted as dyskinesis (DK) in 5 pts, akinesis (AK) in 9 pts and hypokinesis (HK) in 4 pts.

All contrast ventriculographic studies were performed 24 h after the
equilibrium gated radionuclide evaluation. Both analyses were carried out
in postprandial periods and without premedication. Data for the radionuclide
method was collected and processed using a CGR gamma camera and a 64 K-word
16-bit Simis III Informatek central memory computer. The cardiac cycle was
decomposed into 16 frames using a 64×64 matrix. Each frame contained
500,000 counts. The superimposing of cardiac cycles was synchronized using
the peak of the R wave. Following cycles presenting a deviation of 10 % from
the mean were rejected.

5. TRANSFORMS
5.1. Karhunen-Loeve (2) (3)

The Karhunen-Loeve transformation (KL transformation) has been shown to
be the most efficient linear transformation in the field of information
compression. Because of its theoretical optimality, KL transformation appears
to be an attractive way of reducing the number of significant parameters
when dealing with multidimensional data. Actually it became a standard in
many areas of image processing, e.g., in remotely sensed data for earth
resource studies. The aim of this study is the application of the KL transformation to the set of images consisting of scintigraphic sequences. Such
sequences are considered as multitemporal data whose variance is controlled
by a few statistical parameters. The KL transformation is capable of extracting them. We will illustrate this result.

5.1.1. Principles. The KL expansion allows the description of a phenomenon, measured in a basis whose elements are correlated, by means of uncorrelated parameters in another basis with the same size. In our case the original basis is a temporal one; the sequence of images is obtained by a discrete time sampling of the behaviour of the object. A linear filtering of
the sequence considered as a time function will allow the extraction of the
dominant information. This is obtained by a change of basis.

This new basis is that of the eigenvectors of the covariance matrix of
the initial data. These new basic vectors are ranked according to a decreasing variance order. Significant parameters are therefore selected by keeping
vectors associated to a maximum amount of variance. Then, an effect of information compression is obtained by expanding the initial sequence of images
onto the most significant vectors of this new basis. These projected images
are called "principal images" in the following.

5.1.2. <u>Principal image determination</u>. The intensities $B_i(t)$ of the different pixels i (i = 1. N) of each sequential image at time t_i ($t_i = t_1 . t_n$) form the initial data basis. The terms of the covariance matrix are given by :

$$C_{pq} = \left[B_i(t_p) - m(t_p) \right] \left[B_i(t_q) - m(t_q) \right] \qquad 5.1.1$$

p = 1,n and q = 1,n

$$m(t_p) = \left[B_i(t_p) \right] = \frac{1}{N} \sum_{i=1}^{i=N} B_i(t_p) \qquad 5.1.2$$

where brackets denote a group average and $m(t_p)$ denotes the average intensity of the p-th sequence of pixels.

The more important the lateral terms of the covariance matrix, the less convenient the data system in describing the phenomenon. The definition of a new uncorrelated data system imposes, therefore, the diagonalization of the covariance matrix.

Information scattered on the covariance matrix is reorganized and concentrated on elements of its diagonal form, which is the case of the KL technique. These diagonal elements are the eigenvalues of the covariance matrix. Therefore, the eigenvalues describe the variance of the phenomenon, when projected upon the associated eigenvectors of the covariance matrix.

Ranking the eigenvalues in decreasing order helps determine the number of eigenvectors necessary to keep a given part of information.

Using the KL transformation, each sequential image $B_i(t)$ can be expressed by means of a set of orthogonal functions $\psi_k(t)$ (k = 1,n) :

$$B_i(t) = \sum_{k=1}^{k=n} a_{ik} . \psi_k(t) \qquad 5.1.3$$

The $\psi_k(t)$ are the eigenvectors of the covariance matrix. Using the property of orthogonality, the a_{ik} coefficients are defined by the scalar product :

$$a_{ik} = \sum_{t=t_1}^{t=t_n} B_i(t) . \psi_k(t) \ (i = 1,N) \qquad 5.1.4$$

The a_{ik} (i = 1,...,N) coefficients make up the k-th principal image.

The properties of these principal images, as well as their contribution
to be display of clinical and useful information, are discussed in what
follows.

5.2. <u>Fukunaga-Koontz</u> (4) (5) (6)

In the case of two linearly separable classes it is possible to define
orthogonal axes associated with each class, such as the projections of the
members of one class upon its own axis exhibit a maximal variance while
that of the members of the other class upon the same axis is minimal.

5.2.1. <u>Principle</u>.
Let C1 and C2 be the covariance matrices of each class,
that of their mixture being :

$$C = C1 + C2 \qquad\qquad 5.2.1$$

where C1 is defined by :

$$C1 = B1 \; . \; B1^t \qquad\qquad 5.2.2$$

where B1 is the data matrix. Let V and Λ be the matrix of eigenvectors and
eigenvalues of C, respectively :

$$CV = \Lambda V \qquad\qquad 5.2.3$$

A first rotation is performed upon the two data matrices :

$$B1 \; : \; \Lambda^{-\frac{1}{2}} \, V^t \, B1$$
$$B2 \; : \; \Lambda^{-\frac{1}{2}} \, V^t \, B2 \qquad\qquad 5.2.4$$

The covariance matrices of the rotated classes become :

$$C'1 = \Lambda^{-\frac{1}{2}} \, V^t \, B1 \, B1^t \, V \, \Lambda^{-\frac{1}{2}}$$
$$C'2 = \Lambda^{-\frac{1}{2}} \, V^t \, B2 \, B2^t \, V \, \Lambda^{-\frac{1}{2}} \qquad\qquad 5.2.5$$

Let 1 and 1 be the eigenvector and eigenvalue matrices of C'1, respectively :

$$C'1 \; \Phi1 = \Gamma1 \; \Phi1 \qquad\qquad 5.2.6$$

Using this equation and 5.2.1 leads to :

$$C'2 \; \Phi1 = (I - \Gamma1) \; \Phi1 \qquad\qquad 5.2.7$$

where I denotes the unitary matrix. The result of this rotation is that
both rotated classes share the same eigenvectors but in reverse order. Consequently the first eigenvector of 1 carries in the same time the maximum
variance relative to the first class, and the minimum variance relative to
the second one. This is just the opposite when dealing with the last vector

of $\Phi 1$. Therefore the Fukunaga-Koontz transform, which consist of rotating any data, D, according to 5.2.4., and projecting them upon the first eigenvector of $C'1$:

$$D : \Lambda^{-\frac{1}{2}} V^t D V_1 \qquad\qquad 5.2.8$$

offers the opportunity of reducing the multidimensional data analyses to a one-dimensional projection, fitted to a two-class problem. The well-known techniques of decision theory apply straightforwardly because one deals only with scalar quantities.

The geometric interpretation of this transform is given as follows (see Fig. 5.2) :

- a first change of axes is performed which selects the directions of principal variances of the mixture of the two classes (e.g. B1 becomes $V^t B1$) ;

- the two classes are whitened so that their present the same variances ($V^t B1$ becomes $\Lambda^{-\frac{1}{2}} V^t B1$) ;

- the rotated classes are projected upon the new axis of one of the two classes (giving $\Lambda^{-\frac{1}{2}} V^t B1 \ V1$).

The Fukunaga-Koontz transform has been validated by using a mathematical model, and next applied to gammacineangiography in order to improve the separation between atrial and ventricular behaviours in the overlapping areas.

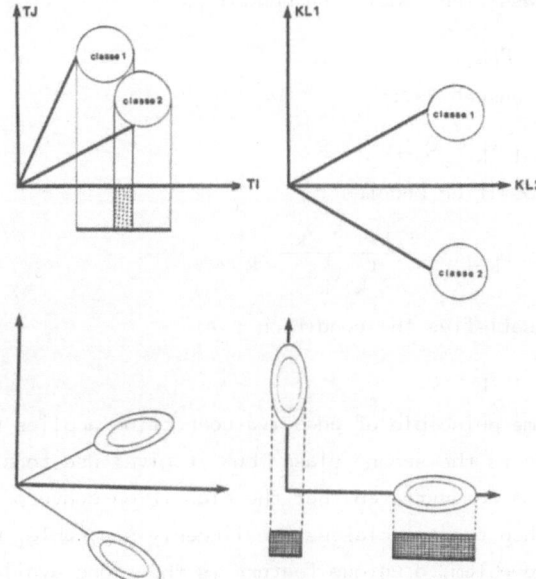

FIGURE 5.2.1

5.3. Perceptron (7)

The algorithm of the recursive trainable classifier called perceptron has been applied to the problem of discriminating the superimposition areas between atrium and ventricle. This two-class problem is addressed from a deterministic point of view, assuming that estimated prototypes of each temporal behaviour are available (the question of the optimal estimation will be discussed in the next section). Let us recall the principle of this algorithm. Originally suggested by the Mac Culloch-Pitts model of the neuron (1943), it describes a multiple input-single output machine. Nowadays it is just considered as a TLU (threshold logic unit). The goal is a vector p such that :

$$p^t y_i > 0 \quad , \text{ if } y_i \text{ belongs to the class 1}$$
$$p^t z_i < 0 \quad , \text{ if } z_i \text{ belongs to the class 2}$$

5.3.1

This vector is built by a recursive procedure based upon the reward-punishment concept. Given two training sets belonging to the two classes, at the step k the classifier is fed by the data y_k. Its current state is p_{k-1} (see fig. 5.3.1). If y_k belongs to class 1, and if the answer is :

$$p^t_{k-1} y_k > 0$$

5.3.2

the classifier remains unchanged :

$$p_k = p_{k-1}$$

5.3.3

If the answer is :

$$p^t_{k-1} y_k < 0$$

5.3.4

the classifier becomes :

$$p_k = p_{k-1} + \frac{p^t_{k-1} \cdot y_k}{y^t_k y_k} y_k$$

5.3.5

which satisfies the condition :

$$p^t_k \cdot y_k > 0$$

5.3.6

The same principle of adaptive correction applies when the kth training data belongs to the second class (but it gives use to a negative response). It has been demonstrated that the classifier converges towards a unique solution when the two classes are linearly separable. When dealing with a two-class problem, a unique feature is therefore available, which can be used

as a TLU. This feature is nothing else but the normal to the hyperplane separating the two classes. When dealing with a N class problem, as many hyperplanes are required as there are couples of classes.

FIGURE 5.3.1

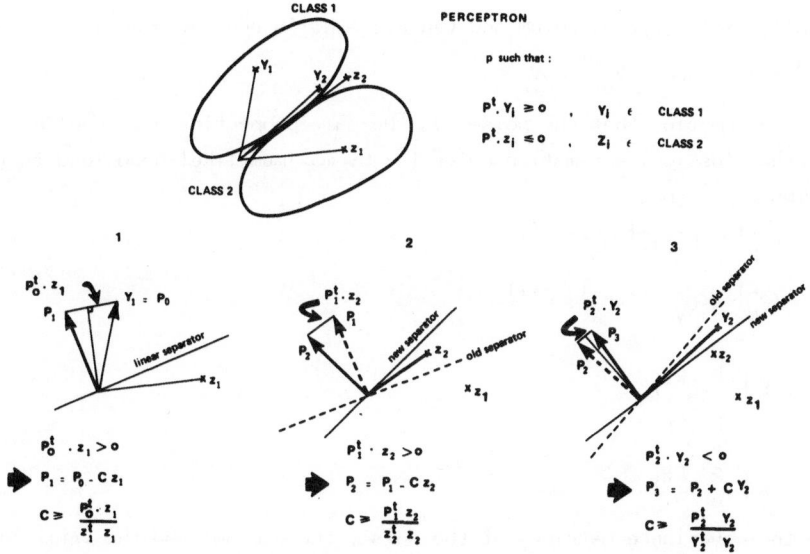

5.4. Estimating the temporal behaviours

The simplest method of supervised classification consists of giving the
prototypes of the temporal behaviours that are to be recognized. As the
scintigraphic sequence is made up from 16 images, each prototype is a 16-
dimensional vector. The vector associated to each pixel is then compared
to the prototypes.

The very root of the method is the acquirement of "good" prototypes. In
our case we restricted the study to three temporal behaviours characterizing
the atrium, the ventricle, and the background noise, respectively. To this
end three ROI's are defined. Our model presents :

- in the ROI of the noise : $N^{(i)}$, $(i = 1,...,n_N)$ the activity of the ith
noise pixel ;

- in the ROI of the atrium : $\omega^{(i)} = A_t^{(i)} + N^{(i)}$, $i = 1,...,n_A$
the activity of the ith atrium pixel ;

- in the ROI of the ventricle : $\zeta^{(i)} = V_e^{(i)} + N^{(i)}$, $i = 1, \ldots, n_V$
the activity of the ith ventricle pixel ;

where $N^{(i)}$, $\omega^{(i)}$, $\zeta^{(i)}$, $A_t^{(i)}$, and $V_e^{(i)}$ are n-uple vectors. Different
assumptions can be made on the homogeneity of these ROI's, leading to different optimal estimation schemes :

a) If all pixels of the atrium and ventricle ROI's are homogeneous, it comes :

$$A_t^{(i)} = A_t \quad \text{and} \quad V_e^{(i)} = V_e$$

With the assumption that the noise has the same properties all over the image, the classical estimation rules (8) by maximum likelihood lead to the following prototypes :

$$\hat{A}_t = (C_N^{-1} + C_{At}^{-1})^{-1} \, C_N^{-1} \, \omega^{(i)}$$
$$\hat{V}_e = (C_N^{-1} + C_{Ve}^{-1})^{-1} \, C_N^{-1} \, \zeta^{(i)}$$

5.4.1

where

$$C_N = E\{N^k \, N^{kt}\}$$
$$C_{At} = E\{A_t^k \, A^{kt}\}$$
$$C_{Ve} = E\{V_e^k \, V_e^{kt}\}$$

5.4.2

denote the covariance matrices of the noise, the atrium, and the ventricle, respectively.

b) If all pixels of the atrium and ventricle ROI's are not homogeneous, an average temporal behaviour can still be estimated from each ROI, using a recursive scheme :

$$\hat{A}_t^{(i)} = \hat{A}_t^{(i-1)} + D_1^{(i)} \, C_N^{-1} \, (\omega^{(i)} - \hat{A}_t^{(i-1)}), \quad i = 1, \ldots, n_A$$
$$\hat{V}_e^{(i)} = \hat{V}_e^{(i-1)} + D_2^{(i)} \, C_N^{-1} \, (\zeta^{(i)} - \hat{V}_e^{(i-1)}), \quad i = 1, \ldots, n_V$$

5.4.3

with :

$$D_1^{(i)} = \text{var}\{A_t^{(i)} - \hat{A}_t^{(i)}\} = (C_N^{-1} + D_1^{(i-1)})^{-1}$$
$$D_2^{(i)} = \text{var}\{V_e^{(i)} - \hat{V}_e^{(i)}\} = (C_N^{-1} + D_2^{(i-1)})^{-1}$$

5.4.4

where $\hat{A}_t^{(i)}$ denotes the estimate of $\hat{A}_t$ computed from the ith pixel of the ROI.

The two assumptions have been successively applied, and the corresponding estimates of the temporal behaviours of atrium and ventricle were found to show only slight differences. These estimates are used in the following implementations.

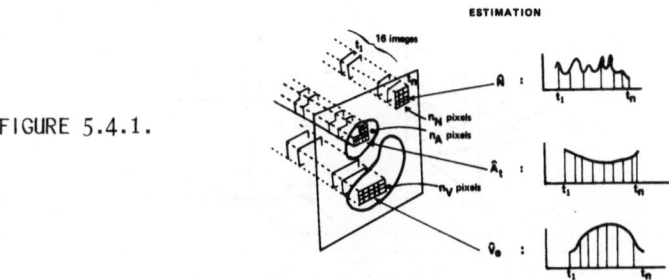

FIGURE 5.4.1.

5.5. <u>Supervised classification by cross-correlation</u>

Each pixel of the image is a vector (B) (see fig. 5.5.1). Its cross-correlation function with the estimated prototypes is given by :

$$C_A(t_j) = \sum_{i=1}^{n} B(t_i) \, \hat{A}_t \, (t_i - t_j)$$ 5.5.1

for example. The degree of resemblance of B and $\hat{A}_t$ is readily assessed by $C_A(0)$, which is the dot product of these vectors.

A decomposition of the pixel-vector B on the basis of the three estimated behaviours is obtained by the normalized coefficients :

$$a_1 = C_A(0) \, / \sqrt{C_A^2(0) + C_V^2(0) + C_N^2(0)\}}$$

$$a_2 = C_V(0) \, / \sqrt{C_A^2(0) + C_V^2(0) + C_N^2(0)\}}$$ 5.5.2

$$a_3 = C_N(0) \, / \sqrt{C_A^2(0) + C_V^2(0) + C_N^2(0)\}}$$

Three images are built from this decomposition ; each one represents the spatial fluctuations of one coefficient accross the whole image. Moreover the quality of the method is illustrated by the error-image, defined by the squared modulus of the difference between the sequence of successive activities of a pixel and the corresponding value reconstructed from the above coefficients :

$$\epsilon^2 = \sum_{i=1}^{-n} \left| B(t_i) - \sum_{j=1}^{3} A_j \, V \, (t_i) \right|^2$$ 5.5.3

with $V = \hat{A}_t, \hat{V}_e$ and $\hat{N}$. This quantity is computed for each pixel.

214

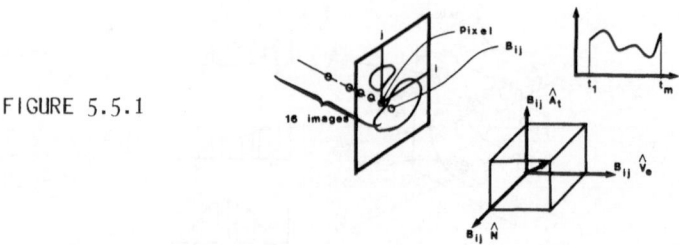

CORRELATION

FIGURE 5.5.1

5.6. Positive components

The feature vectors are the estimated temporal behaviours registered in a previous section. The positivity constraint stems from a double consideration : (1) only physiological factors are allowed in describing the activity vector, V, of each pixel ; (2) this activity is the sum of these registered factors, with positive coefficients. One has to find an estimate, $\hat{V}$, of V, such that :

$$\hat{V} = \sum_{i=1}^{I} w_i \, C_i, \text{ with } |V - \hat{V}|^2 = \min \qquad\qquad 5.6.1$$

where I denotes the total number of factors C_i, and w_i must satisfy :

$$w_i > 0 \qquad\qquad 5.6.2$$

The fulfilement of the positivity constraint is readily achieved by letting :

$$w_i = \alpha_1^2 \qquad\qquad 5.6.3$$

Then, define the unknowns vector X whose components are the $\{\alpha_i\}$, and F the equations vector :

$$F = \begin{cases} |V(t_1) - \sum_{i=1}^{I} a_i^2 \, C_i(t_1)|^2 \\ \quad\cdot \\ \quad\cdot \\ |V(t_n) - \sum_{i=1}^{I} a_i^2 \, C_i(t_n)|^2 \end{cases}, \quad X = \begin{cases} \alpha_1 \\ \alpha_2 \\ \alpha_3 \end{cases} \qquad 5.6.4$$

This set of non linear equations is written :

$$F(X) = 0 \qquad\qquad 5.6.5$$

.t is solved by a classical Newton-Raphson iterative technique, which starts from an initial condition :

$$F(X_0) \neq 0 \qquad 5.6.6$$

and define, by a Taylor expansion :

$$F(X_0 + \Delta X) \simeq 0 \qquad 5.6.7$$

giving :

$$\Delta X = - \left(\frac{\partial F}{\partial X}\right)^t \left(\frac{\partial F}{\partial X}\right)^{-1} \left(\frac{\partial F}{\partial X}\right)^t F(X_0) \qquad 5.6.8$$

that allows the iterative process until (5.6.7) is satisfied. As a result it is possible to decompose the activity of a pixel as a sum of estimated factors with positive weights. Notice that in this case (see fig. 5.6.1) the solution does not always exist, and that the error, eventhough minimal, can be very important. The comfort brought to the image interpreter by handling physiologically designed factors is obviously impaired by the rising of the quadratic error initiated by the positivity constraint.

FIGURE 5.6.1

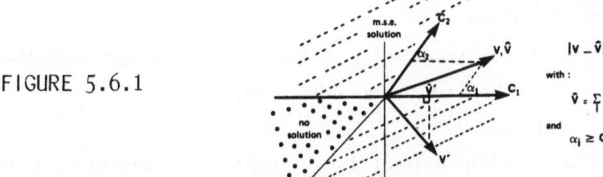

5.7. Gram-Schmidt

The factors estimated from the ROI's are not orthogonal. The quadratic error committed when using this oblique basis can be reduced, and the data can be reconstructed with a better accuracy. To this end one has, first, to relax the positivity constraint, and, second, to allow the basis to be orthogonal (see fig. 5.7.1). Starting from the oblique basis (A_t, V_e, N), an orthogonal basis (G_1, G_2, G_3) is obtained by the Gram-Schmidt process (9) :

$$G_1 = A_t$$

$$G_2 = V_e - \frac{A_t^t V_e}{A_t^t A_t} A_t \qquad 5.7.1$$

$$G_3 = N - \frac{A_t^t N}{A_t^t A_t} A_t - \frac{G_2^t N}{G_2^t G_2} G_2$$

The philosophy of this transformation is the following : The vector G_1 is identical to the first factor ; consequently, because of the correlation of the factors that make up the oblique basis, we expect to find significant components of almost all the pixels upon this "new" basis vector. The vector G_2 represents what in V_e is orthogonal to G_1 (i.e. $\dot{A}_t$). It will be specific, and located on the ventricular area of the heart as well as the other areas which have the same behaviour. A simple rule proceeds from this remark : choose as the first vector of the orthogonalized basis the factors you are not interested in.

The activity vector V of each pixel becomes :

$$V = \sum_{i=1}^{I} \gamma_i \, G_i, \text{ with : } \quad \gamma_i = G_i \, t \, V \qquad\qquad 5.7.2$$

As the coefficients γ_i are no longer positive, the quadratic error :

$$|V - \sum_{i=1}^{I} \gamma_i \, C_i|^2 \qquad\qquad 5.7.3$$

is allowed to take a lowest value.

When compared to the positive components technique, the Gram-Schmidt orthogonalized basis presents the following advantages :

- it is computed once and for all ;

- the coefficients of a pixel are given by a simple, dot product, without any recursion ;

- the quadratic error is lower ;

- the orthogonal factors specifically match the temporal behaviours (because of the retention of their orthogonal parts).

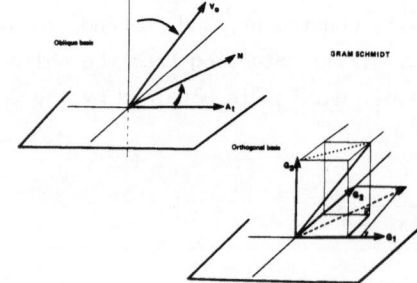

FIGURE 5.7.1

6. RESULTS - DISCUSSION

The different methods have been applied to 21 patients. All the corresponding acquired sequences have been smoothed using a spatial filter 3 x 3 points with weighting, and zoomed. The last two images of each sequence are kept or not, according to the mean energy of the first 14 images.

The processed images produced by the different methods have been discussed according to three criteria :
- the contour accuracy ;
- the evidencing of the regions of superimposition ;
- the capacity of analyzing wall motion abnormalities.

The first criterion has been implemented by rating the images given by each method by 1 or 0, depending on their ability of separating left and right ventricles at the lowest part of the septum. The results are summarized in table 1 :

	F	KL	PERC	GS	COR	PC
EDGE RATE/21	7	7	1	20	1	20

As to the problem of the regions of overlapping, the capacity of sorting the left and right atria from their respective ventricles is rated 1 or 0 as the extracted contours correspond or not to those, whose location is determined in sequential mode (Table 2) :

	F	KL	PER	GS	COR	PC
OVERLAPPING AREA RATE/21	0	0	3	21	0	21

The third criterion first refers to the capacity of pointing a wall motion abnormality -without taking into account its magnitude- with respect to the reference angiography. The performances have been studied on all the patients in order to determine the sensitivity and the specificity of the methods (Table 3) :

	ANG	F	KL	PER	GS	COR	PC
Normals	3	5	3	3	3	3	3
Abnormals	18	16	17	15	12	14	14
Sensitivy		88%	94%	83%	66%	77%	77%

Then the capacity of the methods of assessing the magnitude of the wall
motion abnormalities has been studied with respect to the reference angiography (Table 4). Notice that because of the possible difference between
the incidences in angiography and scintigraphy, some abnormalities attested
by one investigation may not be seen by the other.

	ANG	F	KL	PER	GS	COR	PC
NK	3	3 1 1	3 1	3 2 1	3 3 1 2	3 3 1	3 3 1
HK	4	3 3	3 4	0	1 7 2	2 3	1 7 2
AK	9	5 2	5 1	1	1	2	1 2
DK	5	3	4	2 7 5	1	2 5	1

Examples of the results obtained with different methods are shown next
page for a patient with an antero-septal dyskinesis and lateral and apico-
lateral hypokinesis (a : KL image – b : F.K – c : Per. – d : G.S – e : COR.
f : P.C).

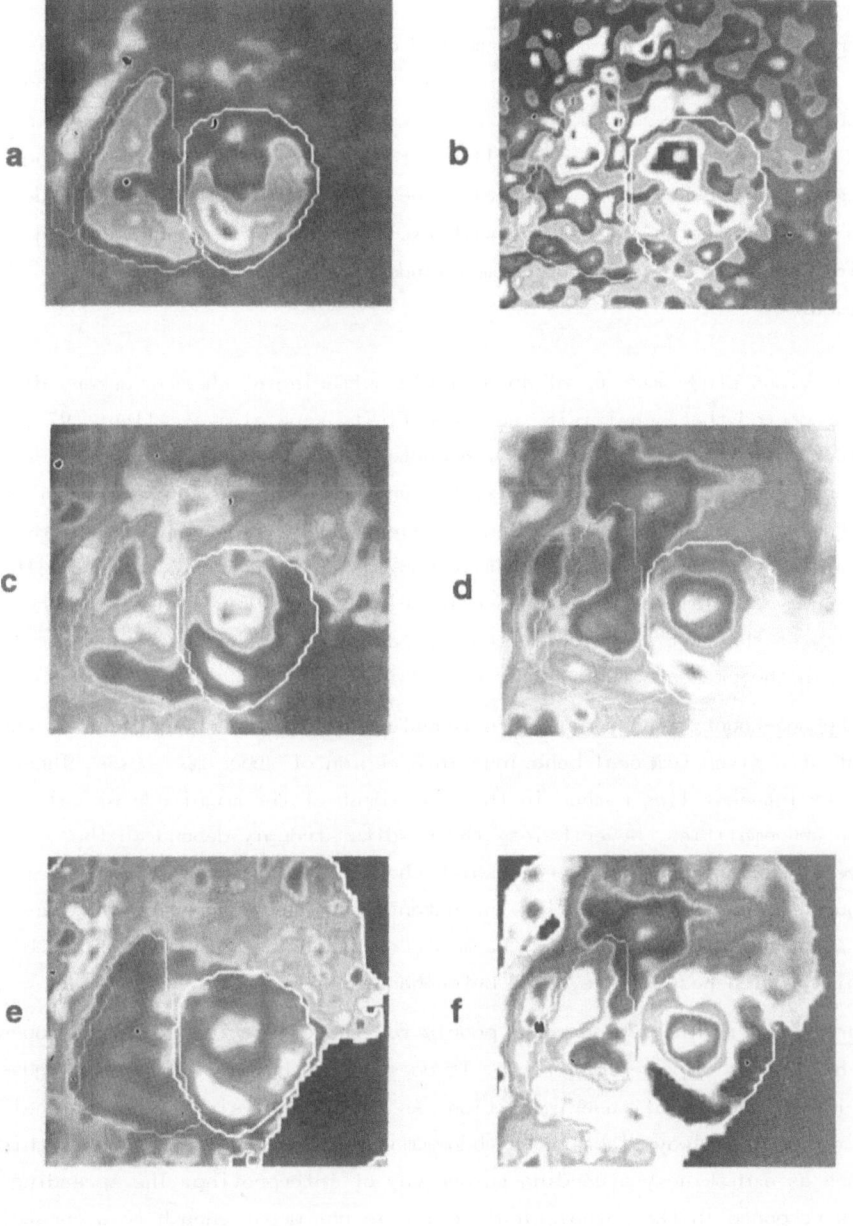

Discussion

Karhunen-Loeve transform : This method does not well determine ventricular and atrial contours, and does not evidence the regions of superimposition. As the processed images it produces carry most of the temporal information in the sequence, it is allowed to classify each pixel according
to its temporal behaviours. Especially the first principal image, KL1, detects the wall motion abnormality with excellent specificity (100 %) and
sensitivity (94 %). Moreover, the magnitude of the abnormality is well
assessed.

A previous study made up of 46 patients suffering of chronic artery disease reported that sensitivity and specificity were also excellent (97 %
and 100 % respectively). This study reported that the matching with the
reference angiography is about 85 %. KL1 underestimated the intensity of
regional wall motion abnormality in 3 patients suffering from inferior myocardial infarction. One false negative was observed also in a patient with
inferior myocardial infarction whose inferior segment was akinetic on the
RAO view of the left ventricular contrast angiography. We note the same
things in the present study.(10)

Fukunaga-Koontz transform : This transform allows the recognition of the
amount of a given temporal behaviour in a region of superimposition. Therefore its interest lies rather in the assessment of the magnitude of wall
motion abnormalities. Nevertheless the results strongly depend on the
choice of the regions of interest which characterize the two temporal behaviours to be recognized. Being inconstant, this method applies in a second step for the refinement of the measurement of the magnitude of an abnormality which has been revealed beforehand.

Perceptron : This method works poorly for the extraction of the contours
and the regions of superimposition. It does not much improve the image quality in the regions of superimposition. As to the analysis of the regional
wall motion, it always labels the abnormality as an atrial behaviour ; this
appears as a diskinesy according to our way of interpreting. The spreading
of its response in the pathological region is not great enough to accurately
assess the magnitude of the abnormality. Because of its rapidity, this method desserves to be improved, e.g. by introducing a 3-class problem scheme
(atrium, ventricle, background), and by sharpening the training set.

Positive components and Gram-Schmidt : Both methods give almost the same results. They work well for the evidencing the contours of atrium and ventricle, which appear well individualized in their respective associated images —even in the regions of superimposition. All the normal patients are recognized as normal, but there are some false negatives. In the other cases, these methods allow the recognition of the extension of the abnormalities, but without being able to specify their magnitude, which is generally undervalued despite the use of the time/activity curves. The results obtained for the analysis of the regional wall motion are still insufficient ; they should be improved after modifying the estimates of the temporal behaviours. These methods are of interest when designing a program for the automatic recognition of contours (the needed training curves being also automatically matched to the temporal behaviours). As to the choice between the two methods, it appears that Gram-Schmidt presents a lowest computational burden.

Correlation : The results are comparable in the aggregate with those obtained by Fourier or Karhunen-Loeve ; but the sensitivity in the assessment of the magnitude of the abnormalities is lower.

CONCLUSION

Comparing the different methods according to the above defined criteria, it appears that the Karhunen-Loeve transform is the most sensitive to the magnitude of the wall motion abnormalities. Paradoxically the supervised methods, which need a training, do not well assess the magnitude of these abnormalities. This result do not solely originate from the difficulties the operator encounters when determining the training areas. It also proceeds from the fact that these methods emphasize the activity of the pixel to the detriment of the shape of its temporal behaviour.

As to the determination of the extension of the regions of superimposition, the Positive Components and Gram-Schmidt lead to a better delimitation of the region under study. About the supervised methods, the performances can be improved by imposing a constraint upon the shape and amplitude of the temporal variations. They will therefore be well suited to the automatic determination of contours.

REFERENCES

1. Andrews HC. 1972. Introduction to mathematical techniques in pattern recognition. Ed. Wiley - Interscience.
2. Watanabe S. 1965. Karhunen-Loeve expansion and factor analysis. Trans. 4th Prague. Conf. Information Theory.
3. Verdenet J, Cardot JC, Baud M et al. 1983. A computer program for compression of dynamic studies. Computer Programs in Biomedicine, 1983, 16, 77-82.
4. Fukunaga K. 1972. Introduction to statistical pattern recognition. Ed. Academic Press.
5. Verdenet J, Cardot JC, Baud M et al. 1983. La transformation de Fukunaga-Koontz appliquée aux gammacinéangiographies à l'équilibre. Colloque de Médecine Nucléaire de Langue Française, Luxembourg.
6. Verdenet J, Cardot JC, Baud M et al. 1982. Apport de la transformation de Fukunaga-Koontz dans la détermination des zones de superposition des cavités cardiaques en imagerie nucléaire. Colloque National G.B.M. Toulouse.
7. Tou JT, Gonsalez RC. 1974. Pattern recognition principles. Ed. Addison-Wesley Pub. Co.
8. Van Trees HL. 1968. Detection, estimation and modulation theory. Ed. John Wiley.
9. Strang G. 1976. Linear algebra and its applications. Ed. Academic Press.
10. Berthout P, Cardot JC, Faivre R et al. 1983. Apport de la transformation de Karhunen-Loeve à l'analyse de la cinétique ventriculaire gauche. Colloque de Médecine Nucléaire de Langue Française, Luxembourg.

Acknowledgments : We are indebted to H. Dupraz for his expert assistance in the english translation, M.L. Allemandet for her expert secretarial assistance and E. Bernard for performing radionuclide imaging.

A COMPARATIVE REVIEW OF METHODS OF OBTAINING AMPLITUDE/PHASE AND RELATED
IMAGES FOR GATED CARDIAC STUDIES

A.S. HOUSTON AND M.A. MACLEOD

1. INTRODUCTION

In recent years, single-harmonic Fourier amplitude/phase imaging has
been used extensively in the analysis of gated cardiac studies (e.g. 1-6).
However, doubt has been cast on the validity of the method since the
underlying assumption that pixel curves (dixels) may be approximated by
one harmonic of a Fourier series is not generally true (7-10).

Several alternatives, which attempt to overcome this criticism, have
been postulated. These include parametric images, related to amplitude
and phase, based on multi-harmonic curve-fitting (8, 9), and the use of
transformations to enable easier interpretation of images obtained from
factor analysis (10,11).

In this study, these alternatives are compared with the original
method and with each other using both statistical and perceptional
considerations.

2. MATERIALS AND METHODS

2.1. Data collection

Gated cardiac studies are performed in the anterior, LAO, and
(occasionally) RAO positions using a Siemens LFOV camera (later upgraded
to ZLC) interfaced to a Nodecrest NMS-80 minicomputer. A bolus of
890MBq (24mCi) of 99m-Tc-pertechnetate is injected using semi-in vitro
labelling (12). Five million counts (10 million for ZLC) are collected
with a temporal resolution of 16 frames/cycle and stored in a 32x32 array
covering one-quarter of the available field of view.

Several different techniques were used to produce amplitude/phase
images for 32 patients including 16 normals. The 16 abnormal studies
were chosen as a representative sample of the various pathologies which
present, including hypokinesis, aneurysm, and valvular incompetence.
Both normal and abnormal groups contained 10 studies obtained on the

original LFOV (5 million counts) and 6 obtained with the ZLC upgrade (10 million counts). Only one RAO view, obtained on a normal control on the original LFOV, was included.

2.2. Techniques compared

2.2.1. Single-harmonic Fourier analysis. This method (1-6) assumes that each dixel can be approximated by the first harmonic of a Fourier series, i.e.

$d(t) = a/2 + b \cos (wt) + c \sin (wt)$ $(0 \leqslant wt < 2\pi)$

or, in polar form,

$d(t) = a/2 + r \cos (wt-p)$

where a is a mean value, r is amplitude, and p is phase.

Amplitude and phase images are formed by displaying the spatial distribution of parameters r and p.

2.2.2. Multi-harmonic Fourier analysis. This method (8, 9) allows the use of higher harmonics in the Fourier series i.e.

$d(t) = a/2 + r_1 \cos (wt-p_1) + r_2 \cos (wt-p_2) + ----$

Amplitude may then be defined as the difference between maximum and minimum values on the fitted curve, while phase may be considered equivalent to time-to-maximum (or minimum) on a cyclic scale.

For the purposes of this study, two, three and four harmonics were compared, as was the use of either definition of phase. The method of weighting higher harmonics (8) was also considered. In this case four harmonics were given weights 1.0, .853, .5 and .146, the aim being to reduce the effect of oscillations caused by higher harmonics.

2.2.3. Factorial amplitude/phase imaging. The first two (or some-times three) non-trivial components of a factor analysis (13) are generated and compared with cosine and sine functions. In a manner analogous to the single-harmonic Fourier case, a polar transformation of the co-efficients of cosine and sine-like components yields factorial amplitude and phase images (10).

The training set used to generate the components was formed in one of two ways:

(a) by using dixels from the study under examination only; or,

(b) by using dixels from a fixed series of studies, which may or may not include the study under examination.

In case (a), the matrix size was reduced to 16x16 by combining 2x2 blocks. Regions were drawn round the heart in all views and dixels within these regions combined to form the training set.

In case (b), eight studies (5 normals, one hypokinesis, one aneurysm, and one valvular incompetence) obtained on the original LFOV were used. Only anterior and LAO views were included, thus producing a total of 16 views. The matrix size was reduced to 8x8 by combining 4x4 blocks. Again, a region was drawn round the heart in each view and dixels within the regions combined.

The two methods will be referred to as factor (a) and factor (b).

2.2.4. <u>Factorial images obtained using an oblique transformation</u>. An oblique transformation (11) is applied to the initial components of a factor analysis to produce factors and co-efficients which contain no negative values. Since physiological curves always demonstrate this property, these factors may be thought of as the underlying physiological factors which combine to form each dixel. Hence, each factorial image, formed from the appropriate co-efficient distribution, may be regarded as the contribution of the corresponding physiological factor (11, 14, 15). As in the previous case, two different methods ((a) and (b)) were used to form the training set.

3. METHODS OF COMPARISON

3.1. <u>General comments</u>

It was felt that the comparison of the various methods should concentrate on phase images rather than amplitude images. From the literature (1-10), it appeared that these were more frequently used for diagnostic purposes. Also, from a statistical viewpoint, it was felt that certain parameters which could be derived from phase images, such as standard deviation across the left ventricle, would be more useful in a comparison than any equivalent amplitude parameter.

Several problems arose concerning the oblique factor images. First of all, it was decided to use two components in their generation. The use of the first two components was compared with the use of cosine and sine-like components when these were not the same. With two components, each view will produce three oblique factors with corresponding factor images. Although these may be combined using different colours for each factor and different brightnesses for each co-efficient range, it was not felt that our display could supply sufficient variation in each colour to produce good quality images. Hence, each factor image was viewed independently. As such, it was decided that no statistical parameter could be derived for this method, and it was not included in the observer experiment.

3.2. Subjective comparison

Before the various methods were subjected to a statistical analysis and observer trials, the images were first examined by the author (ASH), who did not subsequenly take part in the trials. Any obvious anomalies were examined and an explanation attempted. Points specifically examined included goodness-of-fit of individual dixels (although this parameter was not quantified), uniqueness of parameters such as time-to-maximum for a multi-harmonic fit, the occurrence of cosine and sine-like factors among the principal components, and the oblique factors and factor images. The latter were given special attention since this method did not figure subsequenly in the experiments.

The influence of factors such as count statistics and pathology on the occurrence of anomalies was also considered.

3.3. Statistical analysis

For the purposes of a statistical analysis, only points within the left ventricle on the phase image were used. The left ventricle was defined in each case by drawing a region on a view summed over the cardiac cycle.

Several parameters were then derived for each phase image, including mean phase (m) and population standard deviation (s). A perfect cosine curve peaking at frame 1 was defined to have zero phase. In the calculation of mean phase, all phases were defined to lie in the range $180^\circ < p \leqslant 180^\circ$. In the definition of standard deviation, no deviation from the mean was allowed to exceed 180°. As a means of determining if real, structured, phase variations occurred, the auto-covariance function, $A(d)$, was calculated as a function of distance between pixels. It should be noted, however, that this function will also contain the effects of noise texture (16), and should therefore be treated with caution. In order to obtain adequate statistics, distances were divided into one pixel ranges, so that d=1 corresponded to 0.5 to 1.5 pixels, d=2 to 1.5 to 2.5 etc. In particular, $A(0)=s$ and $A(1)$ is the co-variance between adjacent (including diagonally adjacent) pixels.

Initially, these parameters were derived for the 5 normal studies included in the composite training set used for factor (b). Since, for a given patient position, these may reasonably be considered to be from the same sample, it is valid to combine the variances to produce an estimate of the normal population standard deviation. Combining values of A(d), however, is not valid, particularly for large values of d, since different left ventricular (LV) sizes would tend to cancel out any systematic effects. A reasonable argument could be made, however, for combining values of A(1), producing a composite value for the co-variance between adjacent pixels. The ratio $r = A(1)/A(0)$, where these are composite values, will be referred to as "structure", it being a measure of the non-randomness of adjacent pixels (although it will clearly contain a noise contribution which could be large).

From these values, it may be possible to eliminate certain methods at an early stage, particularly if they produce very high standard deviations with little or no apparent "structure".

Composite values of s and r were then calculated for each remaining method in each of the following groups:

(i)   10 normals obtained in anterior view using 5 million counts;

(ii)   6 normals obtained in anterior view using 10 million counts;

(iii) 10 normals obtained in LAO view using 5 million counts;

(iv)   6 normals obtained in LAO view using 10 million counts;

Individual values of s and r were obtained using each method for all views of abnormal patients and for the single RAO view.

The mean value ($\bar{m}$) and population standard deviation (m_s) of the mean phase over the left ventricle was calculated for each position using the 16 normal studies.

3.4. Observer trials

All methods remaining after the initial elimination process (5 in total) were included in a perception experiment. A single observer (MAM) was presented with a randomly ordered series of Polaroid films, each containing four images. These were the anterior and LAO phase images of two patients, each obtained, for simplicity, using the same method. A cyclic scale with 30 colour levels was used to display the images. The LV outline, used in the statistical analysis, was superimposed on each image. In all 80 Polaroids (16 per method) were presented. The observer

was informed that 50% of the images were of normal patients and was
asked to rate the pairs of images (anterior and LAO) according to a standard
rating system (17), i.e.

1. Almost certainly normal;

2. Probably normal;

3. Equivocal

4. Probably abnormal

5. Almost certainly abnormal;

The observer was asked further to classify suspected abnormals (rated
4 or 5) into one of the following classes:

A. Wall motion defect (hypokinesis)

B. Wall motion defect (aneurysm)

C. Filling and/or emptying defect (shunt, valvular incompetence etc.)

Patients were also classified clinically into one of these categories
by studying case histories at least two months post-examination. It was
necessary to include a category AB for four cases of hypokinesis, two
with suspected aneurysms and two with small aneurysms confirmed by
angiography and ventriculography.

The observer ratings were then analysed using receiver operating
characteristic (ROC) analysis (e.g. 18-20), while the number of correct
pathology classifications for each method was also calculated. A sample
size of 32 is clearly too small for definitive conclusions to be reached,
but it was hoped that some useful indications might be revealed as a
prelude to further perception experiments involving larger sample sizes
and more observers.

4. RESULTS

4.1. Subjective comparison

An examination of curves fitted to dixels using the various methods
revealed that only the single-harmonic Fourier could be regarded as a
poor fit. For all regions of importance such as the left ventricle, two,
three and four (weighted) harmonics gave acceptable fits, while four
harmonics (unweighted) showed a slight tendency to follow pixel noise for
studies obtained using 5 million counts. Fig. 1 shows a typical LV
dixel for such a study with fits obtained from one, two, three and four
unweighted harmonics.

Examples of phase images for the anterior view obtained using four
methods are shown in Fig. 2. The methods involved are single-harmonic

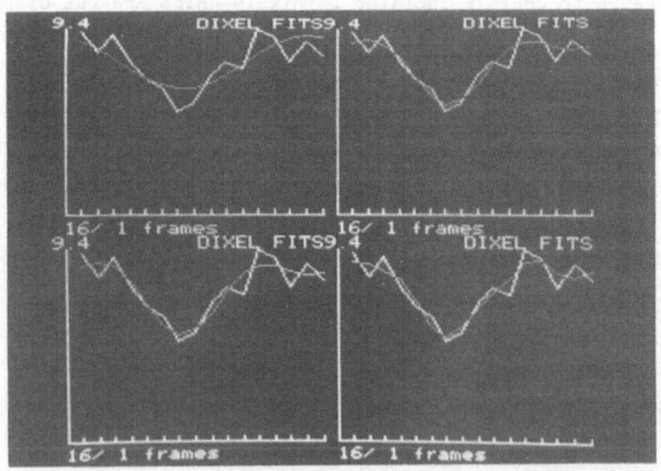

FIGURE 1. A typical LV dixel with fits obtained using 1 (upper left),
2 (upper right), 3 (lower left), and 4 unweighted harmonics.

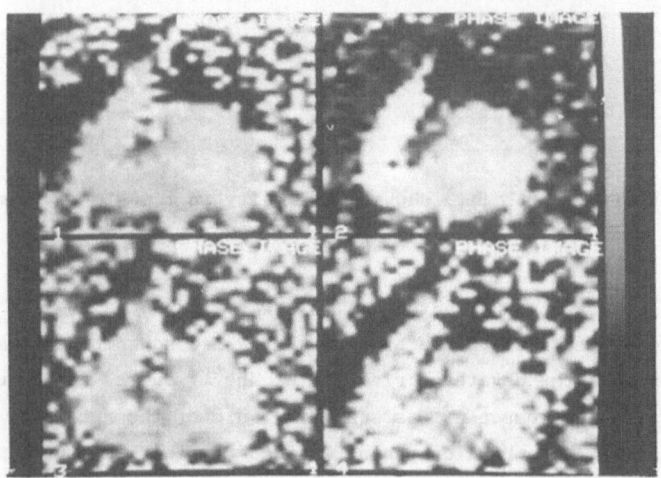

FIGURE 2. Phase images obtained using 1 harmonic (upper left), factor (a)
(upper right), 4 harmonics weighted (time-to-min.) (lower left), and 4
harmonics weighted (time-to-max.).

Fourier, factor (a), and 4 harmonics weighted (times to min. and max.).
The latter appears to contain isolated LV pixels which are out of phase
with their neighbours. An examination of such a pixel curve (with fit)
reveals an ambiguity regarding the time-to-maximum (Fig. 3). This
problem occurred frequently when time-to-maximum methods were used.
Fourier methods produced greater noise outside the cardiac region than
did factorial methods, particularly when more than one harmonic was used
(see Fig. 2). Since these regions can be masked off, this is not
regarded as a major disadvantage.

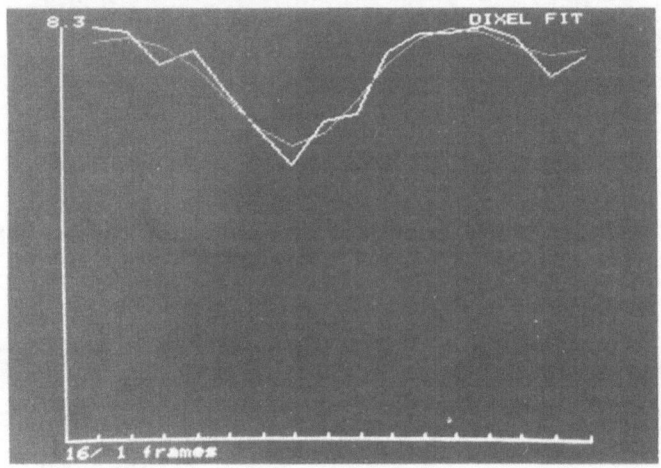

FIGURE 3. LV dixel (with fit) showing ambiguity in time-to-maximum.

The first component of a factor analysis was always cosine-like but
contained the asymmetries of the LV curve. The second component was
sine-like (or like the negated derivative of the LV curve) in 25 out of
32 cases. The third component was sine-like in 6 of the remaining cases.
For the last case, the third component was deemed sine-like purely because
it was more so than the second component. Examples of cosine and sine-
like components, including the rogue example, are shown in Fig. 4. Of
the seven cases where the third component was used, only two (including
the rogue) were abnormal patients, and three (again including the rogue)
were obtained using 10 million counts. Furthermore, the components, in
general, seemed to be no less noisy for normal compared to abnormal, or
for high counts compared to low counts.

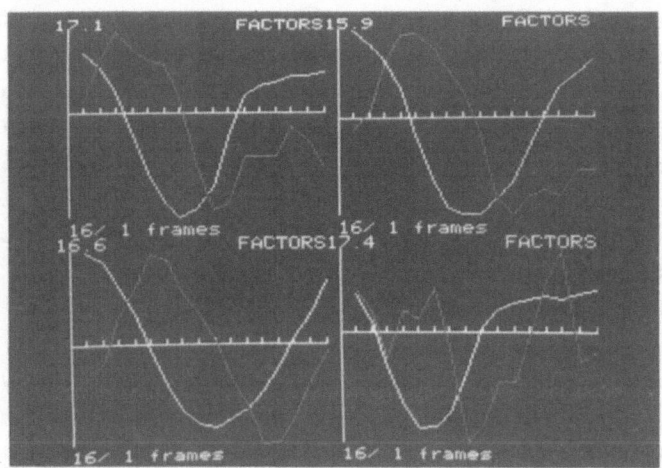

FIGURE 4. Cosine and sine-like components obtained in four cases. The rogue example is on the lower right.

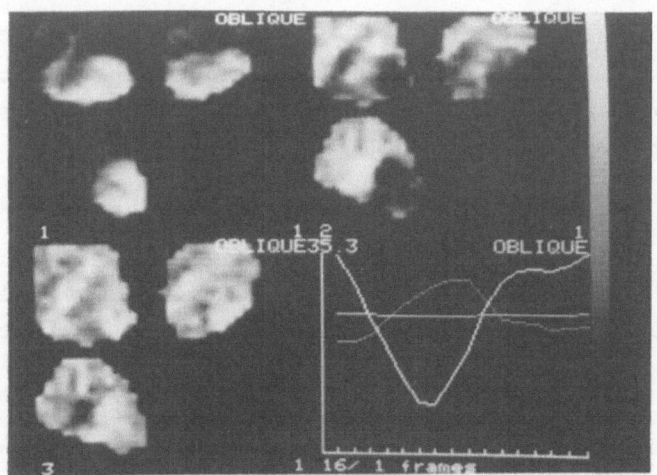

FIGURE 5. Oblique factors and factor images for a normal study:
The LV factor images are shown in the upper left quadrant, the inverse LV factor images in the upper right, and the background factor[*] images in the lower left. The three images in these quadrants correspond to anterior, LAO, and RAO views.[*] ERRATUM: The background factor has subsequently been found to be due to a programming error. The third factor is, in fact, different from patient to patient and generally represents a third phase value. The first two factors and the three factor images are unaffected by this error, except that the third image does not correspond to background.

The oblique factors for a normal patient are shown in Fig. 5. In every case, these took the form of an LV factor, an inverse LV factor peaking fractionally after end-systole, and a background factor. The factor images corresponding to these factors are also shown in Fig. 5. In the cases where the third component was sine-like, the first two components produced better results than the first and third. However, two cases, where the factors were slightly irregular, belonged to this group. A parameter corresponding to ejection fraction could be calculated from the LV factor. Since this varied from 34% to 100% in normals and from 9% to 100% in abnormals, it did not appear to be related, in any way, to LV ejection fraction.

When a composite training set was used (as in factor (b)), the oblique factors were similar to those in Fig. 5, except that the LV factor had a minimum value close to zero. The advantage of using a composite set is that factor images from different patients can be directly related, while the disadvantage is that the factors might be unrepresentative of cases where the LV curve is dissimilar in shape to the LV factor.

4.2. Statistical analysis

Composite values of LV phase standard deviation (s) and "structure" (r) for 5 normal studies are shown in Table 1 for 11 methods. Results for the single RAO study are included.

Table 1. Values of s and r for 5 normal studies.

	Factor			Time-to-maximum					Time-to-minimum			
	(a)	(b)	1h	2h	3h	4h	4hw	2h	3h	4h	4hw
Ant											
s	15.0	14.7	12.8	39.8	39.4	41.8	35.8	15.7	21.8	24.6	18.3
r	7.2	7.2	4.8	6.7	-0.7	-2.7	1.5	6.0	4.0	6.7	4.1
LAO											
s	20.2	19.8	16.4	42.8	44.4	43.6	40.0	16.8	23.7	25.1	19.8
r	10.3	3.9	6.9	-5.5	-5.1	-2.3	-7.3	9.1	5.6	8.5	7.1
RAO	(one study)										
s	18.2	16.9	14.9	41.7	40.0	39.9	36.6	18.0	21.8	24.3	19.0
r	41.7	33.3	31.4	0.0	3.4	6.2	4.1	19.2	8.2	10.2	13.8

N.B. nh denotes the use of n harmonics, while w implies weighted.

r is expressed as a percentage.

It is clear that time-to-maximum methods give the largest standard deviations and, in general, the lowest "structure" values. This is almost entirely due to the fact that time-to-maximum is ill-defined in many studies. It was decided at this stage to omit these methods. Of the remainder, time-to-minimum methods using 3 and 4 harmonics (unweighted) consistently produce the largest standard deviations without any significant improvement in "structure". Because of this, it was decided to omit those methods, thus restricting the number of methods for subsequent analysis to five.

The large values of r for the single RAO study are interesting. However, the results of a single study cannot be considered in any way significant, and indeed, a subsequent normal LAO study, obtained admittedly using 10 million counts, gave values of the same magnitude.

The values of s and r for all normal studies are shown in Table 2. The studies are grouped as defined in section 3.3.

Table 2. Values of s and r for all normal studies.

| | Five million counts (10 studies) | | | | | Ten million counts (6 studies) | | | | |
| | Factor | | | Time-to-min | | Factor | | | Time-to-min | |
	(a)	(b)	1h	2h	4hw	(a)	(b)	1h	2h	4hw
Ant										
s	16.6	15.4	13.3	14.3	16.7	16.6	16.0	13.9	14.6	16.6
r	11.5	10.5	11.2	9.6	8.2	20.1	8.3	7.6	13.8	13.2
LAO										
s	23.1	21.1	17.0	18.3	21.2	22.2	21.3	16.2	21.3	23.7
r	9.1	6.8	8.3	9.6	6.5	18.3	13.9	17.1	3.0	2.7

Surprisingly, there appears to be little difference between the standard deviations obtained using different count levels, although it should be stressed that the change in count level coincided with a gamma camera upgrade. For the only patient repeated in the full sample (a normal collected at both count levels), s was greater using ten million counts for every method and patient position.

From Table 2 it is seen that the single-harmonic Fourier method gave the lowest value of s in every case, while factor (a) produced relatively high values of r. Whether this is due to inherent phase structure being revealed, or whether the method merely produces large noise blobs, is not known at present.

Table 3 shows the mean and standard deviation for 16 normals of the average phase across the left ventricle.

Table 3. Values of $\bar{m}$ and m_s for 16 normals

| | Factor | | | Time-to-minimum | |
	(a)	(b)	1h	2h	4hw
Ant					
$\bar{m}$	-3.8	-12.8	-41.1	-46.8	-44.4
m_s	2.9	21.8	19.2	20.6	21.3
LAO					
$\bar{m}$	-2.3	-8.2	-39.0	-44.5	-41.7
m_s	6.0	23.9	19.0	18.6	19.8

Clearly, $\bar{m}$ is closest to zero for factor (a), which also has the lowest values of m_s. The former will result in a systematic phase shift for the other methods and is of little importance. However, a large value of m_s will result in colour differences among normal left ventricles, a situation which has been reported (10). This non-uniformity among normals could clearly lead to confusion. While it might be possible to reduce this effect by calculation LV curve assymetries and adjusting the phase values accordingly, this will involve more processing time.

Let us define the normal range of each parameter to be the actual range of values found for the 16 normal studies. Standard deviations lay outside the normal range for the five cases involving an aneurysm and for six out of nine cases of hypokinesis using every method. Two cases of hypokinesis had values of s within the normal range for all methods. The remaining case showed s outside the normal range in the LAO view every time, but inside in the anterior view for all methods except the double-harmonic where it was marginally outside. Insufficient clinical data was available to explain this situation. For the two cases of valvular incompetence, one had values of s close to the normal limit in both views, while the other showed normal in the anterior view and close to the limit in the LAO. This was consistent with the fact that the incompetence concerned the aortic valve in the former case, and the mitral valve in the latter. The various Fourier methods seemed to be marginally superior to the factorial methods in discriminating valvular incompetence from normal using LV standard deviations.

Although "structure" values were increased in some abnormals, this parameter did not appear to be very useful in discriminating either normal from abnormal or among the three pathological classes. Values of r were generally greatest using factor (a) for both normals and abnormals.

Not unexpectedly, mean phase was a poor discriminatory parameter. However, for factor (a), 10 abnormals in the anterior view and 12 in the LAO lay outside the normal range, suggesting that the small normal range found using this method might be useful diagnostically.

4.3. Observer trials

The results of the ROC experiment are shown in Fig. 6. No curve fits have been attempted. No false positives were found at levels 3 and 4, and only 3 overall were found at level 3. Therefore, for clarity, only the maximum true positive rate corresponding to a zero false positive rate is shown for each method in Fig. 6. Because of the small sample size and the lack of false positives at levels 5, 4, and 3, there is little conclusion to be drawn, except perhaps that the single-harmonic Fourier method might be poorest.

Table 4 shows the numbers of each pathology detected (Dt) and correctly classified (Cl) at the 4 or 5 level. Class AB was considered to be correctly classified if either A or B was reported.

Table 4. Classification of pathology.

| | | Factor | | | | | | Time-to-minimum | | |
| | | (a) | (b) | | 1h | | 2h | | 4hw | |
	No.	Dt Cl	Dt Cl		Dt Cl		Dt Cl		Dt Cl	
A	9	5 3	5 2		3 0		6 2		5 1	
AB	4	4 3	4 4		4 4		4 2		4 2	
B	1	1 0	1 0		1 0		1 0		1 0	
C	2	0 0	0 0		0 0		0 0		0 0	
Total	16	10 6	10 6		8 4		11 4		10 3	

All cases where an aneurysm was confirmed or suspected were detected as abnormal at the 4 or 5 level using every method; both cases of valvular incompetence were always missed (although these were usually picked up at the 2 or 3 level); while the detection of hypokinesis had a moderate

degree of success. The factorial methods gave slightly better classification than the Fourier methods, but clearly larger sample sizes are
necessary for confirmation, or otherwise, of these findings.

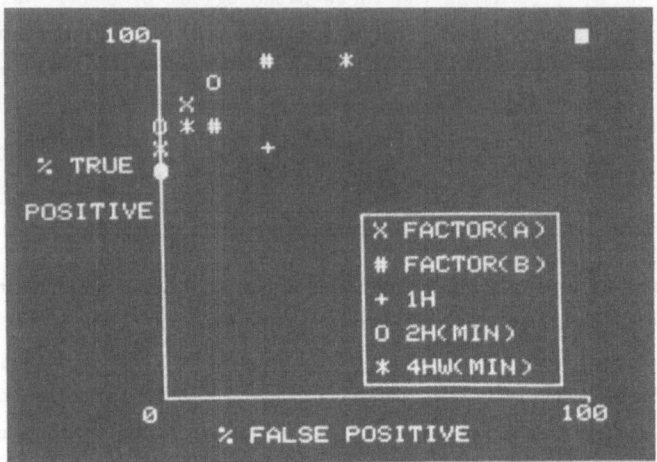

FIGURE 6. ROC analysis comparing five methods.

5. CONCLUSION

Of the various methods considered, time-to-maximum imaging following
multi-harmonic dixel-fitting gave the poorest results, due to the fact
that maximum dixel value, in the presence of noise, is not restricted to
a small range of possible values. Time-to-minimum imaging gave better
results, especially when only two harmonics were used, or when the
harmonics were appropriately weighted. However, it has not been
demonstrated conclusively that this technique is an improvement on the
use of a single harmonic.

Factorial phase imaging appears to have several advantages over
Fourier phase imaging. Although standard deviations in the LV region
are slightly up when compared with the single-harmonic, the value of the
"structure" parameter also increases suggesting, possibly, that the
deviations may represent real changes. Noise outside the cardiac region
is reduced, and the use of an internal training set (factor (a)) aligns
mean phase values within normal left ventricles.

The results of the perception experiment, although inconclusive due to
poor statistics, indicate that factorial phase imaging is at least worthy

of further investigation, particularly when differential diagnosis is
involved. Further perception experiments are at present being designed.

The role of factorial imaging using oblique transforms is, as yet,
undetermined. Bias, due to display methods, observer preferential training, etc., means that the design of perception experiments involving
factorial amplitude/phase and oblique factor images is difficult. However,
provided the same components are used in each case, we are merely
transforming the original factorial images, which have interpretation
problems, into two representations of the same information. The only
difference between the methods, therefore, is one of image interpretation.

REFERENCES

1. Geffers H, Adam WE, Bitter F, Sigel H, Kampmann H. 1977. In Proc.
   5th conf. Information Processing in Medical Imaging, Nashville, ORNL/
   BCTIC-2.
2. Links JM, Douglass KH, Wagner HN. 1980. J. Nucl. Med., 21, 978.
3. Mena I, Fain J. 1981. Nucl. Med. Commun., 2, 93 (abstract).
4. Pavel D, Byrom E, Swiryn S, Meyer-Pavel C, Rosen K. 1980. In Medical
   Radionuclide Imaging 1980. STI/PUB/564 Vienna:IAEA.
5. Vos PH, Vossepoel AM, Beekhuis H, Pauwels EKJ. 1980. Nucl. Med.
   Commun., 1, 10.
6. Bacharach SL, Green MV. 1982. IEEE Trans. on Nuclear Science, NS-29,
   1343.
7. de Graff CN, van Rijk PP. 1980. Nucl. Med. Commun. 1, 19.
8. Wendt RE, Murphy PH, Clark JW, Burdine JA. 1982. J. Nucl. Med., 23,
   715.
9. Maeda H, Takeda K, Nakagawa T, Yamaguchi N, Taguchi M, Konishi T,
   Hamada M. 1982. In Proc. 3rd World Congress of WFNMB, Paris.
10. Houston AS, Elliott AT, Stone DL. Phys. Med. Biol., 27, 1269.
11. Cavailloles F, Bazin JP, Di Paola M, Chassat C, Di Paola R. 1982. In
    Proc. 3rd World Congress of WFNMB, Paris.
12. Sokole EB, Vyth A, Raam CFM, van der Wieken LR, van der Schoot JB.
    1981. J. Nucl. Med. 22, P10 (abstract).
13. Schmidlin P. 1979. Phys. Med. Biol., 24, 385.
14. Barber DC. 1980. Phys. Med. Biol., 25, 283.
15. Bazin JP, Di Paola R, Tubiana M. 1979. In Proc. 6th conf. Information
    Processing in Medical Imaging, Paris, INSERM vol. 88.
16. Metz CE, Beck RN. 1974. J. Nucl. Med., 15, 164.
17. Goodenough DJ, Rossmann K, Lusted LE. 1974. Radiology, 110, 89.
18. Green DM, Swets JA. 1966. Signal Detection Theory and Psychophysics.
    New York, John Wiley and Sons. Reprinted with corrections (1974),
    Huntington NY, Robert E Krieger.
19. Metz CE. 1978. Seminars in Nucl. Med., 8, 283.
20. Swets JA. 1979. Investigative Radiology. 14, 109.

RAPID AUTOMATIC FUNCTIONAL IMAGING OF THE HEART AND THE APPLICATION OF TIME IMAGES

N.J.G. BROWN, S.R. UNDERWOOD, S. WALTON, P.H. JARRITT, M.A. SEIFALIAN, P.J. LAMING.

1. INTRODUCTION

The objectives of data analysis in Nuclear Medicine are firstly the correction of the data for systematic error and secondly, the derivation of clinically useful indices. There are two ways of approaching the problem of finding clinically useful techniques. The first involves applying some established mathematical method and empirically determining its clinical significance. The second is to design the method of analysis in the light of existing knowledge of the system being studied. In the analysis of renography data, the use of compartmental analysis is an example of the first approach, while the use of deconvolution analysis is an example of the second. The known physiology of the kidney giving meaning to the frequency distribution of transit times obtained by the latter method. Corresponding examples in the case of Nuclear Cardiology are the application of Fourier series to obtain the Phase image (implying the assumption that the volume curve is a sinusoid) and time images showing the distribution of the times of occurrence of specific known events in the cardiac cycle.

In this paper we discuss methods of obtaining time images and describe the application of images obtained by the simplest and hence most rapid technique. Particular emphasis will be given to the application of the Time of End Diastole (TED) image, showing the distribution of the time

of maximum count, which has not received much attention in
the literature. This image is convenient as an identifier
of normal ventricle and can show subtle detail not revealed
by the Phase or the Time of End Systole (TES) image (showing
the distribution of the time of emptiest) alone.

2. THE LIMITATIONS OF THE PHASE IMAGE

The widely used Phase image arose from the empirical
application of Fourier Series in the derivation of
parametric images from ECG triggered equilibrium cardiac
data. Amplitude and Phase images were obtained from each of
a number of the lower harmonics of the series but no
significancece could be found in the Phase of any but the
first.

The so called Fourier Phase image is thus effectively
derived from the fitting to the individual pixel count time
curves of a single sinusoid of period ,T, equal to the mean
R-R interval:

$$v(t) = a + b.\cos(x-y)$$

Where v(t) is the count (volume) at time t into the cycle, a
is the zero offset, b is the amplitude and x=2.pi.t/T is the
time expressed as a fraction of the period converted to
radians and y is the off-set of the curve along the time
axis which is again expressed as a fraction of the period
converted to radians.

When the first harmonic phase values, obtained from the
single pixel count time curves which make up the set of
dynamic frames are displayed as a functional image, striking
results are obtained (Fig.1). The image differentiates the
atria from the ventricles and thus provides a valuable aid
in the reproducible definition of ventricular ROIs (1) The

image obtained from the amplitude parameter is also of value
in defining the septum and the free border of the ventricle
by identifying regions of the image which beat.

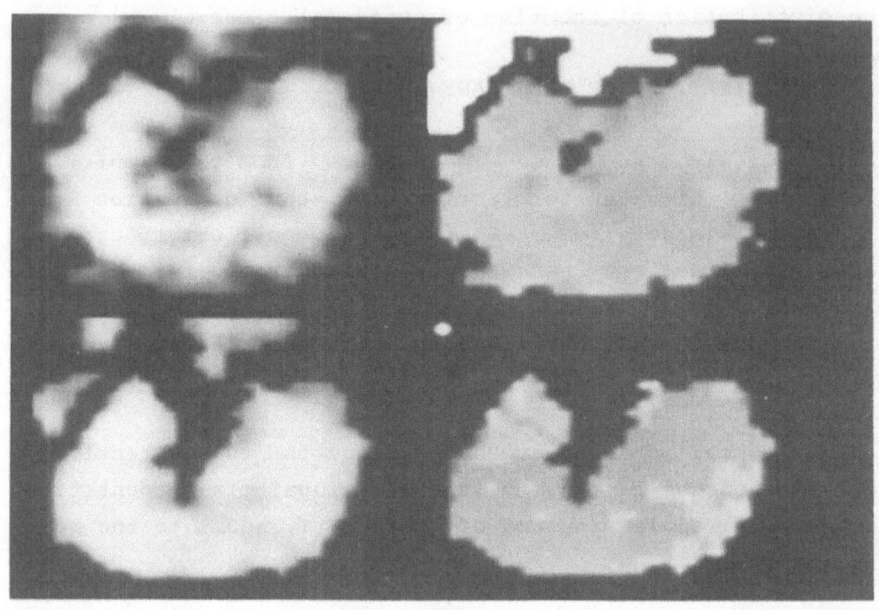

FIGURE 1. Top: Amplitude and Phase. Below Difference and TES

The phase image has gained wide acceptance,not only as an
aid to ROI definition, but also in the identification and,to
some extent, the classification of defects such as
aneurysms. On theoretical grounds its success in the latter
application might be questioned. The disadvantage of the
phase image arises from the fact that the individual pixel
count time curves are not,in fact, perfect sinusoids. The
effect of a given variation in curve shape on the Phase of
the fitted sinusoid is difficult to predict. What is
certain is that a change in any part of the curve will lead
to a change in Phase. This had been elegantly shown for
simulated data by Bacharach et al (2) The most which can be
stated regarding the distribution of the values in the Phase

image is that those parts which have the same value probably have similar shaped count/time curves associated with them, whereas those with different values have different shapes. The successful clinical application of the Phase image may perhaps be explained by the predominance of one pattern of abnormality in the patients studied. However, it may be that a more subtle form of analysis would yield further information of clinical value which has been, up till now, unrevealed.

3. TIME IMAGES

Various parameters are currently derived from the volume curve.   Any of these can in principle be used to obtain parametric images. The most fundamental features of the curve are its points of maximum and minimum. It might reasonably be thought that images based on the amplitude of these points and their times of occurence, would yield the most fundamental information about the distribution of ventricular function.   Brown et al (3) obtained images of the distribution of time of fullest (termed Time of End Diastole or TED) and time of emptiest (termed Time of End Systole or TES), by a very simple method. The image data was first subjected to one space smooth (conventionally weighted 3x3).   Background subtraction was then performed by a modification of the interpololative technique of Goris (4).

The background subtracted images were subjected to two time smooths (1,2,1 between frames) and a routine called which identified the values and frame numbers of the points of maximum and minimum count for each individual pixel count/time curve. Thus for 16 frame data time was measured with an accuracy of one part in 16. When the images are displayed using a scale having 16 discrete colours, clear information about timings is indicated.

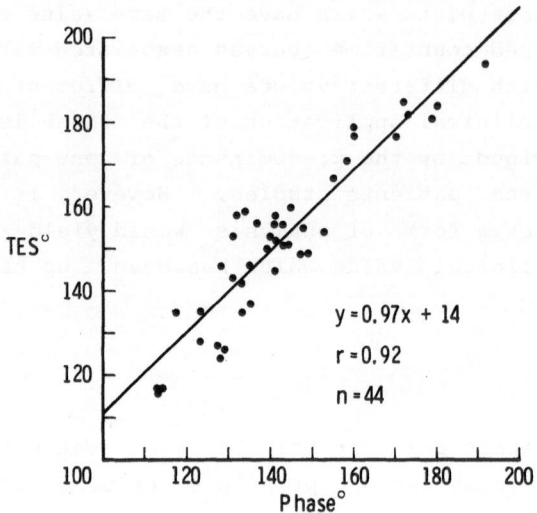

FIGURE 2. Correlation of phase and mean TES for LV

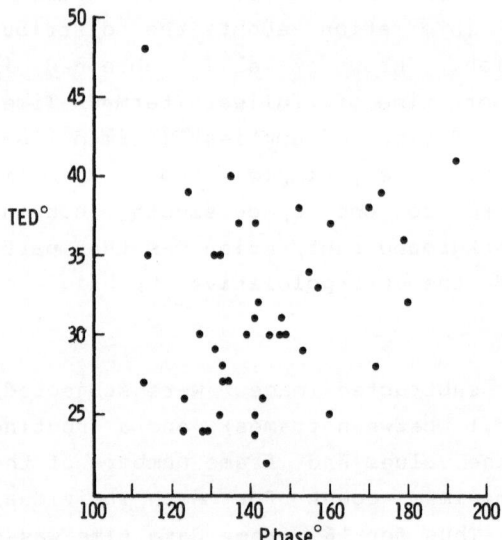

FIGURE 3. Correlation of phase and mean TED for LV

A 15% contour on the difference image obtained by subtracting the minimum from the maximum value was used to mask all images(Fig.1). The difference image was very similar to the Fourier amplitude image (apart from differences due to mask contour level). The TES image was very similar to the Phase image indicating that the latter roughly follows the time of emptiest of the curve. This was not surprising since the trough is the major feature of the curve. Fig.2 shows the correlation between the mean Phase and TES values obtained from the left ventricular region of interest. TES has been expressed in the same units as Phase. Fig.3 shows that there is no correlation between Phase and the Time of End Diastole, or time of fullest mean value.

4. AUTOMATIC DERIVATION OF CONVENTIONAL PARAMETRIC IMAGES

The Time of End Diastole image provides a valuable means of identifying regions of normally functioning ventricle automatically. A normal ventricular pixel is defined as one in which the maximum occurs during the first quarter of the cycle. A contour of the appropriate level of the TED image contains all points within the left and right ventricle which conform with this criterion. The automatically defined ROI based on this contour, can be used to obtain a left+right ventricular count time curve from which the End Systolic frame can be determined. This allows the automatic calculation of paradox and regional ejection fraction (REFI) images.

This technique (using the time of maximum) works well even in the presence of aneurysms, which would not be the case if normal ventricle were defined on the basis of the time of emptiest being within a given range. A machine code program was written which calculated the time images, difference image, paradox and REFI images together with

images showing the rates of maximum filling and emptying and
their times. Its running time when used with 16 frames of
32x32 data which could be held in store concurrently, was
under 10 seconds on a Nodecrest V77 Computer System, the
rate images being obtained following two more time smooths.

5. ALTERNATIVE TECHNIQUES FOR OBTAINING TIME IMAGES

The time images obtained by the method described above
are not so visually pleasing as the Phase image, since they
contain only 16 discrete values, while the Phase values are
continuous. Furthermore it might also be argued that the
statistical accuracy of the data warranted the measurement
of time with an accuracy better than one part in 16 of the
R-R interval. Obtaining parameters from some curve fitted
to the original data might be expected to yield greater
accuracy. Goris et al (5) described the derivation of time
images from data back calculated from Fourier series of 3
harmonics. Bacharach et al(6) have shown that the optimum
number of harmonics to use depends on the parameter sought.
The higher the number of harmonics used, the better the fit
to error free data, but the greater the chance of erroneous
oscillation in the fitted curves in the presence of
statistical error. In their study, statistical error was
added to curves of high accuracy and sample rate obtained
from a probe. A series of two or more harmonics was fitted
and a value for a given parameter, such as time at emptiest
was obtained from the original, virtually error free data,
and compared with the same value obtained from the fitted
curve. A range of differences from near zero up was found
indicating that an excellent fit was obtained on some curves
but not others. Although the average error could be
minimised by choosing the appropriate number of harmonics,
errors in individual cases were still noticeable.

The implication of the latter finding is that a Fourier series cannot provide a good fit to all points of an individual pixel count time curve containing statistical error at a level found in practice. It might be imagined that better results could be obtained for a given parameter by fitting a function to the appropriate part of the curve only, rather than attempting to fit the entire curve as is done by the Fourier technique. Bacharach et al (7) have described the application of a cubic equation to fit the trough of a global volume curve. This technique might be expected to give good results for the TES image and rates and times of maximum filling and emptying images obtained from individual pixel volume curves. However, such a technique would be expensive in computer time by comparison with the simple direct technique described in section 3. It therefore appeared worth while to investigate further the direct method as a means of obtaining clinically useful images.

6. EVALUATION OF THE DIRECT METHOD

It was pointed out above that a major disadvantage of the direct method as applied so far arose from the poor cosmetic appearance of the image as a result of the limitation to 16 discrete levels. This arose from the fact that the data had been collected at this temporal accuracy.It has been shown by Bacharacyh (1980) that to achieve satisfactory accura 10 milliseconds at exercise, should be universally employed. This implies collecting 50 frames for a normal heart rate allowing the direct calculation of time images with more than 3 times the number of levels used so far. Such images might be expected to be cosmetically better but would suffer from greater statistical error. Accordingly data was collected at the higher frame rate and analysed. A 16 frame series was obtained by adding appropriate frames. More detail was seen in the higher frame rate data but the effects of statistics were of course also more apparent.

An evaluation of the effect of statistics on the results
cannot be made using true data since the acquisition time
required to obtain the necessary accuracy is prohibitive.
Similated data was thus required. This was obtained by
adding statistical error to data back calculated from the
coefficients of a two harmonic Fourier series. The data
used for this was as above but without background
subtraction and following a single space smooth. The
parametric image programme was run on the error free and
error added data. No smoothing was applied to the error
free data before calculating the images. More detail was
certainly visible when the image was derived from a larger
frame set. However, the essential information appeared to
be present in the 16 frame data. This may arise from the
smooth nature of the original simulated data. On the other
hand it may be that the extra subtlety added by the extra
frames is of no clinical significance. Furthermore no
improvement in the cosmetics was seen as a result of the
worse statistics.

7. INFORMATION CONTENT OF TIME IMAGES

It might be asked whether the Time images do, in fact,
yield more useful information than the Phase images. Goris
et al (5) found the combination of TED, TES, Time of maximum
rate of emptying and Time of maximum rate of filling images
to be more sensitive in the detection of abnormal wall
motion, than the phase and amplitude images. The possible
mechanisms leading to a given pattern of Time images was not
discussed however. The following examples illustrate our
findings using the 16 frame Time images TED and TES.

Since the phase value depends on other aspects of the
curve than the times of maximum and minimum, it would be

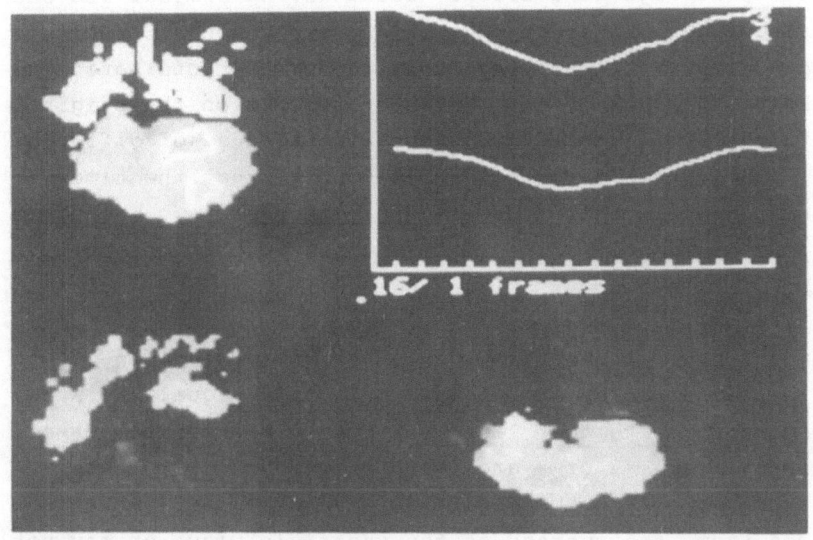

FIGURE 4. Top Phase. Below left TED, right TES. Similar TED
and TES values in the presence of different phase.

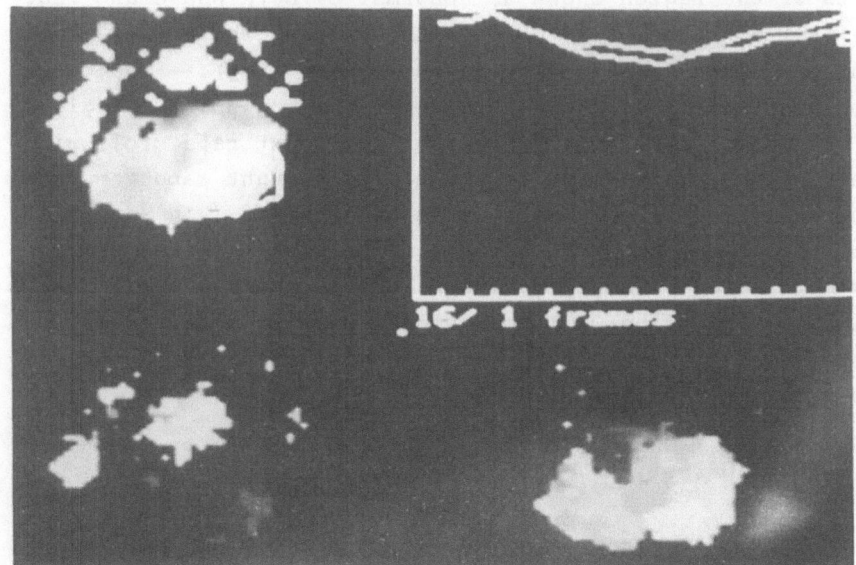

FIGURE 5. Top phase. Below left TED, right TES. Abnormal
TES and phase region containing regions of normal and
abnormal TED.

expected that regions could be found having similar TED and TES values but different phase values. Such a result is shown in Fig.4. It is not possible to see the information as clearly in this grey scale representation as on the original colour images. The two ROIs contain regions of different phase. The curves from these ROIs confirm that the times of maximum and minimum are the same in both regions. The phase difference evidently arises from a difference in the rate of filling.

In patients with normal function, the TED values within the left ventricle are found uniformly equal to that corresponding with the first frame. In abnormal cases, patches of frame 2 or 3 are frequently found but these are not invariably present. Regions of abnormal TES (more than 2 frames from the average of the ventricle) may or may not be accompanied by regions of abnormal TED. An example is shown in Fig.5. The curves have been obtained from equal parts of the region shown as abnormal by both phase and TES. One ROI contains all normal TED values while the other contains late values (shown as lighter grey). The curve from the latter ROI shows a rise at the beginning. Regions of abnormal TED imply increase in count rate following contraction. This must presumably be brought about by the ventricular wall bulging towards the camera. In cases of gross aneurysm, the TED value will be equal to the time of maximum rate of emptying (when the pressure is greatest) while the TES value will correspond with frame 1. It may be that some technique for the classification of aneurysms could be derived from this data.

8. CONCLUSION

The data discussed show that parametric images derived by a simple direct method can give useful results. The TED image does not suffer from the errors which can arise when

Fourier methods are used to obtain a fitted curve. They have the advantage of being more readily understood by the non-specialist than the Phase image, on account of their simple and direct relationship with the physical processes being studied.

REFERENCES

1. Walton S, Jarritt PH, Swanton RH, 1980. Improved reproducibility of the ejection fraction estimation utilizing the phase image: use of the techniqe to determine the heart's response to isometric exercise. Nuclearmedizin 220-224.
2. Bacharach SL. Green MV, DeGraaf CN,et al: 1981 Fourier phase distribution maps in the left ventricle: toward an understanding of what they mean. In Functional Mapping of Organ Systems. Esser PD,Ed.New York,Society of Nuclear Medicine,pp 139-148.
3. Brown NJG, Jarritt PH, Walton S, Ell PJ, 1980 Time of diastole and time of systolic parametric imaging of the heart. Nuc.Med.Comm. 1,163.
4. Goris ML, Daspit SG, McLaughlin P, 1976. Interpolative background subtraction. J.Nuc.Med.17,pp 744-747.
5. Goris ML, Briandet PA. Kriss JP, 1982. Decomposition of the information content of first harmonic phase images. Proceedings of the Third World Congress of Nuclear Medicine and Biology August 29-September 2 Paris, France.
6. Bacharach SL, Green MV, Vitale D, White G, Douglas MA, Bonow RO, Jones AE, 1983. "Fourier Filtering Cardiac Time Activity Curves: Sharp Cutoff Filters". In pro Bruxcelles.
7. Bacharach SL, Green MV, 1982. Data Processing in Nuclear Cardiology:Measurement of Ventricular Function IEEE Transactions on Nuclear Science,Vol.NS-29,No.4
8. Bacharach SL, Green MV, Borer JS,et al: 1979. Left ventricular peak ejection rate, filling rate, and ejection fraction - Frame rate requirements at rest and exercise. J. Nuc.Med.20: pp 189-193.

THE NORMAL HEART: PATTERNS FOR VARIOUS FUNCTIONAL IMAGES
OBTAINED FROM RADIONUCLIDE GATED EQUILIBRIUM STUDIES

D.G. PAVEL, P.A. BRIANDET, R.B'. FANG, K. ZOLNIERCZYK, J. SYCHRA,

INTRODUCTION

An increasing variety of functional images is presently
available for the evaluation of dynamic cardiac studies. Most
commonly these images are used in conjunction with radionuclide
gated equilibrium studies. It has become increasingly apparent
that a major difficulty in interpreting these images is the
relative lack of detailed description of normal patterns and
their variants. Knowledge about the normal pattern is also
essential when trying to decide which of the functional images
to use or in what combination.

In the present paper we have concentrated on the most
proven or promising categories of functional images available.
The methods evaluated were: a) Phase analysis (1-5); b)
Time functional images (6): c) Factor analysis (7-9).

MATERIALS AND METHOD

Large field of view camera, optimized LAO view for best
septum separation, 18-30 mCi Tc-99m labeled RBC (according to
patient's height and weight). The acquisition was done in 64
frames, 32x32 matrix for 200-300/cts/frame.(*) No beat rejection method was used (these were all normal patients).
Tail drop correction of the time activity curve was done by
using either one of two methods: a) the RR duration histogram
was used to compute the weighting factor for each frame or b)
scaling images to the total number of counts corresponding
to the first image.

(*) Computer: SOPHA Development, Simis 3 or 4.

Processing for Phase Analysis

A detailed description of the method has been previously
published (4). Briefly, the original 32x32 matrix is expanded
to 64x64 and followed by one spatial smoothing (1-2-1 filter
first in x then in y direction). Cosine and sine coefficients
of first Fourier component were calculated and used to generate
phase and amplitude images. For phase display the convention
used was to associate the minimum of the sinusoid curve at the
very beginning of the cardiac cycle with the argument value
of 1 degree.

Before quantification of phase image, regions of interest
were determined according to a semiautomatic method previously
described (4). The corresponding phase distribution histogram was generated for these regions and several parameters
calculated before and after outlier suppression (4). The
main parameters used were: standard deviation; Δ mean,
Δ mode (obtained by subtracting right ventricular from left
ventricular values: L-R); skew, calculated by using the root
mean cube deviation and kurtosis calculated by using the
mean of the fourth power deviation divided by the fourth
power of the standard deviation.

Processing for time images

The program used was developed by Goris and Briandet and
partially described in (6). On the original 64 images, corrected for tail drop, the 32x32 matrix was expanded to 64x64,
followed by one spatial smoothing and summed 4 by 4 for to ob-
otain a 16 image sequence. To save memory space and processing
time, the further analysis was restricted to a 45x45 region
containing the heart image. Each pixel's time activity curve
was then filtered by using the first 3 Fourier components.

The corresponding six images, representing the sines and
cosines of the first 3 Fourier components, together with a
360° table of sin ($n\alpha$), cos ($n\alpha$), where n = 1,2,3, were then
used to compute filtered time activity curve F(t) for each
pixel and the corresponding derivatives F'(t), -F'(t) and F''(t)
for t = 1,2,..., 360°. The locations of the minima of these
functions were estimated by successive searches: first, the

total 360° interval was divided into 9 intervals of equal size
and the 9 boundary values of these intervals were computed; the
two intervals that were separated by the smallest boundary value
were then divided into a total of 10 intervals of equal size,
refining the search by a factor of 5 and yielding the interval
width of 8 degrees. This procedure was repeated twice by dividing into 8 and 4 intervals, respectively, to reach the final
interval width of 1°. This search by successive approximations
is justified by the character and smoothness of the filtered
activity curve and their derivatives. By taking this approach,
a significant reduction of processing time has been achieved
as only 31 values of each function were evaluated instead of 360.

As all time values were expressed in degrees, and in order
to simplify comparison of the computed images, an arbitrary
offset of their pixel values was chosen to center their histograms at about 180°. The color scale used for display had the
same sequence of 9 colors previously described (4) but in order
to facilitate the qualitative evaluation, an interval of only
18° was assigned per color and the yellow-brown boundary was
always centered on the peak of the histogram. To encompass the
remaining scale on both sides, up to 360°, the dark blue
color covered a total of 216°. Expressing time values in
degrees, made it also possible to process, display and evaluate
the histograms and related parameter by using algorithms and
software already developed for phase analysis.

In order to achieve an objective comparison of time images
with the phase image, the latter was reconstructed by using the
same preliminary steps as in the case of time images. Parameters of the new phase image were then compared with the
ones computed by our standard method to ascertain that there
were no significant differences.

All the quantifications were based on the regions of interest independently delineated, as previously described (4).

Each image was evaluated qualitatively for patterns and
amount of inhomogeneity and quantitatively by comparing the
standard deviation of the LV frequency distribution histogram
of each type of image. These histograms were not submitted to

any outlier suppression algorithm.

The following images were compared:

T_1 = time of local systole (nadir).

T_2 = time of maximum ejection rate.

T_3 = time of maximum filling rate (measured from origin).

T_4 = time from point of maximum ejection rate to nadir.

T_5 = time from nadir to point of maximum filling rate.

Processing for Factor analysis

The algorithm used was developed by Bazin and DiPaola (7,8) and represents an extension of the principal component analysis approach used by Barber (10). It was applied on a sequence of 16 frames, 64x64 each, obtained from the original 64 frames, as described for time images above.

The principal component analysis (PCA) can be summarized as follows. Let us assume that: P = number of input frames; n^2 = number of pixels/frame; R^p = p-dimensional space; I_k = intensity (count rate) in a given pixel of k-th image; and $[I_1, I_2 \ldots I_p]$ = point in p dimensional space (R^p) representing that pixel value over the whole image sequence. This can be done for all pixels, which are then represented by a set of points in R^p.

The unit vector which has the direction in which this set is dispersed most, is called the first eigenvector. Projecting the set of points on the hyperplane (p-1 dimensional subspace) perpendicular to the 1-st eigenvector results in a new set of points. The 2-nd eigenvector is the unit vector which has the direction of the maximal dispersion of this new set. By continuing in same way we may obtain 3-d, 4-th....q-th eigenvectors that will now define orthogonal coordinate axes of a PCA subspace of R^p, e.g. a q-dimensional subspace (where q = number of orthogonal axes of the subspace) in which the n^2 points are best separated, when compared to all other q-dimensional subspaces of R^p. The origin of coordinates of the PCA subspace coincides with the center of gravity of the intensity point set.

Eigenvectors, in a restricted sense, can be called loading factors or loading curves. This is because each pixel value of m-th PCA image is computed as a linear combination of the corresponding pixel values of the p input images, where the components of the m-th eigenvector are used as coefficients.

The resulting PCA images contain mutually "uncorrelated" information, i.e. the repetition of the same information from image to image that is observable in the input image sequence, is not any more present in the PCA images. PCA performs a data reduction and with every subsequent PCA subspace reduction the respective images contain less information than the previous ones. The number of principal components q is usually given a priori. (ex. 2, 3, or 4)

In order to increase the direct physiologic meaning of PCA, the orthogonal axes have been replaced by a system of oblique axes of a factor analysis, and positivity constraints were added (7,8,10). This restricts the factor components (factor curves) as well as the oblique projections (pixel values of factor images) to non-negative values.

Factor images are then formed from the original images in ways similar to the construction of the PCA images i.e. by using the loading factors representing the amount of contribution of each of the original images to the particular factor image.

In addition, Bazin and DiPaola (7,8) accelerated the convergence of the algorithm used to compute the oblique axes, by the process of successive approximations. Execution of the algorithm is terminated when all values of the principal components and all values of the factor images are positive or when a predetermined maximum of iterations is attained.

However, even the described procedure does not necessarily guarantee a solution that would satisfy the imposed constraints. In practice, if the absolute value of the sum of the negative intensities in ROI exceeds a given percentage of the sum of positive intensities (3% in our study), the factor image is declared as being a "negative" image, and such a solution is rejected together with all corresponding factor images. The processing is continued by requesting the next lower number of factor images (factors).

In its present form, the program leads to occasional failure of the iterative search for factors. In some cases the search ended by an illegal operation (overflow).

Factor analysis was applied on a limited portion of the field by masking out everything that was not included in the region of interest of the two ventricles (this region was the same one mentioned above for phase and time images). A subsequent zooming (x 2) established the final size of the field. The search was conducted based on 8x8 areas called dixels (dynamic study pixel) i.e. the elemental time activity curves for an 8x8 pixel area. The program was requested to search for a maximum of three factors and to use 5 iterations to establish the initial estimate of factors.

The criteria for rejecting the three-factor result were that one (or both)of the following situations was found:
1) presence of a negative image (see definition above)
2) presence of a so called "average" heart image (in fact corresponding to the static blood pool image). Once a three-factor result was rejected, only the two-factor result was considered.

RESULTS

Phase analysis: Overall the images were consistently homogeneous and the patterns of phase progression found are schematically represented in Figs. 1 and 2.

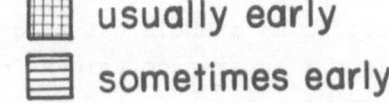
usually early
sometimes early

Fig. 1. Areas in which early phase values were found (represented separately for each ventricle).

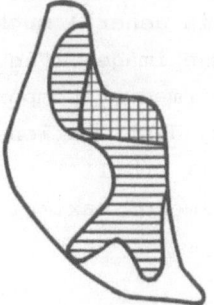 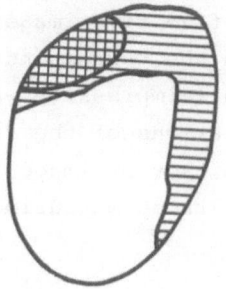

256

Fig 2. Pattern of phase
progression. Three com-
mon patterns were found
within the left ventricle
and are shown in A,B, and
C. The pattern shown in
D was by far the most
common within the right
ventricle.

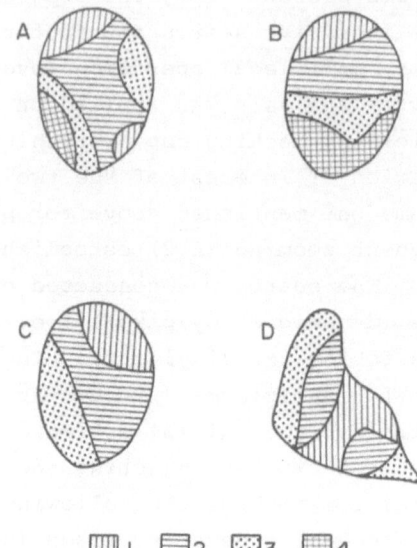

The parametric values obtained are shown in Table I. There
were no significant nor systematic differences between the
parametric values obtaine from the two variants used for
phase image generation. The effect of outlier suppression
on histogram standard deviation was also found to be statist-
cally nonsignificant for this normal population. Overall the
left ventricle as a whole has slightly lower mean and mode
phase values i.e. average values for Δ mean and Δ mode were
negative.

Time images: The qualitative evaluation showed that
all five time images were in general much less homogeneous
than the corresponding phase image. (Fig. 3, A, B). This
visual impression was confirmed by comparing the standard
deviations of the frequency distribution histograms of
each type of image (Table II and III). The noisiest images
were those measuring the time of maximum filling rate (T_3

Table I. Phase image parameters of left and right ventricles (*).

Pt.#	Δmean (L-R)	Δmode (L-R)	LV SD	LV Skew	LV Kurtosis	RV SD	RV Skew	RV Kurtosis
1	-3	-9	7	-4	4.9	11	-9	3.3
2	2	9	5	5	4.5	15	4	3.9
3	-9	-6	6	6	7.2	15	17	5.6
4	-7	-9	6	5	4.2	8	4	3.3
5	-9	-6	8	10	8.4	22	20	5
6	-6	-9	6	5	5.2	10	-9	4.1
7	-2	-6	7	-3	2.5	12	-9	3.1
8	-5	-3	8	6	3.6	12	9	7.5
9	-3	-3	6	5	5.4	8	-2	3.3
10	-5	-3	6	4	3.9	13	-5	7.5
11	-8	-3	8	8	4.3	16	20	7.3
12	1	0	6	7	8.5	9	8	7.1
13	-4	0	7	7	6.4	14	18	8.9
min.	-9	-9	5	-4	2.5	8	-9	3.1
max.	2	9	8	10	8.5	22	20	8.9
mean	-4.5	-3.7	6.6	4.7	5.3	12.7	5.1	5.4
SD	3.5	4.9	1.0	4.0	1.8	3.8	11.3	2.0

95% confidence intervals for means:

	-6.5	-6.6	6.0	2.3	4.2	10.3	-1.7	4.1
	-2.3	-0.7	7.2	7.1	6.4	15.0	11.9	6.6

(*) parameters calculated after outlier suppression (4).

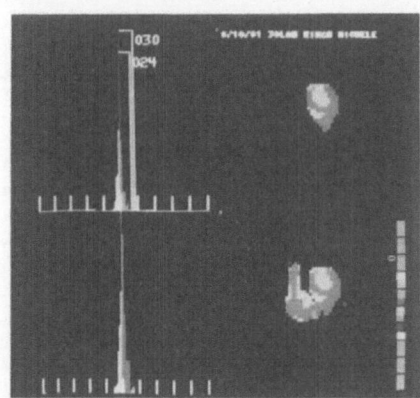

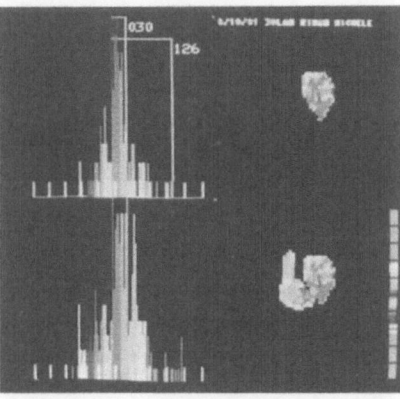

Fig 3A. Phase images with corresponding histograms. Upper half: Isolated left ventricle. Lower half: both ventricles. Note homogeneity of images and narrow histogram.

Fig 3B. T5 image (time from end systole to maximum filling rate). Note extreme inhomogeneity of image coupled with very wide frequency distribution histogram.

Table II. Comparison of Standard Deviation values of frequency distribution histograms for phase (*) and time images

Subject No.	PHASE	T_1	T_2	T_3	T_4	T_5
1	8	21	22	30	15	47
2	8	22	16	42	20	49
3	6	22	21	43	13	52
4	6	20	23	46	15	55
5	12	19	23	44	27	51
6	6	26	24	26	22	43
7	7	12	26	30	25	29
8	8	16	18	37	14	41
9	6	13	28	28	26	33
10	6	14	15	24	14	33
11	12	23	25	33	24	45
12	6	26	26	28	26	38
13	7	16	15	31	5	41
mean	7.5	19.2	21.7	34.0	18.9	42.8
SD	2.1	4.7	4.4	7.5	6.8	8.0

95% confidence intervals for means:

	6.2	16.4	19.0	29.5	14.8	38.0
	8.8	22.1	24.4	38.5	23.0	47.7

(*)phase image obtained after same preliminary processing as time images. No outlier suppression was applied to the histograms. (see text)

TABLE III. Pair-wise comparison of histogram SD from Table II
N = no evidence of significant difference between SC pairs
Y = significant difference between SD pairs for $p < .05$

	PHASE	T_1	T_2	T_3	T_4	T_5
PHASE	-	Y	Y	Y	Y	Y
T_1		-	N	Y	N	Y
T_2			-	Y	N	Y
T_3				-	Y	Y
T_4					-	Y
T_5						-

and T_5). The least noisy was T_4 image, but even this one was
worse than the phase image.

Factor analysis: Out of thirteen normals eight had two
well defined factors and five had three factors. In all cases
the factor image corresponding to the left ventricular function had a very close resemblance to the amplitude image
obtained during phase analysis (Fig. 4). The second factor

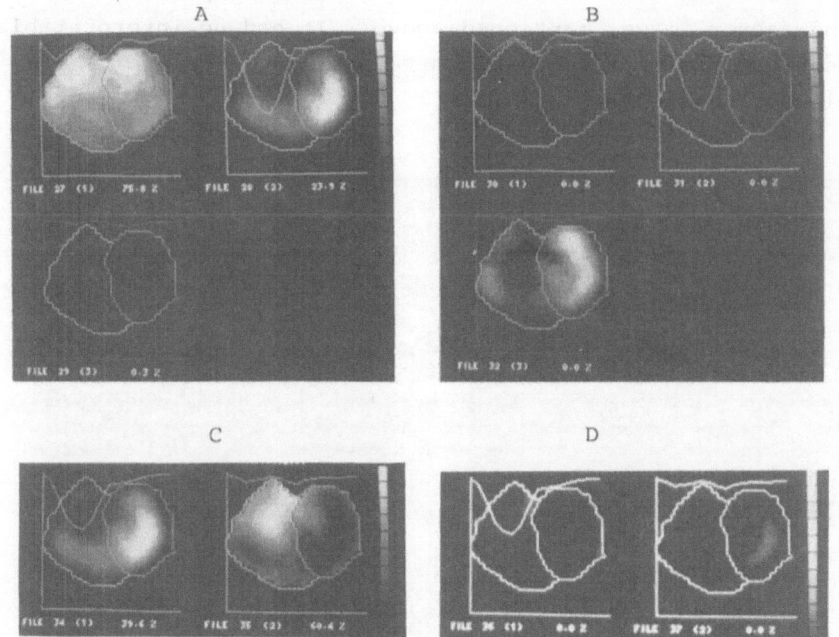

Fig 4. Example of two-factor result. The three-factor
display A has only two positive images while the negative
display B reveals a well defined negative image. Consequently the three-factor result is rejected.
In C the two-factor display identifies a ventricular
factor which appears identical to the ventricular amplitude
image and has a corresponding loading curve very similar to
the ventricular time activity curve. The second-factor
image has highest pixel intensity at the base of both ventricles. In the left ventricle it has a "peninsula" shape.
The corresponding loading curve is illdefined, generally flat.
In D no significant negative intensities are found.

260

image had a corresponding flat loading curve, and in the
region of the left ventricular base had a pattern either
similar to a peninsula, or in some cases simulating a
crescent. This image also identified the area corresponding to the pulmonary outflow tract in the right ventricular
ROI. In those cases where three factor images were obtained,
no further split of the ventricular factor image was found.
The additional third image, resulted from the split of the
second factor image, mentioned above. It had no interpretable
pattern and its corresponding curve was also devoid of
physiologic sense. (Fig. 5).

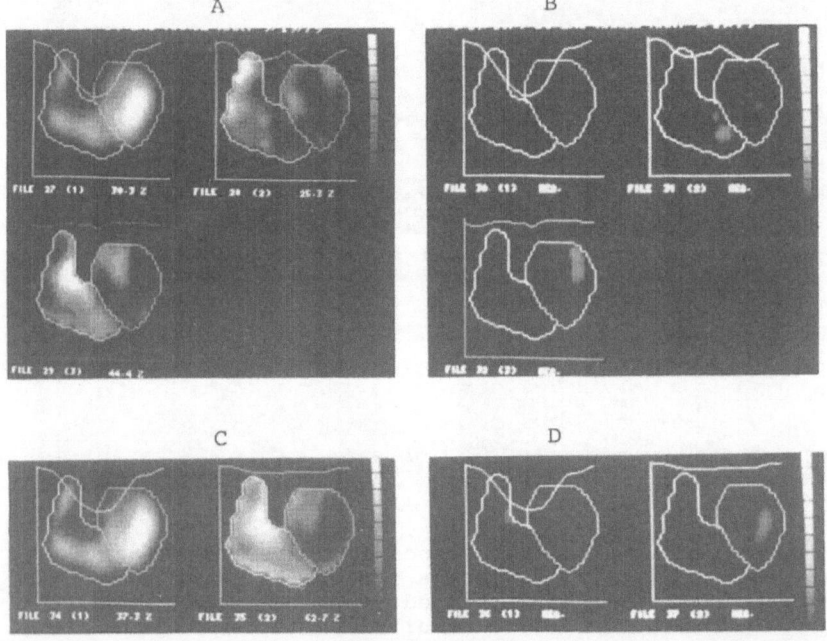

Fig 5. Example of three-factor result. In A, there are 3
positive images, while in B there is no significant amount
of negative image. Note similarity between the ventricular
factor shown in A and C. The additional (third) factor
generated in this case (A: right upper quadrant) was not
the result of a ventricular component split. Its morpho-
logic appearance as well as loading curve are illdefined
and without interpretable pathophysiologic significance
(the curve has several peaks).

DISCUSSION

Among the normal functional images evaluated, the most homogeneous pattern was found in phase images. This is not surprising from the theoretical point of view (5). The homogeneity of such images makes it easy to identify characteristic patterns both qualitatively and quantitatively. (Figs. 1 and 2) The progression of phase values over the ventricular region of interest can be considered to be in accordance with the basic electophysiologic knowledge concerning the sequence of normal ventricular activation (11). While there is a certain amount of normal variation in the phase sequence (Figs. 1 and 2), this is most likely due in part to the impossibility to generate identical two dimensional projections of three dimensional objects (ventricles) known to have great anatomical variability. As a rule the most common early areas are the upper septum in the right ventricle and the base of the left ventricle. Overall the left ventricle as a whole has a slightly earlier phase value as shown by the average values of Δ mean and Δ mode which are negative. (Table I)

For detailed parametric evaluation, an outlier suppression algorithm is necessary to protect against the unavoidable minor imperfections of a semiautomatic region of interest delineation. In a normal population the differences between parameters obtained after or before outlier suppression are not really consequential. For example the pair-wise differences of standard deviations of phase histograms before and after an outlier suppression (from Tables I and II) were not found statistically significant. Nevertheless, considering that the ultimate goal is to separate normals from abnormals the use of outlier suppression is important (4).

The time functional images appeared less homogeneous than phase image on qualitative evaluation and some of them appeared extremely inhomogeneous (Fig. 3). In addition, no consistent pattern and sequence of progression was found for any one of them. Therefore it may be quite difficult to use such images for the detection of anything less than severe

abnormalities. Both qualitative and quantitative evaluation
(Table II) indicated that the least noisy were the T_4 image
which represents the last part of systole (interval between
point of maximum ejection rate and end systole) and the T_1
image (time of local systole). There was no systematic
correlation between their appearance in the same subject: in
some, T_1 is noisier than T_4, in others the reverse is true.
The noisiest by far, were T_3 and T_5 images which are both
related to the time of maximum filling rate (measured from
origin or from end systole). This finding could have important
practical consequences in view of the fact that parameters
related to filling rates are increasingly popular today and
attempts have already been made to evaluate regional filling
rates. The extreme inhomogeneity of T_3 and T_5 may indicate
that local filling rates have to be considered with great
caution and the threshold of abnormality may be difficult to find.

Factor analysis was based on the algorithm of
Bazin and Di Paola (7,8). It became obvious during preliminary
work that the final results can differ to a certain extent,
mainly due to difficulties in controling the large number
of variables involved, during processing as well as during
preprocessing. The most significant variable found was
the field of search used, i.e. the extent of masking and thus
the effect of anatomy and underlying function. For this
reason, the most radical decision made was to consider only
the regions of interest of the two ventricles, (obtained
independently as described in the method section). This fact
has limited the variability of the results but, most importantly,
has enabled the protocol to become essentially operator
independent.

It is intuitively easy to accept that processing a normal
study should result in only two factors: one of them should
correspond anatomically and functionally (loading curve) to
the ventricles (ventricular factor), and the other one to
portions of the base of both ventricles. The fact that the
latter has a correspondingly flat loading curve can be explained by the unavoidable partial superimposition of atria

and great vessels over portions of the ventricular regions
of interest (Figs. 4 and 5). Note that because the major
part of the atria is not included in the field of search there
is no clear atrial type curve found.

In all normal cases the ventricular factor appeared
virtually identical to the amplitude image obtained from
phase analysis. The image had a compact appearance with
well defined high intensity area, generally oval or of inverted C shape. The corresponding loading factor curve was very
similar to the typical ventricular time activity curve.
The second factor image had its highest intensities at the
base of the ventricles: in the right ventricle its appearance
was quite variable, but in the left ventricle it had a fairly
characteristic appearance of "peninsula" or "crescent"
shape. This difference can be explained by the much more
pronounced and unpredictable superimposition of structures
at the right ventricular base.

In 5/13 normals where a three-factor result was obtained,
a close analysis revealed the following guidelines for
"normality". As shown in Fig. 5, the two-factor images correspond to the description above. In the three-factor image it is
apparent that there is still only one ventricular component
(virtually identical to the one in the two-factor image). In
other words, the additional factor did not result from a
split of the ventricular component. The additional third
factor image, and its corresponding loading curve, were not
interpretable from the anatomic and/or pathophysiologic point
of view. It had split anatomical locations within the region
of interes and the curve had several peaks, and thus appeared
indeterminate and/or uninterpretable.

CONCLUSION

Comparing the different functional images it appears that
at the present time the phase and amplitude images should be
considered the center piece of functional interpretation.
Phase image is easy to interpret qualitatively and lends
itself very easily to quantification. Adding time images to

the battery of results may not be of practical help, at least
for images based on individual pixel evaluation, because of
their inhomogeneity and variability.

Factor images appear promising because they may ultimately
lead to the next step of interpretation after phase analysis
results have made it possible to obtain a first impression.
There is nevertheless a need for further research concerning
the optimal processing protocol not so much for factor analysis in general, but for factor analysis specifically
applied to gated cardiac studies.

REFERENCES

1. Bitter F, Adam WE, et al: Synchronized steady state heart
    investigations. In Garsou J, Gordenne W, Merchie G (eds):
    Proceeding International Symposium; Fundamentals in
    Technical Progress: Ultrasound, Dose Planning and Nuclear
    Medicine. Vol II. Liege, Presses Universitaires de Liege,
    1979, pp 9.1-9.5.
2. Adam WE, Tarkowska A, Bitter F, et al: Equilibrium (gated)
    radionuclide ventriculography. Cardiovasc Radiol 2: 161,
    1979.
3. Deconinck F, Bossuyt A, et al: A cyclic color scale as an
    essential requirement in functional imaging or periodic
    phenomena. Med Phys 6:331, 1979.
4. Pavel D, Byrom E, et al: Detection and Quantification of
    regional wall motion abnormalities using phase analysis
    of equilibrium gated cardiac studies. Clin Nucl Med 8:315,
    1983.
5. Pavel D, Briandet P: Quo Vadis Phase Analysis. Clin
    Nucl Med 8:564, 1983.
6. Goris M, Briandet P, et al: Decomposition of the inform-
    ation content of first harmonic phase images. In Raynaud
    C (ed): Proceedings 3rd World Congress of Nuclear Medicine
    and Biology, Vol I. Paris, Pergamon Press, 1982, pp 46-49.
7. Bazin JP, DiPaola R: Advances in factor analysis applic-
    ations in dynamic function studies. Proceedings of the
    Third World Congress of Nuclear Medicine and Biology,
    Paris, 1982, p 35-38.
8. DiPaola R, Bazin J, et al: Handling of Dynamic Sequences
    in Nuclear Medicine. IEEE Transactions on Nuclear Science,
    Vol NS-29, No 4, 1982, p 1310-1321.
9. Cavailloles F, Bazin J, et al: Factor Analysis in Dynamic
    Cardiac Studies at Equilibrium. Proceedings of the Third
    World Congress of Nuclear Medicine and Biology, Paris,
    1982, p 2361-2364.
10. Barber D: The use of principal components in a quantitative
    analysis of gamma camera dynamic studies. Physics Med
    Biol 25:283, 1980.

11. Swiryn S, Pavel D, et al: Sequential regional phase
    mapping of radionuclide gated biventriculograms in
    patients with ventricular tachycardia: close correlation
    with electrophysiologic characteristics. Am Heart J 103:

Acknowledgement: We greatfully acknowledge the technical
                  assistance of B. Patel.

FOURIER FILTERING CARDIAC TIME ACTIVITY CURVES: SHARP CUTOFF FILTERS

S.L. Bacharach, M.V. Green, D. Vitale, G. White, R.O. Bonow, M.A. Douglas
A.E. Jones, and S.M. Larson. National Institutes of Health, Bethesda MD,
USA

INTRODUCTION

Several problems may occur when analyzing cardiac left ventricular
(LV) time activity curves (TACs) using the techniques of Fourier analysis.
These difficulties are of course not unique to cardiac TACs, but rather
are representative of the general problems encountered when applying
Fourier analysis to discrete, sampled data. In the case of LV TAC's created
from equilibrium gated blood pool studies, one usually applies Fourier
analysis in an attempt to filter counting statistical noise from the
data. One of the common methods employed to accomplish this goal (albeit
probably the least justified) is to Fourier transform the TAC into the
frequency domain, filter the data with a sharp cutoff filter (i.e.
multiplication in the frequency domain with a rectangular pulse) and
invert the filtered data. The reason for the choice of a rectangular
cutoff filter is usually simplicity. Whatever the reason, using a sharp
cutoff in the frequency domain is identical to describing the data by a
truncated Fourier series. Thus one is able to skip the Fourier transform
step and instead directly calculate only those first few Fourier coefficients
one is interested in. Several concerns need to be addressed. First, are
the two constraints of the sampling theorem satisfied? That is, is the
underlying TAC which has been sampled by the gated equilibrium procedure
band limited, and if so is the sampling rate adequate (at least equal to
the Nyquist rate). Second, what criteria can be used to select the
cutoff frequency of the filter (i.e. how many harmonics should be used)?
Third, what are the practical effects of beat length fall off - that is,
if the TAC is truncated, due to the finite width of the beat length
distribution, how will this effect the filtered data?

The first of these three problems - that of adequately sampling the
TAC, has been investigated elsewhere (1-3). We address here the remaining
two.

CUTOFF FREQUENCY SELECTION

We began with the assumption that a sharp, rectangular shaped frequency filter is to be used (i.e., The TAC is described by a truncated Fourier series). Difficulties with this filter shape will be considered later. Two factors must be considered in the selection of the cutoff frequency - reduction of (counting statistical) noise and preservation of signal content. One approach which has been reported involves measurement of the power spectra of LV volume curves. Spiller (4) for example, reported that greater than 99% of the power spectrum was contained in the first 4 harmonics of the LV volume curves he examined. Fischer (5) reported a different approach, looking instead at the noise content. By plotting amplitudes on probability paper he found a cutoff frequency could be determined as that point above which the amplitudes were normally distributed. Thus amplitudes above this cutoff frequency could not be distinguished from noise. It was recognized, however, that looking at either the power spectrum or the noise spectrum one can not be sure to what extent clinically important information is being eliminated by the filter. Thus, although 95% of the power spectrum of a particular TAC is contained in the first 3 harmonics, it may happen that the 5% contained in the higher harmonics is vital to the calculation of some clinically important parameter. For this reason a different, more empirical, approach has been considered (6). In this approach one calculates what one believes to be the clinically important parameters from an unfiltered LV TAC which is (due to large total counts) as free from statistical fluctuations as possible. By progressively describing this TAC with a Fourier series containing first 6, then 5, etc down to 1 harmonic, one can empirically observe the effect of the filter on each of the clinical parameters. Similarly, by adding Poisson noise to the TAC prior to filtering one can empirically observe the effects of noise reduction on each of the clinical parameters.

This empirical approach has one obvious disadvantage - the results are applicable only to the clinical parameters chosen for study. This is not an unreasonable restriction however, as every portion of a TAC will indeed be influenced differently by filtering. The following three sections present: First, the effect filtering has on parameters calculated from statistically "perfect" TACs - that is, how accurately does filtering preserve the true signal? Second, the influence of filtering on noise reduction; and

finally, a method to combine these two results in order to minimize the
effects of signal loss while maximizing the effects of noise reduction.

Preserving the Signal

The empirical approach mentioned above is illustrated in Figure 1.
Six clinically relevant parameters were chosen: Time to end systole
(TES), ejection fraction (EF), peak ejection rate (PER), peak filling
rate (PFR), and their respective times of occurrence (TPER, TPFR). These
parameters were measured in each of 16 unprocessed time activity curves
(sampled at 100 points per second) chosen to have very high total counts
(4×10^7 total counts on average). Each parameter was measured from the
unprocessed TAC and then from the filtered TACs (with cutoff frequencies
of 1 through 6 harmonics). The difference between the "true" value as
measured from the unfiltered TAC, and the value determined from the
filtered curve, was calculated. Figure 1 shows the absolute value of

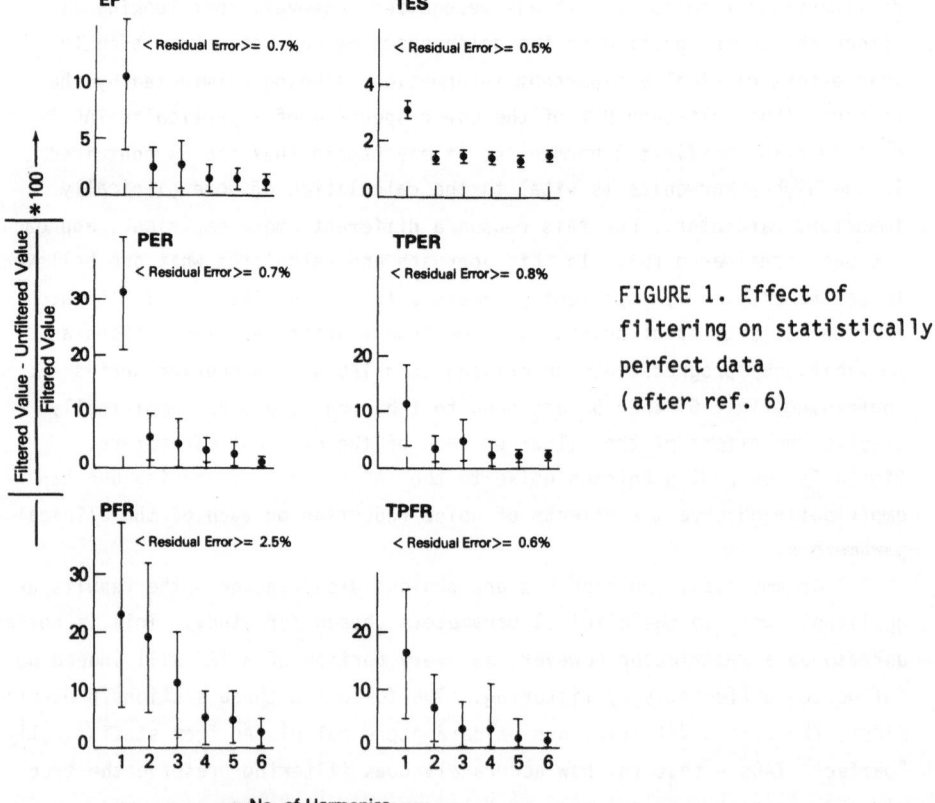

FIGURE 1. Effect of
filtering on statistically
perfect data
(after ref. 6)

this difference (expressed as a percentage), averaged over all 16 subjects. Obviously, some TACs will be nearly unaffected by filtering (e.g. TACs with nearly cosinusoidal shape) while others may be strongly affected. The error brackets in Figure 1 estimate these subject to subject variations (1 standard deviation) in each parameter calculated from the fitted TAC. Looking at filling rate for example, it is seen that a 2 harmonic fit resulted in an error of between 5 and 32% in PFR for two thirds of all the subjects.

Note that the difference between the Fourier filtered values and the "true" values decreases with increasing harmonic number. So, too, do the subject to subject variations. That is, while some TACs are adequately described by 1 harmonic, most require a larger number. The larger the cutoff frequency, the fewer TACs that will be inadequately fit.

If the unprocessed TACs contained an infinitely large number of counts there would be no statistical fluctuations in the observed "true" values for each parameter. The subject to subject deviations shown in Figure 1 would then approach zero as frequency cutoff increased. In fact, the unprocessed TACs, while possessing greater than usual statistical precision, were not perfect. Each parameter calculated from these unprocessed TACs thus could be expected to exhibit small statistical fluctuations due to limited counts. The quantity referred to as "residual error" in figure 1 represents the average values (for all 16 TACs) of these statistical fluctuations. As harmonic number is increased, the subject to subject deviations cannot, therefore, fall below this residual error.

No pattern could be seen as to whether a particular parameter was over or under estimated by a given number of harmonics. Depending on the TAC shape, parameters such as peak filling rate could either be underestimated by using too few harmonics (e.g. in the case of normal individuals with a high filling rate) or overestimated (e.g. in the case of CAD subjects with severely reduced filling).

Reduction of Noise

Figure 1 tells us the degree to which certain clinically important parameters are preserved by describing the TAC with a truncated Fourier series. It does not, however, permit us to judge how well noise has been reduced by the filtering process. Again, one must remember, it is a proper balance between signal (i.e. parameter) preservation and noise reduction, which is sought. To investigate the noise reduction properties of the sharp cutoff filter, the following experiment was performed. A selected TAC was replicated 64 times. Gaussian noise was added to each of the resulting 64 TACs by replacing each point on the TAC with a value drawn at random from a Gaussian distribution (with σ given by the square root of the counts at that point on the TAC). Thus 64 TACs, identical except for the effects of counting fluctuations were produced. Each of the 64 TACs were filtered (using a cutoff which varied from 1-6 harmonics), and the parameters of interest calculated from the filtered TAC. Although all 64 TACs were derived from the same original TAC, the 64 values of each parameter fluctuated, due to the presence of noise. The standard deviation of these fluctuations for each parameter was measured and used as an indicator of the degree of noise reduction achieved by each filter. Figure 2 illustrates this. The ordinate gives the standard deviation of each parameter (as measured from the fluctuations), averaged over all 16 subjects. The abscissa is the cutoff frequency used. For each parameter, the 3 curves represent 3 different levels of noise. As expected, the

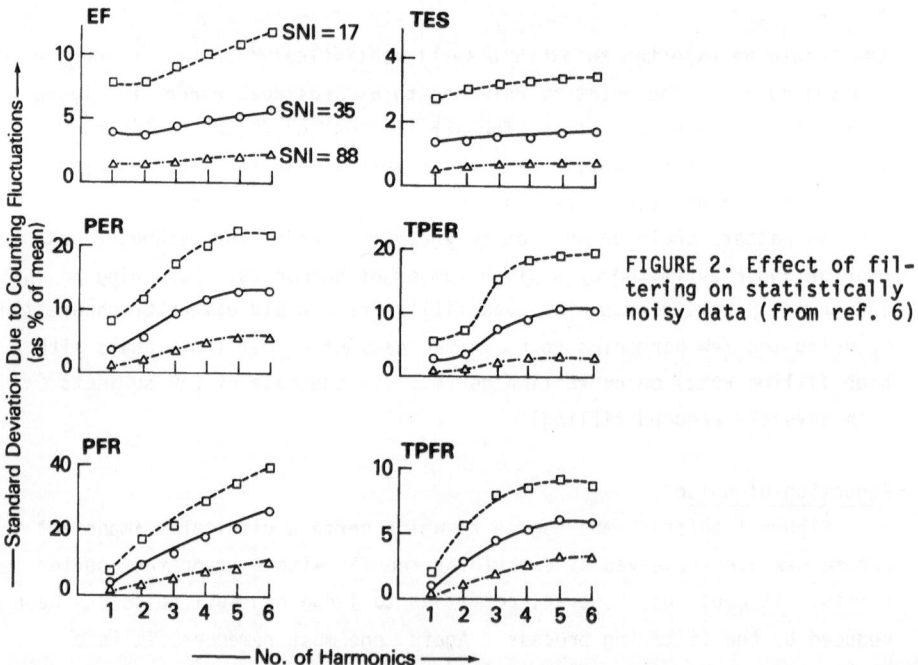

FIGURE 2. Effect of filtering on statistically noisy data (from ref. 6)

higher the cutoff frequency, the greater the fluctuations in each parameter due to noise.

An index was sought to describe the effects of statistical fluctuations on the calculation of parameters from the TAC. Each parameter is of course influenced by statistical noise in a different manner, dependent both upon the parameter and the algorithm used to calculate it. Ideally, then, an expression would be derived for each parameter giving the standard deviation of that parameter as a function of the noise level (i.e. counts) present in the TAC. For parameters such as EF it is quite straight foward to do this. For the timing parameters such as TPFR, TES, etc. it is more difficult. To avoid the need to calculate an error expression separately for each parameter, and to make the results which follow more generally applicable a single descriptor was sought. Several possible descriptors, indicative of both signal and noise content of the TACs, were examined. Since each parameter's error expression is in general different, it was recognized in advance that one single descriptor could never accurately describe the error for every parameter. It was hoped, however, that one of these descriptors might at least allow estimation of the error in all the parameters. The parameter usually referred to as the signal to noise ratio was one of those examined.

$$S/N = \frac{\text{Signal}}{\text{Noise}} = \frac{A_1}{[1/n \sum [LV(i) - Cm(i)]^2]^{1/2}}$$

$$\cong \frac{A_1}{\sqrt{<Cm>}}$$

Where

A_1 is the first harmonic amplitude
n is the number of points in the TAC
$LV(i)$ are the "true" counts at point i
$Cm(i)$ are the measured counts at i
$<Cm>$ are the average counts per point in the TAC

The first harmonic amplitude is indeed an adequate estimator of signal content (7). Likewise, the square root of the mean counts per point in the TAC is a reasonable approximation to the variance about the "true" unbackground corrected TAC (since the unbackground corrected counts do not change by more than about 30%-40% from ED to ES). Unfortunately, S/N

272

does not behave properly with respect to changes in sampling rate. Gated
equilibrium studies use a sampling aperture whose width is T/N where T is
the cardiac period and N the number of samples per cardiac period. Thus
the definition of S/N will increase by $\sqrt{2}$ simply by halving the frame
rate (A_1 will double, $\sqrt{<Cm>}$ will increase by $\sqrt{2}$). To alleviate this
problem, and to take into account the fact that most parameters are
estimated by using a region of the curve, not a single point, the S/N was
modified by replacing the square root of the variance in the denominator
with the standard error. The resulting expression, referred to here as
signal to noise index (SNI) is thus:

$$SNI \; = \; \frac{A_1}{(<Cm>/n)^{\frac{1}{2}}}$$

and is seen to be independent of frame rate. A test was made to ascertain
how well SNI predicted the actual calculated parameter standard deviations.
The ordinate of Figure 3 shows the actual calculated parameter errors

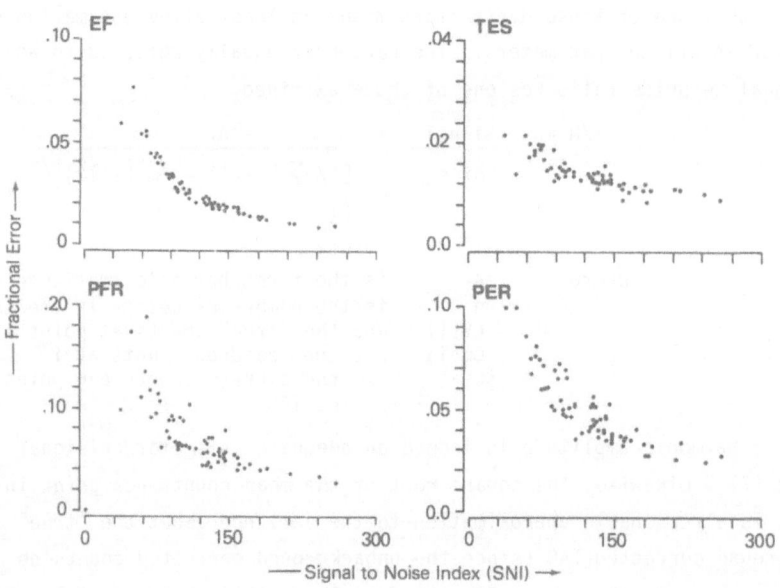

FIGURE 3. Measured noise as a function of SNI

(one standard deviation) as a function of SNI, for 66 randomly selected
TACs chosen to span a range of SNI values. It can be seen that there is
a strong relationship between SNI and the calculated error in each of the
parameters. Thus one can estimate the expected error in a parameter due
to counting fluctuations by computing SNI and using Figure 3. The estimate
of the error will be quite good for parameters such as EF and TES and
considerably more uncertain for PFR.

Optimizing Signal Retention and Noise Reduction

The preceeding two sections have demonstrated: (1) The error which
occurs in measuring a clinical parameter from a Fourier filtered TAC as
opposed to direct measurement from a (nearly noise free) TAC, and (2) How
fourier filtering reduces the fluctuations in clinical parameters when
counting fluctuations are present in the TAC. These two results can both
be considered an error due to filtering - in the first case an error
which decreases with increasing cutoff frequency and in the second case
an error which increases with increasing cutoff frequency. This suggests
that one may think of combining these two "errors" in some way. Since
the two errors respectively increase and decrease with respect to cutoff
frequency, a minimum in the combined error may exist. The cutoff frequency
at which this minimum combined error occurred could then be considered an
"optimum" choice of harmonic number.

It is not clear how one should combine the two error terms. For some
parameters (e.g. filling rate) the two errors are probably not wholly
independent. For example it is not unlikely that TACs with a very straight
and rapid filling would be both poorly described by a low cutoff filter
and less susceptible to counting fluctuations. Despite their possible
dependence, the two errors were combined as:

$$E_t = [E_1^2 + E_2^2]^{1/2}$$

Where E_t is the total combined error and
E_1 and E_2 the two errors discussed above.

When figures 1 and 2 are combined to form a total error, a minimum does
indeed occur. In figure 4, the mean values of figure 1 and 2 were combined
to produce the total error shown. Each parameter's minimum error is

shown for several values of SNI. It is seen that, for noisy TACs (low
SNI values) the minimum is often pronounced. That is using either fewer
or more harmonics causes the total error to increase significantly.

TAC TRUNCATION

Effects of Leakage

All the time activity curves considered here used the technique of
reverse framing (8) in an attempt to reproduce the late diastolic portion
of the TAC. Whether or not this method is always valid, the procedure
does produce TACs with no discontinuities, and which are periodic with a
period T equal to the average R-R interval length. In contrast, many
computer systems produce curves with notable fall off at the end of the

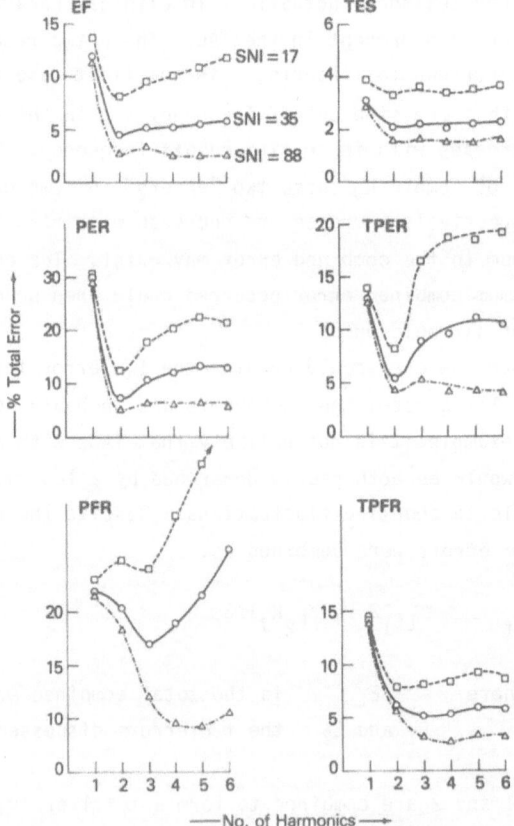

FIGURE 4. Total error as function of cutoff frequency

cardiac cycle, due to fluctuating R-R interval lengths. One approach to this problem has been to truncate such TACs at a time equal to the shortest R-R interval occuring in the study. Such truncation, at other than the natural period of the cardiac cycle, produces a periodic function with sharp discontinuities. It is well known (9) that truncation in the time domain will result in additional frequency components in the frequency domain. The effect of multiplying the TAC by a rectangular truncation function in the time domain is, of course, the same as convolving the TACs frequency function with the function

$$A \frac{\sin(2\pi T f)}{\pi f}$$

where T is the truncation period.

This "leakage" of high frequency terms into the TACs frequency function is a well known phenomenon. Its practical implications in nuclear cardiology however, have not been investigated. Again an empirical approach has been taken. Three TACs from among the 16 high count rate curves mentioned previously were chosen for study. These three were chosen as representative of 3 distinct TAC shapes which are often encountered. Figure 5 shows the TACs as well as their Fourier spectra. The three TAC categories are (A) a "usual" resting TAC, with noticeable diastasis period and small atrial contraction, (B) a TAC with no diastasis period, and in which atrial contraction has blended in with rapid filling to form a nearly linear filling period, and (C) a TAC with reduced magnitude of early filling in which atrial contraction contributes greater to the stroke volume.

Examining the Fourier spectra of these three TACs one notices that A and C possess larger amplitude at high frequency (e.g. 2 through 4 harmonics). This is expected since TAC B does not have the sharp slope changes which are present in A and B at the junction of rapid filling and diastasis.

Each TAC was filtered with a rectangular cutoff filter with a cutoff of first 1, then 2 etc. up to 6 harmonics. All the clinical parameters mentioned previously were then calculated from each of the six filtered TACs. The TACs were then truncated by one time point and again filtered with from 1 to 6 harmonics. The ratio of the parameters calculated from

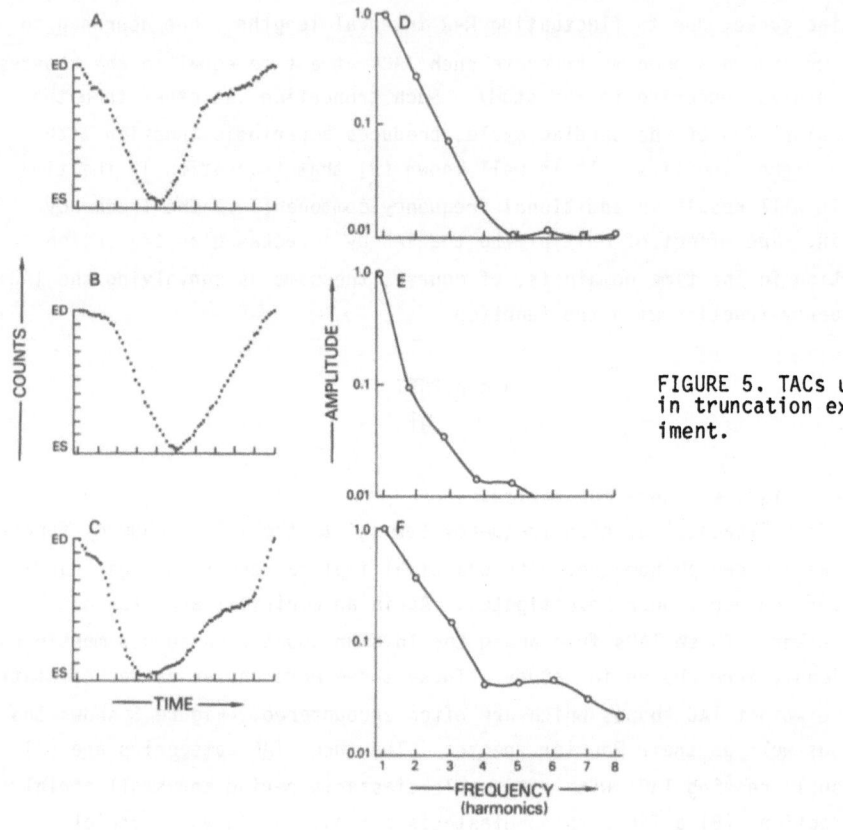

FIGURE 5. TACs used in truncation experiment.

the truncated filtered TACs to the non truncated filtered TAC was calculated for each cutoff filter frequency. The TACs were then truncated by 2 time points and the calculation repeated. Each time the ratio

$$R^n = \frac{P_t^{\,n}}{P^n} * 100\%$$

was calculated.

Where $P_t^{\,n}$ is a parameter calculated from a TAC truncated to t seconds and filtered with an n harmonic cutoff frequency and P^n is parameter calculated from the untruncated TAC filtered with an n harmonic cutoff.

This ratio, then, shows the effects produced only by the truncation. Since the comparisons are made only between parameters calculated from

filtered TACs the a-priori effects of filtering the unprocessed TAC are
eliminated.

One can speculate about the expected results of this experiment.
First, in a TAC with a long diastasis period and no noticeable atrial
contraction, the ratio R^n will be nearly unity for all cutoffs greater
than 1. Truncation will not produce any discontinuity at all in such a
TAC. The only effects will be those of shortening the diastasis period.
Because such shortening will alter the curves symmetry, R^1, the ratio of
the first harmonic parameters, will vary as a function of t, the truncation
interval. In fact, it is for this reason that "phase", derived as it is
from a 1 harmonic cutoff filter, is not a reliable indicator of any of
the clinical parameters chosen. Parameters calculated from truncated,
filtered TACs possessing different shapes (as in figure 5) may be expected
to be influenced differently by the truncation and associated leakage. The
effects observed for the three TACs shown are summarized below, and in
Figure 6. Figure 6 is a plot of R^n (the ratio of the untruncated parameter

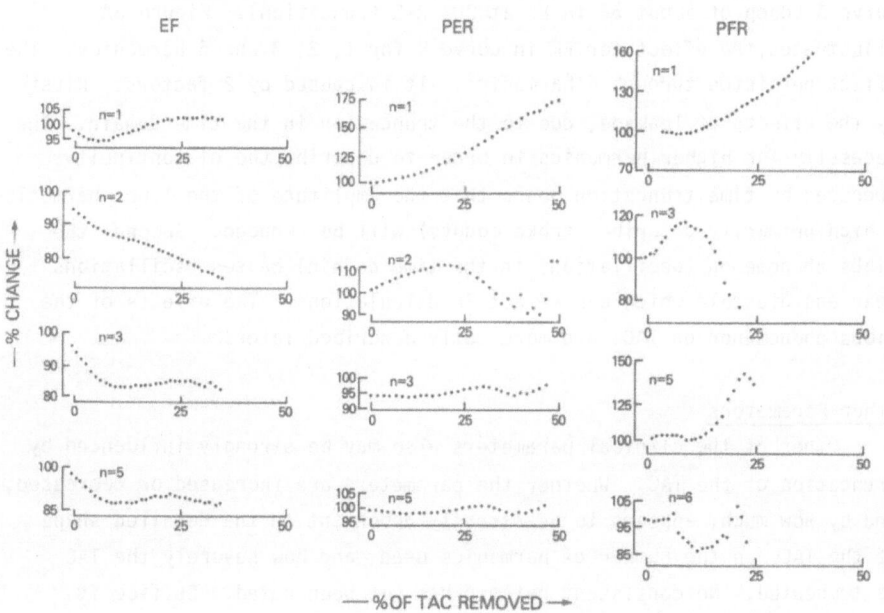

FIGURE 6. Effects of truncation on filtered TAC parameters

to the truncated parameter after filtering with a cut off of n harmonics)
as a function of the percentage of the TAC which has been truncated.
Thus the abscissa is expressed as a percentage of the cardiac period
which has been eliminated. TAC truncations were performed by successively
deleting 10 msec points, until the cardiac cycle had been shortened by
about 30% or more.

TES

For curve 5A, TES did not vary more than 3 or 4% as a function of
truncation width (0 to 40% of the curve truncated) for all harmonics
studied (1-6). TES did vary for all curves for 1 harmonic since
truncation alters symmetry.

EF

Ejection fraction fell as the amount of TAC truncation increased. The
effect was more pronounced in TACs 5B and 5C (EF dropped about 15% when
20% of the cardiac cycle had been truncated), but was also noticeable for
curve A (drop of about 5% in EF at 20% R-R truncation). Figure 6A
illustrates the effect for EF in curve B for 1, 2, 3 and 5 harmonics. The
effect persisted through 6 harmonics. It is caused by 2 factors: First,
by the effects of leakage, due to the truncation in the time domain. The
necessity for higher harmonics in order to describe the discontinuity
produced by time truncation means that the amplitude of the lower harmonics
(which primarily describe stroke counts) will be reduced. Second, the
Gibbs phenomenon (oscillations in the time domain) causes oscillations
near end diastole which can effect EF calculations. The effects of the
Gibbs phenomenon on TACs are more fully described later.

Other Parameters

Other of the clinical parameters also may be strongly influenced by
truncation of the TAC. Whether the parameters are increased or decreased,
and by how much, appears to be strongly dependent on the detailed shape
of the TAC, on the number of harmonics used, and how severely the TAC
is truncated. No consistent pattern has yet been noted. Suffice it
to say that truncating a TAC, even by a relatively small amount, can
seriously affect the usual clinical parameters when calculated from data
filtered with a sharp cutoff.

In the cases shown in Figure 6 we see PER increasing by 11% with a
20% truncation at 2 harmonics. At higher harmonics the influence of TAC
truncation is considerably reduced. PFR increases dramatically after
even slight truncation at low harmonics. Use of higher harmonics (up to 5)
does not improve the situation.

Discussion

Two phenomena have conspired to produce the results above: truncation
in the frequency domain (i.e. use of a truncated Fourier series) and
truncation on the time domain (i.e. truncating the TAC itself). If the
TAC is not truncated (e.g. reverse framing is used, or any other technique
employed in order to approximately reproduce the end of the cycle) then
one is left only with truncation in frequency space. Such truncation
still may produce oscillations in the time domain. These oscillations
occur primarily at discontinuities in the TAC, or, to a much reduced
extent at discontinuities in the derivitive of the TAC. If the TAC is
not truncated, there are no major discontinuities. The only discontinuities
occur due to the slight time delay in the gating process due to the R
waves not occurring at exact multiples of time tics. In the TACs of
Figure 6 this time delay is, on average, 5 msec, causing no noticeable
discontinuity in the TAC but producing a slight discontinuity in the
derivitive. The relatively smooth "discontinuity" at the junction of a
rapid diastolic filling period and a flat diastasis period may also cause
very small ripples near the transition from filling to diastasis. Such
effects, however, are usually masked by the effects of counting fluctuations.

If one truncates the TAC, however, a very sharp discontinuity in the
time domain is produced. This, coupled with the frequency domain
truncation, causes very noticeable rippling in the TAC. The structure
of the ripples is such that its points of 0 derivitive should occur at:

$$t_{peak} \text{ and } t_{valley} \text{ at } \frac{j\pi}{2n} \quad j=1,2....(2n-j)$$

where j is an integer as shown, and
n=the cutoff harmonic in the filter

Thus the higher the cutoff frequency, the higher the ripple frequency.
This can easily be demonstrated to occur in truncated TACs. In Figure 7
TAC B of Figure 5 has been truncated by 22% (i.e. 150 msec), and then
filtered with a 2, 4, 6 and 10 harmonic cutoff filter. For comparison

the non-truncated TAC is shown filtered with the same cutoff frequencies. Note the huge, broad peak at 2 harmonics, which gets narrower at 4 harmonics (at which time a second ripple appears) and still narrower (with still more ripples becoming evident) at 6 and 10 harmonics. The frequency of the "ripples" roughly corresponds with that predicted by theory.

The situation can be understood by realizing that a sharp frequency cutoff filter will not affect the data from curves from Fig. 5 because these TACs have band limited Fourier spectra. Temporal truncation of the TAC, however, causes "leakage" of high frequency components into the Fourier spectrum - thus the TACs are no longer band limited and so are now adversely affected by a sharp cutoff filter in the frequency domain.

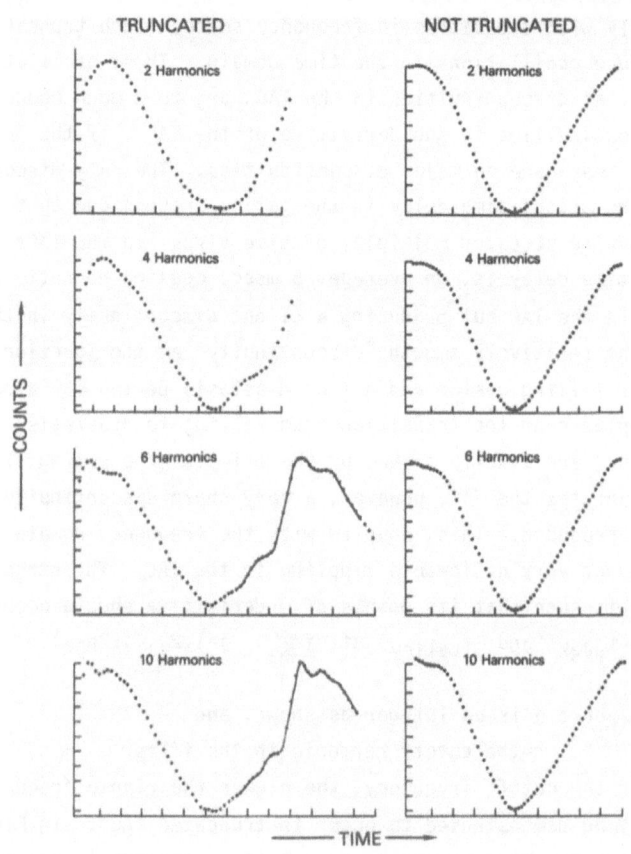

FIGURE 7. Effects of TAC truncation: production of oscillations.

Both of these related problems - that of the Gibbs phenomenon and leakage, can of course be avoided. In both cases, the solution is to not use such a sharp cutoff filter (in either the frequency or the time domain: i.e. to avoid truncation of the TAC.)

CONCLUSION

The popular method of sharp cutoff Fourier filtering (that is, fitting a TAC with a truncated Fourier series) can be employed successfully to reduce the noise in a TAC without a significant reduction in the ability to accurately calculate clinical parameters from the filtered TAC. To achieve this goal one must carefully select the number of harmonics employed. The error minimization technique discussed here is one technique by which one can make this selection. Even though frequency domain truncation has been employed, no significant deleterious effects are observed in clinical parameters calculated from the filtered TAC. This is probably due to the lack of high frequency components in most TACs (c.f. figure 5) and due to the fact that the TACs were sampled uniformly over the entire cardiac cycle (and thus were periodic with no large discontinuities). If, however, time domain truncation is performed, either for practical reasons or in a desire to filter, for example, only a limited portion of the curve, the effects of frequency domain truncation may become severe.

REFERENCES

1) Bove, A.A., Ziskin, M.C., Freeman, E., et al., Invest. Radiol., 5:329-335 (1970).
2) Hamilton, G.W., Williams D.L., Caldwell, J.H., in "Nuclear Cardiology: Selected Computer Aspects", p.p. 75-83, Soc. Nuc. Med. New York (1978).
3) Bacharach, S.L., Green, M.V., Borer, J.S., et al., J. Nuc. Med., 20:189-193 (1979).
4) Spiller, P., Quantitative Laevokardiographie, Urban Und. Schwarzenberg, Muchen (1978).
5) Fischer, P., Knopp, R., Bruel, H.P., Nucl. Med. 18:167-171 (1979).
6) Bacharach, S.L., Green, M.V., Bonow, R.O., et al., Journal of Nuclear Medicine, (in press).
7) Douglas, M.A., Bailey, J.J., VanRijk, P.P., et al., Computers in Cardiology, p.p. 315-318. IEEE 82CH1814-3 (1982).
8) Bacharach S.L., Green, M.V., Borer, J.S., Seminars in Nuc. Med. 9:257-274 (1979).
9) Brigham, E.O., "The Fast Fourier Transform", Prentice Hall, New Jersey.

DATA PROCESSING IN NUCLEAR VENTRICULOGRAPHY : ASSESSING CARDIAC FUNCTION FROM NOISY DATA

R. LUYPAERT and A. BOSSUYT

1. INTRODUCTION

In nuclear ventriculography, the equilibrium distribution of an intravascular tracer in the cardiac blood pool is monitored as a function of time during the heart cycle. Making use of ECG gating, computerized acquisition, processing and display, sequences of scintigrams spanning the entire cardiac cycle are obtained. The resulting data (Fig. 1) typically consist of some 65000 integers, each originating from a counting procedure and therefore subject to (usually quite large) statistical fluctuations. In order to be able to make quantitative assessments of the information contained in these data it is necessary to achieve considerable data reduction, introducing ventricular function quantifiers such as ejection fraction or 1st harmonic amplitude and phase. When doing this, two important questions must be answered:

1. In how far do the selected quantifiers contain the relevant information present in the original data ?
2. What is the effect of the statistical fluctuations in the original data ?

With these questions in mind, we have studied the extreme case of the synergy indices. These indices were developed in our hospital in view of quantifying

regional wall motion anomaly (1).
Using a computer model of EGNA observations the effect
of physiologic conditions and statistical noise were
evaluated. Strategies for neutralizing noise-induced
systematic errors were developed and tested.

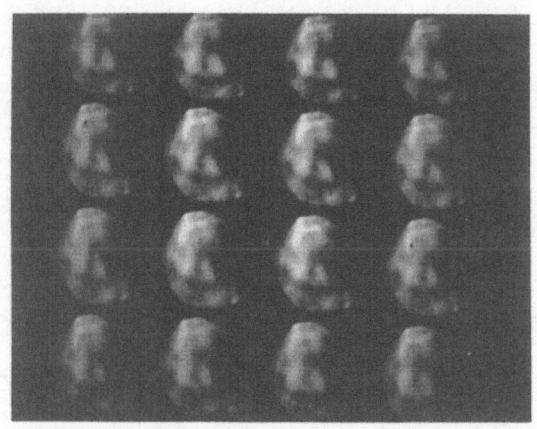

FIGURE 1. Typical nuclear ventriculography data set.

2. SYNERGY INDICES

The synergy indices aim at discovering asyner-
gic motion in the heart by comparing local and global
time-activity curves (TAC) for a certain region of
interest (ROI), for instance the left ventricle (LV).
They are defined as follows :

$$CI = \frac{ED - ES}{ED - MIN}$$

$$FI = \frac{ED - ES}{MAX - ES} \tag{1}$$

284

$$EFF = \frac{ED - ES}{MAX - MIN}$$

where ED represents the maximum of the global ROITAC,
ES the minimum of the global ROITAC, MAX the sum of the
maxima of the TACS of the pixels within the ROI and MIN
the sum of their minima: MAX = $\Sigma \, max_i$ and MIN = $\Sigma \, min_i$.
In fact, these expressions compare the pumping
contributions located at the individual pixels with the
net result in global pumping yield and give an idea of
the efficiency with which all parts cooperate in order
to generate the desired pumping action.

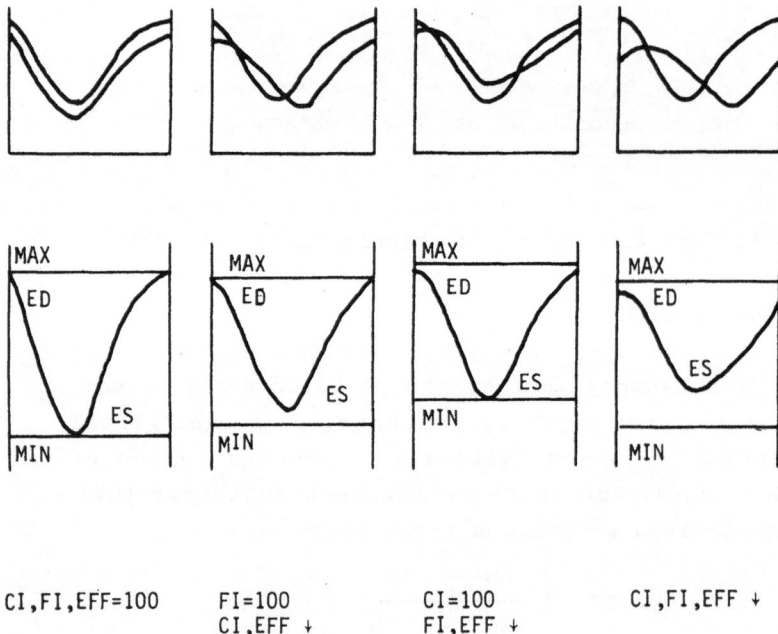

| CI,FI,EFF=100 | FI=100
CI,EFF ↓ | CI=100
FI,EFF ↓ | CI,FI,EFF ↓ |

FIGURE 2. Two-pixel examples: comparison of local and
global TACs and corresponding index response.

The way these indices work is illustrated in Fig. 2 for the 2-pixel case. In an ideal heart all parts of the LV cooperate and, consequently, global and local extrema coincide, leading to indices of 100 %. As soon as cooperation is broken somewhere along the cardiac cycle, however, a discrepancy between local and global extrema develops and at least two of the indices drop below 100 %.

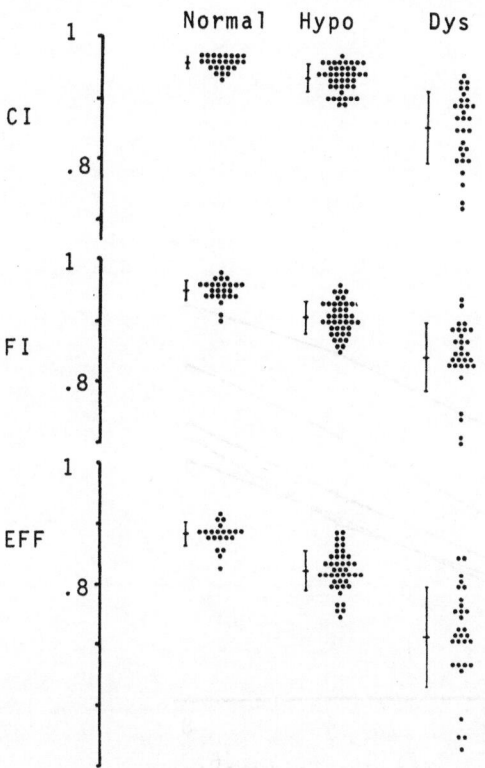

FIGURE 3. Relationship between indices and ventricular status.

Preliminary clinical investigations predicted
the synergy indices to be promising for assessing structural ventricular disorders (Fig.3). Additional tests,
however, collecting data sets at a number of different
counting statistics have subsequently shown their merit
to be jeopardized by large noise-induced systematic
errors (Fig.4); whereas at fixed counting statistics
the indices are well-defined, problems arise when comparing results obtained at different statistics.

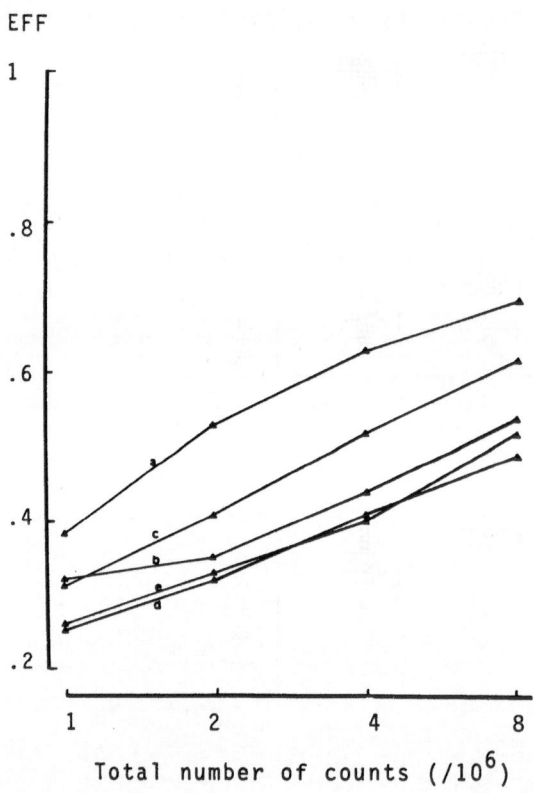

FIGURE 4. Dependence of measured EFF on counting
statistics (5 patients).

3. INDEX CHARACTERISTICS

The problem of characterizing and neutralizing this undesirable aspect as well as getting an idea of the quantitative behaviour of the indices was addressed here in the context of a computer model of EGNA observations. Equilibrium gated nuclear angiocardiographies were modeled in our computer by a 3D matrix containing localized, 16 frames/cycle TACs $f_{ij}(t)$ constructed on the basis of a truncated Fourier representation $s_{ij}(t)$ of the noise-free data and normally distributed, random noise $n_{ij}(t)$:

$$f_{ij}(t) = s_{ij}(t) + n_{ij}(t)$$
$$s_{ij}(t) = A0_{ij} + Cl_{ij} \cos(\omega t + \phi 1_{ij}) + \ldots \qquad (2)$$
$$n_{ij}(t) = \text{rand} \{ N (\text{Mean} = 0, \text{S.D.} = \sqrt{s}_{ij}(t) \}$$

By choosing appropriate sets of Fourier coefficients and phases and including or omitting the noise term it was possible to simulate various patient and data acquisition characteristics and estimate the effect of counting-statistical fluctuations. For conciseness we have only discussed EFF here : other indices behave analogously.

Two types of results were obtained using this approach. In simulations of the first type, the effect of simple motion deficiencies was investigated by introducing subregions of interest with pixels having a first harmonic amplitude smaller than that of the healthy pixels (C1 → C1/ ΔA) or exhibiting a first harmonic phase shift (Δφ) or a combination of both deficiencies. Some of the results have been summarized in Fig. 5. As expected, a lack of synchronicity between various wall segments is translated by lowered synergy indices. In fact, in contrast to the now widely accep-

288

ted phase/amplitude analysis, asynergy detection is not restricted here to 1st harmonic effects: any factor disturbing the synergic motion of the ventricle wall will lower the pumping efficiency and the indices. On the other hand, pure amplitude effects will not affect cooperation between segments and will therefore not influence synergy indices based on noise-free data. The decrease in index values noted in figure 5b must therefore be entirely due to the presence of noise.

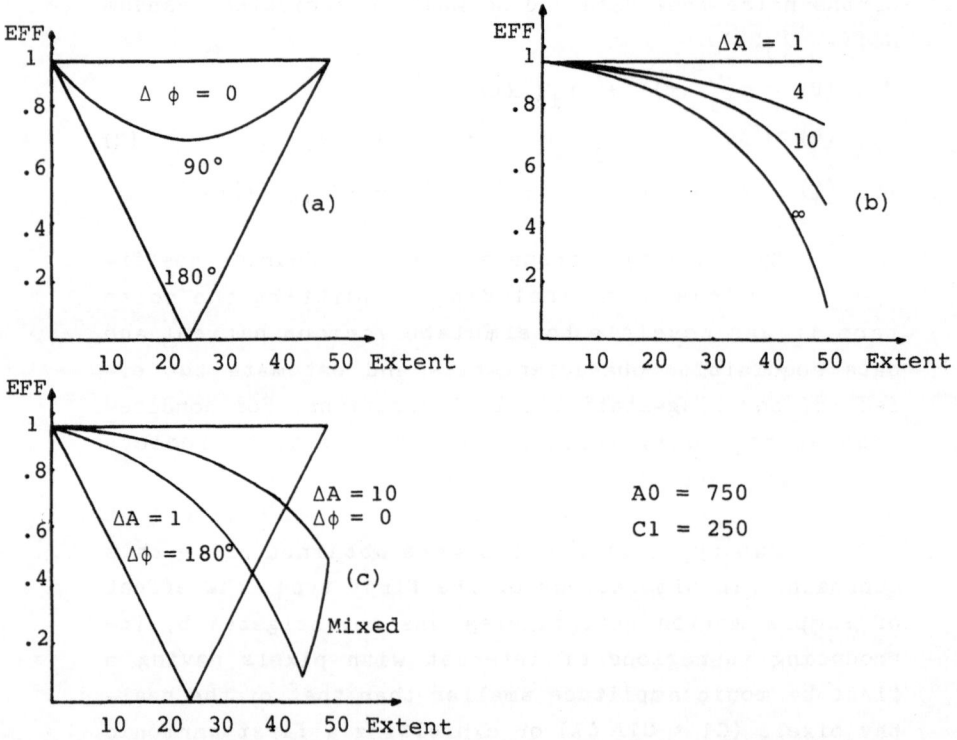

FIGURE 5. Relationship between EFF and lesion extent (ROI contains 50 pixels) for simple physiological deficiencies: a) timing effects, b) amplitude effects, c) mixed.

This may be further understood when contemplating the second type of results. In graph 6, the effect of changing levels of statistical noise in different situations is illustrated. It was found that counting-statistical fluctuations in the TACs entail large systematic errors in the indices (due to overestimating maxima and underestimating minima).

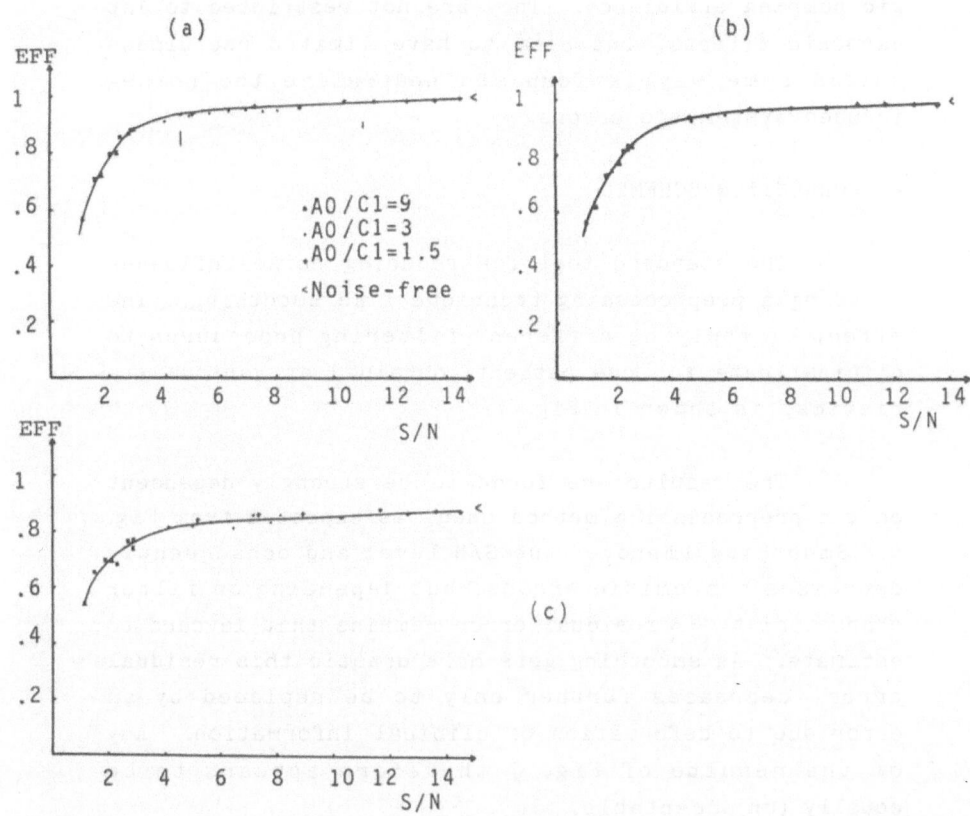

FIGURE 6. EFF as a function of counting statistics: a) complete synchronism, b) amplitude defect (ΔA = 2 in 7/50), c) phase defect ($\Delta\phi$ = 90° in 7/50).

As shown in the figure, the signal-to-noise ratio (S/N), as measured by C1 / SQRT (AO) (2), provided a suitable parametrization for the noise behaviour : TACs of widely different shapes but the same S/N yield very nearly equal systematic errors.

The preceding results show that the synergy indices have some quite attractive characteristics : they provide objective hemodynamic quantities, measuring synergic pumping efficiency. They are not restricted to 1st harmonic effects, but seem to have limited usefulness unless some way is found to neutralize the noise-induced systematic errors.

4. CORRECTION SCHEMES

The standard tool for reducing noise influence is using a preprocessing technique like smoothing. The effect of applying different filtering procedures to clinical data for one patient, obtained at various statistics, is shown in Fig. 7.

The results are found to be strongly dependent on the preprocessing method used, as expected from Fig. 6. Smoothing improves the S/N level and consequently decreases systematic errors, but depending on filter characteristics a residual error remains that is hard to estimate. As smoothing gets more drastic this residual error decreases further only to be replaced by an error due to deformation of clinical information. Any of the results of Fig. 7 therefore appears to be equally (un)acceptable.

In order to design a correction method that works, a few further aspects of the noise properties of the synergy indices have to be considered.

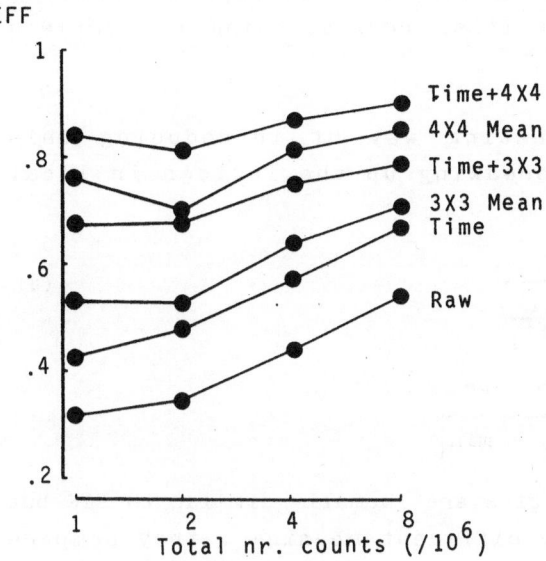

FIGURE 7. The effect of smoothing on dependence EFF vs counting statistics (1 patient).

First, the measured (i.e. including systematic error) value EFF* may be described by :

$$EFF^* = EFF + \Delta EFF \qquad (3)$$
$$= EFF \left(1 - \frac{\Delta(MAX - MIN)}{MAX - MIN}\right)$$

where systematic errors are denoted by Δ signs.
EFF contains the synergy information and is free of noise, while the expression inside the brackets is, to a good approximation, only dependent on S/N for the different pixels : since

$$\Delta(MAX - MIN) = \Sigma \, \Delta(max_i - min_i)$$

the systematic errors are determined by 1-pixel statistics and therefore not affected by asynergy. As a consequence, the average behaviour f(S/N) of pixels with a known S/N is described by Fig. 6a (case of identical 1-pixel TACs, corresponding to complete synergy and EFF = 1).

Secondly, an interesting way of introducing this information is breaking up the indices in local contributions :

$$EFF = \frac{1}{\Sigma \frac{1}{eff_i}} \qquad (4)$$

where

$$eff_i = \frac{ED - ES}{max_i - min_i}$$

These local quantities are formally similar to EFF but have a completely different meaning : they compare single-pixel stroke volume to the global stroke volume and therefore yield information on motion amplitude rather than synchronism. As a consequence of (4), the systematic error on EFF may be traced to a systematic error on eff_i with a known dependence f(S/N), providing a basis for correcting EFF^* via well-defined corrections of eff_i^*.

Finally, since akinetic segments do not influence noise-free synergy indices while contributing strongly to the noise effects, it may be advantageous to eliminate low amplitude parts before correcting. This may be done, for instance, by introducing a lower limit to local S/N or requiring a minimum C1/AO (connection between both criteria : Fig. 8), eventually after changing effective S/N by spatial smoothing.

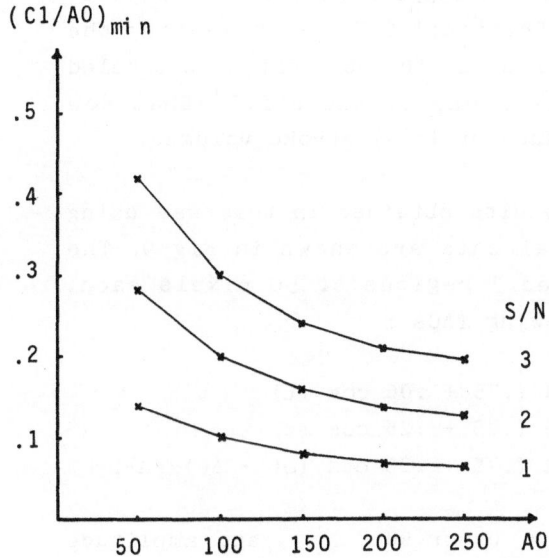

FIGURE 8. Comparison between akinesis and "akinesis".

Taking these points into account, the correction scheme that was finally adopted uses following steps :

1. Preprocessing with 9 point spatial smoother;
2. The effective S/N of each pixel within ROI is calculated;
3. Pixels with S/N < 1 are rejected and labeled "akinetic";
4. For all accepted pixels eff_i^* is calculated and corrected via

$$eff_i = \frac{eff_i^*}{f(S/N)} \qquad (5)$$

5. From the corrected local indices a corrected global index EFF is derived.

The results may be supplemented by a new parameter, the "akinetic fraction" (AF), representing the
relative number of points in the ROI that were labeled
"akinetic" and also by a map of the eff_i^{-1} that now
provide a correct measure of local stroke volumes.

Examples of results obtained in this way using
simulated and clinical data are shown in Fig 9. The
simulated LV contained 3 regions of 50 pixels each,
characterized by following TACs :

Region 1 : a_1 (t) = AM (.75 + .06 cos ωt)
Region 2 : a_2 (t) = AM (.75 + .25 cos ωt)   (6)
Region 3 : a_3 (t) = AM (.75 + .25 cos (ωt + $\Delta\phi$)/ΔA),

where phase shift $\Delta\phi$ = 0 or 90 °   and amplitude
attenuation ΔA = 1 or 2 in region 3.   In Fig. 9a the
original and corrected values are plotted together with
the true values (no noise) for a number of counting
statistics. As shown, the corrected indices afford a
good approximation to the true ones. These findings
were confirmed by the clinical results of Fig.9b. Here
a small dependence on statistics remains, due to the
changing region of points labeled "akinetic". The
resulting indices nevertheless provide a correct
description of the accepted segments for all counting
statistics. The effect of correction on the indices
quantifying local stroke volume is illustrated in Fig.
10. Again the corrected values provide a good appoxima-
tion of the true values. Fig. 11 shows analogous
results based on clinical data from a healthy and a
disturbed heart (the black region between two ROI boundaries is "akinetic").

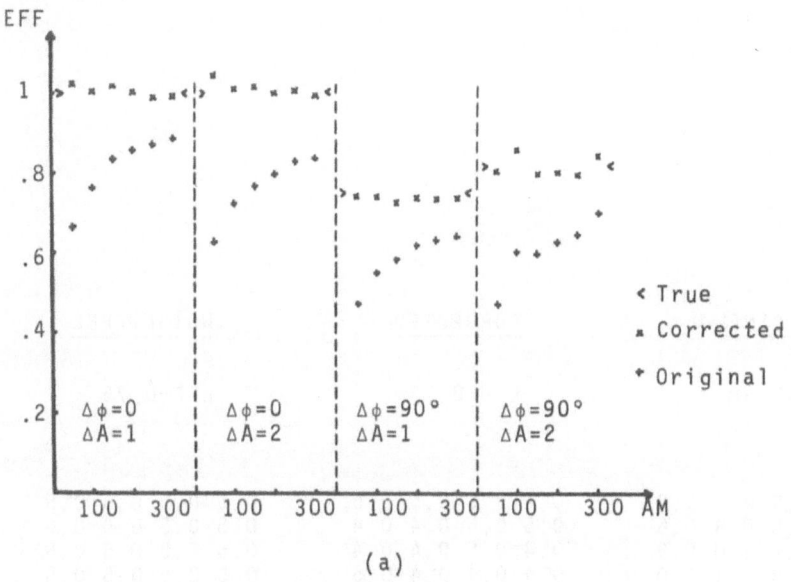

(a)

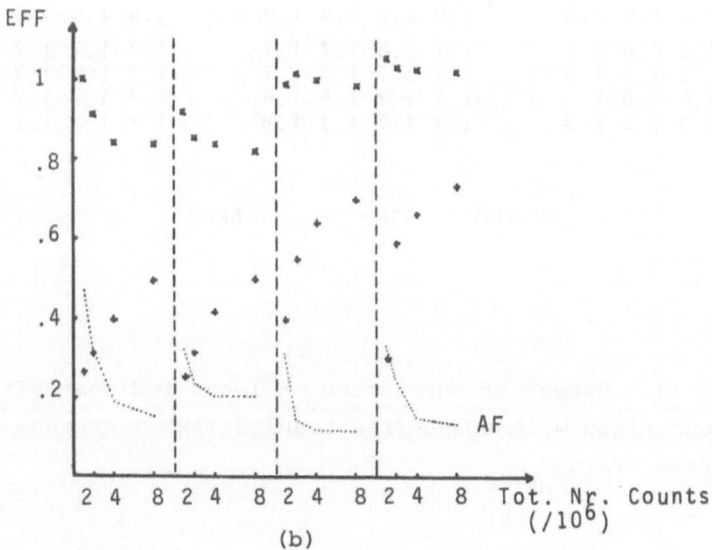

(b)

FIGURE 9. EFF vs counting statistics before and after correction: (a) simulated data,(b) clinical data (4 patients)

ORIGINAL	CORRECTED	NOISE-FREE
EFF=0.58	EFF=0.73	EFF=0.75

```
0.9 0.9 0.8 1.0      0.4 0.5 0.5 0.5      0.5 0.5 0.5 0.5
0.9 0.8 0.9 0.6      0.5 0.5 0.4 0.4      0.5 0.5 0.5 0.5
1.0 1.2 1.0 0.9      0.4 0.5 0.4 0.4      0.5 0.5 0.5 0.5
0.7 0.9 1.1 1.0      0.4 0.4 0.4 0.5      0.5 0.5 0.5 0.5

2.1 1.8 2.3 2.8      2.0 1.9 1.8 1.9      1.9 1.9 1.9 1.9
2.0 2.2 2.7 2.2      1.9 1.9 1.9 2.0      1.9 1.9 1.9 1.9
2.1 2.2 2.2 1.6      2.0 2.0 2.1 2.0      1.9 1.9 1.9 1.9
2.5 2.1 1.9 1.0      2.0 2.0 2.0 1.9      1.9 1.9 1.9 1.9

2.0 2.2 2.0 2.3      1.7 1.8 1.7 1.7      1.7 1.7 1.7 1.7
1.9 2.5 1.9 1.8      1.7 1.7 1.7 1.7      1.7 1.7 1.7 1.7
1.7 2.0 2.0 2.3      1.7 1.7 1.6 1.6      1.7 1.7 1.7 1.7
1.8 1.9 1.8 2.3      1.7 1.7 1.7 1.8      1.7 1.7 1.7 1.7
```

AM=150   ASN=7.8   AF=0

FIGURE 10. Effect of correction on local indices (eff_i^{-1}) and comparison with noise-free results (ASN = average effective S/N).

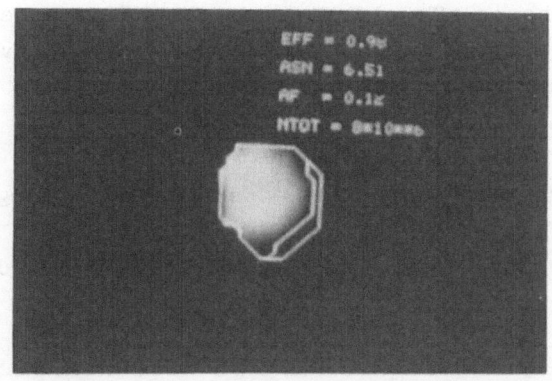

(a)

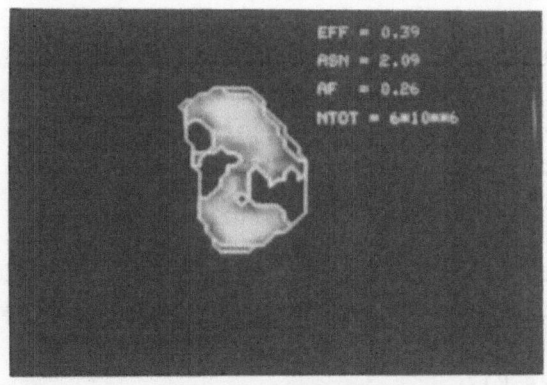

(b)

FIGURE 11. Complete set of results for 2 patients : a) healthy, b) disturbed.

5. CONCLUSIONS

On the basis of a computer model of EGNA measurements we have developed a procedure for quantifying regional wall motion. When completely carried out, the procedure yields following information:

1. Noise-corrected global indices expressing synergic pumping efficiency;
2. Noise-corrected local indices providing a measure of relative local stroke volume;
3. The fraction of "akinetic" pixels.

Clinical investigations of the sensitivity and relative merit of these parameters are under way.

REFERENCES

(1) Bossuyt A, Deconinck F 1982. Radionuclide indices of cardiac function related to structural ventricular disorders. In : Digital Imaging - Clinical Advances in Nuclear Medicine. Ed. P. Esser. SNM, New York.

(2) Bacharach SL, Green MV et al. 1983. Optimum number of harmonics for fitting cardiac volume curves. In: Proceedings of 30th Annual Meeting SNM, J. Nucl. Med. 24 P17.

THE DEFINITION OF A SINGLE MEASURE OF REGIONAL WALL MOTION ABNORMALITY IN
SCINTIGRAPHIC VENTRICULOGRAPHY

MICHAEL L. GORIS
Stanford University School of Medicine

ABSTRACT

We undertook this study to investigate if a single measure of focal
or regional wall motion abnormalities could be devised. Since it can be
shown that the global ejection fraction does not necessarily decrease
until a substantial fraction of the myocardium has been damaged, and
since global parameters are easily influenced by non-myocardial variables
such as after-load, pre-load and heart rate, it seemed that a more
precise measure of focal damage was needed.

Our approach is based on the hypothesis that in the absence of
focal damage, each myocardial segment has a constant relative contribution to the global ejection fraction. While global, non-cardiac factors
which influence the global ejection fraction will also influence all
segments, they will not influence the relative (amongst segments)
contraction of the segments. Hence, all data could be normalized to a
"normal" global ejection fraction.

The first step of the method is analogous to the circumferential
profile methods in Thallium myocardial perfusion scintigraphies; after
the (automatic) delineation of the left ventricular borders and the
isolation of left ventricular activities by interpolation from those
borders, 255 radii evenly spaced over 360 degrees are defined, originating
in the center of mass of the left ventricle computed in the end-diastolic
frame. Along those radii counts are integrated over the outer half, between
center and border, in the end-diastolic image, and over the identical pixels
in the end-systolic image. From those data 256 radial ejection fractions
are computed.

From 12 middle-aged volunteers a normal resting and a normal stress
profile is then computed, with a standard deviation value for each radial
value. The index of regional or focal wall motion abnormality is computed
from the cumulative difference between corresponding points in the test

cases versus the "normal" profile, expressed either in absolute units or
in fractions of the local standard deviations.   The difference, however, can
be either the sum of the absolute differences, the sum of the square, or
the cubes of the differences. Those definitions favor, respectively, wide
or deep abnormalities.

To test the feasibility (and not yet the clinical efficacy), we studied
8 patients with infarction who for two years had no further cardiac problems,
and 8 patients chosen from the same cohort but who did have a medical cardiac
event during the same time. Both groups differ significantly from the "normal"
and to some extent from each other.

INTRODUCTION

Focal cardiomyopathies can affect regional ventricular contractility
without affecting global ventricular function. Indeed, in myocardial infarction
the global ejection fraction (EF) does decrease in larger infarctions, but it
can be shown that the decrease of EF is not linearily proportional to the size
of the insult (1). Recently interest has been expressed in using scintigraphic
ventriculography to estimate the effect of an intervention aimed at reducing
infarct size. The study would include lateral comparisons (treated vs.
untreated group) and longitudinal comparisons, eventually with pre- and post
treatment evaluation. It is unlikely, however, that the global EF could yield
sufficiently precise results to exclude small treatment effects, since, in
addition to yielding a non-linear relation with infarct size, the EF is also
influenced by non-myocardial factors such as pre-load and after-load.

Until now, however, no single quantitative measure of focal dyskinesis
or hypokinesis has been accepted.

MATERIALS AND METHODS

1.   The definition of the WMAI

While it is not difficult to detect focal hypo- or dyskinesis and
while descriptive evaluations do exist (2,3), it is not intuitively clear
how one would QUANTIFY a lesion. The difficulty arises in part from the
ambiguity between size and depth: how can one comapre a large hypokinetic
region with a small dyskinetic region? Furthermore, the very definition of
"focal" fails as large focal abnormalities merge with diffuse abnormalities.

The first aim is to separate global from purely regional ventricular
function. This is made difficult by the fact that global function is the
sum of regional function and that factors which affect global function can
affect the expression of regional (dys) function. In that respect, it

should be noted that in the classical angiographic interpretation regional hypokinesia can be present in all segments, which results in confusion between global function and focal injury.

The second aim is to quantify regional or focal dysfunction with a single numeral, which should remain distinct from the EF, even though the latter is a function of the former. Furthermore, this single numeral must be derived in a manner which allows accounting for SIZE and DEPTH of the dysfunction.

To overcome the conceptual difficulties associated with those aims, it is necessary to clarify the semantics:

We redefine a focal contractility abnormality (or Focal Wall Motion Abnormality - FWMA) as lesser contractility than expected for the location in relation with the EF. If $X(J)$ is the measure of wall motion at location J, then $X(J)$ is compared to a "normal value" $E(J)$, following a normalization by the global EF value. The normalization is somewhat arbitrary and yields $Y(J)$.

The expected measure of wall motion in location J is $E(J)$. $E(J)$ is computed as the average of $Y(J)$ values from a set of "normal" patients, and represents the average normalized normal value at J, and is associated with a standard deviation $S(J)$.

The FWMAI describes the degree to which the test profile $Y(J)$ differs from the "expected normal" profile $E(J)$. Less obvious is the need to modulate by $S(J)$. In the normal $S(J)$ is not zero, nor constant for different J's. One could therefore compute $SUM((Y(J))**2/S(J))$, to reduce the effect of "natural variation". The degree to which the FWMAI favors deep abnormalities or wide abnormalities depends on the manner of registration of the difference between $Y(I)$ and $E(I)$. The "zero" moment which is $SUM(ABSOLUTE(Y(J)-E(J)))$ favors wide abnormalities, the higher moments (e.g., $SUM(ABSOLUTE(Y(J)-E(J))**3)$ favors deep abnormalities.

2. Computations

The data are obtained from scintigraphic ventriculographies, either first pass (FPNA) or Equilibrium ECG Gated (EGNA). In both cases the acquisition algorithm (in EGNA) or the preprocessing algorithm yields an "image" of a representative cardiac cycle, mapped in a three dimensional array of count rate densities $A(k,l,i)$. This image consists of 16 frames ($i=1, 16$), with the ED data mapped into frame 1 and 16, and the end-systolic (ES) mapped in a frame close to frame 8. Each frame has a resolution of 64 x 64 (k and I = 1,64).

Processing includes the definition of a left ventricular sampling region or Region of Interest (LVROI) (4) in non-interactive mode. Following this an image of the "isolated left ventricle" is produced, from the original, filtered and thresholded data, by the application of an interpolative background subtraction (5), which uses the LVROI as reference. This image of the isolated left ventricle, $IA(k,l,i)$, has the same structure as $A(k,l,i)$ but only those counts which originated from the left ventricle are assumed to be included.

A radial approach is used to compute $X(J)$. The image of the "isolated left ventricle" $(IA(k,l,i)$ is first transformed from Cartesian to polar coordinates, with the origin at the center of mass of the ventricle and 0 degree at the apex. In the transformed data set $IB(lr, j,i)$ lr represents the distance from the center, j the angle number and i the sequence number in the data set or the temporal coordinate. To avoid oversampling at the center, the row values are sampled from $IR1$ to $IR2$ where $IR1=IR2/2$ and $IR2$ is the outer edge of the end-diastolic ventricle at that angle. The row sum of $IB(lr,j,ED)$ is $BS(J,ED)$ where ED is the sequence number of end-diastole, and $BS(J,ES)$ is the corresponding value for end-systole. Therefore $X(J)=BS(J,ED)-BS(J,ES))/BS(J,ED)$. For N angles we define N+1 $X(J)$ values, $X(N+1)$ being computed from the image elements not included in the row-sum.

The selection of N is not arbitrary, but is based on the resolution of the data set. For a 64 x 64 frame, the value of N needed to avoid undersampling is 256 (6).

The alignment of the apex at angle 0 and 360 is a simple translation in the polar image (6,7).

The EF to which $X(J)$ will be normalized to obtain $Y(J)$ is found from the integrated counts in the Cartesian image $IA(k,l,i)$ which yield a time-activity vector $T(I)$. Since the data are uncontaminated left ventricular data, the GEF is simply $(T(i)max - T(i)min)/T(i)max$.

The normal angular values $E(J)$ are computed from measured values in a set of normal cases, $Y(I,J)$, where I is the patient number and J the angle number as before: for N patients $E(J) = SUM (Y(I,J))/N$ summated over I only. The variation is computed as a standard deviation $S(J) = SQRT ((SUM(Y(I,J)**2)-SUM(Y(I,J))*E(J))/(N-1))$, summated over I only

(SQRT = square root).

The FWMA index is computed as SUM (ABSOLUTE ((Y(J)-E(J))/W)**P) summed over J and with values of P varying from 1 to 3 and with W either equal to 1 or to S(J).

RESULTS AND DISCUSSION

The computational method used is a deliberate compromise between the linear analysis associated with cineangiography, which favors the detection of "peripheral" abnormalities, and the densitometric analysis, associated with scintigraphic studies, and recently with digital angiography, which approached the image as a three-dimensional rendition of volumes (x, y and the count rate density). To avoid having all values unduly influenced by the behavior of the central portion of the ventricle, we start the radial summation away from the center. The radial ejection fractions computed in this way do therefore tend to favor peripheral events.

Amongst various methods to normalize, we found empirically that the relation Y(J) = X(J) + (75.-0.5*EF) was the most effective. To have simply normalized by 1/EF would have resulted in an artificial increase in the range of the radial ejection fractions. Indeed, the index became almost totally a function of the normalization factor.

Even so, the index is not totally independent of the EF, and by linear regression analysis we found that the index computed with W=S(J) and P=2. was related to the EF as FWMAI = 14.82 - 0.179* EF. The correlation coefficient was -0.87 and the F ratio (1,17) was 57. But this correlation appeared as an artifact of the data set, in which all low values of the global EF were in patients with large infarcted areas.

On the other hand, as shown in Table 1, the index is larger in patients with documented infarction, and tends to be larger and increase with exercise in those with presumably residual ischemia.

Since no objective measure of the index exists independently, its value will have to come from clinical validation, or its predictive value. The number of (arbitrary) alternative methods to measure such an index make the evaluation particularly difficult. Yet, this work demonstrates that the approach can lead to a discriminating index, whose independent value remains to be established.

REFERENCES

1. Goris ML, Hung J, Vanhaecke J, Barat JL, Paldi JH and DeBusk RF: The correlation between ventricular function and the quantitative analysis of exercise and rest Thallium myocardial scintigraphy. Clin Nucl Med 6: (suppl.) 450, 1981.
2. Adam WC, Tarkowska A, Bitter F, Stauch H, and Geffers H: Equilibrium (gated) radionuclide ventriculography. Cardiovasc Radiology 2: 161-173, 1979.
3. Maddox DE, Holman BL, Wynne J, Idoine J, Parker JA, Uren R, Neill NM, and Cohn PF: Ejection fraction image: A non-invasive index of regional left ventricular motion. Am J Cardiology 41: 1230-1238, 1978.
4. Goris ML, McKillop JH, Briandet PA: A fully automated determination of the left ventricular region of interest in nuclear angiocardiography. Cardiovasc Interven Radiology 4: 117-123, 1981.
5. Goris ML, Daspit SG, McLaughlin P and Kriss JP: Interpolative background subtraction. J Nucl Med 17: 744-747, 1976.
6. Goris ML, Sue J and Johnson MA: A principled approach to the circumferential method for Thallium myocardial perfusion scintigraphy quantitation. In: Non-invasive Assessment of the Cardiovascular System. Ed. EB Diethrich. John Wright PSG Inc., pp 273-276, 1981.
7. Goris ML and Briandet PA: A Clinical and Mathematical Introduction to Computer Processing of Scintigraphic Images. Raven Press, New York, NY, pp. 206-208.

Table 1: WMA Index Values in Three Subgroups of Patients

	REST		L1		L2		EP		RECOV	
	AV	SD	AV	SD	AV	SD	AV	SD	AV	SD
Normal	2.1	3.3	2.9	3.7	1.7	1.3	0.9	1.0	0.5	0.7
Group 1	5.3	4.9	7.4	6.5	6.9	6.4	7.2	7.8	5.3	6.7
Group 2	6.3	3.8	9.7	5.9	9.7	5.2	11.0	5.0	9.5	9.1

The tabulation is given for normals (not used to determine the normal
distribution) and two groups of patients with infarction, the second
with a poor outcome within three years, but otherwise both groups taken
from the same cohort.

The results are given for the resting state and three levels of stress,
including the last level reached (EP) and the immediate post-exercise
period (recovery)

The data are given as average (AV) and standard deviation (SD), this
latter in contradistinction to the standard error of the mean, which
would be smaller. Student's t test would not be appropriate, since the
variances are significantly different between normal and the infarct
groups. The infarct groups do not differ significantly.

The increase of the WMA index at the last level corresponds with a
separate observation that healthy well motivated volunteers tend to
exercise until the ventricular reserve is reached. In this case P=2 and
W=S(J) (see text).

IMAGE ANALYSIS –TOPOLOGICAL METHODS.

A. Toet, J.J. Koenderink, P. Zuidema, C.N. de Graaf.
Department of Medical and Physiological Physics and Institute of Nuclear Medicine, State University Utrecht, The Netherlands.
Mailing address: Physics Laboratory, Princetonplein 5, 3584 CC Utrecht, The Netherlands.

ABSTRACT.

The aim of image analysis is to provide a symbolic description of the image structure, that can serve to supply information about the image for all kinds of different tasks.

We will give a complete description of the topological structure of images, studied simultaneously at all levels of resolution. This can be achieved through the artifice of embedding an image into a continuous family of images that can be uniquely generated by it. We will show how the representation of the image structure on different levels of resolution may be linked in a logical manner, so that features existing at different levels of resolution get related to each other.

Our method explains the succes of recently introduced 'pyramid' algorithms and is of value for the study of image morphology per se. Furthermore, it is not at all limited to two-dimensional images.

INTRODUCTION.

1.1. The aim of image analysis.

In this article a distinction will be made between image processing and image analysis. With <u>image processing</u> we refer to all those methods that have the original picture as input, and give another picture as output, for example methods like thresholding, filtering and distorting. The output is thereafter studied by a human observer, and the transformation is valued for its capability to accentuate or suppress certain properties of the original input image. When the transformation is irreversible certain features of the original input picture are discarded and the resulting image will have less structure than the original one. This can be very useful when there are a priori reasons to consider certain properties of a picture as irrelevant ('noise'). Image processing is trivial in the sense that the proper interpretation of the contents of a picture is left to the observer. When the character of the desired information changes, it is necessary to go back to the original picture and apply a different kind of transform to it.

With <u>image analysis</u>, the input structure is also a picture, but the outcome isn't. The problem is not so much to eliminate noise, as to seperate events at different scales arising from different physical processes. Here the desired result is a symbolic description of the image structure. Such a description can serve as a datum for automatic diagnostic decision procedures. If such a symbolic description is to have a general applicability there should be no need to return to the original input image if the character of the desired information alters. So what we are looking for is a general description of the structure of an image, that can serve to supply information about that image for all kinds of purposes.

1.2. Towards a hierarchical description of the structure of images.

A symbolic description of the structure of an image should be as <u>compact</u> as possible, and its elements should correspond as closely as possible to meaningful objects or events in the signal forming process. It should be <u>natural</u> in the sense that partial descriptions (e.g. truncations) should be simpler than the original and should have the character of a logically filtered image. Local deletion of detail should not affect global description (figure 1). We will show that the level lines through the critical points of the image induce a unique organical decomposition thereof into a collection of juxtaposed and superimposed blobs of low and high function value, by which the basic differential topological structure of the image is revealed.

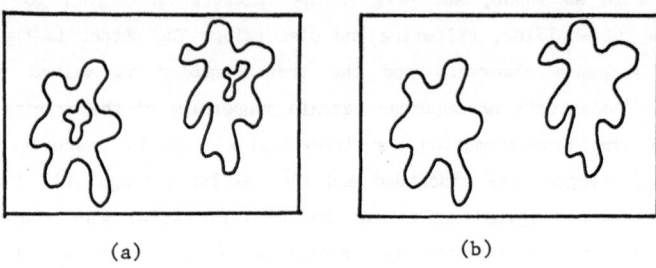

(a)   (b)

Figure 1. (a): Arbitrary image. (b): Local deletion of detail does not
          affect the global decription of (a).

It is important to realize that the structure of an image depends on aperture size, and that sampled (=real) images, obtained with different resolving power, yield different maps of the same region as it were, none of which is intrinsically more interesting or important than the others. For instance for different resolving power fig. 2 may be interpreted as a line piece, squares, circles or points. We will show that image structure, described in terms of a foliation through level lines, changes at discrete values of the resolving power. The set of all structural formulae, ordered with respect to resolving power, will be called the aperture spectrum of the image.

Thus the dependence of image structure on resolving power introduces an ambiguity that is inherent and inescapable. Merely computing the image structure for multiple levels of resolution is clearly of no avail to reduce this ambiguity. By relating the resolution levels to each other we get a hierarchical description of the image structure which enables us to deal

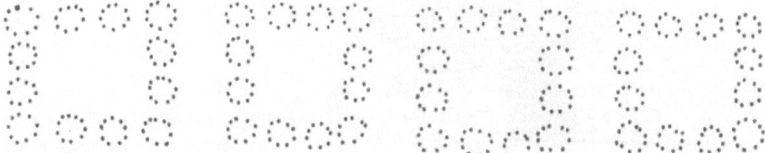

Figure 2. Illustration of the resolution dependency of image structure.

effectively with this problem. Parts of an image that look interesting on low levels of resolution may be subjected to a closer examination on higher levels of resolution, without having to waste time with the examination of irrelevant details outside the interesting regions.

There remains the problem of finding a relation between the description of image structure on different levels of resolution. Work done in this area has led to the development of so called "pyramid" or "cone" algorithms [1]. However, no unique criteria for constructing them have been developed. We will show that the artifice of embedding an image into a continuous family of images that can be uniquely generated by it, provides a way to link images on different levels of resolution in a logical way. We propose to use the method of projection along steepest descent curves on levels of constant function value to convey information obtained at low levels of resolution to higher resolution levels.

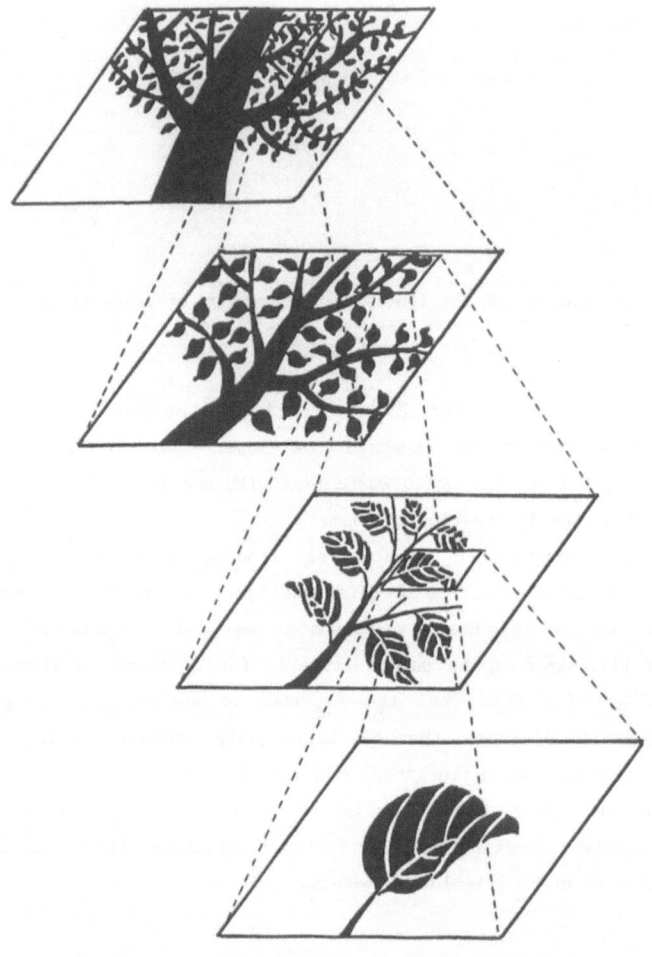

Figure 3. The linking of descriptions of image structure at multiple levels of resolution allows for zooming in on relevant details.

2. IMAGE STRUCTURE AT A SINGLE LEVEL OF RESOLUTION.

In the context of this paper an 'image' is a two-dimensional scalar field (e.g. luminance, photographic desity , etc.) denoted $\phi(\vec{r})$ (or $\phi(x,y)$, where x,y are Cartesian coordinates in the image plane). In the sequal we restrict the discussion to analytic functions $\phi(\vec{r})$. In the next section it will turn out that this is no real restriction, however.

First we consider the <u>local</u> structure of the image. Any analytic function can locally be approximated with its Taylor series, we write

$$\phi(\vec{r}+\vec{\delta r}) = \phi(\vec{r}) + \vec{\nabla}\phi(\vec{r}).\vec{\delta r} + \vec{\delta r}.H\vec{\delta r} + \ldots$$

with

$$\vec{\nabla}\phi(r) = (\frac{\partial\phi}{\partial x} , \frac{\partial\phi}{\partial y}) \quad , \text{ the gradient}$$

and

$$H = \begin{pmatrix} \dfrac{\partial^2\phi}{\partial x^2} & \dfrac{\partial^2\phi}{\partial x\partial y} \\ \dfrac{\partial^2\phi}{\partial x\partial y} & \dfrac{\partial^2\phi}{\partial y^2} \end{pmatrix} \quad , \text{ the Hessian matrix.}$$

Depending on the vanishing of terms in the Taylor series we distinguish three main cases:

<u>regular points</u>: at a regular point the gradient term does not vanish $(\vec{\nabla}\phi.\vec{\nabla}\phi \neq 0)$.

<u>critical points</u>: at a critical point the gradient term vanishes $(\vec{\nabla}\phi.\vec{\nabla}\phi = 0)$, the behaviour is described by the second order terms (det $H \neq 0$) . The value of the function at the critical point is called a critical value.

<u>degenerated critical points</u>: at degenerated critical points both the gradient and the determinant of the Hessian matrix vanish $(\vec{\nabla}\phi.\vec{\nabla}\phi = $ det $H = 0)$.

A 'Morse-function' or 'generic function' ϕ is distinguished through the fact that:

  - it has no degenerated critical points;
  - its critical points are isolated, thus there can be only finitely many critical points in an image of finite extent;
  - all critical values are distinct.

In differential topology [2,3] it is shown that the Morse functions are dense in the space of analytic functions. In other words, almost all functions are Morse. Any non—Morse function has Morse functions infinitesimally near it: so the slightest perturbation is sufficient to make it a Morse function. Thus Morse functions are truely 'generic', real (i.e. known to a finite tolerance) functions are all generic.

Hence the local structure of (generic) images is simple enough: almost all points are regular (thus fairly trivial) and of the 'special' points there exist only a few types. These types can be conveniently distinguished by the sign of the determinant of the Hessian

$$(\frac{\partial^2 \phi}{\partial x^2} \frac{\partial^2 \phi}{\partial y^2} - (\frac{\partial^2 \phi}{\partial x \partial y})^2) \qquad \text{and the sign of its trace}$$

$$(\text{tr } H = \frac{\partial^2 \phi}{\partial x^2} + \frac{\partial^2 \phi}{\partial y^2} = \Delta\phi, \text{ that is the Laplacian of } \phi) .$$

You have:
  - det $H < 0$ a saddle point (e.g. $w(x,y) = x^2 - y^2$ at the origin) .
  - det $H > 0$ an extremum. Of these there are two types:
       - tr $H > 0$ a pit (e.g. $\phi(x,y) = x^2 + y^2$ at the origin);
       - tr $H < 0$ a peak (e.g. $\phi(x,y) = -x^2 - y^2$ at the origin).
Regular points, saddle points, pits an peaks exhaust the possibilities of local image structure.

A global structure of Morse images is generated by drawing the level lines of the function (e.g. isophotes, equidensity contours) for its critical values. This gives a foliation of the picture into areas consisting of nothing but regular points. The level lines through the extrema will of course degenerate into points, so that the foliation is in fact completely defined by the level lines through the saddle points. These lines are closed loops with selfintersections (the influence of the boundary is not considered here, it is easy to solve this problem). The selfintersections are the saddle points, and we can name the loops after them. They divide the family of level lines into equivalence classes of homotopic curves (curves that can be continuously deformed into each other), that are simple closed loops (without selfintersections) or that end on the edge of the image. The loops are oriented: they either enclose a region of higher or of lower functional values. If a critical level line has a high level compared to a loop that just encloses it, we call it a pseudo—peak, otherwise a pseudo—pit. Both pseudo

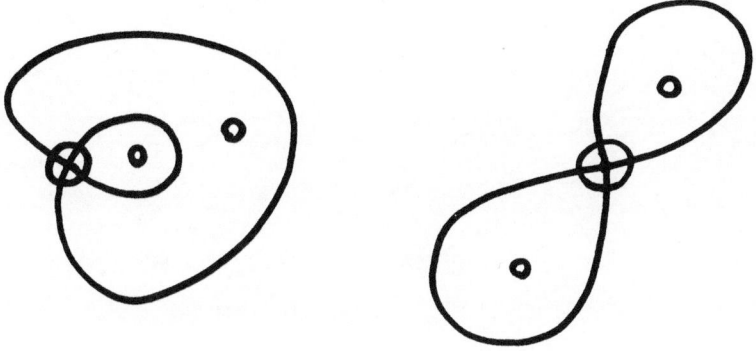

Figure 4. Level lines for the critical values of a two dimensional scalar function.

extrema occur in two varieties: the loop can have a figure eight shape (figure 5) or it may encircle some points twice (figure 6). In the first case a pseudo-pit contains two (pseudo-) pits (similar for pseudo-peaks), in the latter case it contains a (pseudo-) pit and a (pseudo-) peak.

The (pseudo-) extrema occur juxtaposed and can be nested to arbitrary depth (figure 7). This representation of the global image structure is particularly convenient, because it treats pits and peaks on the same footing, and it explicitly shows a (partial) order of critical levels.

When minima are represented by round, and maxima by rectangular parentheses, then the qualitative structure of an arbitrary image can be represented by a parentheses formula (e.g. figure 8a: $([A]((D)([B](C))_\gamma)_\beta)_\alpha$ or in words: a light spot A and a dark spot β consisting of a dark spot D and a dark spot γ consisting of a light spot B and a dark spot C embedded in a dark spot α).This is a unique description of the qualitative structure of the image. The parentheses formula may be augmented in a variety of ways with

314

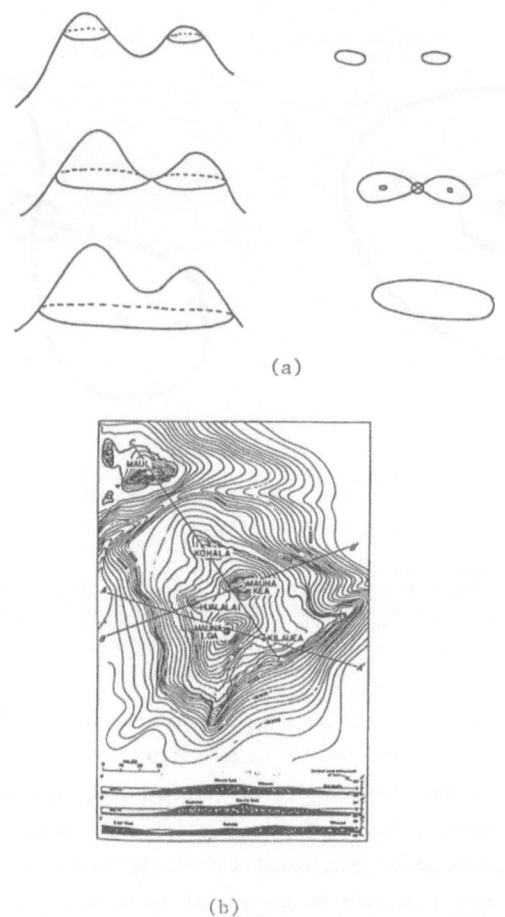

(a)

(b)

Figure 5. Examples of level lines with a figure eight shape. (a): The general structure near a level line with a figure eight shape. (b):Figure eight shape of a contourline in a map of contourlines of the isle of Hawaii.

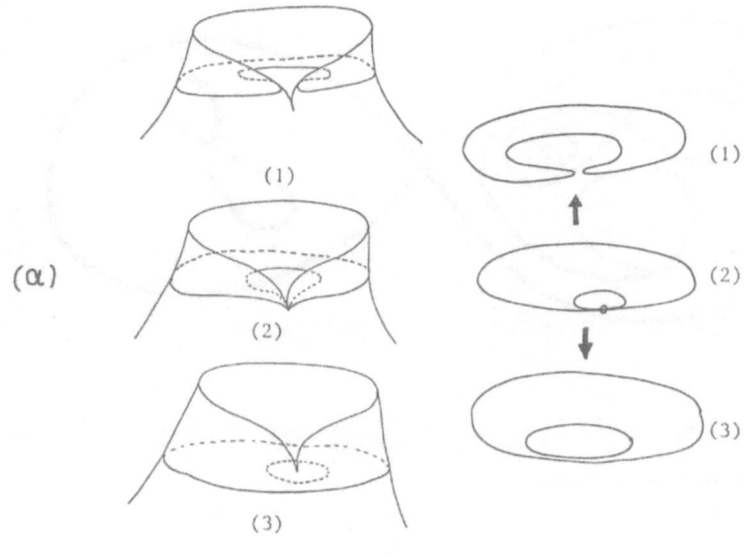

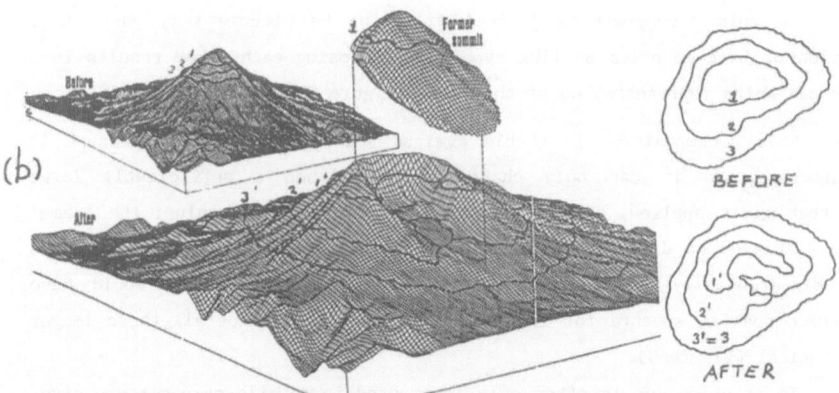

Figure 6. Examples of level lines with an inverted figure eight shape. (a):
The general structure near a level line with an inverted figure eight shape.
(b): Mount St. Helens before and after the eruption. After the eruption the
level line with the inverted figure eight shape (2') divides the family of
contour lines into two equivalence classes of homotopic curves, while previous
to the eruption all level lines were homotopic : the eruption clearly resulted
in a change of structure of Mount St. Helens.

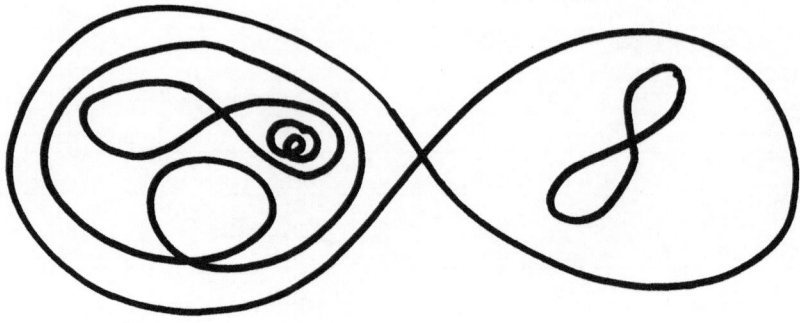

Figure 7. The nesting of extrema.

metrical information about the contrast between the extrema, formparameters of
the loops etc.

In this decomposition logical filtering has become very easy. E.g.
deletion of bracket pairs of like type just enclosing each other results in a
black and white representation of the image (figure 8b).

This decomposition is stable against small perturbations, because it
is discrete, so it can only change suddenly when a sufficiently large
perturbation is applied. This is of considerable practical value: the 'same'
image displayed on different TV sets would be differently warped spatially as
well differentially deformed in gray scale. Thus these images would have
different spatial spectra for instance. Yet the structure of all these images
is identical (figure 9).

In practice one is often only interested in details of a certain size,
and smaller and larger details may be omitted. Lowpass filtering is not
appropriate because this deteriorates the definition of the bigger details
(blurring). If one is interested in the vertices of trees, one doesn't want to
see leaves, but clear cut vertices (figure 10).It is obvious that the
parentheses formula has to be weeded, in other words we want to get rid of
loops that are too small. The fact that it is only possible to give the exact
location of a vertex in a lowpass filtered version of the image suggests the

317

study of the dependence of the parentheses formula on the level of resolution. Relevant parentheses can be tracked down on low levels of resolution and thereafter be projected down to levels of higher resolution. In order to do so we first have to describe the structure of an image on all levels of resolution simultaneously, and find relations between these levels.

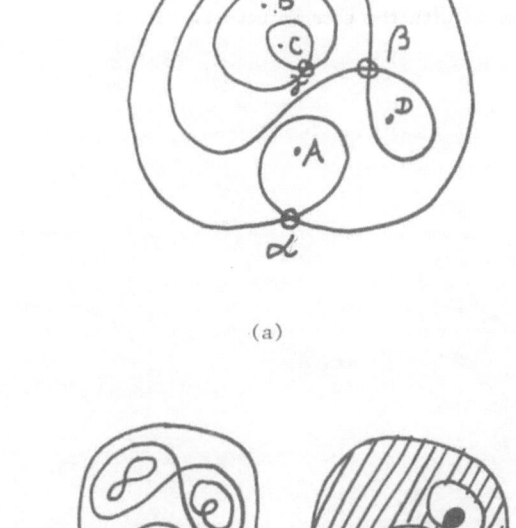

(a)

(b)

Figure 8. (a): An arbitrary image.

(b): Simplification of an image to its black and white representation.

318

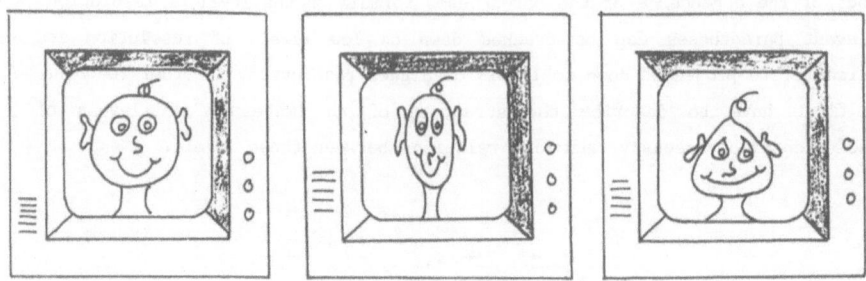

Figure 9. Deformed images with the same structure.

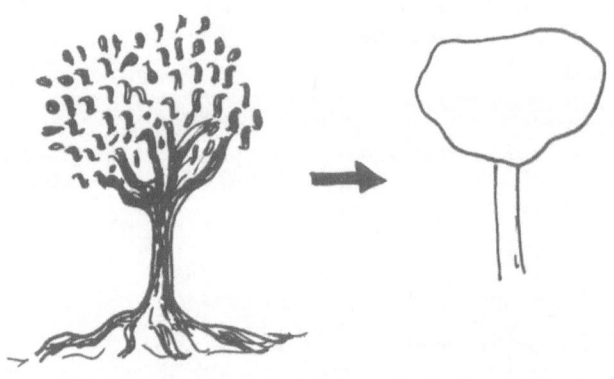

Figure 10. Determination of the vertex of a tree.

3. HOW TO EMBED AN IMAGE INTO A FAMILY OF IMAGES, GRADED WITH RESPECT TO RESOLUTION.

A 'defocussed image' is an image that has been convolved with some point spread function (PSF) $\psi(\vec{r};t)$. Suppose the PSF has the following properties:

1. semi-definite positiveness : $\psi(\vec{r};t) \geqslant 0$

2. normalization : $\int \psi(\vec{r};t)d^2r = 1$

3. central symmetry : $\int \psi(\vec{r};t)\vec{r}d^2r = 0$

4. isotropy : $\int \psi(x,y;t)x^2 dxdy = \int \psi(x,y;t)y^2 dxdy = t$
   $\int\int xy\psi(x,y;t)dxdy = 0$

Semi-definite positiveness is necessary to keep the convolution product of the PSF and the input image positive. Normalization is necessary to prevent overall attenuation or amplification. The symmetry property seems obvious enough. The width of the PSF is defined by the last property. These properties represent the main features of what is instinctively meant by "blurring". None of these restrictions is really necessary, but the convenience of this choice will become clear in a moment.

Now consider a sequence of images, each one obtained from its predecessor through progressive defocussing with the same PSF $\psi(\vec{r};t)$. In $(\vec{r};t)$ space this sequence can be represented by a discrete stack of images with a resolution spacing depending on the value of the width of the PSF.

On a level t=constant in $(\vec{r};t)$ space a low-pass filtered version $\Phi(\vec{r};t)$ of the input image $\phi(\vec{r})$ can be found , the resolution being determined by the value of t ($\Phi(\vec{r},0) = \phi(\vec{r})$: the original input image). Because of the constraints on the PSF we have

$$\lim_{t\to 0} \psi(\vec{r};t) = \delta(\vec{r})$$

In this limit (and with the use of property (3) : $\psi(-\vec{s};t) = \psi(\vec{s};t)$) the discrete stack passes on to the continuous one

$$\lim_{t \to 0} \int \Phi(\vec{r}+\vec{s};u) \; \psi(\vec{s};t) \; d\vec{s} = \Phi(\vec{r};u)$$

and

$$\lim_{t \to 0} \frac{\partial \Phi(\vec{r};u+t)}{\partial t} = \frac{\partial \Phi(\vec{r};u)}{\partial u} \tag{1}$$

On the other hand, Taylor expansion of the defocussed image $\Phi(\vec{r};u+t)$ in powers of t

$$\Phi(\vec{r};u+t) = \int \Phi(\vec{r}+\vec{s};u) \; \psi(\vec{s};t) \; d^2 s$$

$$= \Phi(\vec{r};u) \int \psi(\vec{s};t) \; d^2 s$$

$$+ \vec{\nabla}\Phi(\vec{r};u) \int \vec{s} \; \psi(\vec{s};t) \; d^2 s$$

$$+ \frac{\partial^2 \Phi(\vec{r};u)}{2 \; \partial x^2} \int x^2 \psi(x,y;t) \; dxdy$$

$$+ \frac{\partial^2 \Phi(\vec{r};u)}{2 \; \partial y^2} \int y^2 \psi(x,y;t) \; dxdy$$

$$+ \frac{\partial^2 \Phi(\vec{r};u)}{\partial x \partial y} \int xy \; \psi(x,y;t) \; dxdy + \cdots\cdots$$

$$= \Phi(\vec{r};u) + \Delta\Phi(\vec{r};u).t + \cdots$$

Thus

$$\lim_{t \to 0} \frac{\partial \Phi(\vec{r};u+t)}{\partial t} = \Delta \; \Phi(\vec{r};u) \tag{2}$$

and from (1) and (2) we see that

$$\frac{\partial \Phi(\vec{r};u)}{\partial u} = \Delta\Phi(\vec{r};u) \tag{3}$$

holds on all levels of the continuous stack. Because of the boundary condition $\Phi(\vec{r};0) = \phi(\vec{r})$ we have

$$\lim_{u \to 0} \frac{\partial \Phi(\vec{r};u)}{\partial u} = \lim_{u \to 0} \Delta\Phi(\vec{r};u) = \Delta\Phi(\vec{r};0) = \Delta\phi(\vec{r})$$

So we have shown that a unique family of defocussed images can be assigned to each input image $\phi(\vec{r})$ by means of a second order partial differential equation. From (3), which is the well-known diffusion of heat flow equation, can be deduced that $\Phi(\vec{r};u)$ may be obtained directly from $\phi(\vec{r})$ by a convolution with Green's function

$$G(\vec{r};u) = \exp(-\vec{r}^2/4u) \;/\; 4\pi u$$

In the sequal we will show that a logical way to define links between different levels of resolution is provided by the constraints put on the family $\Phi(x,y,u)$ by the diffusion equation.

4. PATHS OF PROJECTION: THE VERTICAL STRUCTURE OF THE CONTINUOUS STACK.

We start with the diffusion equation and study the structure of level surfaces of Φ in (x,y,u) space. First consider the absolute value of Φ. You have

$$\frac{\partial}{\partial u}|\Phi|^2 \;=\; 2\Phi\,\frac{\partial \Phi}{\partial u} = 2\Phi\Delta\Phi$$

This expression is positive for pits (respectively peaks) with positive (respectively negative) function values of the function Φ, and negative for pits (peaks) with negative (positive) values of the function Φ. In other words: when $\Phi > 0$ peaks are eroded (Φ decreases with increasing u) and pits are filled in (Φ increases with increasing u) through defocussing, when $\Phi < 0$ the reverse holds. Defocussing always decreases the variation of Φ. Only on the surfaces $\Delta\Phi(x,y,u) = 0$ does the value of Φ remain invariant under defocussing: such surfaces may be called 'neutral tubes'. (For the Green's function the tube is $x^2+y^2=t$.)

A link, or projection between images at different levels of resolution can be obtained as follows: look for paths in (x,y,u) space with the property that Φ is constant, whereas $\frac{d\vec{r}}{dt}$ is minimal. These steepest paths are found (by way of Lagrange's multipliers) to be defined through:

$$\frac{\partial \vec{r}}{\partial u} = -\;\frac{\Delta\Phi}{\vec{\nabla}\Phi.\vec{\nabla}\Phi}\;\vec{\nabla}\Phi$$

On the neutral tubes this expression vanishes, and the paths run in the u-direction ('vertical'), whereas on the critical points of the images ($\vec{\nabla}\Phi.\vec{\nabla}\Phi = 0$) the method breaks down. Note that — except for the critical points — this expression defines a smooth vector field in (x,y,u) space, and thus a family of paths that link one image to the other.

5. SINGULAR FEATURES OF THE FAMILY OF STEEPEST PATHS.

Whenever $\Delta\Phi \neq 0$ defocussing changes the character of the image locally and the projection of one image on another (which is merely a translation $(x,y,u) \rightarrow (x,y,u')$ for harmonic images) becomes complicated. In many cases projection is merely a deformation, without changes in the image structure. Because we are mainly interested in those cases in which image structure does change, we will now study the singular features of the family of projection paths. For instance we need to know whether paths can end (in that case you may never reach the projection level and no relation between features at different resolution levels can be defined) or whether paths can bifurcate (in that case the projection is no longer unique), etc.

We will start with the introduction of several important geometrical loci in (x,y,u) space, closely connected with the structure of images:

- the locus of critical points. This locus is a set of <u>curves</u>, because we have two equations: $\dfrac{\partial\Phi}{\partial x} = \dfrac{\partial\Phi}{\partial y} = 0$;
- The locus of degeneracy. This is the <u>surface</u> defined through the vanishing of the Hessian determinant $\left(\dfrac{\partial^2\Phi}{\partial x^2}\dfrac{\partial^2\Phi}{\partial y^2} = \left(\dfrac{\partial^2\Phi}{\partial x\partial y}\right)^2\right)$;
- the bifurcation set. This is a set of <u>points</u> defined through the three conditions

$$\frac{\partial\Phi}{\partial x} = \frac{\partial\Phi}{\partial y} = \frac{\partial^2\Phi}{\partial x^2}\frac{\partial^2\Phi}{\partial y^2} - \left(\frac{\partial^2\Phi}{\partial x\partial y}\right)^2 = 0.$$

These loci are closely connected with the level surfaces of Φ in (x,y,u) space. Consider the surface $\Phi(x,y,u) = \Phi_0$ at a point where $\vec{\nabla}\Phi$ (as always we mean $\left(\dfrac{\partial\Phi}{\partial x}, \dfrac{\partial\Phi}{\partial y}\right)$ in the image plane) vanishes. There we take orthogonal coordinates (p,q) instead of (x,y), such that Φ_{pq} vanishes. Then the Gaussian and mean curvatures of the surface are conveniently calculated with standard methods [5] to be:

$$K = \frac{\Phi_{pp}\Phi_{qq}}{\Delta\Phi^2} = \frac{\det H}{\Delta\Phi^2} \qquad \text{the Gaussian curvature}$$

$$H = -\tfrac{1}{2} \qquad \text{the mean curvature.}$$

These formulas have several important consequences:

- only if K = 0 is the point a bifurcation point,

- let the point be an extremum (K>0). Then both principal curvatures of the surface have equal sign. But because the mean curvature is negative , both curvatures must be negative. Thus the shape of the surface is that of a peak with the convexity turned to u = + ∞ . So following a steepest path downwards (decreasing u) you cannot get into a hollow in which the path ends (figure 11a).

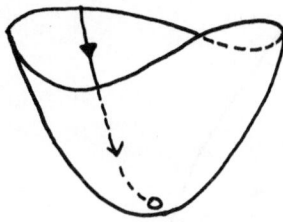 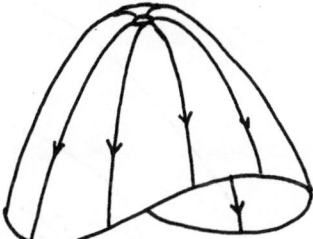

Figure 11. (a): this situation cannot occur. (b): general structure
of extrema of level surfaces of Φ .

Consider points on the locus of critical points for which det H ≠ 0. We treat the cases K>0 (peak of $\Phi = \Phi_0$) and K<0 (saddle of $\Phi = \Phi_0$) seperately.

First let $\vec{\nabla}\Phi.\vec{\nabla}\Phi = 0$ and K>0. Then there are local coordinates (p,q), such that the surface $\Phi = \Phi_0$ can be written (by Morse's lemma [2,3]): $u = u_0 - \frac{1}{2}(ap^2 + bq^2) + \dots$ with a,b>0. So the paths down are not unique, there is a whole 'umbrella' of paths (figure 11b). In this case <u>down-projection</u> is possible (although not unique), whereas <u>up-projection</u> is not possible. This happens because defocussing erodes peaks and fills pits: extreme functional values cannot be traced to layers of lower resolution. A solution would be to ascend by way of the loci of the extrema ($\vec{\nabla}\Phi.\vec{\nabla}\Phi = 0$ curve). This is done by choosing a point 'most like' (but not necessarily of equal value) in the next layer of the stack. (In this context 'next layer' must be understood as a layer infinitesimally close to the point of interest). As will be shown in the sequel, these paths are also useful in case of down-projection: then from each point of the 'improper' path issues

324

an umbrella, resulting in a family of umbrellas covering a whole region, to which a constant value will be assigned in case of down-projection (figure 12).

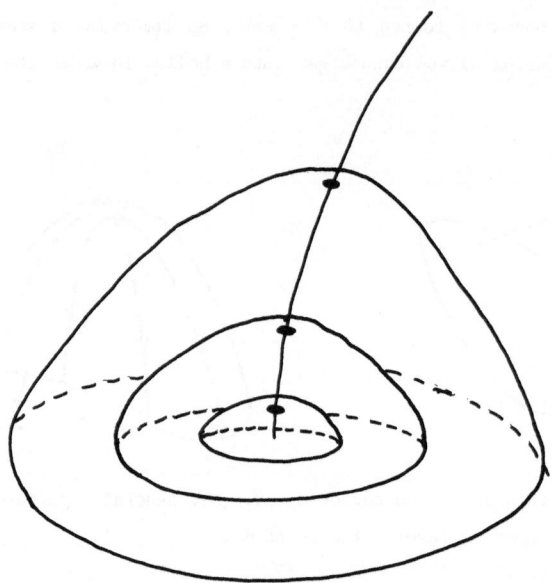

Figure 12. The 'shower-method' of projection.

Next let $\vec{\nabla}\Phi.\vec{\nabla}\Phi = 0$ but $K<0$. Then (again by Morse's lemma) coordinates (p,q) can be found such that

$$u = u_0 + \tfrac{1}{2}(ap^2 - bq^2) + \ldots \qquad a,b>0.$$

We will exclude the trivial case a=b (harmonic function). Then there exist two singular paths impending on the point from opposite directions, whereas two other paths leave it in opposite (and different) directions (figure 13a). Together the singular paths issuing from all points on the curve of saddle points form singular surfaces as shown in figure 13b. The downprojection of a level line of an image results in the change-over of connectivity (fig. 14).

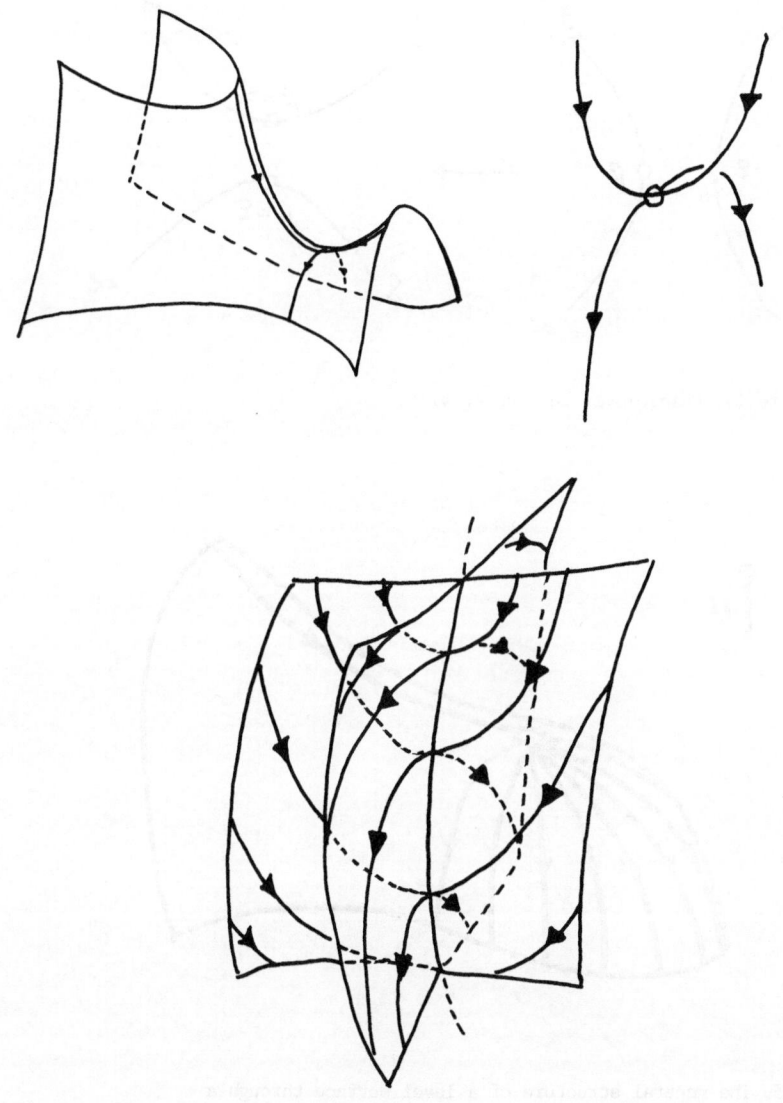

Figure 13.(a): Paths of projection near a saddle point. (b): Singular surfaces.

326

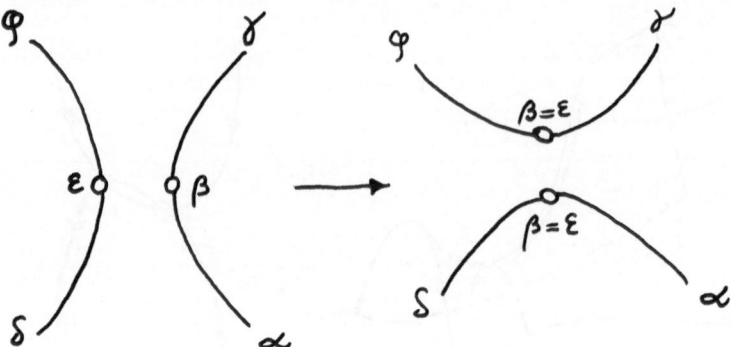

Figure 14. Change-over in connectivity.

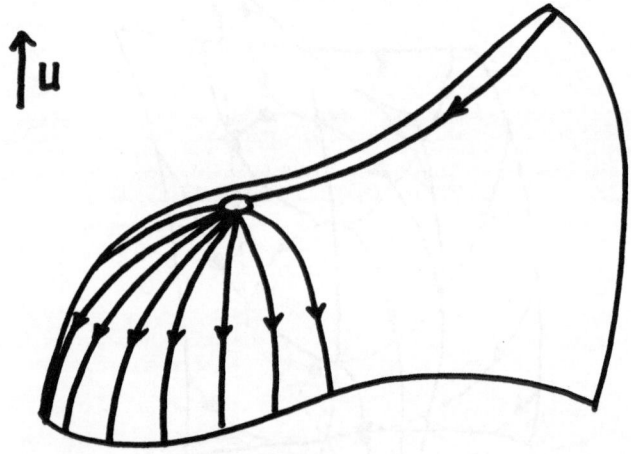

Figure 15. The general structure of a level surface through a
bifurcation point.

Finally consider the case $\vec{\nabla\Phi}.\vec{\nabla\Phi} = K = 0$ which represents the bifurcation set. Catastrophy theory [6,7] tells us that the general structure at such points is always the same (known as a '<u>fold</u>' in differential topology). Therefore this case can be treated at the hand of an example without losing generality. The shape of the surface $\Phi = \Phi_0$ through such a point is shown by fig. 15. The family

$$\Phi(x,y,u) = \frac{x^3}{6} - \frac{y^2}{2} + xu - u$$

with $\vec{\nabla\Phi} = (\frac{1}{2}x^2 + u , -y)$; det $H = -x$; $\Delta\Phi = x-1$ (i.e. $\neq 0$ in a neighbourhood of the origin). The locus of critical points is $x = \pm \sqrt{(-2u)}$, $y=0$. There are no solutions for $u>0$, and two solutions for $u<0$. The branch $x= + \sqrt{(-2u)}$ describes the locus of a saddle point of the image, the branch $x= - \sqrt{(-2u)}$ the locus of a peak. With increasing u (decreasing resolution) the saddle point and the peak approach each other, and at u=0 they meet and annihilate (fig. 16).

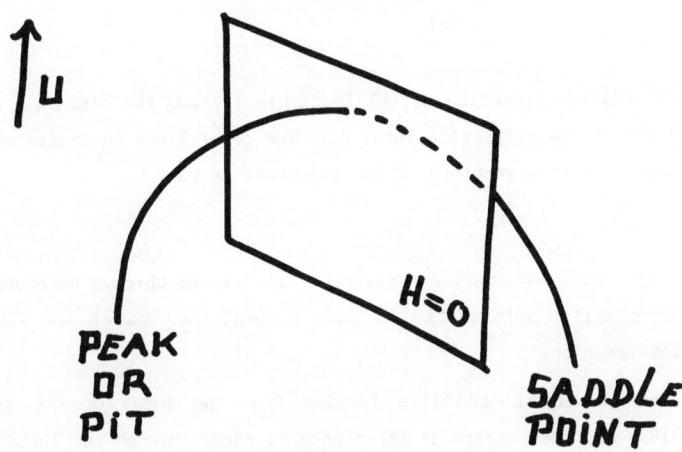

Figure 16. The annihilation of a (peak,saddlepoint) pair.

This is quite general: along such a locus u is never stationary, except at a
bifurcation point where a pit - saddle point or a peak - saddle point pair
annihilates (for increasing u) or is created (for decreasing u). Figure 17
shows the level lines in an image near u=0.

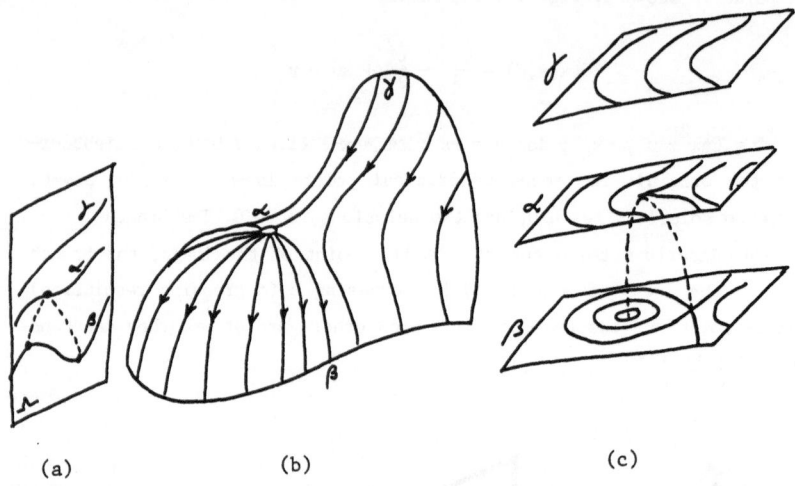

(a)   (b)   (c)

Figure 17. (a): Intersection of (b) (= figure 15) and the surface Λ defined
by the paths of the critical points. (c): The level lines in images near u=0
(= in horizontal intersections of the structure in (b))

This clearly shows how the image structure is removed through defocussing: a
loop with a self - intersection becomes cusped, then smooth and without a
self - intersection.

The shower of umbrellas issuing from the locus of the extremum
(figure 18a) and the surface of interchanging paths through the locus of the
saddle point (figure 18c) interleave and merge at the bifurcation point
(figure 18b). Because it represents the general singularity, we will now
have a close look at the structure of the family of projection paths near
the bifurcation point.

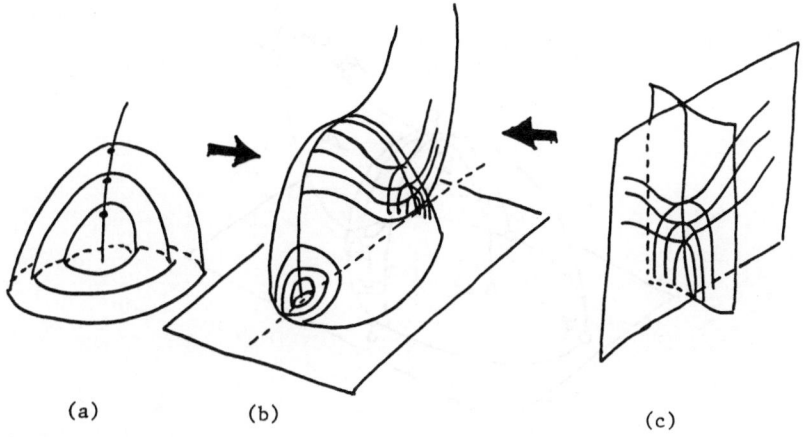

(a)   (b)   (c)

Figure 18. The composition of the family of projection paths near a bifurcation point.

Let $0 = (0,0,0)$ be the bifurcation point, Γ a plane $u = -\varepsilon$ ($\varepsilon > 0$; fig. 19a). The locus of critical points is the hairpin curve $\alpha\eta o\beta$ ($o\beta$ the saddle point, $o\eta\alpha$ the extremum). The path μo reaches the bifurcation point. From there it splits up into a 'semi-umbrella', with boundary $o\delta$ and $o\gamma$ (figure 19b). (The path $o\zeta$ is a member of the semi-umbrella. All these paths end on $\delta\zeta\gamma$.) All paths in the surface Λ end on the locus of the saddle point ($o\beta$) . There these paths split into two branches, lying in the Ξ, Ξ' . One branch ends on $\beta\delta$,the other on $\beta\gamma$ (figure 19c). The umbrellas issue from points on the locus of the extremum ($o\eta\alpha$) . For points on $\eta\alpha$ these umbrellas end on a closed loop in the plane Γ , surrounding α (figure 19d). For points on ηo there is one path (within Σ) that ends on the locus of the saddle point and branches off in two paths in Ξ and Ξ' (figure 19e).

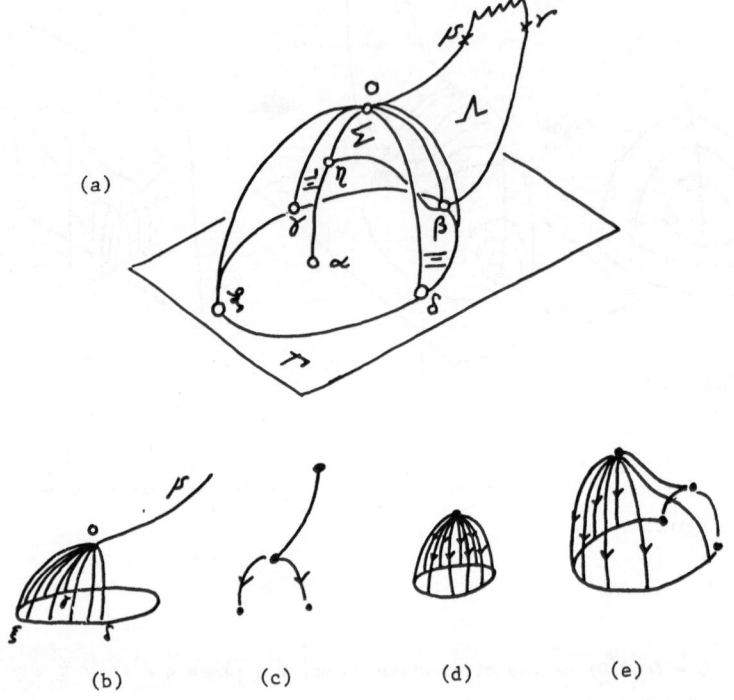

(a)

(b)   (c)   (d)   (e)

Figure 19. The structure of the family of projection paths near a
           bifurcation point.
           (b)-(e): projection paths for points on resp. μo , Λ
                    ηo and ηα.

6. THE STRUCTURE OF THE CONTINUOUS STACK.

Note that the family $\Phi(x,y,t)_3$ contains non-Morse images. An example is the image t=0 for $\Phi(x,y,t) = \frac{x}{6} - \frac{y}{2} + tx - t$. The bifurcation point is a degenerated critical point. This is inherent to the method: slight perturbations of the image can only shift the levels of the non-Morse images somewhat, they cannot be perturbed away. The family as a whole is structurally stable , and is called 'versal' in the language of differential topology.

The critical points can be ordered in (pit, saddle point), (peak, saddle point) pairs, such that the members of a pair annihilate together on defocussing (in the bifurcation points). The resolving power at which the pairs vanish (t values of the bifurcation points) can be put into neat linear order: the pairs are annihilated one by one (or the family wouldn't be structurally stable or versal). The proces of defocussing changes the hierarchy of nested and juxtaposed figure eight and inverted figure eight critical level lines stepwise (figure 20).

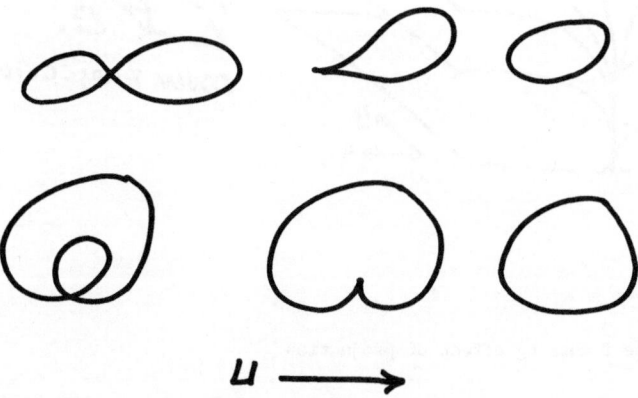

Figure 20. The change of image structure in case of defocussing.

The structure of the image (and thus the organical decomposition thereof into equivalence classes of level lines) changes in discrete steps (at the levels of the bifurcation points) on defocussing. You may speak of an aperture spectrum of the image [8].

The structure of (x,y,u) space is of interest for the proces of 'image segmentation'. To return to our treetop example, suppose a blob in the defocussed image can be identified with a treetop. Defocussing not only removes fine scale features, it also broadens and flattens the features that survive. The 'true' location of the contour of the treetop may be found by projection to the groundplane: this obviously has a 'focussing' effect (figure 21).

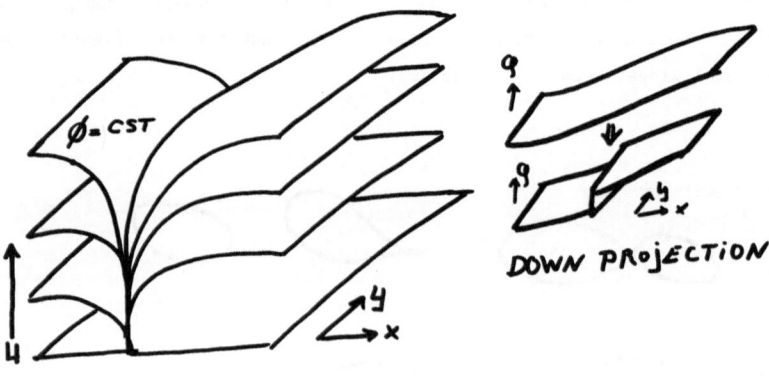

Figure 21. The focussing effect of projection.

Just take the level line in the defocussed image that encircles the blob you call 'treetop' as a segmentation boundary and project that region downwards by means of the family of projection paths (including the improper paths). This indeed 'focusses' the region.

In practice one usually has some prior information about the level of resolution at which relevant details are just discernable (let this level be called t1) and about the resolution one wants the end result to have (let this level be called t2). Down projection will take place from level t1 unto level t2. Simply chosing t2=0 (projection onto the input image) would have caused the segment boundaries to become more frayed than necessary. The level t1 determines the qualitative structure and level t2 the articulation of the level lines in the end result.

Yet there are some complications with downprojection: suppose the bundle of projection paths contains a path that meets a bifurcation point: then from that point on you have a 'semi-umbrella' of paths that projects on a open loop and assigns a fixed value to all points of that open loop, while there will remain open spots in the projection level (figure 22).

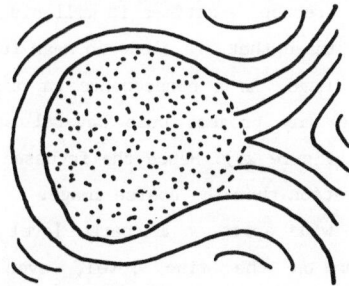

Figure 22. The generation of open spots in the projection level.

The structure of the original image outside these open spots remains unaltered. The method appears to work as a logical filter: certain details are simply left out and replaced by open spaces. The structure originally contained by these open spots obviously couldn't maintain itself at large values of t. These open spots can be filled up with a kind of 'neutral' function for which $\Delta I = 0$ (and so $I_t = 0$, in other words a function which is invariant for blurred representation) with the value of the level lines on the edges of the open spots as boundary conditions. We can also use the 'shower method' which assigns a constant value to a whole region (figure 23). Another complication is the fact that an infinitesimal perturbation of the segmentation boundary in the coarse image will lead to a finite change in the 'projection' (figure 24).

334

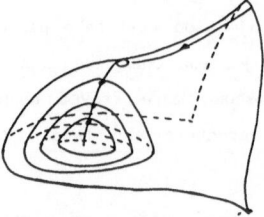

Figure 23. The use of the 'shower- method' in case of projection.

Whereas the projected boundary is 'sharp' (high projected gradient), there remains an uncertainty in its exact location. (Sometimes the projection will reckon a certain leaf to the treetop, sometimes it will discard it.) Spatially separated parts of the input image that are close in mean functional value may be fused in the defocussed image. As a consequence on projection, a single blob in the defocussed image may project unto several spatially separated blobs in the focussed image (figure 25). Hence the focussed image may contain more structure in the segmentation than the coarse image.

Because paths spaced wide apart on a coarse level often converge on regions of steep gradient on the fine level, even quite arbitrary segmentations on a coarse level may reveal the structure of the original image after downprojection. (E.g. let $\phi(\vec{r})$ be a binary (black/white) image, then all paths obviously end on the contours of the original image, no matter where they started from. Any segmentation at all must show at least part of the original contours!) This explains the succes of the 'pyramid' algorithms, in which the image is sampled at $2^N \times 2^N$ pixels, and successive stack layers are obtained by forming sums of 2x2 subimages (thus yielding images of $2^{N-1} \times 2^{N-1}$, ...,2x2 pixels). At the top level (a 2x2 pixel image) the segmentation is forced by the format of the stack (only four different segment values are possible) and has nothing to do with the original image. Yet down projections reveal quite sensible segmentations of the original image. This happens because the structure of the image is coded in the branching of the family of down projection paths. The same holds true for the continuous stack structure: the connectivity of the family of projection paths contains the structure of the hierarchy of (pseudo-) pits and peaks, graded with respect to the level of resolution at which they are created (through focussing) or

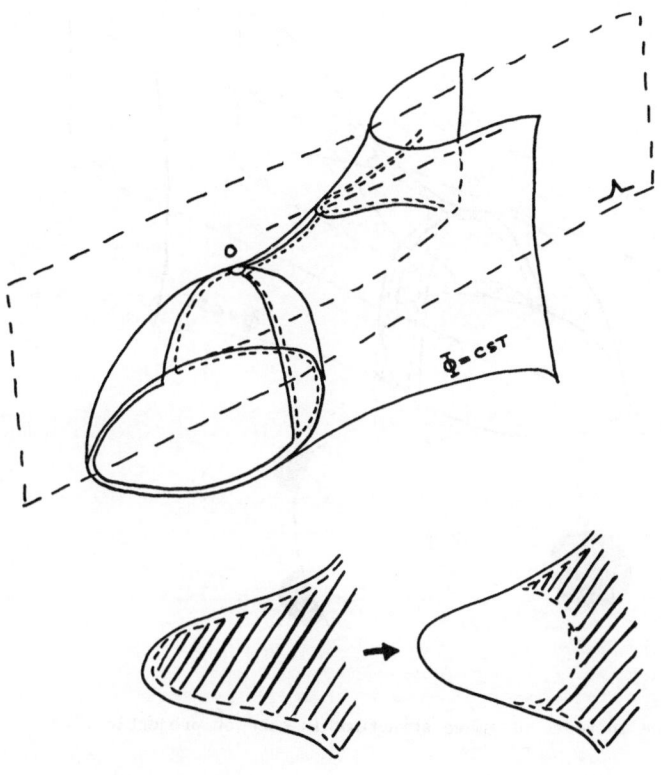

Figure 24. A finite change in the 'projection' caused by an infinitesimal perturbation of the segmentation boundary in the coarse image.

annihilated (through defocussing). In fact the discrete stack (which has the virtue that it is amenable to analytical and differential topological methods) is an excellent and heuristically useful model for the discrete pyramid structures.

336

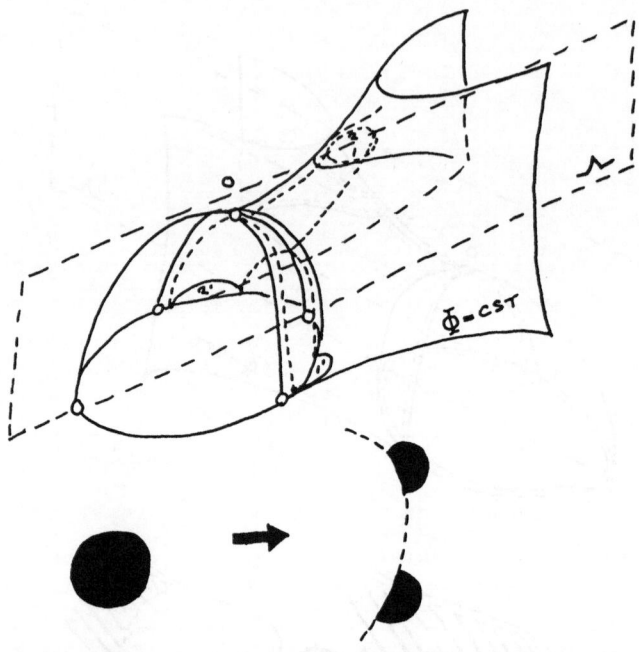

Figure 25. The increase of image structure in case of projection.

7. CONCLUSION.

We have given a complete description of the topological structure of images, studied on all levels of resolution simultaneously. This was achieved by embedding the image in a continuous family of images that can be uniquely generated by it. The structure of the family is determined by a second order partial differential equation, a diffusion (or heat) equation. The constraint this equation puts on the family makes it possible to link the images in a logical manner, so that features existing at different levels of resolution get related (e.g. the treetop and the leaves). The method yields a valuable insight into the functioning of recently introduced 'pyramid' algorithms [1], moreover it is of value for the study of image morphology per se. A discrete implementation of the stack algorithm with a linking procedure is very successful in segmenting images (figure 26).

The general method of embedding an image in a continuous family by means of a partial differential equation with the original image as boundary condition, can be implemented in different ways. If you are interested in multiple resolution images the diffusion equation is the logical choice, but it is equally possible to use the wave equation to obtain a continuous stack of images intermediary between an image and its fourier-transform, etc.

Finally, it may be noted that the method is not at all limited to two-dimensional images. For instance, it is easily applied to one-dimensional images (e.g. functions of time) and we have used it to implement very useful and powerful filters for one-dimensional signals (figures 28 and 29). It can also be applied to three-dimensional images (x,y and time) and thus can supplant image sequence analysis with a more holistic approach that looks directly for spatio-temporal structure [10]. In that case the structure of the family of projection paths has to be derived anew: this structure depends on the dimension. (E.g. in one dimension the generic critical points are only extrema, there are no saddles, thus the down projection consists only of regular paths and umbrellas.)

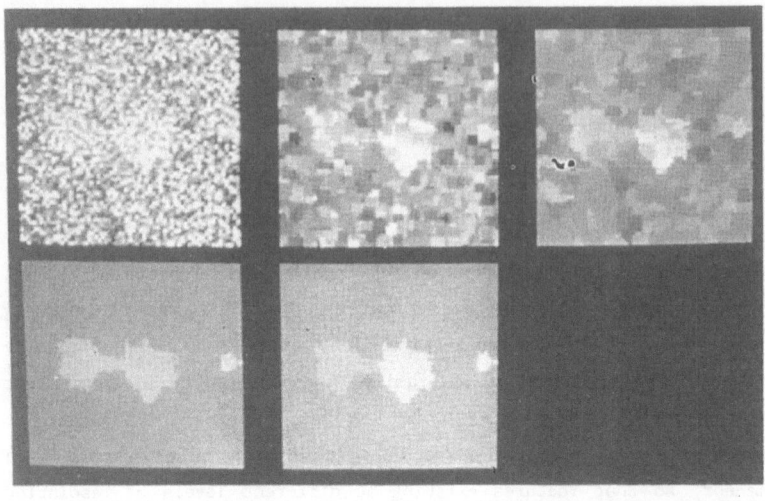

(a)

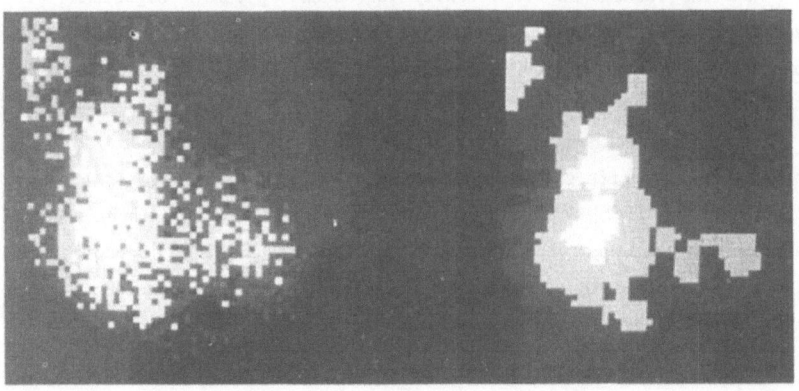

(b)

Figure 26. Application of the discrete stack-algorithm with inter-level linking to image sementation. (a): Artificial 64x64 pixel image, consisting of two circular blobs with a radius of 8 pixelwidths and a mean pixelvalue of 100 for the left and 102 for the right blob, on a background with a mean value of 96 (arbitrary units). From left to right are depicted the projections from resp. the levels 1,3,4,8,96. (b): The segmentation of a heart scintigram by the discrete stack-algorithm. Left the 64x64 input image; right the projection from level 96 in the stack.

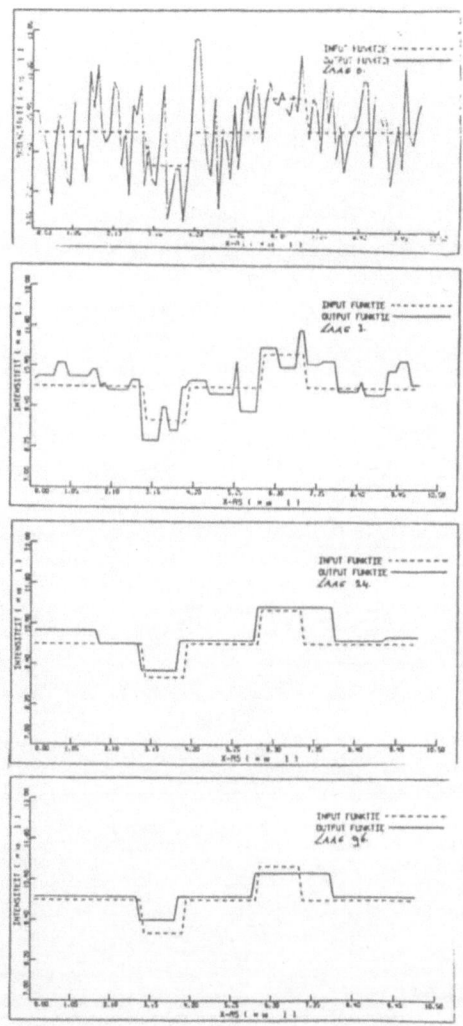

Figure 28. (a): Input function to the stack algorithm, created by means
of a Poisson generator about a prescribed mean (broken
lines) signal level.
(b)-(d): Projections from resp. level 3,24 and 96.

340

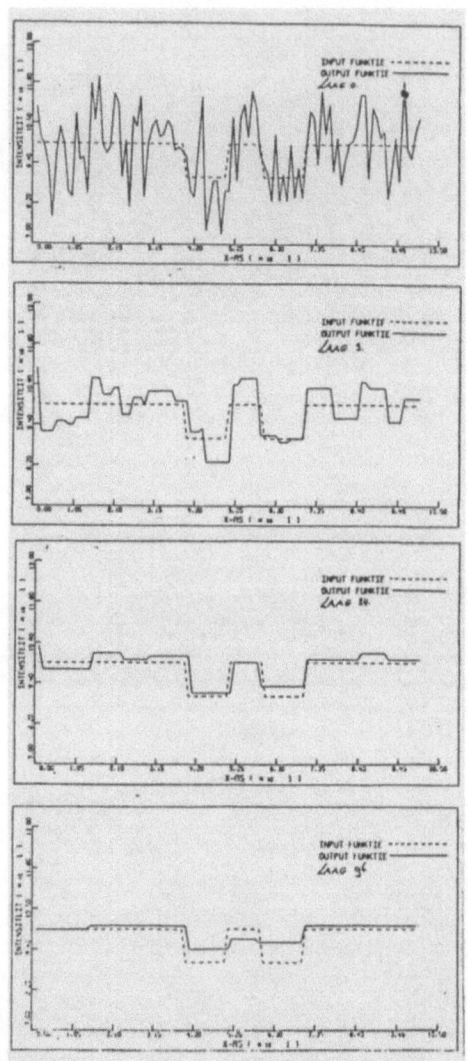

Figure 29. As figure 28, with a different form of the mean signal level.

REFERENCES.

[1] P.J. Burt, Tsai - Hong Hong and A. Rosenfeld, 1981.
     Segmentation and estimation of image region properties
     through cooperative hierarchical computation.
     IEEE Trans. on Systems, Man and Cybernetics, Vol. SMC-11, no. 12,
     pp. 802-809.

[2] M. Golubitsky and V. Guillemin, 1973.
     Stable mappings and their singularities.
     Springer Verlag ; New York - Heidelberg - Berlin.

[3] J. Eells, Jr., 1967.
     Singularities of smooth maps.
     Gordon and Breach, New York.

[4] M. Spivak, 1975.
     A comprehensive introduction to differential geometry. Vol.III.
     Publish or Perish, Inc., Berkely, Calif., U.S.A.

[5] R. Thom, 1972.
     Stabilité structurelle et morphogénèse, essai d'une théorie
     générale des modèles.
     W.A. Benjamin Inc., Reading, Massachusetts

[6] T. Poston and I. Stewart, 1978.
     Catastrophy theory and its applications.
     Pitman Publ. Ltd., San Fransisco.

[7] J.J. Koenderink and A.J. van Doorn, 1979.
     The structure of two-dimensional scalar fields with applications
     to vision.
     Biol. Cybernetics, vol. 33, pp. 151-158.

[8] A. Toet, 1982.

Hierarchical image segmentation.

M.Sc. Thesis, University of Utrecht, The Netherlands.

[9] J.J. Koenderink, C. Huys and A. Toet, 1983.

Resolution dependent structure of images.

Submitted for publication to IEEE Trans. on Inf. Theory.

[10] C.N. de Graaf, A. Toet, J.J. Koenderink, P. Zuidema, P.P. van
Rijk, 1983.

Some applications of hierarchical image processing algorithms.

Proc. 8th Conf. Information Processing in Medical Imaging.

Ed. F. Deconinck, Brussels. (this book)

SOME APPLICATIONS OF HIERARCHICAL IMAGE PROCESSING ALGORITHMS

Cornelis N. de Graaf, Alexander Toet, Jan J. Koenderink, Peter Zuidema,
Peter P. van Rijk. Institute of Nuclear Medicine and Department of Medical
Physics, University of Utrecht, The Netherlands *)

1. INTRODUCTION

   Within the past few years considerations concerning the structure of the
human retina and the perceptual system have led to increasing interest into
hierarchically organized image description schemes (1). Such a hierarchical
organization allows for controlling the simultaneous processing of information,
on low levels of resolution, by information that itself was acquired on a high
level of resolution. For example, the investigation of a certain object in an
image can be established in an efficient way by determining the spatial location
of that object on low resolution levels, followed by detailed analysis on
higher resolution levels. In these and related techniques the resolution decreases with increasing height in the hierarchy and vice versa. As a side-
effect the amount of noise may be reduced, or superfluous details suppressed.
A degree of similarity of spatial distributions can be obtained from a comparison of their descriptions throughout a range of resolution levels. The greater
the resolution range in which spatial distributions match, the greater is the
degree of similarity between these distributions.

   During the last ten years a whole family of hierarchical algorithms has been
proposed. They have in common the attempt to break the image down into
"segments", which are connected or unconnected groups of pixels that are
approximately equal in intensity, or in another sense. These segments can be
traced to all levels of resolution to which the image may have been reduced:
usually they are connected ("linked") through a hierarchical tree-structure.
The most interesting members insofar medical image processing is involved are:
- Quadtrees (2-5), by which images are represented as labeled trees with a
  fixed degree (usually 4) of branching. This representation is related to the
  below mentioned structure of pyramids, in that pyramidal branches are pruned
  and horizontal element linkages are eliminated.

---

*) Mailing address: AZU k.73038, Catharijnesingel 101, Utrecht, The Netherlands

- Cones (6,7), are hierarchical data networks to which different processors can be applied in a flexible way.
- Regular decompositions (8): the topological decomposition of an image into segments that can be organized in a tree-structure.
- Pyramids (1,9-23): are ideally suited for the processing and analysis of an image on various levels of resolution simultaneously, and allow for processing upon multiparametered data.
- Stacks (24-26): are similar to pyramids, do not establish remote linkages, and are less overrelaxated with respect to convergence.

Recently (27,26) it has been shown that most of these structures can be considered as discrete approximations to continuous structures, which can be described and analyzed by using the methods of differential topology. In this way some of the properties of these structures can be explained.

The construction of pyramid and stack structures usually is a bottom-up process, followed by iterative or non-iterative down-projection. Regular decompositions involve top-down processing. The socalled local split-and-merge processes that are applied in pyramids and quadtrees are a combination of these.

The purpose of this paper is to make a global exploration of these hierarchical segmentation techniques and investigate their potentials in the processing of medical image information, viz. scintigraphic material and NMR images. This is accomplished by applying two of these techniques, the pyramid and the stack, to several different study types. Also some enhancements to the pyramid are proposed, such as segment edge smoothing, as well as extending its structure to facilitate the processing of threedimensional images. In the next sections the mechanisms of pyramid and stack are globally outlined, followed by a description of, and discussion on several experiments that were carried out.

2. THE PYRAMID

2.1. General description

A pyramid is a layered arrangement of N square arrays in which each array is half as long and wide as the next array below it (figure 1). The bottom level contains the image to be processed. A son-father relationship is defined between elements in adjacent levels. This relationship is not fixed and may be redefined at each iteration. For each element at level $0<k<N+1$ there is a 4x4 subarray of candidate sons at level $k-1$. The element itself, if on level $-1<k<N$, is a member of four such subarrays for elements on level $k+1$. On each iteration the element is linked to a single one of these four higher level

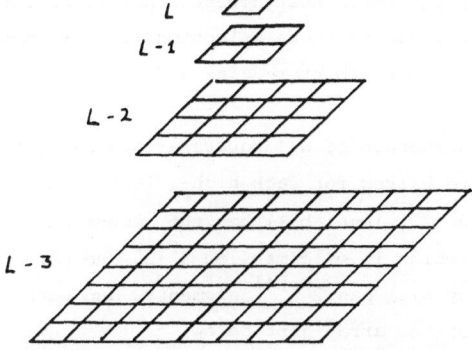

FIGURE 1. The top four levels of a pyramid: level L of 1x1 pixel, and levels L-1 to L-3 of 2x2, 4x4, and 8x8 pixels, respectively.

candidate father elements. After linking, each element will possess between 0 and 16 "legitimate" sons. The son-father links then define segments in the image and ultimately the image segments. The window for a given element is the union of its sons' windows. Image segments are represented by son-to-father links which form tree structures within the pyramid (Figure 2). The local value of the image property is computed within each tree (and not across segment

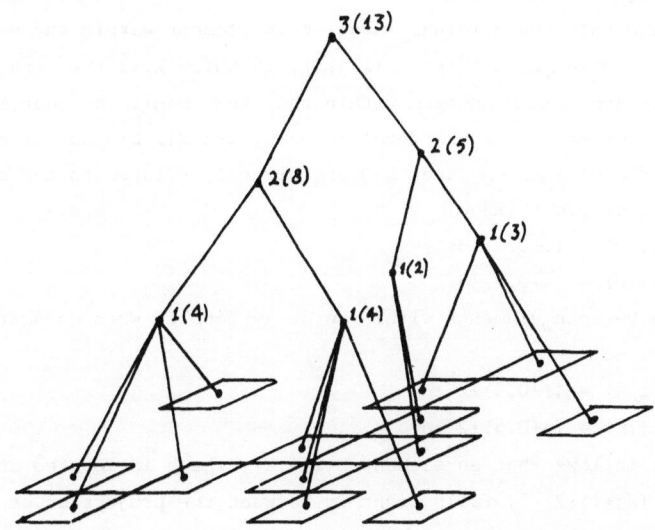

FIGURE 2. The formation of son-father linkages within a pyramid for one segment or part of a segment. Each element is labelled with its level number (the ground level is numbered 0), and with the total area of its ground level descendants.

boundaries). Segmentation is guided by the rules that direct links to be formed between equally valued pyramid elements. Due to these selection rules segments tend to correspond to homogeneous regions of arbitrary size and shape.

2.2. Pyramid structure

A pyramid of order N is a layered structure of N+1 square arrays b(0), b(1), ,..., b(N). Linear array dimensions are halved for each higher level. The ground level b(0) has the dimensions $2^N \cdot 2^N$, level b(1) has the dimensions $2^{N-1} \cdot 2^{N-1}$, and so on until level b(N) which is of dimension $2^0 \cdot 2^0$ and hence consists of just one element. So, array b(k) has 2^{N-k+1} elements, and each array has ¼th the number of elements of the array just below.

Each array element b is a record of four items:

c: the local image value,

p: the area (in units of ground level pixelsize) over which the value c was computed,

f: (father) a link to a father on the next higher level, e.g. the index of that father, and

s: segment value: the average value of the whole segment to which the element b belongs.

The local image values of the elements on the ground level are equal to the pixel values within the original image. Each element within the pyramid structure is indexed by a triplet (i,j,k), in which k is the array level, and i and j are row and column numbers within the array b(k). The coordinates of an element with respect to ground level geometry are X(i,k) and Y(j,k). The location of the elemnts on level k=0 are directly related to the size d of the pixels in the original image:

$$X(i,0) = (i+0.5) \cdot d$$
$$Y(j,0) = (j+0.5) \cdot d$$

The distance between elements within an array doubles when going to a next higher level, so:

$$X(i,k) = (i+0.5) \cdot 2^k \cdot d$$
$$Y(j,k) = (j+0.5) \cdot 2^k \cdot d$$

From this it follows that an element b(i,j,k), which is located at $(2i+1) \cdot 2^{k-1}, (2j+1) \cdot 2^{k-1}$, falls right in between the projection of its four nearest neighbours b(2i,2j,k-1), b(2i,2j+1,k-1), b(2i+1,2j,k-1), and b(2i+1,2j+1,k-1). See Figure 3.

For each element b(i,j,k) that is not located at the edge of an array, there is on level 0<k<N a 4x4 subarray of candidate sons on level k-1: in Figure 3 each circle is surrounded by four groups of four dots. This subarray is

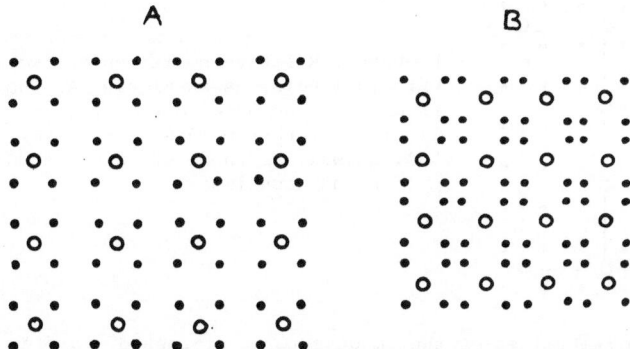

FIGURE 3. A: The relative spatial positions of pixels in two adjacent levels of a pyramid. Circles: father pixels; dots: son pixels. In B the son level is deformed to illustrate that each father is surrounded by 16 candidate sons, whereas each son is surrounded by 4 candidate fathers.

centered around the (X,Y) location of $b(i,j,k)$, which is $(2i+1,2j+1) \cdot 2^{k-1} \cdot d$, and thus contains the elements $b(i',j',k-1)$ for which:

$$i'+0.5 = 2i\pm0.5;\ 2i+1.5;\ 2i+2.5$$
$$j'+0.5 = 2j\pm0.5;\ 2j+1.5;\ 2j+2.5$$

or:

$$i' = 2i\pm1;\ 2i;\ 2i+1$$
$$j' = 2j\pm1;\ 2j;\ 2j+2$$

Similarly each non-edge element on level $k<N-1$ is a potential son for four candidate fathers on level $k+1$, indexed $(i'',j'',k+1)$, for which:

$$2i''+1 = (i+0.5)+0.5\pm1$$
$$2j''+1 = (j+0.5)+0.5\pm1$$

or:

$$i'' = 0.5 \cdot \text{Entier}(i\pm1)$$
$$j'' = 0.5 \cdot \text{Entier}(j\pm1)$$

All computations within the pyramid are on a local basis, in the sense that all record items associated with an element are computed from the corresponding items of fathers and sons of that element. In the following, by "upward processing up till k" is meant a process for all elements on the successive levels 0 to k inclusive, and similarly by "downward processing from k" processing of all elements in k to 0 inclusive.

2.3. Pyramid initialization

The initialization of a pyramid is an upward process in which the item c of each element gets the average of values c of its sons. On level 0 items c are

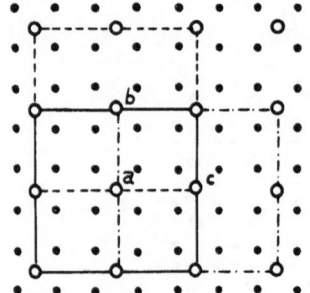

FIGURE 4. Relative positions of two adjacent pyramid levels, as in Figure 2A. The detection areas for candidate sons of father $\underline{a}$ (drawn line) and father $\underline{b}$ (dash line) overlap for 50%, as well as those of father $\underline{a}$ and father $\underline{c}$ (dot and dash line).

equal to the pixel values of the image z to be processed. So:

$$c(i,j,0) = z(X(i,0),Y(j,0))$$

$$c(i,j,k) = Sum(c(i',j',k-1))/16 \quad for \ 0<k<N$$

The initialization of the pyramid is equivalent to the convolution of image z with operators of increasing size. The operators are centered around the elements and overlap by 50% both horizontally and vertically (see Figure 4).

Following the initialization an iterative process takes place. It should be mentioned here, that the pyramids described in (1,9-23) may notably differ in structure and processing. The pyramid described here resembles most that proposed by Burt (14), which was later refined by Hong (20).

2.4. Iteration phases

Each iteration consists of three phases: the upward establishment of son to father links f, the upward recomputation of element values c and areas p, and the downward projection of segment values s. In the establishing of links each son may choose from four candidate fathers the one whose item c differs least from the son's item c. In case two or more equal minimum differences exist, the link of the previous iteration is maintained if it was associated with one of these minimum differences, else a random choice is made. Edge elements deserve special attention. Burt and Hong (14,20,21) fold the array outward over the edge, whereas in the pyramid designed by the authors the selection window for candidates is shifted inward into the array.

The upward computation of local image values c and areas p is carried out by using the newly established links f. On level 0 all area items are equal to 1, and values c are unaltered. On higher levels 0<k<N+1 the area f of each element is (see Figure 2):

$$f(i,j,k) = Sum(f(i',j',k-1))$$

If f is greater than 0, the local image value c is set equal to the average of the values c of the element's sons, weighted over the areas f associated with these sons:

$$c(i,j,k) = Sum(f(i',j',k-1) \cdot c(i',j',k-1))/f(i,j,k)$$

Else, if $f(i,j,k)=0$, and hence the element has no sons at all, its c value is set equal to the weighted average of its 16 candidate sons.

In the third phase of an iteration, segment values are projected downward along the links that were established in the first phase. On the level L from which onwards downprojection must take place, the segment values s are set equal to the local image values c. In a process downward from L-1 the segment value of each element is set equal to that of its father:

$$s(i,j,L) = c(i,j,L)$$
$$s(i,j,k) = s(i'',j'',k+1) \qquad \text{for } -1<k<L$$

in which $b(i'',j'',k+1)$ is the single father of $b(i,j,k)$ as is established by link $f(i,j,k)$.

At the end of the third phase the array $s(0)$ represents the segmentation achieved in the current iteration. Changes in son to father links in a given iteration step, result into changes of local image values of pyramid elements, which in a next iteration can lead to alterations in the links of those elements, so that after downprojection new segments may differ both in value and size from the old ones. Since such alterations shift segments in directions so, that their contents become more homogeneous, this iteration process is guaranteed to converge (22,27). For the segmentation of a 256x256 image usually 6 to 14 iterations are needed.

2.5. A priori information and special pyramids

At one stage in the above described process some a priori information is needed, namely when the number of segments desired is to be selected. If this number is a power of 4, e.g. 4^n, phase 3 can start by $s(L)=c(L)$ for all elements on level $L=N-n$. Else, a level must be selected that contains a number of elements that is equal to the next higher power of 4 compared to the desired number of segments, and in the initialization process an appropriate number of elements on that level is set to an "impossible" value (20), so that no links will ever be established to those elements. The last word about this aspect has not been said yet, however, because it turns out that in certain circumstances the output of the pyramid depends on the choice of the elements to which impossible values are assigned.

A pyramid for threedimensional images, in the following called a 3D-pyramid (although this essentially is a 4D structure), is very much alike the 2D-pyramid, except for the rate by which the pyramid tapers off towards the top. A 2D-pyramid for an image of 4096 pixels (64x64) consists of 7 levels,

whereas a 3D-pyramid for an image of 4096 pixels (16x16x16) consists of 5
levels. A 3D-pyramid element has 8 candidate fathers and 64 candidate sons. The
degree of overlap for adjacent elements is, as in the 2D-pyramid, 50%.

2.6. Size and speed

The total number of elements within a pyramid is approximately $4^{N+1}/3$.
Items c and s need one byte per element; p and f each need two bytes. So the
amount of memory needed for the storage of the pyramid equals $2 \cdot 4^{N+1}$ bytes,
e.g. 32 Kbyte for the processing of images of 64x64, 128 Kbyte for 128x128. In
the processing of a 64x64 image, the time needed for one iteration is in the
order of 5 sec (on a standard minicomputer); usually 5 to 10 iterations are
required.

3. THE STACK

3.1. Structure

Koenderink and Toet's stack (25,26) is a discrete version of a continuous
stack-model (24,27) that was proposed to identify image extrema. It can be
imagined as a pile of equally sized matrices, in which every element represents
a detector of a certain aperture size. Within each matrix (or "layer") the
aperture size is constant, but increases when going upward within the stack,
that is: when increasing the layer number. The ground layer is identical to the
image that is to be segmented. Within the ground layer (or layer 0) the
detectors are in (aperture) size equal to the layer elements (or image pixels).
In higher layers, detectors grow successively in size, and are all centered
around layer elements. Hence, a detector in a higher layer may encompass
several detectors from a lower layer. The input of a layer above the ground
layer is the convolution of the next lower layer with an operator, which is a
3x3 submatrix of weight factors. This operator (or "aperture function") must be
positive definite, normalized to 1, and (usually) symmetrical.

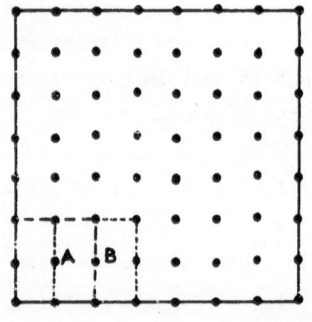

FIGURE 5. The primary selection windows of
two adjacent fathers, A and B, overlap by 67%.

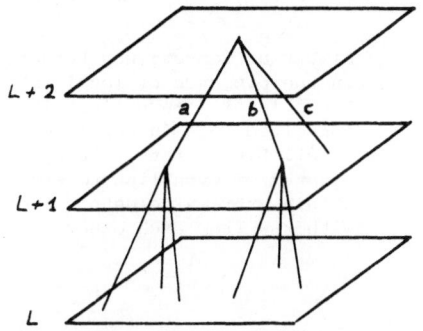

FIGURE 6. Branches <u>a</u> and <u>b</u> of an element in layer L+2 are linked through to layer L, whereas branch <u>c</u> comes to a dead end in layer L+1.

3.2. Stack linking processes

As in the pyramid, also in the stack son-father relations (links) are established between adjacent layers. Since the detector size grows as directed by the aperture function when going from a layer (k-1) to the next higher layer (k), each layer element in k has a 3x3 submatrix of candidate sons (the "primary selection window", Figure 5) in layer k-1, and likewise itself is part of nine 3x3 submatrices of candidate sons within k for k+1, or, in other terms, has nine candidate fathers at k+1. After establishment of the links (similar to the first phase in a pyramid iteration), each element points to one father, and, in layers k>0, possesses between 0 and 9 sons (Figure 6). A special type of processing was included in the father-selection to make certain that fathers tend to be located in regions of low local contrast: within the primary selection window those fathers that show a relatively high deviation (absolute difference) to their own sons, are excluded from the linking process. As a result of this, convergence within the stack is induced by the structure of the image itself. Figures 7 and 8 demonstrate the local convergence tendencies in

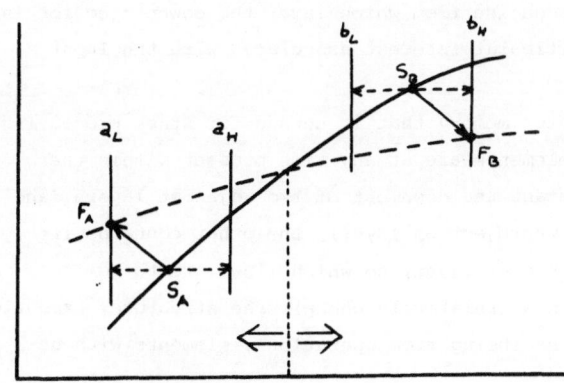

FIGURE 7. The development of a convergence tendency. The son layer represented by the drawn line, is convolved to the father layer, represented by the dash line. Son S_A is linked to father F_A, which of all candidate fathers within the selection window a_L-a_H deviates less from S_A. Similarly S_B links to F_B.

352

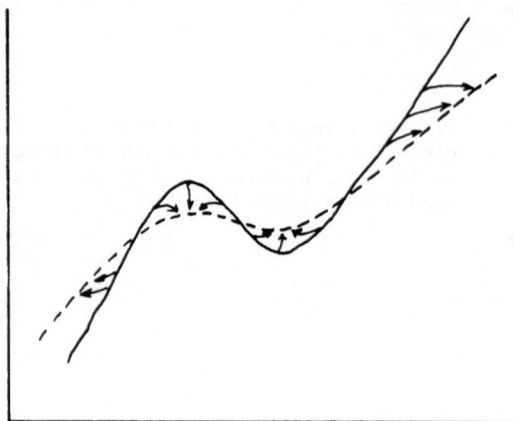

FIGURE 8. Convergence tendency in the presence of local extrema. A son layer (drawn line) is convolved to a father layer (dash line). Linked fathers tend to cluster or even link together within extrema; clusters tend to withdraw from each other.

the presence of continuous slopes and of extrema, respectively. Elements within a distribution near an intersection of that distribution with its convolved version (as in sloped curved planes), will be imaged onto that convolved distribution farther from the intersection away (Figure 7). Element links between two intersections tend to converge towards the local extremum within such an interval (Figure 8). At repetitive convolution the local extrema will average out, and convergence proceeds towards more global extrema. In contrast to the pyramid, where the number of segments is restricted by the level number, the stack shows no imposed relation between the height within the structure and the maximum number of elements corresponding to segments in the input distribution.

3.3. Downprojection, tree structure

The final stage of stack processing consists of downprojection of segment values to the ground layer along the established links. As in the pyramid, a priori information is needed to decide from which layer the downprojection is carried out, to satisfy the particular interest associated with the input distribution.

To limit the amount of computer memory that is needed for stack processing of images, only two layers of elements are at any time present within the memory. One contains at any instant the downmost of two adjacent layers (and serves at the final stage as downprojection layer); the other contains its convolved version, or the next higher layer, to which links are to be established. Links are stored in a (relatively cheap) tree structure. Execution time is saved by flagging, and excluding from operations, elements without descendants (Figure 6).

3.4. Size and speed

With each layer two arrays are associated: for data and for pointers. If pointers are coded as index offsets, one byte per pointer is needed, so that the storage of one layer element requires two bytes. If the suggestion in section 3.3. on the limitation of required memory is followed, the stack needs 2^{2N+2} bytes of memory for the processing of images of order N, else $(k+1) \cdot 2^{2N+1}$ bytes are needed, k being the layer number from which the segments are downprojected. On a standard minicomputer the time needed to build layer 1 from layer 0 is in the order of 15 sec, at higher layers this figure decreases exponentially, dependent on the complexity of the input image.

4. EXPERIMENTS AND RESULTS

The purpose of the experiments to be described was to investigate the performance of segmentation techniques in a range of prospective applications as wide as possible. These study types are:
- Very noisy image information, i.e. one frame out of a dynamic renography kidney transplant study with I-131.
- Parametric image information, i.e. phase maps from Fourier analyzed multiple gated blood pool studies.
- Very detailed image information, i.e. an NMR image.
- Image in which special structures are to be identified, i.e. ribs in a bone scan.
- 3D image information (x-y-z), i.e. myocardium ECT study.
- 3D image information (x-y-t), i.e. dynamic 1st pass study of heart and lungs.
In all of these types one or more studies were chosen randomly, and appropriate segmentation algorithms were applied. No attempt was made to analyze the results extensively, in terms of evaluation of lots of patient studies, comparison to other techniques, ROC analyses, and so forth.

4.1. Noisy image information

Figure 9A shows a 20 sec frame of dimension 64x64 out of a I-131-hippuran dynamic study of a kidney transplant. The transplant is expected to be located somewhat right below the center of the image, whereas the bladder is at the bottom of the image. This image was input to a regular 2D-pyramid to be separated into two segments. This segment image is shown in Figure 9B, in which the high values (white) segment is supposed to represent the hippuran absorbing structures. The edges of these segments were smoothed (as is displayed in Figure 9C), by mapping the segments in array s(1) - that is the 32x32 segment matrix of level 1 - into two different "binary matrices" (that is, of one bit

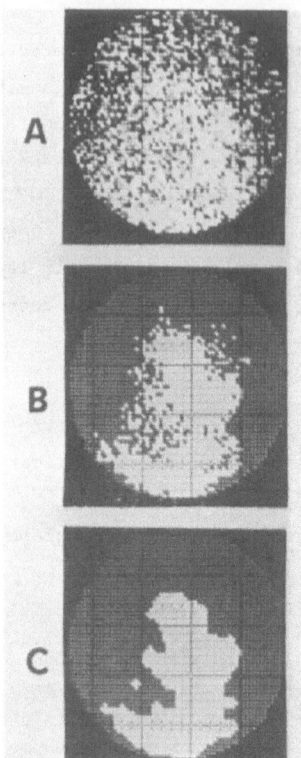

FIGURE 9. Noisy scintigraphic image (SNR 0.5 to 2) of kidney transplant and bladder (A), taken from a I-131-hippuran dynamic study. B: Result of pyramid segmentation with A as groundlevel into 2 segments. C: Segments of B after edge-smoothing; transplant and bladder are contained in the high segment (displayed white).

per pixel). The information in these matrices was smoothed by repetitive region shrinking and growing operations, and mapped back to s(1), followed by further downprojection to s(0).

The same transplant image also underwent processing by a regular 2D-stack. In Figure 10B the downprojection from layer 75 is shown. Although it looks as if the apparent transplant kidney is mapped by one segment, in fact this region is made up by several (4) different, but equally valued segments; the same is true for the bladder.

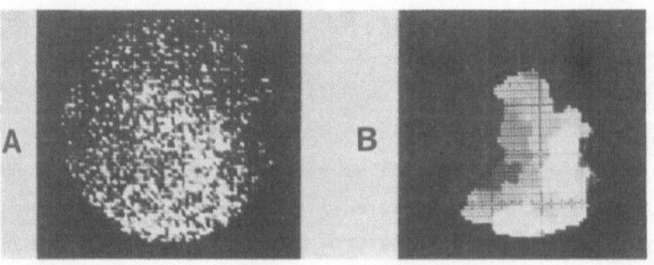

FIGURE 10. A: is identical to Figure 9A. B: layer 75 ot the stack applied of A as layer 0. Transplant and bladder can easily be recognized as the two whitest segment blobs.

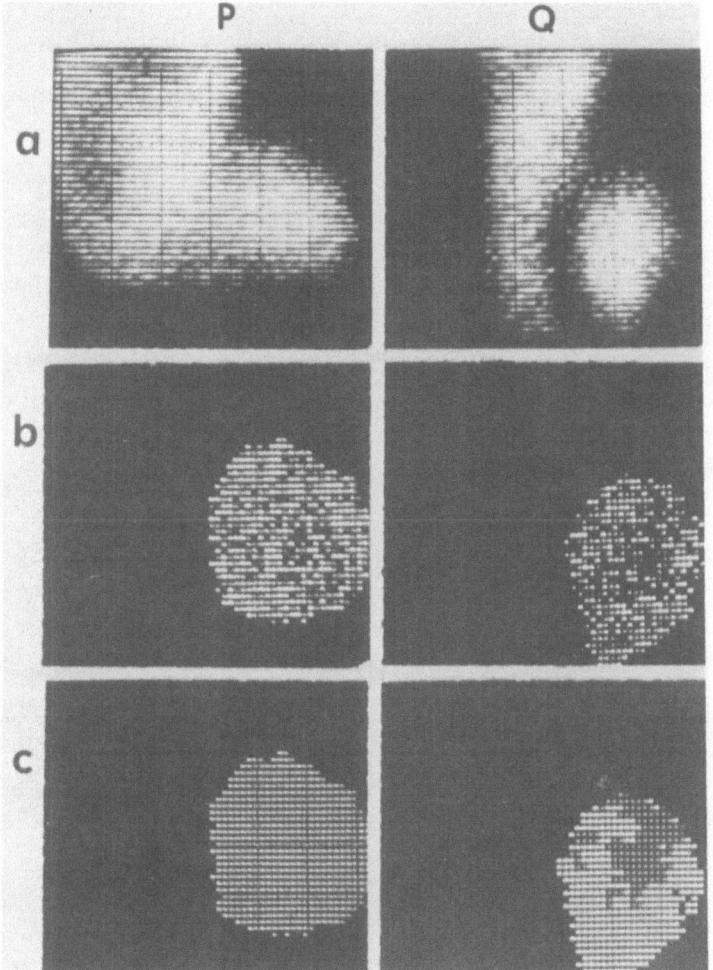

FIGURE 11. P and Q̄ are obtained from cardiac blood pool studies of a patient with a normally functioning heart and a patient suffering from aorta stenosis, respectively. a = end-diastolic images; b = left ventricle (LV) phase maps; c = results of pyramid segmentation with b as ground level into 2 segments. Notice that the segments in Pc are merged into one.

4.2. Parametric image information

Cardiac phase maps were created in a fashion similar to a procedure (28) for investigating phase distribution functions. Figure 11 shows two patient studies, P (normal cardiac function) and Q (aorta stenosis). Images a show the end-diastolic frames, b the left-ventricular (LV) phase maps, and c the outputs of a regular 2-segment pyramid. The algorithm has merged the segments of study

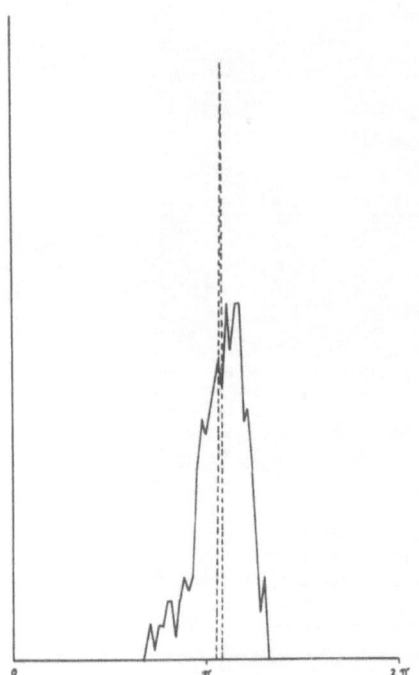

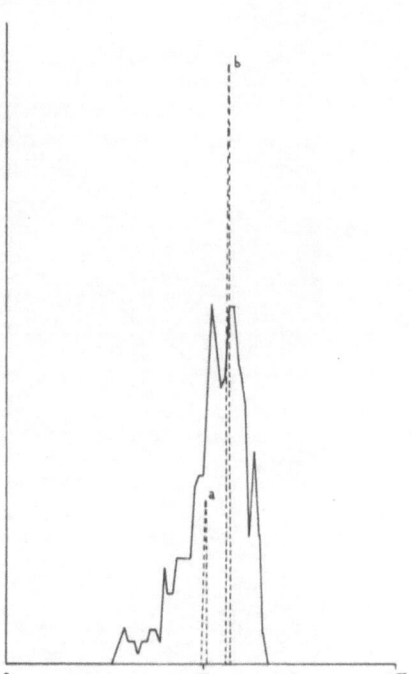

FIGURE 12. Phase distribution functions (PDF) of the phase map of Figure 11Pb (drawn line) and the segmented phase map of Figure 11Pc (dash line, peak height divided by 10). Phase=π is of a normally contracting LV, higher phase values correspond to delayed contraction.

FIGURE 13. PDF's similar to those in Figure 12 of patient Q of Figure 11. Peak a corresponds to the darkest, peak b to the witest of the 2 segments in Figure 11Qc.

P into one, whereas in study Q two distinctly different segments are visible. Figures 12 and 13 show the phase distribution functions related to studies P and Q, both of the unprocessed phase maps and of the segmented versions.

In Figure 14 the unprocessed and segmented (2 segments) LV phase maps of four different randomly chosen patient studies are shown. In study A the pyramid output is merged into one segment, in study B two segments are formed that differ very little in value. In studies C and D two distinctly different segments are formed, notice however, that in D the high (white) segment consists of two regions that have been remotely linked within the pyramid.

4.3. Detailed images

Figure 15A shows a 64x64 section out of a 256x256 saturation recovery 1st spin echo NMR image (29) of the lower abdomen of a female. A regular pyramid

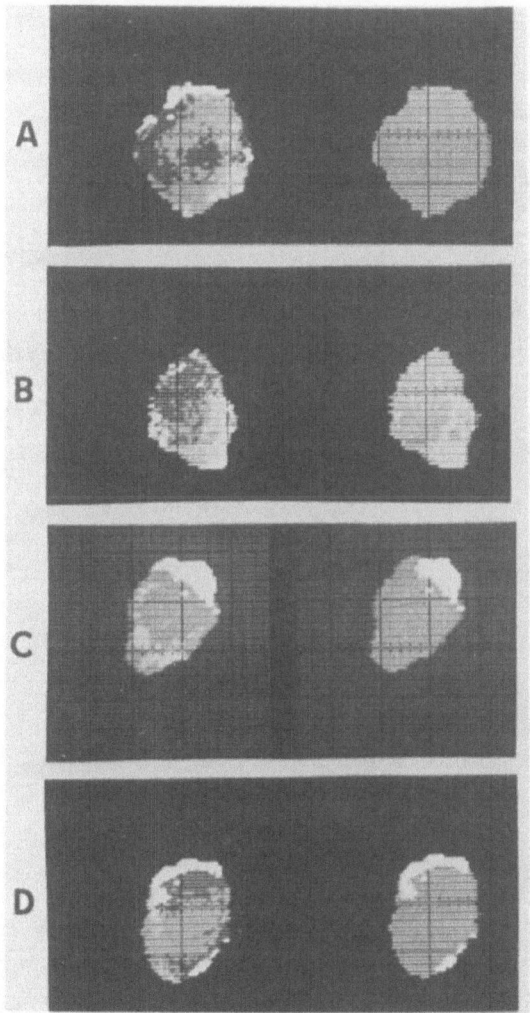

FIGURE 14. Left: phase maps of
four different patients A-D;
right: outputs of a 2-segment
pyramid.

was set up to separate this image into a range of different numbers of
segments, Figures 15B-F. Notice that the 16-segment image resembles very much
the original image. Notice also that some structures (e.g. the femoral caput)
suddenly come up at a certain number of segments, and are further split-down at
higher levels of segmentation.

The same NMR sub-image was input to a regular stack. Figures 16B and C show
the downprojection from layers 27 and 57, respectively. In Figure 16D the
edges of the segments in the downprojection from layer 57 are mapped together.

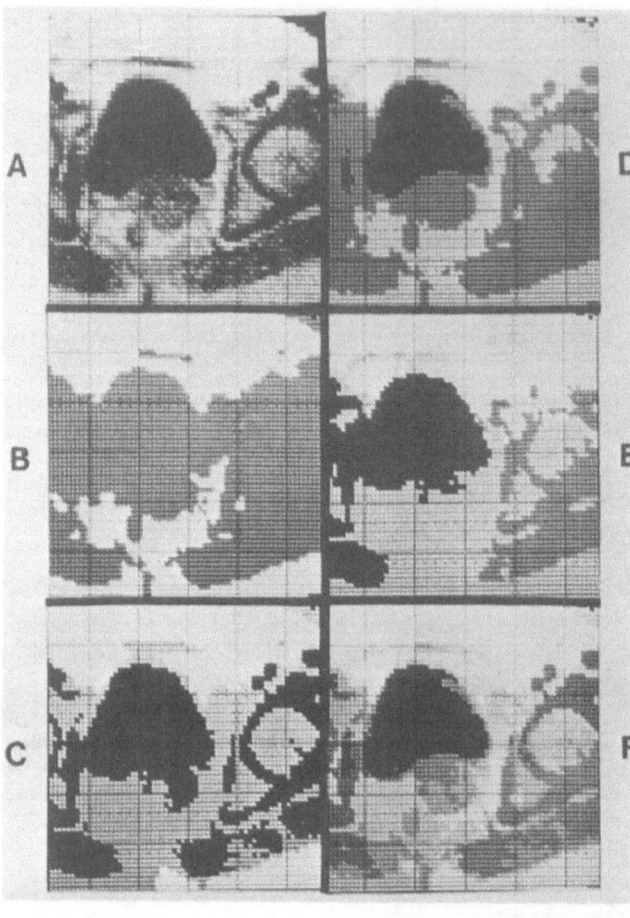

FIGURE 15. A: section of
an NMR-image of the lower
abdomen. B-F: output of
the pyramid with A as
ground level into 2, 3,
4, 8, and 16 segments,
respectively.

Notice that in regions with high contrast there are many small segments,
whereas in regions with low contrast a small amount of large segments are
formed.

4.4. Identification of structures

The standard 2D-pyramid was slightly altered to facilitate structure
identification. After the initialization step a routine was inserted that
transformed all arrays c(k) in such a way, that the desired structure can be
locally identified. In the case, for example, that one wishes to identify
saddle points within the image (and on several levels of resolution
simultaneously), the pyramid arrays can be treated by a "cross operator". This
operator consists of four perpendicular legs, two horizontal ones and two

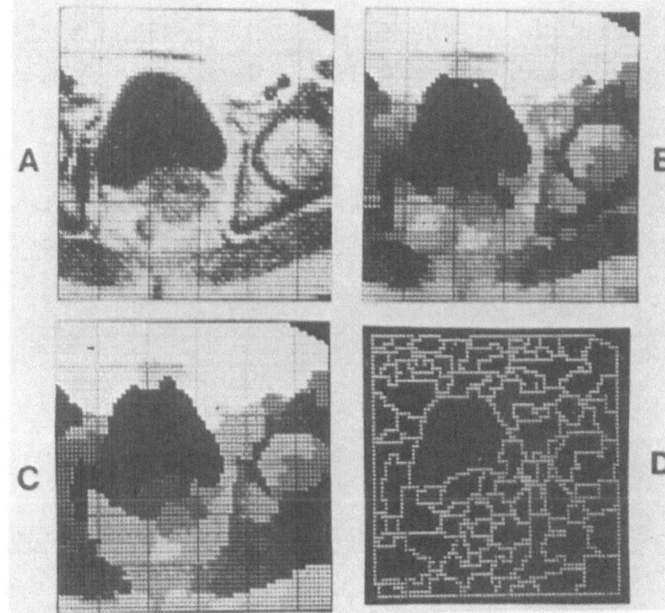

FIGURE 16. A: is identical to Figure 15A. B,C: stack downprojection from layers 27 and 57, respectively. D: segment-edges of C.

vertical ones. At every pyramid element the neighbour elements are scanned along these legs, and a score is computed for the degree to which the data within the cross resemble the shape of a saddle, for example by adding the pixel range over which values decrease in the horizontal legs and the range over which the values increase in the vertical legs. By rotating this cross over 180 degrees in a certain number of steps, and assigning the maximum returned score to the element under consideration, this figure is independent to the orientation of a saddle. After regular pyramid processing of this transformed data, different segments identify different resolution levels for existing saddle points. The three images in Figure 17 show an artificially made-up image (made-up to include a fair amount of saddles of different "sizes"), with superponed on them, in A, B, and C, respectively, the three highest valued segments from the pyramid described above. Notice that in Figure 17A only one point is intensified: this is the major saddle point of the image. Since within the cross-operator both "increase" and "decrease" included "equal to", there is a tendency to identify, apart from saddles, also ridges and valleys, which is clearly visible in Figure 17B and even better in Figure 17C.

A more practicle example of this type of processing is shown in Figure 18. The cross-operator was set-up to identify ridge-like structures, i.e. ribs and

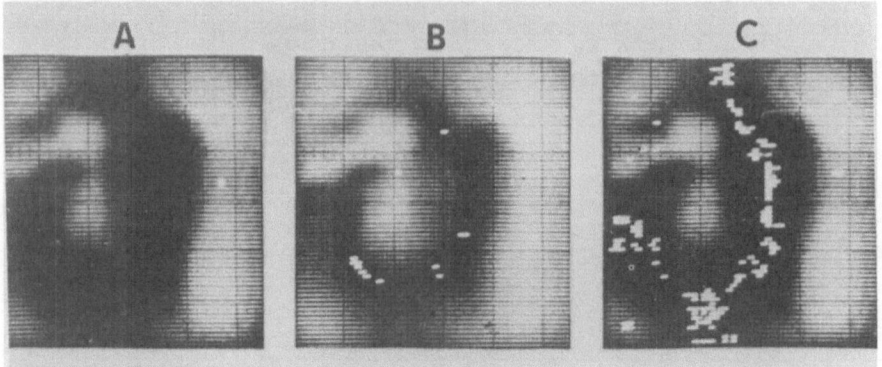

FIGURE 17. Made-up image to be searched for extrema and saddle-points. A-C: saddle-points intensified at increasing levels of resolution, obtained from a range of levels in a pyramid, that was initialized by a saddle-identifying operator.

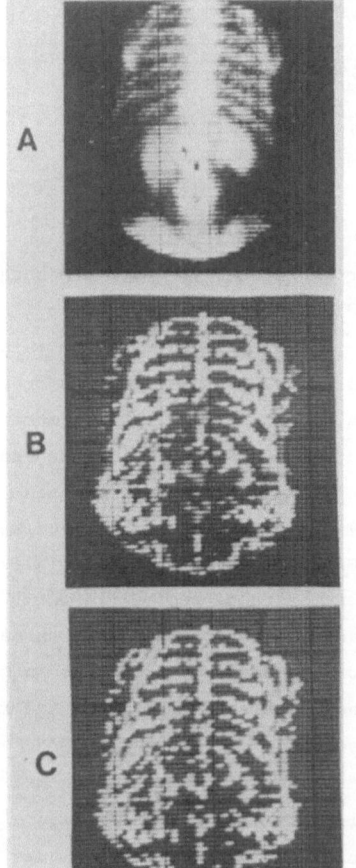

FIGURE 18. A: scintigraphic bone scan. B: output of a 3-segment pyramid that was initialized by a ridge-identifying operator. C: output of a similar 2-segment pyramid.

suchlike, by letting it score for constant value in one direction in
combination with decreasing values in the perpendicular direction. Figure 18A
is a bone-scan of the lower thorax and lumbal region, and 18B and 18C are the
outputs of the "ridge-pyramid" in 3 and 2 segments, respectively.

4.5. 3D images (x-y-z)

A 3D-pyramid was used to segment ECT myocardium Tl-201 data (figure 19).
These images were acquired with a seven pinhole collimator, and tomographic
slices were obtained by ART3 reconstruction including attenuation and
slice-depth/voxel-size correction (30). For certain purposes the seven pinhole
data were acquired as a multiple gated study, but for the experiments described
in this section, only the end-diastolic reconstructed data were taken. The
output of the reconstruction, an image of 20x20x8, was transformed to a
16x16x16 image, to be input to a regular 3D-pyramid. The transformation
algorithm ascertains that within this 16x16x16 image the resolutions are the
same in all dimensions. The output of this pyramid was transformed back to
20x20x8 to be displayed in the same format as the original ECT image. Figure 19
shows a case of slightly diminished uptake in the inferoseptal area.

Similarly, Figures 20 and 21 show the end-diastolic data obtained from a
patient suspected for an ischaemic area in the lateral wall. Notice that this
area lacks uptake in the exercise study and fills in at redistribution, visible

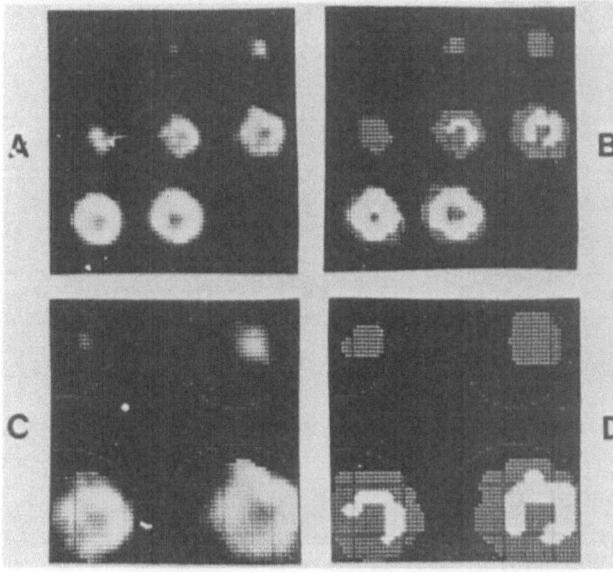

FIGURE 19. A,B: input to
and output from a 2-segm-
ent pyramid for 3D-images.
A contains the 8 tomogr-
aphic slices obtained from
an end-diastolic multiple-
gated seven-pinhole Tl-201
myocardium study that
together form a 20x20x8
image. These slices show
the activity distributions
perpendicular to the axis
of the LV, from apex (top
left, slice 1) to basis
(bottom middle, slice 8),
in the picture running from
left to right and top to
bottom. Within each slice
the anterior wall is at the
top, the inferior wall at
the bottom, septum left,
and lateral wall right.
C,D: top-right sections of
A and B with slices 2,3,5,6.

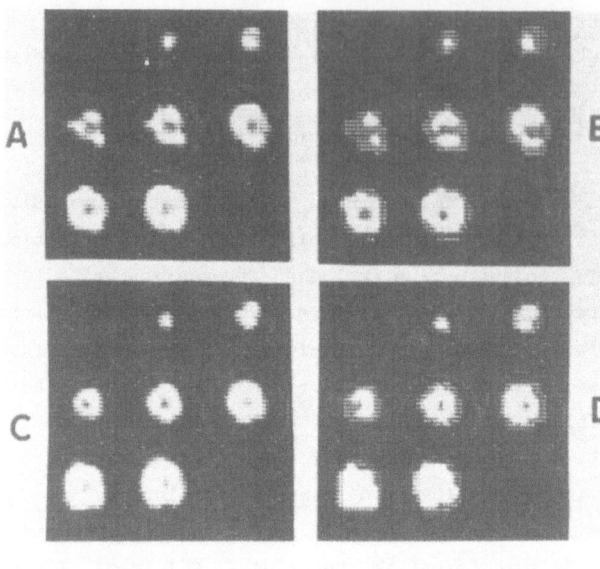

FIGURE 20. A,B: input to and output from a 2-segment pyramid in the format of Figure 19A,B, on data from an exercise study. C,D: similar data from the redistribution study of the same patient.

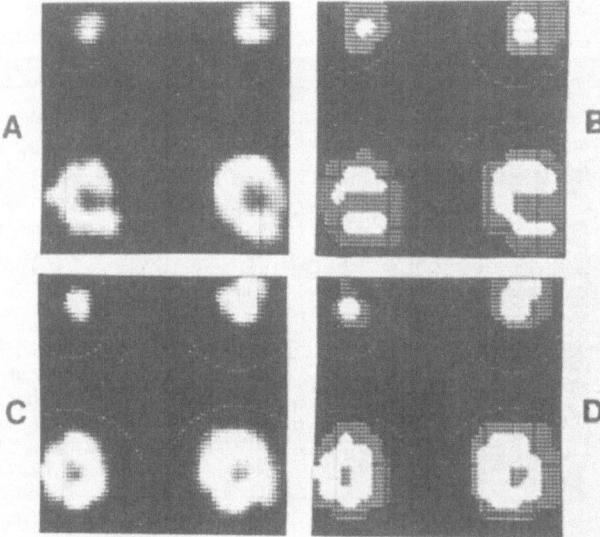

FIGURE 21. A-D: top-right sections (each including slices 2,3,5,6) of Figures 20A-D.

both in the unprocessed and (more clearly) in the segmented images. Notice also, that (Figures 20A,B and 21A,B) the activity blob visible near the septum in the redistribution study in slices 4 and 5, is not assigned to the high, but instead to the low segment. Apparently, the pyramid links voxels in this area in the z (depth) direction, rather than in the x-y direction, and hence this area might possibly be considered as to be a reconstruction artifact.

4.6. 3D-pyramid on x-y-t image information

A "cascade pyramid" was designed to visualize the "wave-front" of activity entering the thoracic vessels in a first-pass study with Tc-99m-pertechnetate (e.g. a left-to-right shunt quantitation study, Figure 22). This pyramid (again 3D, see discussion on how to match the temporal dimension to the spatial

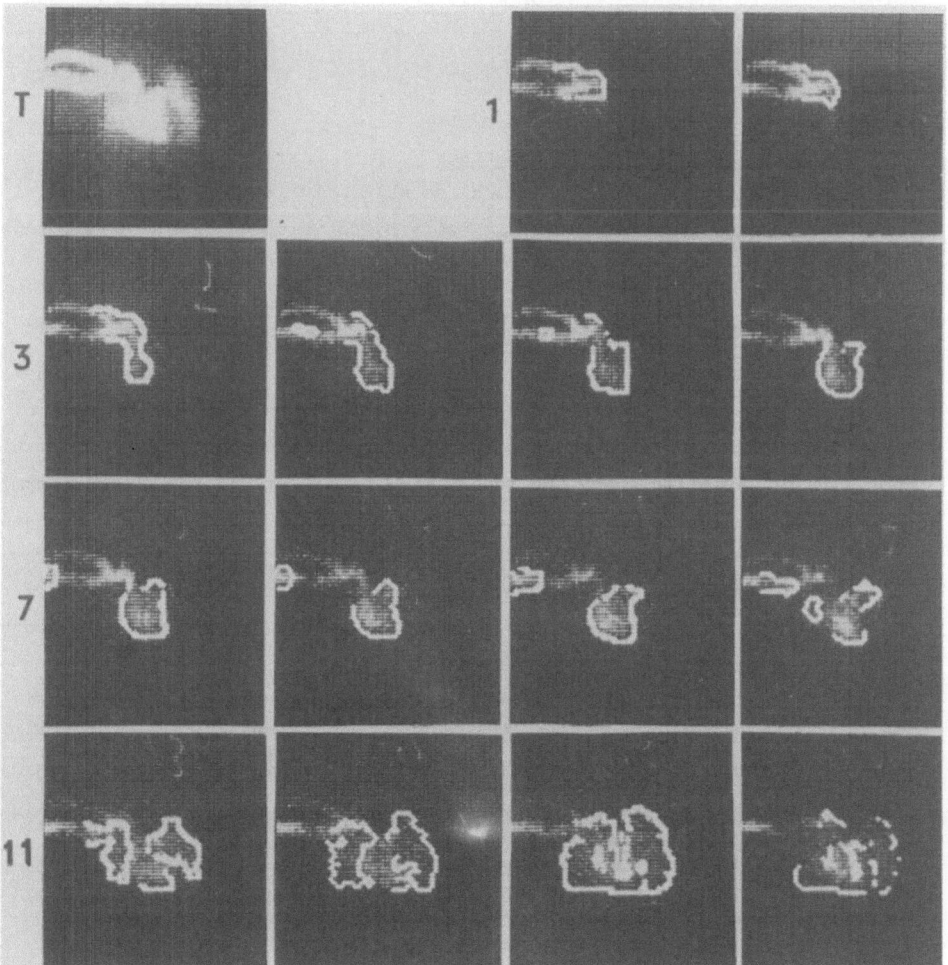

FIGURE 22. T: sum of a sequence of frames in a left-to-right shunt detection study in an infant. Frames 1-14: successive activity distributions sampled at 0.2 sec intervals, in each of which the cascade pyramid ouput is superimposed.

dimensions), operated in two stages. In the first stage it was initialized by the positive time-derivative at each (x,y,t) location, by local linear least-squares fitting. By the term "local", local both in space and in time is meant here. By this initialization process, all elements get a value that reflect the local "upslope" of activity (downslopes, or negative derivatives are set to zero). In the second stage the same initialization process is carried out upon the segment output of the first stage. In both stages the 3D-pyramid separates the data down to two segments. The output of the second stage reflects the wave-front of activity as it extends both in space and time, see Figure 22. Notice also, that from frame 7 onwards a second bolus of activity enters the thorax.

5. DISCUSSION

5.1. Relation between pyramid and stack

In fact the pyramid and the stack resemble only in the initial phase, in which each next level (or layer) is built by convolution of the previous one. In contrast to the stack, in which all layers contain the same number of elements, and convergence properties are determined by the data and the computational process only, in the pyramid convergence is imposed by the structure itself. Going upward, each next array contains a quarter of the number of elements of the previous one, so that a son chooses not from 16, but from 4 candidate fathers, which guarantees rapid convergence, also when this is not directly legitimated by the input image distribution (20,27). Furthermore, pyramid processing represents, due to its iterative nature, not a very natural model of the signal processing within the visual perception system (as the stack does). However, the structure of the pyramid facilitates the realization of the before mentioned goal: a hierarchical image segmentation at low cost of computer memory and execution time.

The most apparent difference between the two segmentation algorithms is in the shape of the segments that are produced. Figures 9B and 10B demonstrate that stack segments are coherent, unsplit, and show relatively smooth edges, whereas (unsmoothed) pyramid segments usually are fragmented (see also Figure 14D): they provide for remote linking of image sections.

5.2. Variations

Burt's pyramid (14) can be varied and extended in numerous ways, as has also been pointed out by Pietikäinen (17) and Hong (20). It is worth to investigate, for example, what the effect is of altering the rules for the selection of fathers for sons, the nature of the description of the image on each level, the rate by which the pyramid tapers off, the degree of overlap of adjacent candidate sets, and so forth. Burt and Hong proposed a technique of filtering on levels k>0 and iterating between levels k>0 and k<N to smooth segment edges. In section 4.1. (Figure 9B,C) it is demonstrated that this can also be achieved by simple region shrinking and growing techniques without extra iterations.

Other variations are shown in the examples in sections 4.2. and 4.4., in which the pyramid does not operate upon image information itself, but on derived data, i.e. phases from Fourier analyzed multiple gated studies, and saddle and ridge scores obtained from static images, such as bonescans. In sections 4.5. and 4.6. an altered pyramid structure is introduced to facilitate the segmentation of 3D-images, and in section 4.6. a "cascade pyramid" is described, that operates by successive stages of complete iteration cycles and feed-back of the output to the input.

Also in the stack the method of building the structure can be varied in many ways. By including neighbour linking, as in Pavlidis' pyramid (10,12), the process can be accellerated, and, additionally, remote linking can be accomplished, although one loses some of the stack's potentials for the identification of extrema.

5.3. Structure identification

Apart from the effect of the segmentation of information derived from images, rather than the images themselves, the experiments described in section 4.4. demonstrate the usefulness of the identification of image structures at several levels of resolution simultaneously. An experiment, for example, not actually carried-out, but easily imaginable, would be to segment the bonescan in Figure 18 for different ridge-widths (similar to the saddles in Figure 17 shown in a range of resolutions), which supposedly may break the image down to the complete anatomical range of ridge-shaped structures it contains. The usefulness of the image in Figure 18C is that it is an almost graphical representation of the structures of interest in 18A, and hence is suitable as input to various analysis algorithms for graphical pictures.

Another useful example of the potentials of segmentation algorithms in structure identification has been demonstrated in section 4.6. The structure to be identified is here of mixed spatial and temporal dimension: a wave-front as it extends in space and propagates in time (Figure 22). This structure, once it is defined completely by its (x,y,t) coordinates, allows (in a first pass study) for quantitative measurement of transit times, for example. In a multiple gated cardiac blood pool study, it might help in the establishing of

regions of interest of the LV throughout the study, and allows for spatial
quantitation of motility.

5.4. Quantitative analyses

In the quantitation, on a pixel-by-pixel basis, of parameters ρ, T1 and T2
in NMR tomography data (29), there are several problems involved with the
iterative solution of (nonlinear) Bloch equations. One is that it is difficult
to approximate, on the basis of the noisy dataset of one single pixel, the
zero-crossing time of magnetization; another is the difficulty in establishing
proper initial guesses for the iteration process. Zero-crossing times and
ρ/T1/T2 parameters are spatially variant throughout the image, however, are
almost spatially invariant in regions of uniform tissue characteristics. To
locate the size, shape, and extent of these regions gives better estimates for
zero-crossing times and ρ/T1/T2 guesses for the pixels in these regions, but
seems to be almost impossible without a priori (anatomical) information. The
results of the experiment described in section 4.3. suggest that the segments
produced by a stack, as applied to such an NMR image (Figure 15), may very well
be suited to act as regions of uniform characteristics. The stack was chosen
here rather than the pyramid, since remote links were to be avoided. The
process of the computation of ρ/T1/T2 parameters can now entirely be
accomodated within the stack structure: at an appropriately high layer
parameters are computed for a restricted number of segments, and are
downprojected as initial guesses to a lower layer with a larger number of
segments, and so on until the ground layer. In this process the tree of
father-son linkages guide the downprojection of parameter estimates.

Another example of using segmentation methods as processors or preprocessors
for quantitative measurements has been described in section 4.2. Bacharach (28)
has proposed a technique to quantify LV wall motion abnormalities by the
analysis of cluster- and variance-weighted distribution functions of Fourier
phase maps, obtained from multiple gated cardiac blood pool studies. This
technique involves three inconveniences: elaborate processing is needed to
evaluate the error propagation in Fourier analysis to obtain local phase
variance figures, the same is true for obtaining cluster weight factors in
building the distribution function, and, finally, the thus produced histogram
cannot be described by an appropriate model, and hence is to be split up in
peaks in a rather arbitrary way. Segmentation techniques can be helpful to
overcome at least two of these inconveniences. In the first place, when a
two-segment pyramid (or a stack involving downprojection from a high layer) is
applied to an image, in which the pixels contain variance values obtained from

local sampling (rather than elaborate error propagation evaluation), it will split the image up into "cardiac" and "peripheral" pixels. If then the phase image, from which the non-LV (by the LV region of interest) and "peripheral" pixels are removed, undergoes two-segment pyramid analysis, a picture is produced, the histogram of which contains only one (no motility defects) or two (motility defect) peaks (see Figures 11,12,13), which, in the course of quantitation, can be cluster-weighted in a very simple way, due to the binary nature of the segmented phase image (see Figure 14).

5.5. 3D-images

The results of the segmentation of ECT myocardium studies, as shown in section 4.5., suggest that defects that are visible in the original images become somewhat better visible in the segmented images, and that possibly reconstruction artifacts are suppressed to a certain extent.

Much more is to be said about the result of a cascade 3D-pyramid, as applied (section 4.6., Figure 22) to a first pass study. In building a 3D image from a time-series of frames, the question is how to match the temporal dimension to the spatial dimensions. Since the linkage candidates within a 3D-pyramid (and 3D-stack) are supposed to be at equal distances in all three dimensions, and, in the initialization process, each higher level is a convolved version of its son level, at least the coherency of the information should be approximately the same in all directions. In the pyramid, with its remote linking power, a lack of coherency is not necessarily a problem, but in a stack such a lack could mean that no linkages are established in the time direction at all. If the coherency in a direction can, in this sense, be described by the distribution of ranges by which structures extend in that direction, one has to take care that if, for example, a wave-front is S pixels wide, the time resolution must be chosen so, that this wave-front can also be observed, at a certain spatial location, during a number of time intervals in the order of S. This means that the time spacing within a 3D-pyramid or -stack should be chosen rather narrow, which unfortunately leads to huge data structures once a fair time-interval of frames is to be investigated. Notice that Figure 22 represents only 2.8 seconds of a study.

REFERENCES

1. S. Tanimoto, T. Pavlidis: A hierarchical data structure for picture processing. Comp Graph Im Proc 4 (1975) 104-119.
2. G.M. Hunter, K. Steiglitz: Operations on images using quadtrees. IEEE Trans PAMI 1 (1979) 145-153.
3. H. Samet: An algorithm for converting rasters to quadtrees. IEEE Trans PAMI 3 (1981) 93-95.

4. H. Samet: Computing perimeters of regions in images represented by quadtrees. IEEE Trans PAMI 3 (1981) 683-687.
5. T. Dubitzki, A.Y. Wu, A. Rosenfeld: Parallel region property computation by active quadtree networks. IEEE Trans PAMI (1981) 626-633.
6. L. Uhr: Layered "Recognition Cone" networks that preprocess, classify, and describe. IEEE Trans Comp (july 1972) 758-768.
7. L. Uhr, R. Douglass: A parallel-serial recognition cone system for perception: some test results. Patt Recogn 11 (1979) 29-39.
8. R. Tremolieres: The percolation method for an efficient grouping of data. Patt Recogn 11: 255-262 (1979)
9. S.L. Tanimoto: Pictorial feature distortion in a pyramid. Comp Graph Im Proc 5 (1976) 333.
10. S.L. Horowitz, T. Pavlidis: Picture segmentation by a tree traversal algorithm. J Ass Comput Mach 23 (1976) 368-388.
11. S.L. Tanimoto: Regular hierarchical image and processing structures in machine vision. In "Computer Vision Systems", A. Hanson, E. Riseman (Eds), Ac Press, New York (1978).
12. P.C. Chen, T. Pavlidis: Segmentation by texture using a co-currence matrix and split-and-merge algorithm. Comp Graph Im Proc 10 (1979) 172-182.
13. T. Ichikawa: A pyramidal representation of images and its feature extraction facility. IEEE Trans PAMI 3 (1981) 257-264.
14. P. Burt, T.H. Hong, A. Rosenfeld: Segmentation and estimation of image region properties through cooperative hierarchical computation. IEEE Trans SMC 11 (1981) 802-809.
15. M. Pietikäinen, A. Rosenfeld: Image segmentation by texture using pyramid node linking. IEEE Trans SMC 11 (1981) 822-825.
16. J.D. Browning, S.L. Tanimoto: Segmentation of pictures into regions with a tile-by-tile method. Patt Recogn 15 (1982) 1-10.
17. M. Pietikäinen, A. Rosenfeld, I. Walter: Split-and-link algorithms for image segmentation. Patt Recogn 15 (1982) 287-298.
18. M. Pietikäinen, A. Rosenfeld: Grey level pyramid linking as an aid in texture analysis. IEEE Trans SMC 12 (1982) 422-429.
19. H. Antonisse: Image segmentation in pyramids. Comp Graph Im Proc 19 (1982) 367-383.
20. T.H. Hong, K.A. Narayanan, S. Peleg, A. Rosenfeld, T. Silberberg: Image smoothing and segmentation by multiresolution pixel linking: further experiments and extensions. IEEE Trans SMC 12 (1982) 611-622
21. T.H. Hong, M. Shneier, A. Rosenfeld: Border extraction using linked edge pyramids. IEEE Trans SMC 12 (1982) 660-668.
22. S. Kasif, A. Rosenfeld: Pyramid linking is a special case of Isodata. IEEE Trans SMC 13 (1983) 84-85.
23. M. Shneier: Using pyramids to define local thresholds for blob detection. IEEE Trans PAMI 5 (1983) 345-349.
24. J.J. Koenderink, A.J. van Doorn: The structure of two-dimensional scalar fields with application to vision. Biol Cybernetics 33 (1979) 151-158.
25. A. Toet: Hiërarchische beeldsegmentatie (Hierarchical image segmentation). M.Sc. Thesis. University of Utrecht, The Netherlands (1982).
26. A. Toet, J.J. Koenderink, P. Zuidema, C.N. de Graaf: Image analysis - topological methods. Proc 8th Conf Information processing in medical imaging, Ed: F. Deconinck, Brussels (1983). This book.
27. J.J. Koenderink, C. Huys, A. Toet: Resolution dependent structure of images. Submitted for publication, IEEE Trans Inf Theory (1983).
28. S.L. Bacharach, M.V. Green, R.O. Bonow, C.N. de Graaf, G.S. Johnston: A method for objective evaluation of functional images. J Nucl Med 23 285-290 (1982).
29. C.J.G. Bakker, C.N. de Graaf, O Ying Lie: Optimal choice of pulse sequence

    parameters in NMR imaging. Proc 2nd Ann Meeting Society of Magnetic
    Resonance in Medicine (1983) 19-20.
30. J.W. van Giessen, C.N. de Graaf, M.A. Viergever: Application of ART3 to
    seven pinhole tomography. Delft Progress Report (1983) In press.

ACOUSTO-OPTIC DECONVOLUTION SYSTEM FOR REAL-TIME ECHOGRAPHY

J.C. SOMER and F.H.M. JONGSMA

1. INTRODUCTION

All ultrasound pulse-echo imaging systems suffer from limitations of both lateral and axial resolution due to beam-width and
pulse-length respectively. Therefore a point-target will always be
depicted as a blurred dot.

In essence only deconvolution of the system's impulse-response (or
smear-function or blurring) could provide further improvement.

An optical system is described which is potentially capable to
process the echo-signals as received by a phased-array pulse-echo
system in real-time and in two dimensions.

A holographic method can be used to produce a complex spatial
filter for a particular reference-target which performs to some
extent inverse filtering or deconvolution.

2. PULSE-ECHO IMAGING

The beam-shape of an ultrasound-transducer is essentially determined by the aperture-size expressed in wave-lengths. The larger the aperture, the longer the near-field of the radiation pattern and the narrower the diverging main beam in the far-field,
and reversed.

Since ultrasound absorption in tissues increases very rapidly with
frequency, imaging to a certain range sets the upper limit of the
ultrasound frequency. For abdominal imaging a frequency of 2.5 MHz
is standard. This represents a wave-length of 0.6 mm. Roughly the
near-field length is given by $n^2.\lambda/4$ where n = the number of wave-
lengths of the aperture and λ = the wave-length. Table 1 shows that
e.g. an aperture size of 24 mm would result in a near-field which
exceeds even the required depth of scanning and the narrow beam in

Table 1

aperture-size in mm	n	near-field length in mm	far-field −3 dB width in degrees
6	10	15	5.07
9	15	34	3.38
12	20	60	2.54
18	30	135	1.69
24	40	240	1.27

the far-field will be of no use. The near-field beam has a width comparable to the aperture-size all over the depth-range.

At an aperture-size of 6 mm the near-field would be very short, but the far-field main beam would be diverging in such a way that the width at the upper range would as well be considerable.

It will be appreciated that cross-sectional images are obtained by scanning the beam over the area of interest and receiving the echoes of reflecting objects. A point-reflector would then reflect sound as long and as strongly as corresponds to beam-width and beam-strength.

This implies that the lateral resolution is directly related to beam-width. The choice of the aperture-size will therefore always be a compromise in order to achieve as uniform a beam-width as possible over the required depth. The resulting lateral resolution must then be taken for granted. Only at a relatively large near-field range acoustical focussing can be applied which is then fixed for a certain range. Electronic range-dependent focussing at reception is possible but very complicated.

Similarly, the axial resolution depends on the length of the pulses as transmitted by the transducer. Also this pulse-length depends on the wave-length since the minimum Q of the transducer is relatively high due to its resonance behaviour. It always contains some two to five wave-lengths which is here between 1 and 3 mm long. There are no means for improvement like there is focussing for the beam-width.

As a conclusion: both lateral and axial resolution are limited to a number of wave-lengths. There is no way, after having done all the possible by beam-focussing and transducer-damping, to increase resolution any further in a direct way. The next chapter will describe the alternative possibility for resolution enhancement.

3. PRINCIPLE OF DECONVOLUTION

It has implicitly been pointed out in the previous chapter that an ultrasound imaging system can be considered a network-system having a transfer-function. When using a point-target, it serves as a spatial delta-function, being the input-function of the system. The output-function is a blurred image: it is the blurring function, smear-function, or better, the impulse-response of the system.

The lower part of Fig. 7 shows the electrical equivalent. When applying a delta-function $\delta(t)$ to the input, the output-signal $s_r(t)$ then is the impulse-response $h(t)$ of the network, speaking in terms of time-domain. In the frequency-domain equivalently $S_i(\omega) = 1$ is the input-spectrum, so $S_r(\omega)$ is the output-spectrum, identical to the frequency transfer-function of the system.

If a second network could be realized having a frequency transfer-function $1/H(\omega)$, then an input-function $s_r(t) = h(t)$, with the spectrum $S_r(\omega) = H(\omega)$, would cause an output of the second network being again a delta-function. The second network is then an ideal inverse filter and a complete deconvolution of the blurred signal $s_r(t)$ is obtained.

Of course, when the only goal is resolution-enhancement, inverse filtering (frequency-domain) or, equivalently, deconvolution (time-domain) is the way to go.

Alternatively, if signal-to-noise ratio is to be optimized, so-called matched filtering, also indicated in Fig. 7, is the proper procedure. The latter will not be treated here any further.

In practice ideal inverse filtering is not possible. The signal band-width is always limited and noise is always present. At the edges of the band where spectral amplitudes are small, mainly noise would be amplified by the inverse filter leading to signal degradation rather than improvement.

Therefore, depending on signal-to-noise ratio, only a limited frequency-band can be "flattened", which will lead to a sort of sinc-function as the deconvolver-output, since a sinc-function is the inverse Fourier-transofrm of a rectangular spectrum. The wider this rectangular spectrum, the narrower the main lobe of the sinc-function, ultimately approximating the delta-function.

Of course, a deconvolver can only be designed and applied when a priori knowledge about the impulse-response of the system is avai-label and, ideally, about the noise conditions as well.

In conclusion: the larger the available signal-frequency band-width and the better the signal-to-noise ratio, the greater the resolution-improvement by proper deconvolution will be.

4. OPTICAL DECONVOLUTION

4.1. Motivation

There are a number of logical steps which lead to the adoption of the concept of optical deconvolution for improving echography.

Firstly, real-time performance should be possible. Real-time pulse-echo systems are invaluable for visualizing dynamic struc-tures like the heart, the vascular system, the fetal movements etc. For us it is therefore an absolute requirement to preserve this facility when applying deconvolution techniques. This ex-cludes digital-computer techniques and only analogue methods have to be considered.

Secondly, the option of two-dimensional filtering[*] simultane-ously draws the attention towards optical methods.

Thirdly, the necessary condition for inverse filtering (as well as for matched filtering) is the cancellation of phase from which the idea emerges of using optical holography for the realization of the complex spatial frequency filter.

---

[*] Ideally, 3-dimensional filtering would be required since also in azimuth beam-shape affects resolution. Here only filtering in the scanning-plane is considered.

4.2 Optical computer

4.2.1. Introduction. Several publications on Fourier optics (1) and on optical computing have appeared during the last two decades (2,3,4).
In earlier papers (5,6,7,8) we already presented the basic principles of optical deconvolution in conjunction with a phased-array puls-echo imaging system. In the following, we will briefly summarize the main features of the overall system but the holographic process will be dealt with in some depth.

4.2.2. Block diagram. Our optical computer is an analogue computer which performs a limited number of operations in real-time and in two-dimensions simultaneously. Fig. 1 is a schematic presentation of the basic elements of an optical computer. The plane indicated as 'Input plane' is uniformly illuminated by monochromatic and spatially coherent normally incident light.

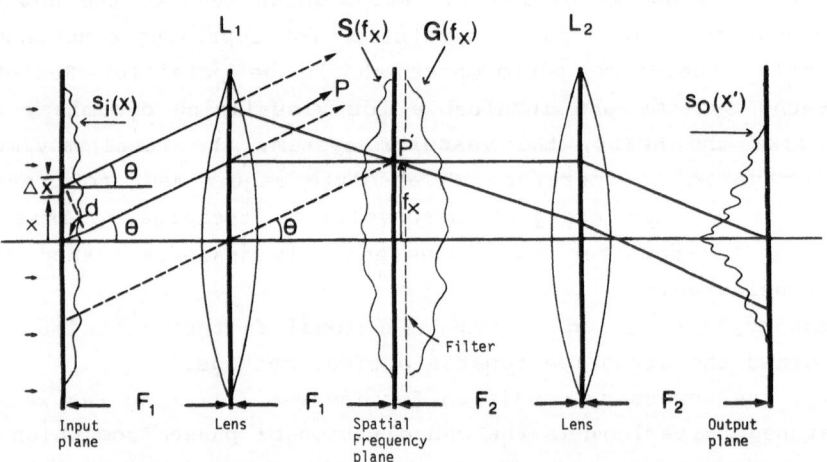

FIGURE 1. Basic elements of an optical computer.

Let us assume that an input signal $s_i(x)$ is represented by an amplitude and/or phase distribution as a transmission function. Under these conditons the light distribution immediately behind the input plane is $s_i(x)$. Now, without the lens, the resulting light distribution at far distance (Fraunhofer-pattern) would be the Fourier-transform of the aperture distribution.

It will be appreciated from Fig. 1 that an element Δx of the input plane contributes to the distribution in a far point P as follows.

$$\Delta s_p(x) = s_i(x).e^{j2\pi d/\lambda}.\Delta x \qquad \text{with } d = x \sin \theta$$

Thus the far field distribution yields

$$S(f'_x) = \int_{-\infty}^{+\infty} s_i(x).e^{j2\pi x f'_x} dx \qquad \text{with } f'_x = (\sin\theta)/\lambda$$

in which we recognize the well-known <u>Fourier-transform</u>.

Analogous to electric theory, where frequency is the number of cycles per second in the time-domain, here the spatial frequency f'_x is the number of cycles per meter in the input plane.

Since P is at far distance all contributions $\Delta s_p(x)$ are in the same direction θ which means that all these contributing rays are in parallel. Therefore, with the lens L1 the calculated far-field distribution appears as $S(f_x)$ in its second focal plane, indicated as 'Spatial frequency plane'. The relationship between f'_x and f_x is found to be

$$f_x = F_1 \tan(\arcsin \lambda f'_x)$$

Usually the angles are small enough to allow the approximation

$$f_x = F_1\lambda f'_x \qquad \text{or} \qquad f'_x = f_x/(F_1\lambda) \tag{1}$$

The expression for the distribution in the spatial frequency plane now becomes

$$S(f_x) = \int_{-\infty}^{+\infty} s_i(x).e^{j2\pi x f_x/(F_1\lambda)}dx \tag{2}$$

or in the two-dimensional form

$$S(f_x,f_y) = \iint_{-\infty}^{+\infty} s_i(x,y)e^{j2\pi(xf_x+yf_y)/(F_1\lambda)}dxdy \tag{3}$$

It is obvious that a second lens L_2 which has the spatial frequency plane in its first focal plane will again Fourier-transform the frequency spectrum $S(f_x,f_y)$. Therefore, the distribution $s_o(x',y')$ in the second focal plane of L_2, the output plane, is identical to $s_i(x,y)$ except for reversed signs of the co-ordinates. Thus, this second Fourier-transform by lens L_2 can be regarded as an inverse Fourier-transform.

A transparency with a transmission characteristic $G(f_x,f_y)$, placed in the spatial frequency plane, multiplies the function $S(f_x,f_y)$ with $G(f_x,f_y)$. The light distribution immediately behind this transparency is then given by

$$S_o(f_x,f_y) = S(f_x,f_y) \cdot G(f_x,f_y) \qquad [4]$$

The output-function $s_o(x',y')$ now represents the 'inverse' Fourier-transform of Eq. [4]

$$s_o(x',y') = F^{-1}\{S(f_x,f_y) \cdot G(f_x,f_y)\} = F^{-1}\{S_o(f_x,f_y)\} \qquad [5]$$

4.2.3. Optical filtering. The signals in the input plane, $s_i(x,y)$ should represent the instantaneous spatial and temporal functions of the returning echoes of a real-time two-dimensional ultrasound imaging system and modulate the light properly. Then the device enables the filtering of echoes in real-time and in two dimensions simultaneously.

We now assume, according to what is said in chapter 3 about the determination of the impulse-response by using a delta-function as input, to receive the echo from an isolated and very small point-target in a 'noise-free' situation, e.g. a very small sphere in a watertank, called reference-target. Its representation[*] in the input plane of the optical computer may be $s_{ir}(x,y)$. In the spatial frequency plane we obtain the Fourier-transform $S_r(f_x,f_y)$ of $s_{ir}(x,y)$ according to Eq. [3]. For ideal resolution we would like to have a filter-function (see also chapter 3)

---

[*] The conversion of the electrical echo-signals to optical input-signals is described in chapter 6.

$$G(f_x,f_y) = 1/S_r(f_x,f_y) \qquad\qquad [6]$$

which, according to Eq. [4] and [5], would result in an output-function as a response to the input $s_{ir}(x,y)$ being

$$s_{or}(x',y') = F^{-1}\{1\} = \delta(x',y') \qquad\qquad [7]$$

We would then have a complete deconvolution for the 'blurring' caused by pulse-length and beam-width. As mentioned before this is called <u>inverse filtering</u> and the very small reference-target as described will be imaged in the output plane as a very small spot. It should again be emphasized that ideal inverse filtering does not exist due to the limitations described in chapter 3.

If it is allowed to consider an arbitrary reflecting object as a superposition of point-targets these are all 'blurred' in the same way. Since a translation in the xy-domain is expressed as phase-shifts of the spectral components in the spatial frequency-domain, the filtering with one and the same filter keeps the relative phase differences intact. This implies that the relative locations of the input-signals are restored in the output plane.

5. THE COMPLEX SPATIAL FILTER

5.1. The Holographic process

Already in 1964 VanderLugt published a method for producing a complex filter by means of a holographic process (2). A holographic plate is illuminated by an object beam and a reference beam simultaneously, see Fig. 2. It is assumed that both beams originate from the same laser source in order to ensure the light to be

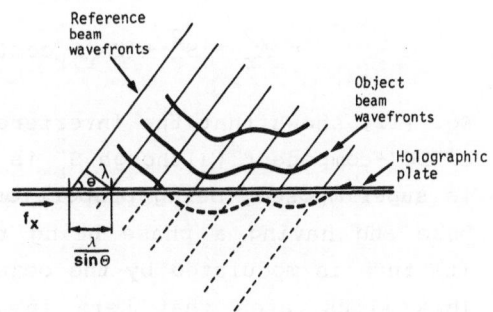

Figure 2. Realization of a hologram.

monochromatic and spatially and temporally coherent. Here, the object beam is the spectrum $S_r(f_x, f_y)$ of the reference-target, of which both amplitude and phase are functions of f_x and f_y. At the surface of the holographic plate the complex function can be expressed as

$$\bar{S}_r = S_r(f_x, f_y) e^{j\phi(f_x, f_y)} = S_r e^{j\phi} \qquad [8]$$

We require the reference beam to have a constant amplitude and an angle θ with the f_x-coordinate only.
It can be found from Fig. 2 that on the plate its complex amplitude can be described as

$$\bar{A}_r = A_r e^{-j\alpha f x} = A_r e^{-j\psi} \qquad \text{where} \quad \alpha = (2\pi\sin\theta)/\lambda \qquad [9]$$

The total amplitude at the plate is now

$$\bar{A}_T = \bar{A}_r + \bar{S}_r = A_r e^{-j\psi} + S_r e^{j\phi} \qquad [10]$$

Since photographic emulsions respond to intensity, rather than to amplitude, we calculate the intensity, which is

$$I_T = \bar{A}_T \cdot \bar{A}_T^*$$

$$= A_r^2 + S_r^2 + A_r S_r e^{j(\psi+\phi)} + A_r S_r e^{-j(\psi+\phi)} \qquad [11]$$

$$= A_r^2 + S_r^2 + 2A_r S_r \cos(\psi+\phi) \qquad [12]$$

Eq. [12] shows that the interference intensity-pattern consists of a "DC"-component (although S_r^2 is a variable) on which a modulation is superimposed, being proportional in amplitude with the object-beam and having a phase being the reference-beam phase which on its turn is modulated by the object-beam phase, since always $\phi \ll \psi$. This illustrates that here in an intensity-function still both amplitude and phase are preserved, due to the use of a reference beam.

If the photographic emulsion would respond to the impinging

light-energy such that the amplitude transmission of the developed plate would be a linear function of this energy, the amplitude transmission would also be expressed by Eqs. [11, 12]. An impinging reference-beam at zero angle would then fall apart into three beams as follows: $(A_r^2+S_r^2)$ at zero angle, and two beams proportional to S_r at angles $+\theta$ and $-\theta$, according to Eq. [9].

On the other hand, if in this special case the object-beam would impinge on the developed plate, the transmitted beams would be proportional to:

a. $(A_r^2+S_r^2).S_r e^{j\phi}$, being a distorted object beam at "zero" angle

b. $S_r^2 e^{j(\psi+2\phi)}$, being the squared amplitude object-beam with distorted phase at an angle $+\theta$.

c. $S_r^2 e^{-j\psi}$, being again the squared amplitude object-beam with cancelled phase under an angle $-\theta$.

5.2. Holographic "inverse" filter

In chapter 3 and in paragraph 4.2.3. it was pointed out that the filter should have a transfer-function, now written in complex notation,

$$\bar{G} = 1/\bar{S}_r = 1/(S_r.e^{j\phi}) = (1/S_r).e^{-j\phi} \qquad [13]$$

In paragraph 5.1 was found that in the $(-\theta)$-diffraction component of the hologram this negative phase is present (leading to the phase-cancellation as in case c), so this aspect is allright. However, instead of $1/S_r$, the amplitude transfer-function of the hologram in par. 5.1 is S_r so that for obtaining an inverse filter the amplitude transmission-function of the holographic plate as a function of the exposure energy should definitely not be linear as was assumed in par. 5.1[*].

Fig. 3 shows a realistic amplitude transmission curve T_a as a function of E=It, the exposure-energy, with t=exposure-time. It

---

[*] In fact, in par. 5.1 we found the way to realize a matched filter (see Fig. 7).

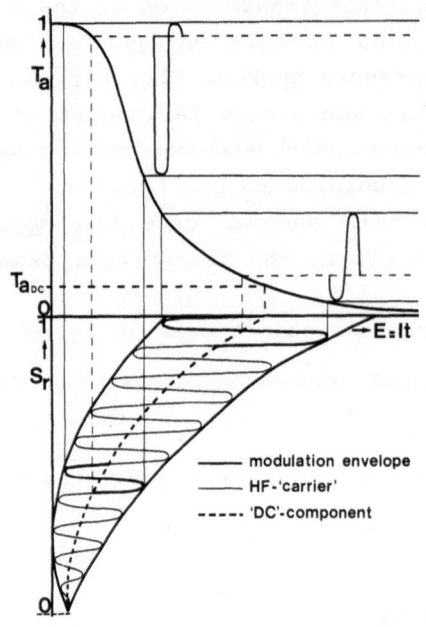

modulation envelope
HF-'carrier'
----- 'DC'-component

Figure 3. Realization of a complex spatial "inverse" filter.

also shows the intensity-function according to Eq. [12]. Here, S_r runs linearly from 0 to 1 and the ratio A_r/S_{rmax} is less than 1. Due to the very non-linear T_a-curve a high modulation-amplitude causes a low transmission-modulation and reversed.

Qualitatively this is just what we wish to achieve. However, to which extent the obtained transmission-modulation function approximates the actually wanted $1/S_r$ (according to Eq. [13]), will be further investigated.

5.3. Evaluation of a model

The result as shown in Fig. 3 suggests that, given a particular T_a-E function, the two possible parameters which can be varied are the beam-amplitude ratio

$$R_a = A_r/S_{rmax} \qquad [14]$$

and the T_{aDC}-value, being the transmission corresponding to the maximum DC-component value, see Fig. 3.

Alteration of R_a causes considerable variation of the DC-component as a function of S_r. The T_{aDC}-value can be adjusted by proper estimation of the exposure-time t.

The process as shown in Fig. 3 can be investigated further by fitting the measured T_a-curve of a particular type of photographic material under particular development-conditions by a mathematical function.

A suitable expression was found in

$$T_a(E) = \{a_4 E^4 + a_3 E^3 + a_2 E^2 + a_1 E + 1/(1-T_\infty)\}^{-1} + T_\infty \qquad [15]$$

providing a rest-value $T_a = T_\infty$ at $E = \infty$ and $T_a = 1$ for $E = 0$, according to reality. From the measured, T_a-E characteristic T_∞ and four different pairs of T_{ai} and E_i values (i = 1...4) should be taken at regular intervals covering the whole significant portion.

Then solving the four corresponding simultaneous equations yields the coefficients $a_1...a_4$ and the fitting function has been determined.

The exposure-energy E can be found from Eqs. [12] and [14], together with stating that $S_{rmax}=1$ (for convenience), as follows

$$E = I.t = \{R_a^2 + S_r^2 + 2R_a S_r \cos(\psi + \phi)\}.t \qquad [16]$$

where t = exposure-time.

In practice θ, the angle of the reference beam, is always taken large enough to let $\psi = \alpha f_x = (2\pi \sin\theta . f_x)/\lambda$ (see Eq. [9]) be much greater then ϕ (Eq. [8]). The modulation frequency, therefore, is mainly determined by ψ and is very close to $(\sin\theta)/\lambda$ and in our case approximately 100 cycles per millimeter.

Since for this model the phase of the spectral function S_r is assumed to be zero (again for convenience), we can write

$$E = \{R_a^2 + S_r^2 + 2R_a S_r \cos\psi\}.t \qquad [17]$$

with

$$\psi = 2\pi . 100 f_x \qquad [18]$$

where f_x is measured in mm on the holographic plate.

Substitution of Eq. [17] into Eq. [15] yields

$$T_a = T_a (\psi) \qquad [19]$$

with the parameters R_a as the beam-amplitude ratio, S_r as the spectral amplitude of the input-function to the system and t as the exposure-time to obtain the required T_{aDC}-value.

From Fig. 3 we will appreciate that the original cosine-function of Eq. [17] is highly distorted by the non-linear T_a-E characteristic, resulting in an oscillating function with many harmonics ψ, 2ψ, 3ψ etc.

Illuminated by a beam this grating pattern will accordingly split it up in diffractions at $+\theta$ and $-\theta$, $+2\theta$ and -2θ, $+3\theta$ and -3θ etc. At using such a grating as a complex spatial filter only the first order diffraction at $-\theta$ is selected out.

In our mathematical model we assume that S_r is varying very slowly with the co-ordinate f_x, which means that at every position f_x the spectral amplitude S_r can be considered to be constant over several grating-oscillations. This makes $T_a(\psi)$, as represented by Eq. [19] to a periodic function with ψ as the only variable and thus $T_a(\psi)$ can be expressed as a Fourier-series

$$T_a(\psi) = A_o + A_1\cos\psi + A_2\cos 2\psi + \ldots \qquad [20]$$

$$= A_o + \frac{A_1}{2}(e^{j\psi} + e^{-j\psi}) + \frac{A_2}{2}(e^{j2\psi} + e^{-j2\psi}) + \ldots$$

As mentioned above, we are interested in the first order $(-\theta)$-diffraction only so that we merely have to evaluate A_1.
From Fourier-series theory we calculate

$$A_1 = \frac{1}{\pi} \cdot \int_{-\pi}^{+\pi} T(\psi).\cos\psi.d\psi \qquad [21]$$

for several values of S_r.
Herewith we in fact obtain A_1 and <u>thus</u> G as a function of the spectral amplitude S_r, still with R_a and T_{aDC} as parameters.

One should realize that we did not find the transfer-function $G(f_x)$ in the spatial-frequency plane of the holographic complex spatial filter for a spectrum S_r, unless $S_r(f_x)$ is defined.

If for all frequencies $G(f_x) = 1/S_r(f_x)$, which is required for an inverse filter (Eqs. [6, 13]), then $G(f_x).S_r(f_x) = 1$.

Accordingly $A_1.S_r$ should be constant for all S_r. We can now determine the product of spectral amplitude and filter-function as a function of the spectral amplitude, in other words

$$A_1.S_r = f(S_r) \qquad [22]$$

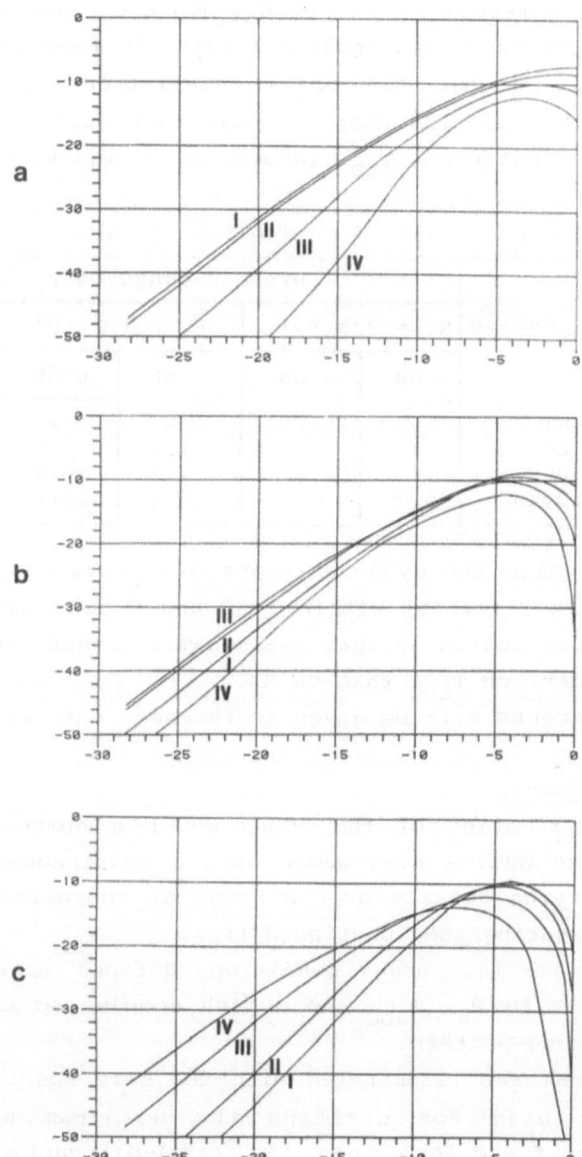

FIGURE 4. Results of model-evaluation of the holographic process.
See Table 2.

The range of S_r over which $A_1.S_r$ is "constant" (within certain limits) then determines the <u>maximum dynamic range</u> of S_r for which the used T_a-E curve can produce a suitable inverse filter.

In Fig. 4 a,b,c the model calculations are presented for R_a = 2/3, 1/2 and 1/3 respectively. Four curves are given representing four different T_{aDC}-values, according to Table 2.

Table 2

Nr. of curve	T_{aDC}-value	Dynamic range of S_r in dB					
		R_a = 2/3 (a)		R_a = 1/2 (b)		R_a = 1/3 (c)	
		3 dB	6 dB	3 dB	6 dB	3 dB	6 dB
I	0.01	–	–	–	–	5.5	7.9
II	0.005	–	–	7.2	–	5.8	8.4
III	0.002	–	–	7.2	10.7	7.2	10.0
IV	0.00135	6.7	–	7.1	10.0	7.6	11.2

In Table 2 also the dynamic ranges of S_r are given for all cases (as far as applicable) within 3 dB and 6 dB limits respectively. The first conclusion is that the dynamic ranges are very small and more dependent on T_{aDC} than on R_a.
Further comments will be given in the next chapter.

5.4. Experiments

For confirmation of the found model a number of experiments were carried out. A grey-wedge with a continuously and logarithmically varying density over a range of approximately 30 dB, was used for creating the function $S_r(f_x)$.
Holograms were made under conditions defined as well as possible with respect to R_a, T_{aDC} and a high enough oscillating frequency of the grating-pattern.
Each hologram was illuminated with the same spectral distribution $S_r(f_x)$ as used for creating the hologram with accurately co-inciding f_x-scales. Then the $(-\theta)$-diffraction was recorded (corresponding with A_1 in the previous chapter), together with the spectral distribution $S_r(f_x)$ itself.
By a computer the data were processed and f_x was eliminated in order to obtain $A_1.S_r$ as a function of S_r, similar to the

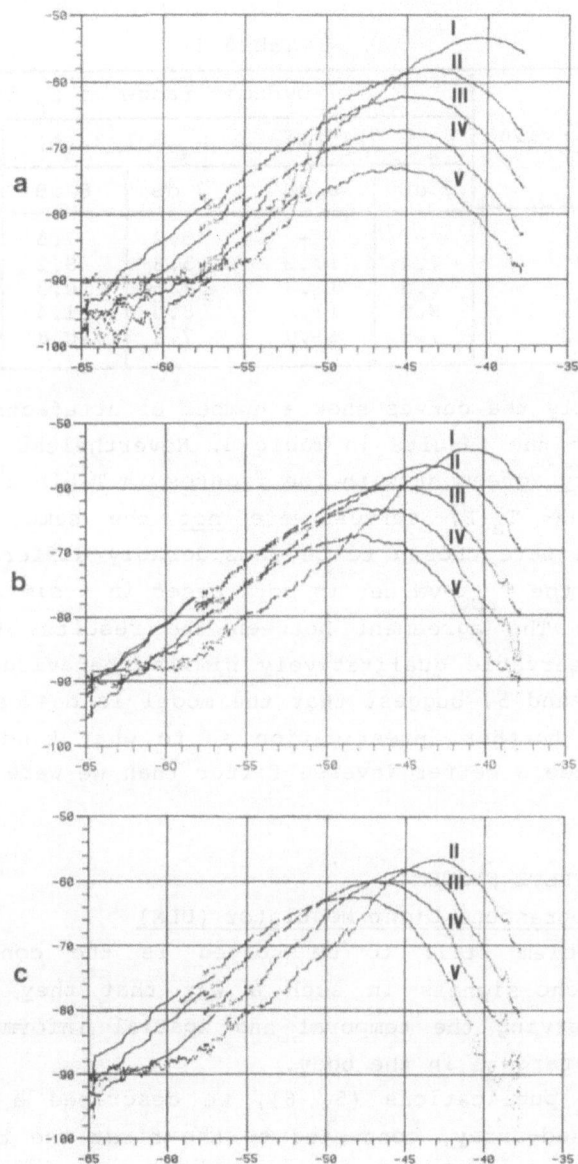

FIGURE 5. Experimental results of the holographic process. See Table 3.

model-evaluation in the previous chapter (Eq. [22]).
The results are given in Fig. 5 a,b,c in combination with Table 3

Table 3

Nr. of curve	T_{aDC}-value	Dynamic range of S_r in dB					
		$R_a = 2/3$ (a)		$R_a = 1/2$ (b)		$R_a = 1/3$ (c)	
		3 dB	6 dB	3 dB	6 dB	3 dB	6 dB
I	0.5	–	–	5.2	7.5	–	–
II	0.2	7.4	11.2	5.8	9.2	5.3	7.3
III	0.1	7.5	11.4	7.5	10.3	5.4	8.0
IV	0.05	8.0	11.4	8.0	11.4	6.1	9.2
V	0.02	7.5	11.0	7.3	10.8	7.3	10.3

Apparently the curves show a number of artefacts, affecting the accuracy of the results in Table 3. Nevertheless there is a very satisfactory agreement with the figures in Table 2.

Since the $T_a(E)$ curves were not the same, also the used T_{aDC}-values were chosen to be considerably different in order to distribute the T_{aDC}-values in both cases in a similar way.
Conclusion: The agreement between the results, together with a clearly observable qualitatively similar behaviour of the curves of Figs. 4 and 5, suggest that the model is basically correct and useful for further investigation as to what kind of $T_a(E)$-curve could provide a better inverse filter than we were able to realize so far.

6. THE COMPLETE SYSTEM

6.1. The Ultrasound Light Modulator (ULM)

The problem still to be solved is the conversion of the received echo-signals in such a way that they modulate light, while preserving the temporal and spatial information about the reflecting targets in the body.
In earlier publications (5, 6), we described a system using a second phased-array, connected to the first one through a set of amplifiers, and radiating in an optical cuvet Medium II, which is placed in the input plane of the optical computer and contains a spherical acoustic reflector for reversing the order of the echoes

before illumination. The sound waves cause refractive-index variations which results in diffraction of light.

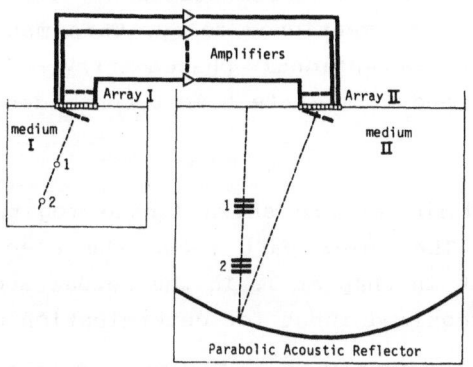

Figure 6. Ultrasound Light Modulator system (ULM).

In Fig. 6 a ULM is represented in which the spherical reflector has been replaced by a parabolic one (7, 8), because the spherical reflector was unable to provide sufficient spatial invariance in the input plane.

In the diagram 'Medium I' indicates the object to be examined, e.g. the body or a watertank with a phantom. The instantaneous amplitude and phase distribution on Array I will be characteristic for a particular target or set of targets and forms simultaneously the transmission-distribution of Array II, radiating in Medium II, the cuvet. The Medium I is ensonified repetitively and non-directionally by short pulses. Since Array II is in the focal point of the paraboloid, after reflection by the reflector all echo-signals will travel along parallel path-ways towards the liquid surface.

The time delay between the transmission of an ensonifying pulse in Medium I and the laserflash of ca 25 ns illuminating the optical cuvet should be 2F/v. Then, the ranges of all received echo-signals with respect to the liquid surface in the cuvet will be proportional to the actual ranges with respect to Array I in Medium I. Angle of direction of a target is converted to lateral displacement in the cuvet, which means that there is no conformal mapping. A minimum of spatial variance has now been obtained at the expense of some image-deformation. This is necessary to cover a wide area of examination with only one holographic filter.

The deformation of the image, as recorded by a TV-camera in the output plane, can easily be restored electronically. The echoes are then displayed at positions corresponding to the pertinent targets.

Due to the non-directional ensonification of Medium I all targets will be "displayed" in the cuvet simultaneously after each transmitted acoustic pulse at the mentioned delay. This makes the system more real-time than conventional phased-array scanning systems since now pulse-rate and frame-rate have become identical.

6.2. Overall block-diagram

The sub-systems described so far are shown linked together in the upper part of Fig. 7. The lower part shows the electrical equivalent already dealt with in chapter 3. In the actual acousto-electro-optical system the required input for determination of the

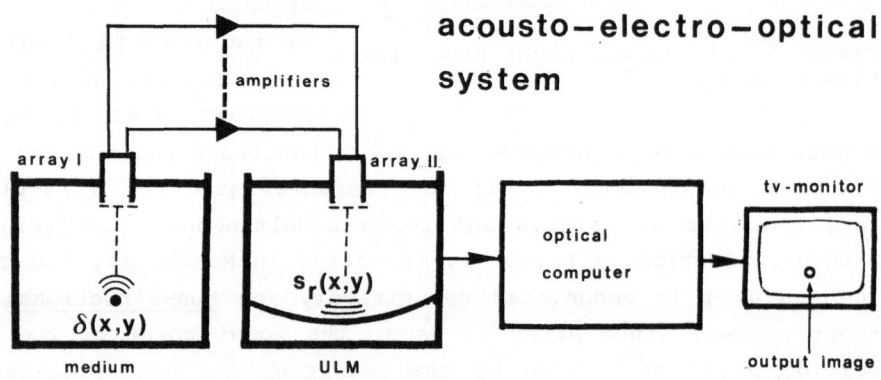

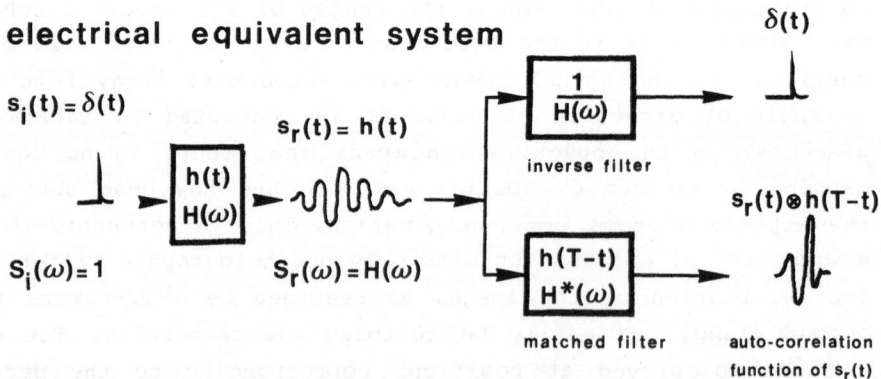

FIGURE 7. Overall-system and the representation of the filtering-process.

impulse-response is formed by a spatial delta-function, being a point-target, as compared to the electrical δ-function in the lower part.

The impulse-response $s_r(x,y)$ appears as an ultrasound grating in the ULM-cuvet and serves on its turn as the input of the optical system for realizing the complex spatial filter in order to perform the deconvolution. Then, once having obtained such a filter and having re-aligned it in the spatial frequency plane, any arbitrarily shaped target can be placed under the primary array-transducer and will be converted to a deblurred image on the television-screen. This is true, provided that any target may be considered to be the sum of an infinite number of spatial delta-functions, like any time-function can be decomposed into delta-functions.

7. PRACTICAL RESULTS

From the investigation of the holographic process in chapter 5 the conclusion was drawn that the dynamic range of the spectrum should be small, e.g. no more than approximately 10 dB. With the set-up as shown in Fig. 7, upper part, two complex spatial filters (A) and (B) were realized for the same point-target in the medium. In the first case (A) the laser-flash delay was made such that the signal $s_r(x,y)$ appeared at a position before reflection against the paraboloid reflector, whereas the second case (B) was the normal situation with the signal $s_r(x,y)$ shown after reflection.

Obviously the flattening of the wave-fronts at reflection against the paraboloid reflector causes a considerable increase of power-concentration through the Fourier-transformation.

Fig. 8 shows case (A) with respectively the obtained spectrum (a), the unfiltered signal supposed to be identical to $s_r(x,y)$ in the input plane (b) and zero and first diffraction orders in the output plane (c).

As explained in par. 5.3 the filter-result appears as the $(-\theta)$-diffraction and is indicated by an arrow in Fig. 8c.

Apparently, a very effective deconvolution has been obtained since this very small spot is depicted at the same scale as $s_r(x,y)$ in (b).

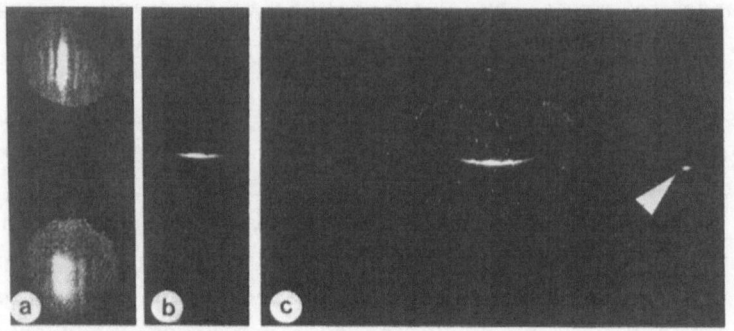

FIGURE 8. Practial results for non-reflected signals.

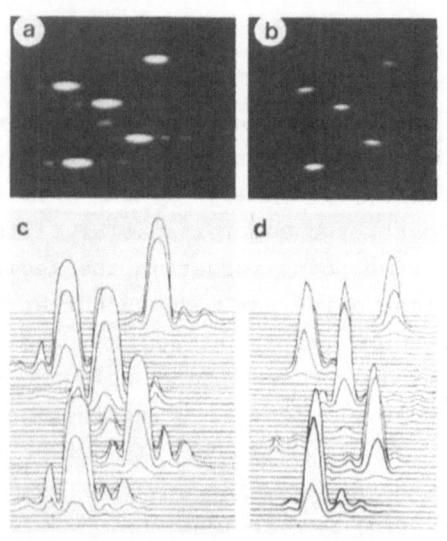

FIGURE 9. Practical results for signals after reflection.

Fig. 9 represents results obtained in case (B). In (a) five signals are shown as they appeared unfiltered in the output plane, again supposed to be identical to the input-signals. The scanned object consisted of five "point"-targets in a rhombus-shaped configuration and the image shows clearly the position-deformation caused by the paraboloid reflector. A filter was realized with only the center-target present in the medium and after installing the filter the corner-targets were mounted at their positions. In Fig. 9b we see the filter-results, being much less spectacular than in case (A). In Fig. 9c and d the signals are shown as measured quantitatively. It is clear that the gain in spatial invariance by using a paraboloid reflector (as a proof showing the five filtered signals in Fig. 9b as being quite similar) has been obtained at the expense of filter-performance because of the increased dynamic range of the spectra. Everything being well in agreement with the results of the model-investigation in chapter 5.

8. CONCLUSIONS

With a ULM-system as described echoes received with a phased-array ultrasounddiagnostic system can be converted to imput-signals for an optical computer. With a complex spatial filter in the spatial frequency plane filtering can be performed. A holographic method has been described to realize such a filter which acts as an inverse filter provided that the spectrum to be processed has a small dynamic range.

A reasonable spatial invariance in the input plane has been achieved at the expense of high dynamic range of the spectrum. Both increasing dynamic range of the filter and compression of the spectrum's dynamic range are the goals of further investigations.

REFERENCES

1. Goodman JW. 1968. Introduction to Fourier Optics. San Francisco, McGraw-Hill.
2. VanderLugt A. 1964. Signal detection by complex spatial filtering. IEEE Trans. on Information Theory, IT-10, p. 139.
3. Stroke GW, Zech RG. 1967. A posteriori image-correcting "Deconvolution" by holographic Fourier-transformdivision. Physics Letters, vol. 25A, p. 89.
4. Preston K. 1972. Coherent optical computers. New York, McGraw-Hill.
5. Somer JC. 1977. Real-time improvement of both lateral and range resolution by optical signal processing. 1977 Ultrasonics Symposium Proceedings, 77CH-1264-1 SU, p. 1002, New York, IEEE.
6. Somer JC. 1978. Real-time improvement of both lateral and range resolution by optical signal processing. Ultrasound in Medicine, Vol. 4, p. 439 (Eds. White D, Lyons EA). New York, Plenum Press.
7. Somer JC, Jongsma FHM, Martens WLJ. 1980. Application of an acousto-optic device in an optical deconvolver for blurred ultrasound-diagnostic images. Proc. 1st spring school on acousto-optics and applications, p. 202, Gdansk, University Physics Institute.
8. Somer JC. 1980. Optical signal processing in ultrasound. Investigative Ultrasonology, vol. 1, Technical Advances, p. 71 (Eds. Hill CR, Alvisi C). Tunbridge Wells, Pitman Medical.

A BAYESEAN ALGORITHM FOR RESOLUTION RECOVERY IN CLINICAL
NUCLEAR MEDICINE.

DOUGLAS A. ORTENDAHL, ROBERT S. HATTNER, LEON KAUFMAN, ELIAS
BOTVINICK, J. WILLIAM O'CONNELL, DONALD FAULKNER AND LOUIS T. KIRCOS

Department of Radiology, University of California, San Francisco,
California 94143

INTRODUCTION

The most commonly used imaging instrumentation in nuclear medicine consists of a position sensitive detector (a gamma camera) and a
parallel-hole collimator. Such a system has four major sources of
blurring: intrinsic detector resolution, spatial distortion, scatter
and depth degradation. This gives nuclear images relatively poor
spatial resolution when compared to modalities such CT or NMR and
limits the utilization of a powerful diagnostic technique. Improvements in instrumentation over the last few years have ameliorated some
of these problems. Spatial distortion is no longer a significant
problem with digitally corrected cameras; at the same time the
improved uniformity makes asymetric high side energy windows practical
for scatter reduction. Intrinsic resolution has also improved, but
progress beyond the current level will be difficult. However little
can be done about the blurring by the collimator of activity at depth.

Digital processing is often applied in an attempt to remove some
of this blurring. While in principle knowledge of the point spread
function (PSF) should allow the calculation of the source distribution
by analytic deconvolution, in practice the noise amplification inherent in the calculation of the inverse filter makes this process
unusable considering the signal/noise of typical nuclear images. The
available signal/noise limits the use of a number of techniques
commonly used in the field of image restoration (1). Attempts to find
suitable modified filters have met with limited success (2). For this
reason the use of image restoration methods in nuclear medicine
remains controversial. We describe a restoration algorithm based on
Bayesean statistics (3). While it suffers many of the problems of
other techniques, we have found it to be very useful in clinical
nuclear medicine.

ALGORITHM DESCRIPTION

The development of this algorithm was motivated by the availability in our laboratory of a small prototype high purity germanium (HPGe) camera (4). This camera with an area of 20 cm² achieves almost total rejection of scatter through an energy resolution of 2.2% at 140 kev. The discrete electronic readout yields an unambiguous 2 mm FW (full width) intrinsic resolution. With a thin-wall square-hole collimator indexed to the camera elements, performance is determined by geometry, a simple and invariant parameter. These unique properties suggested that progress could be made in the problem of depth degradation with parallel hole collimators.

The original derivation of the algorithm did not involve Bayes' theorem at all. Rather the argument involved the use of a weighted back-projection (WBP) method which had been developed for a multi-wire proportional chamber positron camera in our laboratory (5). While not mathematically rigorous this method was the most successful of the algorithms tested (including Fourier techniques) with the high noise limited angle images from the UCSF positron camera. This formulation of deblurring was obtained by tracing rays through the HPGe collimator and weighting each ray appropriately. Such an argument is particularly appealing since once a ray enters the collimator, its position in the HPGe camera is defined exactly by the discrete readout.

It was later realized that this algorithm may be derived directly from Bayes theorem. This theorem may be expressed as

$$P(S|I) = \frac{P(I|S)P(S)}{\sum_C P(I|C) \, P(S)} \qquad (1)$$

$P(S|I)$ is the conditional probability of observing event S given that event I has occurred and $P(S)$ is simply the probability of event S. The sum in the denominator is over all events C which have a finite probability of leading to event I. For our case we are interested in the probability of a source S given an image I. Bayes' theorem gives an estimate of this in terms of the probability of an image given a source. This latter quantity is the point spread function which we denote by A. This leads directly to the iterative relation:

$$S^q_{i,j} = W^{q-1}_{i,j} \times S^{q-1}_{i,j} \qquad (2)$$

where the superscript q refers to the iteration number, the subscripts i,j refer to the pixel, the initial guess S^0 is the original image I and

$$W^q_{i,j} = \sum_{kl} \frac{A_{k-i,l-j} I_{k,l}}{\sum_{mn} A_{k-m,l-n} S^q_{m,n}} \qquad (3)$$

The calculation of the weights is simple sequence of operations. First convolve the result of the previous iteration with the PSF. Divide this pixel by pixel into the original image and then convolve this again. This gives a set of weights with which we multiply the result of the previous iteration, yielding the updated estimate of the source distribution.

In this formulation at each iteration the result is compared to the original image by means of the $I_{k,l}$ in equation (3). The assumption that in equation (3), $I_{k,l}$ may be replaced with $S^q_{k,l}$ leads to what we call the modified Bayesean formulation. This is the same result that was obtained by tracing rays through the HPGe collimator (6). With this formulation subsequent iterations "lose" contact with the original image which has important consequences in terms of convergence.

The assumption that the weights for each iteration may be considered equal gives

$$S^q_{i,j} = [W^0_{i,j}]^p I_{i,j} \qquad (4)$$

where the weight W^0 is raised to the power p. The obvious advantage is an increase in computational speed, since the calculation of the weights (the most time consuming part of the computation) need only be done once. This will be referred to as the power method.

While the deblurred image has better spatial resolution, it also has increased noise. Depending on the clinical problem it is sometimes advantageous to sacrifice some of this improved resolution for reduced noise by convolving once more with the PSF producing an an image called the reprojection. This operation is just a smoothing and could be performed with any size kernel, but we choose to use the PSF since this gives a final image with about the same resolution as the original.

The development of this algorithm was performed independently of the work of Metz and Pizer (7,8) on a Bayesean method which they called iterative biased smearing. While similar to the method described here, there are some important differences. Iterative biased smearing is a true Bayesean technique, since as in equation (3) it compares the result of each iteration to the original image. The authors found it desirable to use a different spread function for each of the convolutions. The convolution kernel in the denominator was chosen to be much broader than the expected point spread function while the convolution of the quotient was performed with a narrower spread function. As in our work they found that additional smoothing was often desirable , but unlike the reprojection step this final smoothing used a gaussian that was very narrow compared to the spread function. One iteration of iterative biased smearing was preferred. Considering the computational expense of the algorithm and their results, the authors concluded that biased smearing held little promise.

CHARACTERIZATION OF ALGORITHM

A complete description of the physical characteristics of the algorithm are given in reference (3), but a few examples are given here. This algorithm will not converge and as such requires that the number of iterations to perform be imposed or a choice of power be made. In figure 1 we show output contrast as a function of iteration or power for cold lesions obtained with the HPGe camera. The direct Bayesean method shows the least improvement in contrast. This is because at each step the result is compared to the original image. Since the modified method compares only to the previous iteration result it gives maximum contrast improvement. But too many iteration will produce output contrast larger than the input leading to artifacts and excessive textured noise. This example suggests a cut-off of 4 iterations or a power of 6. This same cut-off point was obtained by grading processed clinical images. The choice is not critical since a change by one up or down in the number of iterations does not drastically change the results. With this number of iterations or choice of power, for small area lesions we found an increase in contrast with approximately constant signal/noise. Noise increases but signal increases at the same rate. For large areas an increase in the textured noise is seen.

An issue of concern in such an algorithm is the error that can be introduced if the depth of reconstruction is not known. We find that the choice of depth or equivalently, the PSF, is not critical. The effect of overlying and underlying activity will be to reduce the initial contrast and thus the final contrast observed after processing. If there is structure in this over or under lying activity it will of course be enhanced, but there is not a serious problem of over or under correcting because of depth.

Since the modified and power formulations of Bayesean deblurring give similar results we use the power method exclusively for clinical studies because of its speed advantage. Implemented on a PDP 11-34 the deblurring process requires 10 sec for a 64x64 image with an additional 4 sec for the reprojection.

CLINICAL APPLICATIONS

Skeletal Scintigraphy

Skeletal scintigraphy is usually "hot spot" imaging and as such computer processing is not usually required. At our institution such studies are rarely computer acquired. There are specialized applications where processing can be of value. A unique protocol used at our hospital is tempero-mandibular joint arthropathy which is illustrated in Figure 2. The clinically important information in such a study is whether the arthritis is restricted to the socket or extends out into the condyle. This is determined by observing the difference between jaw open and closed. Note in the deblurred image that the activity clearly separates indicating condyle involvement. This diagnosis is more difficult to make in the unprocessed images and was confirmed by other clinical tests. In skeletal images the issue is usually one of resolution rather than noise, as such we have found the deblurred images to be of use, while the noise reduction of the reprojected images is usually not desired.

Liver-Spleen Imaging

In liver-spleen imaging with Tc-99m sulfur-colloid the imaging problem is one of the detection of cold lesions. As such one would expect that Bayesean deblurring could prove useful. In Figure 3 we show a normal liver study which has been both deblurred and reprojected. The original study shows some irregularity of colloid uptake but is otherwise normal. In the deblurred and reprojected images these irregularities are enhanced, in part due to increased textured noise of the Bayesean method. While these irregularities are suggestive of abnormalities, the original images do not support such a diagnosis. In interpreting such processed studies, the physician must clearly raise his threshold for calling abnormalities. This threshold will depend on the unprocessed study. A lower count study is more likely to have such statistical non-uniformities in the image and such regions are more likely to be enhanced. The processed images must be viewed not as a replacement of the unprocessed images but as a supplement.

In Figure 4 is shown a patient with an enlarged liver. The processed images show definite irregularity in the tracer uptake. This is particularly apparent in the reprojected image. However there are no focal lesions. The unprocessed image also shows irregularity. The diagnosis in this case was hepatic parenchymal disease, a common condition for patients with an enlarged liver. It is known that such patients will have an irregular colloid distribution. The processed images allow better visualization of this irregularity.

An example of metastatic disease is shown in Figure 5. In this case the diagnosis from the unprocessed images only, was multiple metastatic lesions in both studies, with worsened disease in the later of the two scans. These findings are well appreciated in the processed images. The later deblurred image especially shows the increased size of the lesions.

While both deblurred and reprojected images provide useful information, in general the deblurred images are preferred for their higher resolution. The count density of liver-spleen images will in general support this higher resolution.

Tl-201 Perfusion Scintigraphy

In this department Bayesean deblurring has been used most extensively in Tl-201 imaging. All Tl-201 images are computer acquired in a 64x64 matrix and are deblurred and reprojected. Since the target to background ratio in Tl-201 imaging can be quite variable, depending on such factors as how well the patient exercised, we have found that the reprojected image is consistently more useful than the deblurred image, mostly for its noise reduction. At readout, the analog images are read first with a very low threshold for calling an abnormality. Suspicious areas are then examined on the reprojected images. This step is not to find additional abnormality, but to confirm the original diagnosis. If the processed images support the conclusions then the confidence of the diagnosis increases. Again the processed images are used as a supplement to the original images. Our experience suggests that reading the processed images alone can be confusing and may well lower observer performance. But with the processed images used in conjunction with the unprocessed images, the diagnostic process is significantly enhanced. In Figure 6 the unprocessed images suggest some reduced perfusion in the septal region. This diagnosis is confirmed in the reprojected images. Note the increased contrast between the interior of the ventricle and myocardium in the reprojected images. For patients who cannot exercise the drug Persantin is often used to simulate exercise by dilating the coronary arteries (9). Useful information about exercise and redistribution is obtained from such studies, but they often suffer from extremely high background. Clinicians have found processing to be very useful in interpreting the results of the studies. In Figure 7 this Persantin study has high background which makes interpretation difficult. The anterior view is particularly difficult, but the reprojected image aids in the conclusion that it is normal. Note the improvement in the LOA45 view. In order to show the effect of the algorithm we have not used any background subtraction in these images. Background subtraction would aid in the interpretation, but it must be emphasized that the image improvement which is observed with the algorithm is not duplicated merely by background subtraction.

Tomography

Another area where the Bayesean technique has shown to be useful
is in limited angle tomography using a rotating slant hole collimator.
It has already been shown that the precise depth of reconstruction
(i.e. the choice of PSF) does not strongly affect the action of the
algorithm. This depth independence suggests that the algorithm might
be used to enhance the projections prior to 3-D reconstruction. In
our slant-hole technique we acquire 6 views, with an angle of slant of
20°. Noise is always a problem in such reconstructions,and prior to
the introduction of this Bayesean algorithm our protocol had always
been to apply a 9-point smooth to the projections prior to reconstruction. We have replaced this 9-point smooth with the reprojection
to obtain the benefits of both noise-reduction and resolution enhancement. Examples of this are shown in Figures 8 and 9. Both studies
show improved resolution and contrast as compared to the conventional
processing. The abnormal study shows a large inferior wall defect
which is easily seen with both methods. In the 13.5 cm depth reconstruction, note the decreased activity probably due to the aortic
outflow tract, seen well in the reprojected images but not in the
images without deblurring.

Automatic Edge Detection

Unlike other areas of nuclear medicine, it is well accepted that
computer processing is essential for the analysis of gated blood-pool
studies. To improve patient throughput automatic determination of the
global volume curve is preferred. At our institution we use a cardiac
analysis package based on the work Verba et al (10). With our protocol we obtain 28 frames in the cardiac cycle and use the first 24 in
the analysis. Both spatial and temporal filtering is performed. The
phase image is used to determine the center of the left ventricle.
The outline of the LV is then determined by searching with an adaptive
second derivative algorithm along 48 rays emanating from LV center.
The boundary along the valve plane is determined primarily by the
phase image, and the free wall perimeter poses no particular problem,
but the perimeter along the septum between LV and RV is determined
only by spatial information. We find that in approximately 15% of

cases, in one or more frames the septum is missed and the edges extend
into the RV as seen in Figure 10. By replacing the spatial filtering
with deblurring and reprojection 75% of these missed edges are corrected as shown. The calculation of the volume curve requires the
subtraction of global background on a pixel by pixel basis. Since
deblurring is a non-linear process, this step would not be correct for
deblurred images. Instead for the calculation of the volume curve we
use the deblurred edges on unprocessed data which has been temporally
smoothed.

The reprojected images when temporally smoothed have also been
shown to be useful for cardiac cine. However, considering the number
of images involved in cardiac studies the computational expense of
deblurring and reprojection becomes heavy. To produce a reprojected
image requires three convolutions per image while the standard filtering requires only one. For this reason we use the Bayesean
algorithm for cardiac analysis only when edges along the septum
between LV and RV have failed. From experience we have determined
that Bayesean processing can do nothing about poor edges near the
valve plane.

DISCUSSION

The results presented here appear significantly better than those
found by Metz and Pizer (7,8). There are several possible explana-
tions for this. Our experience with the direct Bayesean algorithm is
that it was never satisfactory, especially after one iteration. The
amount of improvement didn't justify the effort. The jump to the more
successful modified method is difficult to make without the experience
of the weighted back-projection method derived for the HPGe camera.
The choice of a large convolution kernel in the denominator in biased
smearing meant the potential loss of low contrast objects which is not
a problem in the current formulation. Scintillation cameras are much
improved since biased smearing was completed. The reduction of
textured noise in modern cameras is quite significant considering the
noise propagation from Bayesean deblurring. Finally by raising the
weights to a power we have eliminated the need for any iterations.

A prime motivation for use of this algorithm in our department is

the teaching responsibility of the clinicians, since is often easier
to teach from the processed images. The goal is still to have the
students learn to read the unprocessed studies, but subtle features in
the original images are often better appreciated by students with the
aid of Bayesean processed images. This experience is similar to work
previously published by our department (11). In that study observer
performance for reading Tl-201 images with and without background
subtraction was compared. It was found that the inexperienced
observer found the background subtraction most helpful. We find that
inexperienced observers most appreciate the Bayesean images as an aid
for interpreting the unprocessed data.

CONCLUSION

Bayesean processing has been found to offer improvement in
contrast and resolution without a concomitant loss in signal/noise for
small area lesions. It is a useful supplement to the original images.
Its non-linear features make the interpretation of the Bayesean images
difficult without access to the unprocessed images.

But in conjunction with the original images we have found the
Bayesean images very useful, especially in Tl-201 imaging with high
background. The inexperienced observer appears to benefit most from
the processed images. Teaching is significantly enhanced. Excellent
results have also been obtained using the algorithm for preprocessing
of rotating slant-hole projections and for improved automatic edge
detection for gated blood pool studies.

The main disadvantage of the algorithm is that the deblurring
process requires 2 convolutions with another for the reprojection. As
such it does not qualify as a fast filter (2). While we have not
found this to be a problem for standard static images such as Tl-201
or liver-spleen studies, the increased time for processing 24 frame
gated blood pool images is quite bothersome and may well limit its
application.

ACKNOWLEDGEMENTS

This work is supported in part by USPHS Career Development Award
GM00493 from the NIGMS. The consultation of Drs. Michael Dae and
Barry Englestad is gratefully acknowledged.

REFERENCES

1. Rosenfeld A and Kak AC. Digital Picture Processing. Academic Press, 1982.
2. Todd-Pokropek A and DiPaola R. The Use of Computers for Image Processing in Nuclear Medicine. IEEE Transactions on Nuclear Science NS-29:1299, 1982.
3. Ortendahl DA, Shosa DW, Kaufman L, et al. Resolution and Contrast Recovery at Depth in Planar Nuclear Images. Phys Med Biol 27: 257, 1982.
4. Kaufman L, et al. Imaging Characteristics of a Small Germanium Camera. Investigative Radiology 13:33 1978.
5. Lim CB, Cheng A, Boyd DP and Hattner RS. Stationary Planar Positron Cameras. IEEE Transactions on Nuclear Science NS-25: 196, 1978.
6. Williams S, Cheng AS, Kaufman L and Shosa DW. Elimination of Loss of Resolution at Depth in Single-Photon Nuclear Images. IEEE Transactions on Nuclear Science NS-25:590, 1979.
7. Metz CE and Pizer SM. Nonstationary and Nonlinear Scintigram Processing. Proceedings 2nd International Conference on Data Handling and Image Processing in Scintigraphy, Hanover, West Germany, 1971.
8. Pizer SM, Correia JA, Chesler DA, Metz CE. Results of Nonlinear and Nonstationary Image Processing. Proceedings 3rd International Conference on Data Handling and Image Processing in Scintigraphy. Cambridge, Massachusetts, 1973.
9. Leppo JJ, et al. Serial Tl-201 Myocardial Imaging after Dipyridamole Infusion: Diagnostic Utility in Detecting Coronary Stenoses and Relationship to Regional Wall Motion. Circulation 66:649, 1982.
10. Verba JW, et al. Onset of Mechanical Systole Derived from Gated Radionuclide Techniques and Displayed in Cine Format. J Nucl Med 20:625, 1979.
11. Massie B, et al. Contrast Enhancement of Thallium-201 Myocardial Scintigrams: Improved sensitivity with diminished Specificity in Coronary Disease Detection. American Heart Journal 102:37, 1981.

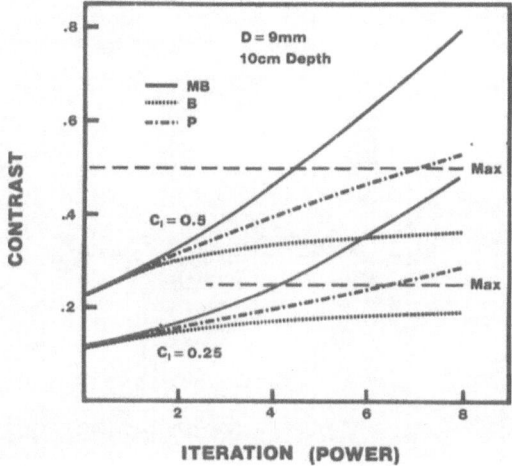

FIGURE 1. Output contrast as a function of iteration or power for cold lesions of 0.5 and 0.25 input contrast obtained with the HPGe camera. MB refers to modified Bayesean, B to direct Bayesean and P to the power method.

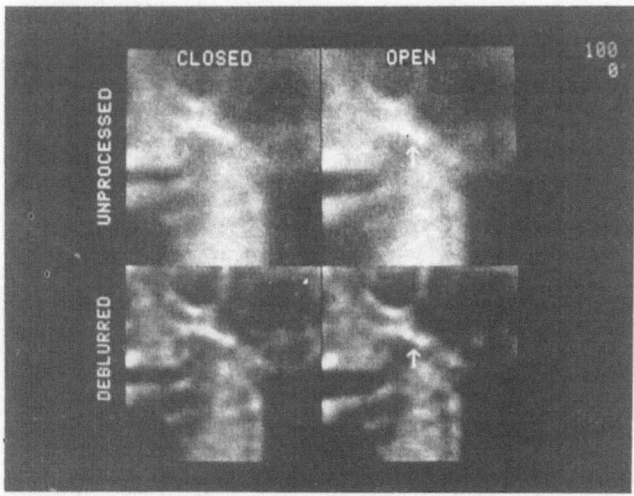

FIGURE 2. Lateral views of a TMJ patient using Tc-99m MDP. The arrow points to the separation of activity between condyle and socket with jaw open.

404

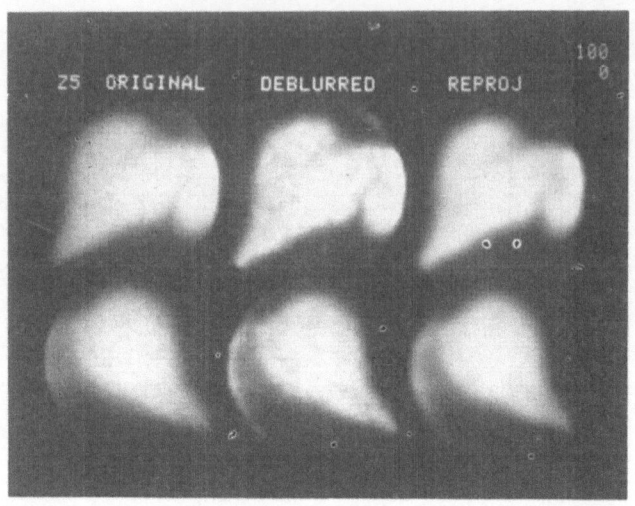

FIGURE 3. Anterior and lateral views of a patient with a normal liver
scan. There is some increase in textured noise in the processed
views.

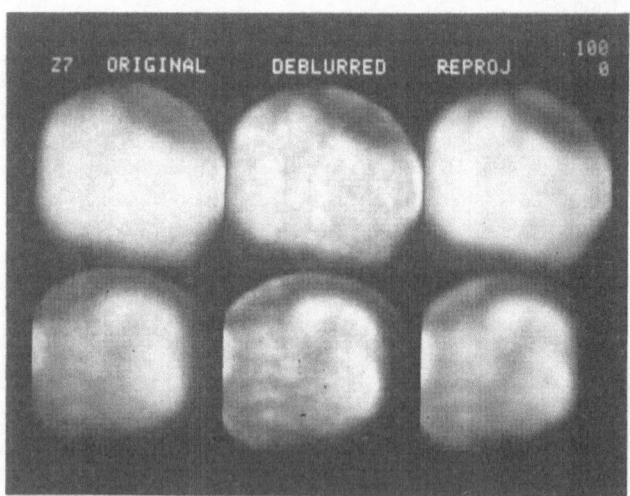

FIGURE 4. Patient with hepatic parenchymal disease. The irregularity
of the colloid labelling is better appreciated in the processed
studies.

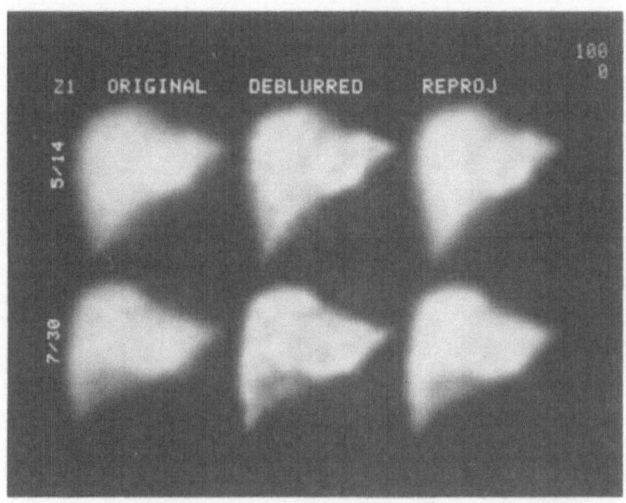

FIGURE 5. Scans two months apart of a patient with metastatic disease. The later scan (bottom) shows worsened disease, clearly apparent with the processed images.

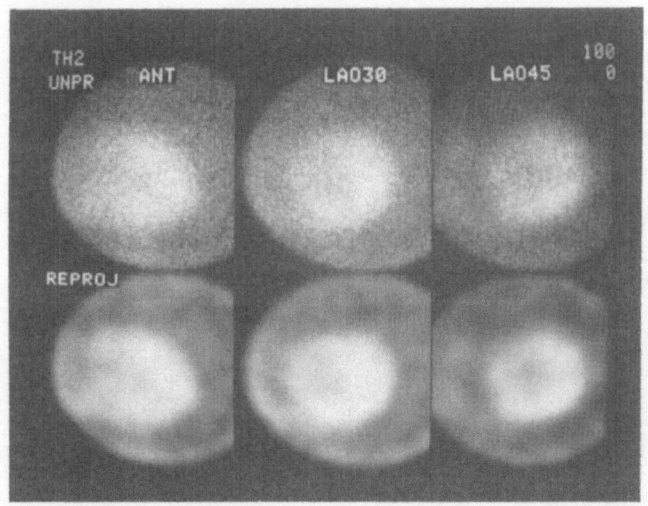

FIGURE 6. Tl-201 exercise study showing reduced perfusion of the septal region. The reprojected images confirm the diagnosis.

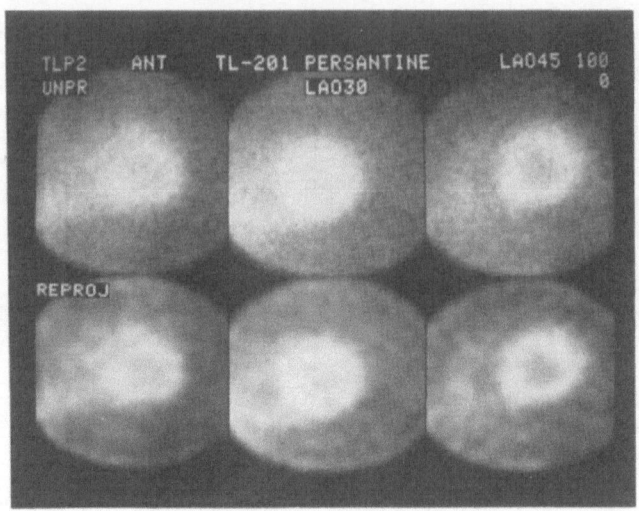

FIGURE 7. Tl-201 Persantin study to simulate exercise. With the relatively high background the reprojected images aid in the diagnosis of a normal study.

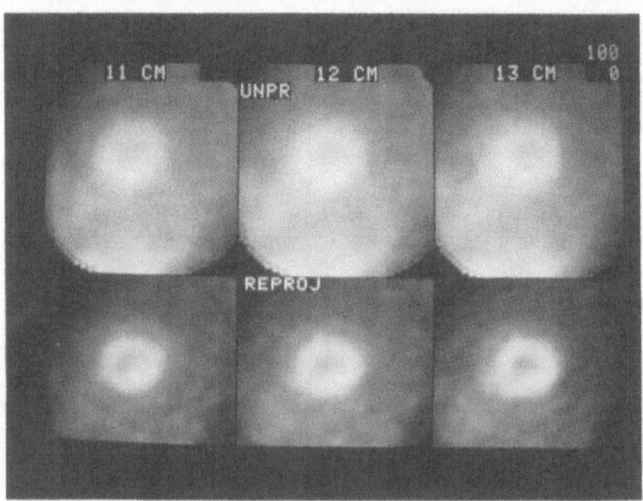

FIGURE 8. Normal Tl-201 rotating slant hole tomograms of the heart with and without deblurring and reprojecting of the six planar projections. Increased contrast is seen with the reprojected images. Depths of reconstruction are indicated. A 9-point smooth of the projections is used for the images labeled unprocessed.

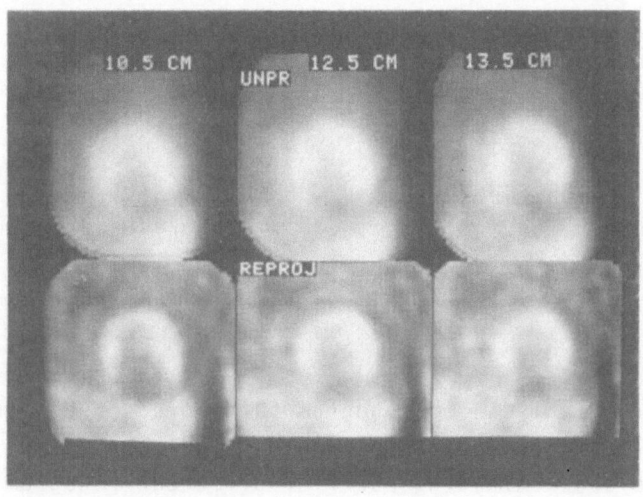

FIGURE 9. Tl-201 rotating slant hole tomograms of a patient with a large inferior wall defect. At the 13.5 cm depth the Bayesean processed images allow visualization of the aortic outflow tract not appreciated in the unprocessed images.

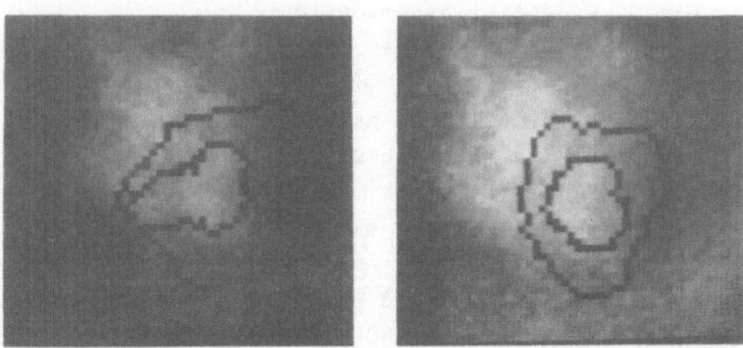

FIGURE 10. Application of Bayesean deblurring to automatic edge detection. (Left) Edges obtained with the standard spatial processing algorithm extend into the RV. (Right) Using the Bayesean reprojection for the spatial processing the edges are confined to the LV.

DISCRIMINANT ANALYSIS OF EXERCISE RENOGRAMS

PETER SCHMIDLIN and JOHN H. CLORIUS
Institute of Nuclear Medicine, German Cancer Research Center,
Heidelberg

ABSTRACT
A quantitative analysis of renogram pattern observed in hypertensive patients during standing and exercise was performed. The discriminating power of different renogram variables was evaluated.

INTRODUCTION
Many hypertensive patients have normal renograms when examined in prone position. These patients are often finally diagnosed as having essential hypertension.

About 20% of all hypertensives have massive bilateral disturbence of intrarenal hippurate transport when examined in standing position. This finding has been called Bilateral Orthostatic Renal Dysfunction (BORD) (1).

About 50% show a similar bilateral hippurate transport disturbence when examined during exercise (Bilateral Exercise Renal Dysfunction, BERD) (2).

To date, all BORD patients showed BERD too, and normotensive patient showed neither BERD nor BORD.

Standing and exercise renography demonstrate existence of transient bilateral tubular dysfunction in many patients with hypertension.

The renogram deformation due to BORD and BERD is easily recognizable by curve inspection (Fig.1). The scintiphotos also demonstrate a typical image sequence. This study presents a quantitative analysis of the data with the following aim:

1. Curve and photo inspection are subjective procedures. Psychological moments can lead to misinterpretations or mis-classifications of the findings. A quantitative analysis proves the objectivity of the decisions of the interpreting physician.
2. It can be shown which variables extracted from the reno-grams are most sensitive to the changes observed in BORD and BERD. This may lead to a simplification of the examination and evaluation procedure in hypertensive patients.
The procedures reported in the following help to assess the discriminating power of variables, i.e. the diagnostic value of evaluations. Their use is independent from the actual problem of BORD or BERD.

MEASUREMENT AND EVALUATION OF RENOGRAMS
The analysis was performed using renogram data of patients reported in the previous study (2). Only patients with com-plete magnetic tape data were used. 42 hypertensives and 12 normotensive controls were included in the study.
Tab. 1 shows the frequency of abnormalities in patients and controls. 9 patients showed BORD, and 23 showed BERD as well as BORD.
All patients and controls had three examinations: prone, standing, and during exercise on a bicycle ergometer.
Tab. 2 shows the variables used for the analysis. They par-tially have been described previously (3). 6 Variables were extracted from each renogram. Alltogether 36 variables were calculated for each patient.

DISCRIMINANT ANALYSIS
The 36 variables were used to evaluate strain sensitivity of renal function. The relative contribution of the variables to this assessment was different. Furthermore, many vari-ables were dependent on each other. A multivariate analysis helped to solve this problem. We used discriminant analysis for this purpose (4).
Discriminant analysis needs a basic set of 'objects' (which

are the patients in the actual case), for which a primary classification is known (which corresponds to the diagnoses). This classification (Tab. 3) was made by the physician using all available data (curve and scintiphoto inpection, renogram variables). The analysis consisted of a computer classification of the objects using all variables. The Mahalanobis distance of each object to the center of each class was calculated, and the object was assigned to the class with the smallest Mahalanobis distance. The Mahalanobis distance of the object ℓ from the centre of each group k is given by

$$d_{\ell k} = \sum_i \sum_j \left(x_{i\ell} - \bar{x}_{ik} \right) \left(\sigma^{-1} \right)_{ij} \left(x_{j\ell} - \bar{x}_{jk} \right)$$

σ is the pooled covariance matrix

$$\sigma_{ij} = \sum_k \sum_{\ell \in k} \left(x_{i\ell} - \bar{x}_{ik} \right) \left(x_{j\ell} - \bar{x}_{jk} \right)$$

where ℓ is a member of group k in the primary classification, and $\bar{x}_{ik}$ and $\bar{x}_{jk}$ are mean values of the variable i and j in group k.

The comparison of primary and computer classification allows conclusions about the quality of both classifications. In case both classifications are in agreement, it can be concluded that the primary classification was objective. In case of disagreement, either the primary classification was not objective, or it was done using criteria which were not expressed in the variables.

If the number of variables is greater than the number of objects, then the covariance matrix is always degenerate, and the calculation of distances is not possible.

If the number of variables is not much smaller than the number of objects, then correlations between variables can lead to a degenerate or quasi-degenerate covariance matrix, which gives meaningless distances. The problem of correlations and sample size is also discussed by Foley (5) and Cochran (6).

In case of degeneration, the analysis must be performed step by step, beginning with the best variables and terminating when the addition of variables fails to improve the result.

There are different ways to select the 'best' variable for each step. These methods also determine the discriminating power, i.e. the diagnostic value of the different variables. We have tested two methods of variable selection:

1. In each step the variable was included which gave the best improvement in the number of correct classified objects. Furthermore, variables were excluded when exclusion improved the classification results.

2. In each step the variable was included which revealed the most significant differences between the classes. The generalized Mahalanobis distance

$$V = \sum_k \sum_i \sum_j u_k \left(\bar{x}_{ik} - \bar{X}_i\right)\left(\sigma^{-1}\right)_{ij}\left(\bar{x}_{jk} - \bar{X}_j\right)$$

with the common means

$$\bar{X}_i = \sum_k u_k \bar{x}_{ik} \Big/ \sum_k u_k$$

was used as criterion of significance (7).

The assignment of patients to different classes according to the values of different variables is a procedure of computer diagnosis. If the covariance matrix is quasi-degenerate because of too many or correlated variables, then the classification procedure yields a perfect classification which however is meaningless for the following reason. An object which does not belong to the basic population may be classified with the same covariance matrix as the basic population. In a nondegenerate case this would lead to a correct classification with the same probability as for the basic population. A degenerate covariance matrix would classify the objects of the basic population, but missclassify the test object.

In the actual study the basic population was small.   It   was
therefore   necessary   to demonstrate the discriminating power
of the variables with a test collective. A test   collective
can   be   simulated using the leaving-one-out method (8).   The
classification of each patient   uses   the   covariance   matrix
calculated from   the   variables of all other patients. This
means a recalculation of the covariance matrix for each patient.   As long as the number of variables and patients is not
excessive, this job is performed in several seconds (VAX11).

RESULTS

The computer classification of the patients of the four groups   is   shown in Tab.   4. All 36 variables were used in the
step-by-step procedure. The significance criterion was   used
for   variable   selection,   and the leaving-one-out method for
classification. The diagonal of the matrix shows the numbers
of patients in each group, for which the computer classification agreed with the physicians classification.   The   table
shows   good   agreement with respect to the statement that the
renal abnormalities exist (last two rows and columns) or   do
not exist (first two rows and columns). There were only four
cases where physician and computer disagreed with respect to
the   existence of abnormalities. Another result is that the
computer was unable to distinguish between controls   and   hypertensives with normal function. This means that the hypertensives with normal function had similar pattern as a   healthy control group.

Tab. 5 shows the results of the step-by-step procedure for
the   two   methods   of variable selection (best classification
and highest significance). For the first variables used, the
classification of the basic population was better when the
best-classification method was   used.   When   more   variables
were   added,   this advantage vanished and, in some cases, was
inverted in favour of the significance method. The superior-
ity of the significance method shows up more clearly in the
results of the leaving-one-out method (31 correct   classified

by best-classification method versus 36 correct classified by highest-significance method). The most powerful variables were the relative amplitudes at 10 and 20 min, in both selection methods.

The similarity of controls and hypertensives without dysfunction suggests that these patients be placed into one group. For this three-group analysis, the highest-significance selection procedure yields 54 correct classified in the basic population and 45 in the leaving-one-out test population, using 11 variables.

The question of existence of dysfunction is answered by placing BERD and BORD patients into one group. This two-group analysis is shown in Tab. 6. The results are comparable with Tab. 4. The relative amplitude at 10 min, observed during exercise, is the strongest variable.

The observed renal dysfunction is a bilateral effect. Therefore the analysis was repeated combining the values of both left and right kidney. This cancels effects of asymmetric renal function or nephroptosis. The results of the analysis with 18 variables are shown in Tab. 7. The variables were selected by the highest-significance procedure. The poor classification rate for the four groups is again due to the similarity of controls and hypertensives with normal function. The sequence of variables shows the importance of the relative amplitude measured at 10 min during exercise. 47 cases can be diagnosed correctly as dysfunction absent or present using the 10min/3min quotient during exercise only.

Finally, the different beheaviour of hypertensives and controls can be verified by combining all 42 hypertensives to one group and testing them vs. the 12 controls. Tab. 8 shows the probabilities for rejection of the null hypothesis obtained with one variable only.

DISCUSSION

The results verify the existence of BORD and BERD in hypertensive patients and the lack of this pattern in normals as well as in part of the hypertensives. Physician and computer

agree in most cases with respect to the existence of the re-
nographic pattern. The instances of disagreement may result
from delayed excretion from the renal pelvis which is not
identified by the computer.

A 10 is the variable with the highest discriminating power for
the BERD resp. BORD renogram pattern. The variables correlated with A 10 (i.e. A 20, T 1) could replace A 10, but with
lower discriminating power. The variable selection procedures help to determine which of closely correlated variables
give the best diagnostic results.

The amplitude relation A 10 in prone position does not contribute to the classification. This is somewhat misleading. In
fact, if more patients with abnormal renograms in prone position would be included in the study, then the variables in
prone position would be needed for decision making.

Discriminant analysis assumes gaussian distributed variables
with equal variances in each group. Quantitative criteria
for normal distribution of the variables cannot be applied
because of the small number of patients. This problem has to
be treated in the future with larger populations. Some patients have values very different of the mean values of their
group. These data seem to disturb the classification procedure. An analysis was performed omitting such run-away data.
The result was not improved, because all distances get smaller, and other patient's data take over the role of run-away
data.

Finally, it should be mentioned that the actual problem really uses continuous data. There is an infinite number of renogram pattern between 'BORD' and 'normal'. This makes a
perfect agreement of different classification procedures unlikely.

Quantitative assessment of variables and methods is frequently needed. The procedures described in this paper are proposed as a possible solution of the problem.

REFERENCES
(1) J.H.Clorius, P.Schmidlin, E. Raptou, W.Huber, P.Georgi,

Hypertension associated with massive, bilateral, posture-
dependent renal dysfunction. Radiology 140,231-235(1981)

(2) J.H.Clorius, P.Schmidlin, The exercise renogram. A new
approach documents renal involvment in systemic hypertension. J.Nucl.Med. 24,104-109(1983)
(3) P.Schmidlin, J.Clorius, Validation of numerical parameters extracted from renograms. VIIth Int.Conf.
Information Processing in Medical Imaging, Stanford,
June 22-26 1981
(4) D.F.Morrison, Multivariate Statistical Methods.
McGraw-Hill 1976
(5) D.H.Foley, Considerations of sample and feature size.
IEEE Trans. Information Theory 18,618-626(1972)
(6) W.G.Cochran, On the performance of the linear discriminant function. Technometrics 6,179-190(1964)
(7) T.W.Anderson, Introduction to Multivariate Statistical
Analysis. John Wiley Sons, 1958
(8) P.A.Lachenbruch, Discriminant Analysis. Hafner Press 1975

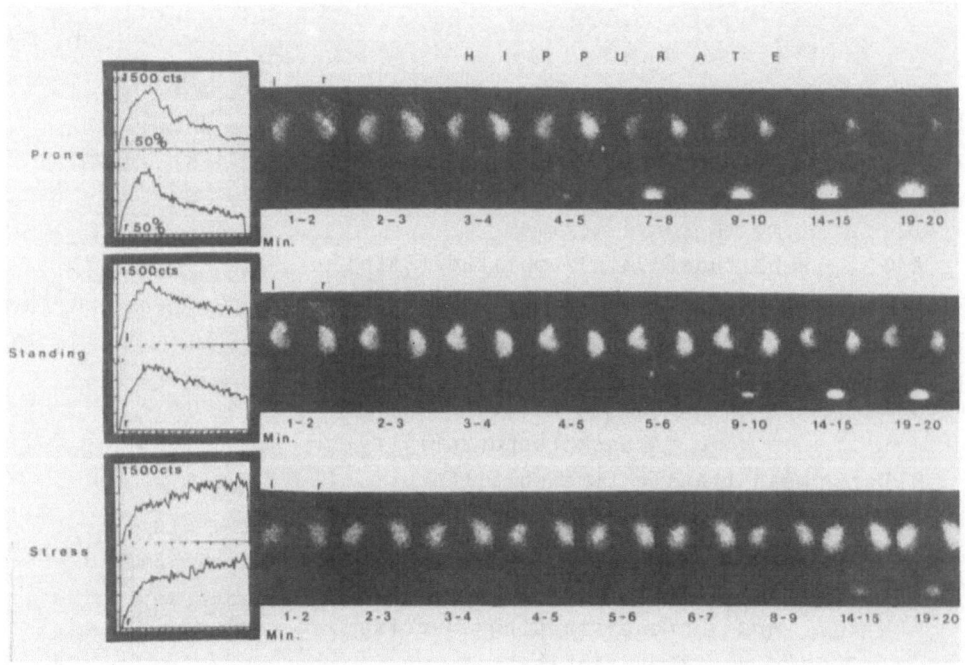

Fig. 1. Renography of a hypertensive patient inprone and
standing position and during exercise.

Tab. 1. Frequency of BERD and BORD in 54 patients

	Examined	Disturbed parench. hippurate transp.		
		prone	standing	exercise
Hypertensives	42	0	9	23
Controls	12	0	0	0
Total	54			

Tab. 2. Variables extracted form renograms

T1	time to curve maximum
A10	amplitude(10min)/amplitude(3min)
A20	amplitude(20min)/amplitude(3min)
AQT	secretion index in relation to background activity
SQT	secretion sum in relation to background activity
MTT	mean transit time obtained by deconvolution analysis

```
all variables    left/right
         and     prone/standing/exercise
           =     36 variables
```

Tab 3. Primary classification for
        discriminant analysis

Group	Description	Number of patients
1	Controls	12
2	HT, normal renogram	19
3	HT, BERD, no BORD	14
4	HT, BORD	9
	Total	54

Tab. 4. Classification table

54 patients
4 groups
15 variables selected from 36
by highest significance
Leaving-one-out

group	assigned to group			
	1	2	3	4
1	9	3	0	0
2	8	9	0	2
3	0	2	9	3
4	0	0	0	9

36 correct classified

Tab. 5. Step-by-step procedure

54 patients
4 groups
Variables selected from 36 variables
by best-classification and highest
significance

No	best-classification Variable	Correct	highest significance Variable	Correct
1	A20 ex l	31	A 10 ex l	24
2	A 10 st l	36	A20 ex l	33
3	T 1 ex l	38	MTT pr l	33
4	A20 st l	41	SQT pr r	34
5	A 10 ex r	42	MTT ex r	41
6	MTT st l	45	MTT ex l	43
7	MTT pr l	47	T 1 pr r	42
8	AQT ex r	47	T 1 ex l	46
9	A20 st r	49	A 10 ex r	46
10	SQT ex r	49	A20 st r	48
11	T 1 ex r	49	SQT pr l	49
12	A20 ex r	49	A20 pr r	49
13	MTT st r	50	MTT pr r	49
14	T 1 st l	51	A20 st l	48
15	MTT ex r	51	A 10 st l	50

Leaving-one-out:

| 15 | 31 | 36 |

Tab. 6. Existence of renal dysfunction

54 patients
2 groups

	best classif.	highest sign.
5 variables used:		
Basic	53	52
Leaving-one-out	50	51 Ⓧ
12 variables used:		
Basic	54	54
Leaving-one-out	44	50

Classification table for Ⓧ :

		assigned to group	
		1	2
Group	1	30	1
	2	2	21

Tab. 7. Sum of left and right kidney

54 patients
Variables selected from 18 variables (left+right added)
highest-significance selection

	4 groups	3 groups 1+2,3,4	2 groups 1+2,3+4		
Sequence of variables	A 10 ex A20 st T 1 pr SQT pr SQT ex	A 10 ex A 10 st A 10 pr SQT st	A 10 ex A 10 pr SQT st T 1 ex	A 10 ex A 10 pr	A 10 ex
Correct class. in basic set	38	45	51	50	47
Correct class. leaving-one-out	32	43	47	50	47

Tab. 8. Test of hypertensives vs. controls

Probability for rejection of null hypothesis

Variable	prone		standing		exercise	
	V	p(%)	V	p(%)	V	p(%)
A 10	.4	~50	5.4	>95	11.4	>99.9
A20	2.3	<90	7.0	>95	13.6	>99.9

V = Generalized Mahalanobis Distance

A STOCHASTIC INTERPRETATION OF THALLIUM MYOCARDIAL PERFUSION SCINTIGRAPHY

Michael L. Goris, Elaine Gordon and D. Kim

ABSTRACT

A method is presented for the quantitative interpretation of Thallium-201 myocardial perfusion studies. The data are planar images collected immediately following the stress injection, and four to six hours later. Data analysis consists of preprocessing, including thresholding of the original data, and data reduction using a variant of the circumferential profile methods.

The profiles are subdivided into segments, and for each segment the difference between the norm and the actual data is computed. This difference is a quantitative symptom, whose size is assumed to be related to the probability of having the disease.

The relationship between the size of the symptom in each of nine segments (three segments/view in three views) and the probability of disease is expressed in a table in which for 30 diseases (combinations of vascular lesions), the sensitivity is described as a Gaussian function whose average and standard deviation is computed from previous validated cases.

Using an arbitrary prevalence, the post testing probability can then be computed using Bayes' formula sequentially. The sensitivities, however, are not expressed as a binary function of the presence or absence of a symptom, but as a distribution function defined by experience.

The method assumes independence of symptoms, which cannot be disproven on the basis of the data available, and relies on the central limit theorem to assume a Gaussian distribution function.

The results are close to the reported results in other methods, but tend to be clustered around extreme probability values, suggesting some symptom interdependence.

INTRODUCTION

The visual interpretation of Thallium myocardial perfusion scintigraphy assumes that the observer decides whether the images at hand differ
significantly from the "expected normal" image, or from an actual reference image appropriate to the case. Since Thallium myocardial scintigraphies have generally low contrast (target/background ratio), various
preprocessing methods have been suggested, either to increase the sensitivity of the study, or to enhance reproducibility (1,2). In early
attempts to objectively evaluate the perceived difference, either fixed
but discrete scaling (3) or area count integration methods (4) have been
described.

The normative evaluation of Thallium myocardial scintigraphies reached
its most advanced format with the various circumferential profile methods.
In the circumferential profile methods the scintigraphic data are reduced
to a set of sampling values in a sampling profile. Each sampling value
represents a characteristic of the image at a certain angle relative to a
coordinate system centered in the center of the heart's cavity (5,6.7).

This approach is in reality based on a polar transformation of the
originally Cartesian coordinate system. If the number of sampled angles
is independent of the data (5,7), the transformation results in an implicit
size normalization. Alternatively, if the number of angles is adapted
to the number of data points along the outside edge of the left ventricular
myocardial area, a size normalization is required explicitly before the
normative evaluation (6).

The result of the polar transformation and the sampling is the
reduction of the image data to a string of values (sampling profile)
which can be compared from case to case, without size of positional
registration problems. Additionally, a set of control cases (verified
normal cases) can be used to produce a "standard profile", which for each
angle defines an expectation value and its variation. The normative
comparison consists of deciding which points of the profile in the case
at hand differ "significantly" from the expected value. Significance in
this case is strictly based on the difference betweeen observed value and
expected value, normalized to the standard deviation (of normal) at that
point. For the diagnostic comparison an arbitrary or optimal limit can
be set to determine clinical significance (i.e., the demonstration of
disease), although for that diagnostic purpose other criteria (e.g., the
number of neighboring points affected) are usually included (7).

Typically, however, the diagnostic criteria are based on a binary limit separating normal from abnormal, and neither the size (depth or width) nor the number and relative position of abnormalities are explicitly used.

In this paper we investigate the possibility of adding a diagnostic step to the normative quantitation, by considering abnormalities in nine regions separately and sequentially, assuming that the specificity increases when the degree of the abnormality increases. We intend to demonstrate that no loss in absolute discrimination (between normal and abnormal) results, but that the method allows one to gauge the confidence of each interpretation. It appears, however, that uncertainty remains even in extreme cases, and an explanation for the phenomenon will be suggested.

MATERIALS AND METHODS

Patient population:

Ninety-seven patients referred to the Division of Nuclear Medicine for an exercise Thallium study are included in this study. Criteria for inclusion are the availability of the results of a coronary arteriogram performed within two months of the scintigraphic study. Patients whose effort on the treadmill was insufficient are not included if the coronary arteriogram was normal, since understressing would favor the classification in a normal group. An acceptable treadmill test ends either with the patient reaching 85% of maximum predicted heart rate, the appearance of ST segment depressions on the ECG, or significant arrhythmias. Twenty-nine patients had reportedly a normal coronary arteriogram, with no vessel showing a constriction of more than 49%. Of those 29, 12 were used to define the normal profiles.

Thallium study:

Ninety seconds prior to the termination of a treadmill test the patient receives an intravenous dose of 1.5 to 2.0 milliCuries of T1-201 CL2. Imaging starts 5 minutes after the injection. Three projections are used: a 45° Left Anterior Oblique view (45 LAO), an Anterior view (ANT), and a 65° LAO view. Imaging is performed in preset time and counts, imaging being terminated after 10 minutes or 600 K counts.

Imaging is performed on a standard scintillation camera, using a converging collimator. The settings are optimized for the 80 kev emissions. The data are collected as 64 square digitized images and stored on a digital computer. The acquisition is repeated 4 to 6 hours after the injection. The data consist therefore of a three view exercise study and a three view delayed study.

Data processing:

Preprocessing consists of a filtering operation in the object domain and interpolative background subtraction (1). The operator identifies the center of the left ventricle and the apex.

Circumferential sampling is performed following an explicit polar transformation of the image from $IA(K,L)$ to $IB(I,J)$, where K and L are the Cartesian coordinates and I the distance from the origin, J the angle. The origin is defined by the identified center, and the zero angle is directed towards the apex. For a 64 x 64 image, the transform uses 256 angles over 360 degrees. It can be shown that this is the minimum required to avoid undersmapling at 32 picture elements of the center (8).

Following this transformation, radial sampling is reduced to sampling along I in $IB(I,J)$. Three values are sampled along I: the maximal pixel value (Max), the sum of pixel values (Int) and the average pixel value (Mean). Processing results therefore in three "profiles" for each view, and each profile is normalized to its maximum value. In each profile three segments are defined: the first segment covers the values from 1 to 32 and from 225 to 256, and represents the apical segment. The second covers the values from 33 to 128, and corresponds to the antero-septal and septal segments in the oblique views and the inferior segment in the anterior view. The third covers values 129 to 224 and corresponds to the posterior wall (45 LAO), postero-inferior (65 LAO) or antero-lateral (ANT) wall.

The standard population profile is computed separately for each sampling value. The data are exercise data obtained from patients (in contradistinction to normal volunteers) who had a negative coronary arteriogram. The normal profiles are stored as sums and sum of squares for each value but used after a conversion to average and standard deviations for each sampling value, at each angle and for all views.

The normative comparison is based on the integration of the differences $(D(J))$ between the test case and the reference profile in each of the nine segments for each of the three sampling values. The reference profile is either the normal population profile or the patient's own redistribution image profile (delayed imaging). The differences are expressed as fractions of the local standard deviation of the normal profile values:

$$D(J) = \sum_{K=1}^{K=3} (R(K,J)-T(K,J))/SD(K,J)$$

where $R(K,J)$ is the reference profile value, $T(K,J)$ the test case sample value and $SD(K,J)$ the standard deviation value of the normal population profile, all at angle J for sampling value K. Each symptom consists of the integration (summation) of the values $D(J)$ in the appropriate segments.

The diagnostic comparison uses Bayes' theorem with distribution functions for the sensitivity of each symptom for each "disease". In this approach diseases are defined as a particular combination of coronary lesions: The coronary tree is schematized to two parallel branching systems, with the main left (ML) branching into the left anterior descending (LAD) and the left circumflex (LCX). Those two vessels, and the right coronary artery (RCA) are further assumed to be branching in two major subdivision. Lesions can be either minor ($50\% < x < 75\%$) or major ($75\% < x < 100\%$). If two dependent branches contain a given lesion, the lesion is assumed to affect the proximal trunk: if only one of the branches is affected, the lesion is reported as one grade lower in the proximal branch. The final diseases are defined in terms of ML, LAD, LCX, RCA. If one includes one disease for normal, the total becomes 30, as shown in Table 1.

A data file is constructed from angiographically verified cases, in which for each disease the sum, sum of squares and number of cases are recorded for each symptom. From this table one can therefore compute the distribution function $H(S(I,L))$ which is the Gaussian distribution of the value of the symptom in segment I for all recorded cases of disease L.

The prevalence of the diseases is arbitrarily set at 50% for all diseases. Furthermore, it is assumed that all coronary lesions have equal likelihood, and the likelihood of a particular disease is derived by computing the probabilities of all lesion combinations which would lead to that disease.

The post-testing or conditional probability of disease L is then computed according to the following expression of Bayes' theorem:

$$P(D(L)/S(I,L),I=1,9) = \frac{P(D(LL)). \displaystyle\prod_{I=1}^{I=9} P(Ha(I,L)/D(L))}{\displaystyle\sum_{K=1}^{K=30} P(d(k)) \prod_{I=1}^{I=9} P(Hx(I,K)/D(K))}$$

where $P(D(L)/S(I,L),I=1,9)$ represents the post-testing probability of disease L, for symptom values $S(I,L)$ for all symptoms; $P(D(L))$ represents the prevalence of disease $D(L)$, and $P(Hx(I,K)/D(K))$ the sensitivity of symptom I for disease K when the value of the symptom = x.

Analysis

For the purpose of this report the method is applied separately (and not sequentially in the Bayesian sense) to each comparison: exercise versus normal population and exercise versus redistribution.

The efficacy of the method is analyzed by using a displacement factor F which is the post-testing probability of being normal divided by the pre-testing probability. Since the prevalence is 50%, this ratio can vary from 0 to 2, with values lower than 1.00 when the analysis favors an abnormal diagnosis.

RESULTS AND DISCUSSION

Table 1 shows the average symptom values and standard deviations for all diseases, in the comparison between the exercise study and the normal population profile. Note that when a particular disease has not been recorded at least five times, the values are the average values for "any or all diseases".

The results of the analysis are presented in Tables 2 and 3: The pertinent observations are the following:

The F values tend to cluster around extreme values (0 or 2). This could be a reflection of the population, if the cases tended to be well differentiated, but is more likely to be due to lack of independence of the symptoms. It is true that the results shown in Table 1 do not support a strong symptom interdependence, but neither do they exclude it. The effect of interdependence is easily understood by assuming the extreme case: If the interdependence (or correlation) is absolute, the observation of two symptoms does not contribute more than the observation of one. In that case, the formulation of Bayes' theorem used in our approach would effectively be equivalent to using the same observation nine times.

The sensitivity of the method is high for LAD and main left domain lesions but low for isolated RCA or LCX, in the small sample available. This is partially explained by the fact that the analysis excludes the observation of right ventricular abnormalities and that the projectional images do not permit isolating LCX from RCA domains effectively. Indeed, the latter explanation is supported by the high sensitivity of the LCX-RCA combination.

The lesser sensitivity of the comparison between exercise and delayed images could be explained by a failure to redistribute in the presence of very high grade stenosis. It should be noted that our analysis does not use absolute washout values (7), which could have improved our results.

In Table 2 the lesser sensitivity for minor disease supports the radiological hypothesis that the degree of stenosis can be used to predict the effect on flow. What is not clear, however, is the presence of two normal cases with extreme pathological F values.

Finally, inspection of Table 1 reveals that the effect of vascular lesions is not additive, and therefore supports the rationale to separate diseases into "combinations" of arterial lesions. The lack of additivity is easily explained by the relative nature of the analysis of Tl-201 myocardial perfusion studies.

REFERENCES

1. Goris ML, Daspit SG, McLaughlin P, and Kriss JP: Interpolative background subtraction. J Nucl Med 17: 744-747, 1976.
2. McLaughlin PR, Martin RP, Doherty P, Daspit SG, Goris ML, Haskell W, Lewis S, Kriss JP, and Harrison DC: Reproducibility of Thallium-201 myocardial imaging. Circulation 55: 497-503, 1977.
3. McKillop JH, Murray RG, Turner JG, Bessent RG: A comparison of visual and semiquantitative analysis of stress Thallium-201 myocardial images in patients with suspected ischemic heart disease. Radiology 136: 187-190, 1980.
4. Lenaerts A, Block P. van Thiel E, Lebedelle M, Becquevoort P, Erbsmann F, and Ermans AM: Segmental analysis of Tl-201 stress myocardial scintigraphy. J Nucl Med 18: 509-516, 1977.
5. Meade RC, Bamrah VS, Horgan JD, Ruetz PP, Kronenwetter C, and Yeh En-Lin: Quantitative methods in the evaluation of Thallium myocardial perfusion images. J Nucl Med 19: 1175-1178, 1978.

6. Burrow RD, Pond M, Schafer W, and Becker L: Circumferential profiles: A new method for computer analysis of Thallium-201 myocardial perfusion images. J Nucl Med 20: 771-777, 1979.
7. Garcia E, Maddahl J, Berman D, and Waxman A: Space/time quantitation of Thallium myocardial scintigraphy. J Nucl Med 22: 309-317, 1981.
8. Goris ML, Sue J and Johnson MA: A principled approach to the circumferential method for Thallium myocardial perfusion scintig-raphy quantitation. In: Non-invasive Assessment of the Cardio-vascular System. Ed. E.B. Diethrich, Littleton, MA: John Wright PSG Inc., pp 273-276, 1981.

Table 1. Average Values of the Symptom Distribution Functions.
(Comparison between stress study and average population profile.)

SEGMENT

NORMAL	199	50	58	85	74	207	23	22	25
RCA MAJOR	209	84	232	227	130	516	2	309	123
LAD MAJOR	1473	223	526	292	792	846	342	176	313
lad minor	323	252	147	309	255	561	157	301	146
lcx minor	30	155	53	82	455	301	5	213	75
RCA-LCX	700	417	1278	925	755	1831	299	719	563
ml-rca	929	362	884	358	533	1321	21	479	495
tvd minor	573	247	829	448	624	1408	276	441	476
All	718	195	495	280	523	881	188	326	304

Capital letters indicated major disease.

The table shows average values only if the disease has been recorded at least five times. Under "All" we tabulate the average for the distribution function of all non-normal cases recorded. In this case it represents the average of 83 cases.

The standard deviations are not shown but are comparatively very large, of the order of magnitude of the averages in all cases.

Table 2: Value of the Displacement Factor "F" as a Function of the Affected Vessel

Comparison of Stress Data to Population Average

		F Values			
		0.00-0.49	0.50-1.00	1.01-1.49	1.50-2.00
Disease:					
LAD	(21)	0.90 (19)	0.04 (1)	0.00 (0)	0.04 (1)
LCX	(4)	0.50 (2)	0.00 (0)	0.00 (0)	0.50 (2)
RCA	(12)	0.41 (5)	0.25 (3)	0.00 (0)	0.33 (4)
LCX-RCA	(5)	1.00 (5)	0.00 (0)	0.00 (0)	0.00 (0)
ML	(9)	0.88 (8)	0.00 (0)	0.00 (0)	0.12 (1)*
MAJOR	(51)	0.76 (39)	0.07 (4)	0.00 (0)	0.15 (8)
MINOR	(17)	0.64 (11)	0.11 (2)	0.00 (0)	0.23 (4)**
NORMAL	(29)	0.06 (2)	0.06 (2)	0.03 (1)	0.82 (24)

LAD   : significant lesion in left anterior descending
LCX   : significant lesion in left circumflex only
RCA   : significant lesion in right coronary artery only
LCX-RCA: significant lesion in RCA and LCX
ML   : significant lesion in main left artery or in LAD and LCX
MAJOR   : any lesion >75%
MINOR   : all coronary lesions are described as resulting in a luminal
          obstruction larger than 50% but less than 75%.

The values in parentheses are the number of patients. The results are expressed as probabilities or fractions P(S/D).

Notes: * : the comparison with the delayed study yielded F=0.51
         ** : in two of those cases the comparison with the delayed study
              yielded F-0.76 and 0.06, respectively.

If one chooses 1.00 as the binary limit, the sensitivity of major disease is 0.83, somewhat lower than reported in the literature.

Table 3. Value of the Displacement Factor "F" as a Function of the Affected Vessel

Comparison of Stress Study to Delayed Study

		F VALUES			
Vessel:		0.00-0.49	0.50-1.00	1.01-1.49	1.50-2.00
LAD	(19)	0.47 (9)	0.10 (2)	0.10 (2)	0.31 (3)
LCX	(3)	0.33 (1)	0.00 (0)	0.00 (0)	0.66 (2)
RCA	(10)	0.50 (5)	0.00 (0)	0.20 (2)	0.30 (3)
LCX-RCA	(5)	0.80 (4)	0.00 (0)	0.00 (0)	0.20 (1)
ML	(6)	0.33 (2)	0.16 (1)	0.16 (1)	0.33 (2)
MINOR	(17)	0.41 (7)	0.11 (2)	0.11 (2)	0.35 (6)
NORMAL	(24)	0.00 (0)	0.00 (0)	0.08 (2)	0.91 (22)

The symbols used are the same as in Table 1.

A NEW APPROACH FOR TESTING THE SIGNIFICANCE OF DIFFERENCES BETWEEN ROC CURVES
MEASURED FROM CORRELATED DATA

CHARLES E. METZ, PU-LAN WANG, AND HELEN B. KRONMAN
Department of Radiology and The Franklin McLean Memorial Research Institute,
The University of Chicago; Chicago, Illinois 60637, U.S.A.

1. INTRODUCTION

Receiver Operating Characteristic analysis is now generally recognized as
the most appropriate methodology for evaluating the diagnostic performance of
medical imaging procedures (1-7). ROC analysis has been used in the field of
psychophysics for three decades, and its theory and experimental methodology
have been developed in considerable detail (8-13). Perhaps surprisingly, the
statistical properties of ROC measures had received relatively little attention
until several years ago, when the limited size of practical data sets in medical applications indicated the need for careful study of this issue. Recent
progress in the statistical analysis of ROC data includes the work of Metz and
Kronman (14,15), who developed a bivariate test for the statistical significance of differences between ROC curves measured from independent data sets;
the work of Hanley and McNeil, who studied the statistical properties of the
area under an ROC curve and developed techniques to predict the number of
cases required to demonstrate the significance of differences between ROC
"Area Indexes" measured from either independent (16) or correlated (17) data
sets; and the work of Swets and Pickett (7), who identified three components
of variation in ROC measures and outlined a general statistical protocol for
testing the significance of differences in the Area Index.

In this paper we describe a new approach to the problem of testing the significance of differences between ROC curves measured from correlated data, and
we show how this approach can be used to perform three distinct statistical
tests. Further, we describe two digital computer programs that perform the
calculations required for the tests and that predict the number of images
required to demonstrate the significance of an actual difference.

2. A NEW "BIVARIATE BINORMAL" MODEL FOR CORRELATED CONFIDENCE-RATING DATA

2.1. The conventional binormal model

ROC curves are usually measured by requiring an observer to choose one of several ratings (1,4,7,12,18) to categorize his confidence that a specified "signal" is present in each of a series of images, some of which actually contain a signal and some of which contain only "noise" (i.e., variable background). The rating data are then used to calculate "maximum likelihood estimates" (19,20) of the parameters of a model that specifies the functional form of the ROC curve. Many functional forms have been proposed (13), but the "binormal" model has been used most widely in medical imaging. According to this model, which includes two adjustable parameters to describe the ROC curve, each curve is assumed to have the same functional form as that implied by two normal (i.e., Gaussian) "decision variable" distributions (1,4,6,12,13) with generally different means and standard deviations. Empirically, this functional form has been found to provide satisfactory fits to ROC data generated in a very broad variety of experiments, and it has the convenient property that all possible ROC curves are transformed into straight lines if they are plotted on "normal deviate" axes (6,12). The two adjustable parameters of the ROC curve can then be taken as the "y-intercept" and "slope" of the transformed ROC. These parameters ("a" and "b", respectively) can be interpreted in terms of an effective pair of underlying normal distributions* as (a) the distance between the means and (b) the standard deviation of the "noise only" distribution, with both expressed in units of the standard deviation of the the "signal present" distribution. By convention, the origin of the decision variable axis is taken as the mean of the "noise only" distribution, and -- perhaps confusingly -- the confidence-rating category boundaries on the decision axis (1,12,19,20), t_i, are expressed in units of the standard deviation of the "noise only" (rather than "signal present") distribution.

The probability that a "noise only" or "signal present" image yields the rating "i" is given by the integral of the appropriate probability density between the boundaries that define the corresponding category of confidence on

---

*A subtle and often misunderstood point requires clarification here. An ROC curve does not uniquely specify the underlying decision-variable distributions; in general, any monotonic transformation of a decision-variable axis yields different underlying distributions but the same ROC curve (9,13). Thus the "binormal" assumption concerns only the functional form of the ROC curve and not the form of the underlying distributions. Parameterization of the binormal ROC curve in terms of an effective pair of underlying normal distributions is simply a convenient convention.

the decision variable axis. Thus (19,20) the probability p_i of obtaining the rating "i" from a "noise only" image is given by $p_i = \Phi(t_i) - \Phi(t_{i-1})$, where Φ is the cumulative standard normal distribution function, and the probability π_i of obtaining the same rating from a "signal present" image is given by $\pi_i = \Phi(bt_i-a) - \Phi(bt_{i-1}-a)$. In these expressions the boundaries t_0 and t_I are taken to be $-\infty$ and $+\infty$, respectively, where I is the number of categories employed in the experiment.

A binormal ROC curve can be fit to a set of rating data by using the "Method of Scoring" (19,20,21) to calculate maximum likelihood estimates of the parameters "a", "b", and $\{t_i: i=1,\cdots,I-1\}$. A simple FORTRAN computer program for this calculation has been published (7). An important benefit of the "Method of Scoring" is that it provides not only maximum likelihood estimates of the desired ROC curve parameters "a" and "b", but also estimates of the sampling variance and covariance of those parameters. These quantities can be used to specify the precision of the estimated ROC curve and to test the significance of apparent differences between ROC curves estimated from independent data sets (14,15).

2.2 The new bivariate binormal model

2.2.1. Correlated rating data. Several common situations in medical image evaluation produce conditionally correlated rating data -- that is, pairs of ratings that are correlated even when ratings from "noise only" images or from "signal present" images are considered alone. For example, if two images of each patient in a clinical ROC experiment are made with different imaging systems, then the ratings from the two images of each patient will tend to agree, even when "noise only" or "signal present" images are considered alone, because any variation in the patient that is shared by the two images (such as lesion size, confusing background structure, etc.) will cause the two ratings to tend to vary together. Similarly, when a single set of images is displayed in two different ways (for example, in an ROC experiment to compare the lesion detectability obtained with different display or image processing methods), the two ratings of each image (from a given state of truth) will tend to agree due to the shared image data. In such situations, the probability of obtaining a particular pair of ratings "i" and "j" is not simply equal to the product of the (marginal) probabilities p_i and p_j or π_i and π_j, and some generalized model is required to describe the rating data.

This need is practically important in testing the significance of differences between ROC curves. The sampling variation shared by the paired ratings causes the two estimated ROC curves to tend to vary together (i.e., both tend to be a-typically "high" or atypically "low"). Thus, when rating data for the measurement of two ROC curves are correlated, a given difference between the measured curves should be interpreted as more significant than if the rating data were independent. Hence, to properly assess the significance of an apparent difference between two ROC curves measured from the same patient sample or the same image sample, the effect of curve covariance on the variance of the difference must be estimated and incorporated into the statistical test.

2.2.2. Bivariate normal densities for the decision variables and their implications for rating data. In the conventional binormal model, the decision variable x is assumed, in effect, to arise from one of two normal probability densities, $f(x|n)$ and $f(x|s)$, corresponding to "noise only" and "signal present" images. As mentioned above, the probability of some rating "i" from a "noise only" or "signal present" image, p_i or π_i respectively, is given by the integral of the corresponding density between the appropriate category boundaries on the decision variable axis. This point of view can be generalized to include two possibly correlated decision variables, x and y, which arise from one of two bivariate normal joint probability densities, $f(x,y|n)$ and $f(x,y|s)$. Each of these densities has generally different means and standard deviations in the x and y directions, and each is characterized by a generally different correlation coefficient, r_n and r_s. The probability of a pair of ratings, "i" and "j", from a "noise only" or "signal present" image, p_{ij} or π_{ij} respectively, is then given by the integral of the appropriate density inside a rectangular region of the decision variable [i.e., (x,y)] plane. Each rectangular region corresponding to a particular pair of ratings (i,j) is defined by the category boundaries t_{i-1} and t_i used on the x-axis (to categorize the decision variable x) and the boundaries u_{j-1} and u_j used on the y-axis (to categorize the decision variable y). This model is illustrated schematically in Figure 1, where the two ellipses represent isopleths of the two bivariate normal densities. The dashed vertical lines and the dotted horizontal lines represent the category boundaries $\{t_i\}$ and $\{u_j\}$ for 5-category rating data (for example) from the first (x) and second (y) observation, respectively. Arbitrarily, the mean of the "noise only" distribution is taken to be (0,0), and the marginal standard deviations of that distribution are taken to be unity in both the x and y directions.

436

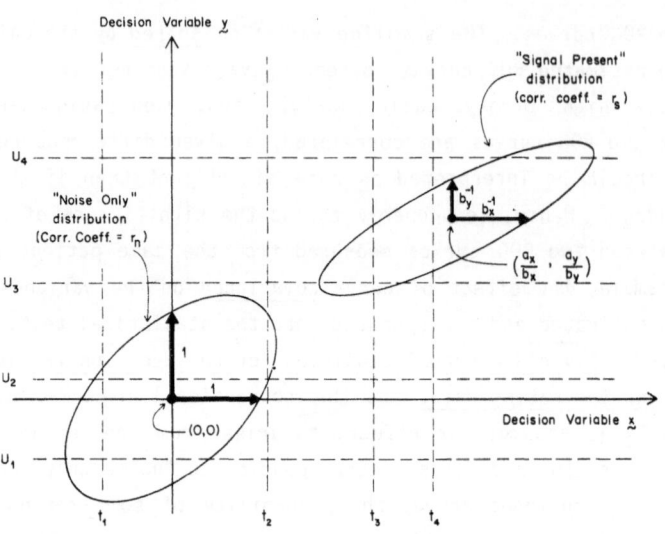

FIGURE 1. Schematic example of the new bivariate model.

This model reduces to the conventional binormal model for a single set of
rating data if either of the decision variables, $\underline{x}$ or $\underline{y}$, is considered alone.
Thus, for consistency with the conventional (univariate) binormal model, the
two coordinates of the mean of the bivariate "signal present" density are taken
to be (a_x/b_x) and (a_y/b_y), respectively, and the marginal standard deviations of
that density in the x and y directions are taken to be $(1/b_x)$ and $(1/b_y)$, where
(a_x,b_x) and (a_y,b_y) are the pairs of parameters that describe the ROC curves
obtained when the first or second observation of each patient or image is
considered alone. These relationships imply that the probability of the rating
pair "i" and "j" from a "noise only" patient or image pair is given by:

$$p_{ij} = L(t_i, u_j, r_n) + L(t_{i-1}, u_{j-1}, r_n) - L(t_{i-1}, u_j, r_n) - L(t_i, u_{j-1}, r_n)$$

where (22):

$$L(x, y, r) = \int_X^\infty dv \int_y^\infty g(v, w, r) \, dw$$

in which

$$g(x, y, r) = [\, 2_\pi \sqrt{1-r^2} \,]^{-1} \quad \exp - [(x^2-2rxy+y^2)/2(1-r^2)]$$

is the standard bivariate normal density. Similarly, the probability of the same rating pair from a "signal present" patient or image pair is given by

$$\pi_{ij} = L(b_x t_j - a_x, b_y u_j - a_y, r_s) + L(b_x t_{j-1} - a_x, b_y u_{j-1} - a_y, r_s)$$
$$-L(b_x t_{j-1} - a_y, b_y u_j - a_y, r_s) - L(b_x t_j - a_x, b_y u_{j-1} - a_y, r_s).$$

2.3.3. Maximum likelihood estimation of parameters. The Method of Scoring (21) can be used to design an algorithm for maximum likelihood estimation of the parameters of the bivariate binormal model described above. With paired rating data in I and J categories, respectively, this model involves (I+J+4) adjustable parameters, or 14 parameters for the conventional situation where I=J=5. A FOR-TRAN computer program for estimation of these parameters ("CORROC") is sketched in Section 4.1 below. It yields, as by-products, estimates of the sampling variance and covariance of the parameter estimates, which can be used to test the significance of differences between the ROC curves estimated from the correlated data, as described next. We mention parenthetically that estimates of the decision-variable correlation coefficients r_n and r_s (which are produced by the program but are not needed for testing differences between the ROC curves) can be used to investigate optimal diagnostic strategies, since they quantify the extent to which two diagnostic tests "x" and "y" yield complementary or redundant information.

3. STATISTICAL TESTS FOR DIFFERENCES BETWEEN ROC CURVES

3.1. A general approach

Often the statistical significance of an apparent difference between ROC curves is of interest. In general, this problem can be approached by a sequence of five steps: (i) selecting an index or set of curve parameters to characterize the sense in which the "similarity" or "difference" of the measured ROC curves is to be judged; (ii) estimating the value(s) of that index or parameter set for each ROC curve and calculating the selected difference(s) between the curves; (iii) estimating the uncertainties and correlation(s) in those indices or parameter sets; (iv) forming a statistic that can be assumed to arise from some standard distribution when the null hypothesis (of no difference in the index or parameters) is true; and (v) calculating the probability ("p-value") that an outcome of the test statistic at least as extreme as that found could have arisen from the assumed standard distribution.

The first step listed here essentially involves choosing a null hypothesis and then relating it to some index or parameter set that can be calculated from the rating data for each curve. The second and third steps can be accomplished by maximum likelihood estimation with the "Method of Scoring" (21). The fourth step may be possible only in the sense that the test statistic follows a standard distribution in some asymptotic limit; in such situations, Monte Carlo simulation can be used to explore the practical implications of departures from the assumed distribution (14,15).

3.2 Application to the bivariate binormal model

The general approach outlined above can be applied to the bivariate binormal model to construct three distinct statistical tests for differences between ROC curves measured from correlated rating data. All three tests are implemented by first calculating maximum likelihood estimates of the two pairs of parameters (a_x, b_x) and (a_y, b_y) that describe the two ROC curves and the maximum likelihood estimates of the variances of and covariances among those parameters. All of these estimates are provided by the Method of Scoring (21) when it is applied to the bivariate binormal model. A test statistic appropriate to each null hypothesis is then constructed on the basis of these quantities and the observation that maximum likelihood estimates approach a multivariate normal distribution in the limit of large data sets (21).

3.2.1 Bivariate Chi-square parameter test. The significance of the difference between two measured ROC curves can be evaluated by testing simultaneously the differences between the two parameters of each ROC curve. [Null hypothesis: The two sets of rating data arose from the same ROC curve -- i.e., $a_x=a_y$ and $b_x=b_y$.] The corresponding test statistic is given in matrix notation by

$$\chi_2^2 = \delta W^{-1} \delta'$$

where δ is the <u>row</u> vector $(\hat{a}_x-\hat{a}_y, \hat{b}_x-\hat{b}_y)$ and W is a 2X2 covariance matrix with elements

$$w_{11} = Var\{\hat{a}_x\}+Var\{\hat{a}_y\} -2\ Cov\{\hat{a}_x, \hat{a}_y\}$$

$$w_{22} = Var\{\hat{b}_x\}+Var\{\hat{b}_y\} -2\ Cov\{\hat{b}_x, \hat{b}_y\}$$

and

$$w_{12} = w_{21} = Cov\{\hat{a}_x, \hat{b}_x\} + Cov\{\hat{a}_y, \hat{b}_y\} - Cov\{\hat{a}_x, \hat{b}_y\} - Cov\{\hat{a}_y, \hat{b}_x\}.$$

In these expressions, the carat ($^\wedge$) indicates an <u>estimate</u> of the corresponding parameter; these and estimates of the various variances and covariances are provided by the maximum likelihood algorithm described in Section 2.3.3. If the null hypothesis is true, this test statistic follows a Chi-Square distribution with two degrees of freedom in the limit of large data sets [i.e., when $\hat{a}_x$, $\hat{a}_y$, $\hat{b}_x$, and $\hat{b}_y$ follow a multivariate normal distribution (21)].

Because rating data in practical medical imaging experiments involve a limited number of images (i.e., ratings), the validity of this test for small data sets must be studied empirically. Using simulation techniques similar to those reported earlier (14,15), we generated 500 sets of correlated rating data involving "m" pairs of "noise only" trials and "m" pairs of "signal present" trials for each of four ROC curves. Data sets were generated with m=50, to represent a typical medical imaging situation, and m=250 to represent typical experiments in psychophysics (and to study the rate at which the asymptotic limit is approached). The four ROC curves used to generate these simulated data involved parameter values typical of those found in clinical ROC data: r_n=0.5; r_s=0.85; b_x=b_y=0.85; and a_x=a_y=1.0, 1.3, 1.7, or 2.0. Because the correlated rating data in any one Monte Carlo experiment arose from the same underlying ROC curve, the fraction of curve-pairs found to differ significantly (f_s) should approximate the "significance level" [i.e., the "critical p-value"] α used for the test if the test performs well. A "worst case" result is shown in Figure 2, which was obtained with the highest ROC curve studied (a=2.0); lower ROC curves gave better agreement between f_s and α. The broken curves indicate the 95% confidence limits for f_s corresponding to the 500 data sets used for each comparison. For the four ROC curves studied, we found that this test causes f_s to be slightly smaller than α in the range $0 < \alpha < 0.1$ for m=50 but to be essentially equal to α for m=250. Thus we conclude that the asymptotic Chi-square behavior of the test statistic is approached very closely with 250 pairs of trials of each kind, but less closely with 50 pairs of each kind, especially for higher ROC curves. Even for 50 pairs of each kind with the highest ROC curve, the test appears to perform satisfactorily, however, yielding about 3% falsely significant results (i.e., Type I error rate) when α=0.05. One should notice that this test is "conservative" in the sense that, for small data sets, it yields Type I errors somewhat <u>less</u> frequently than expected.

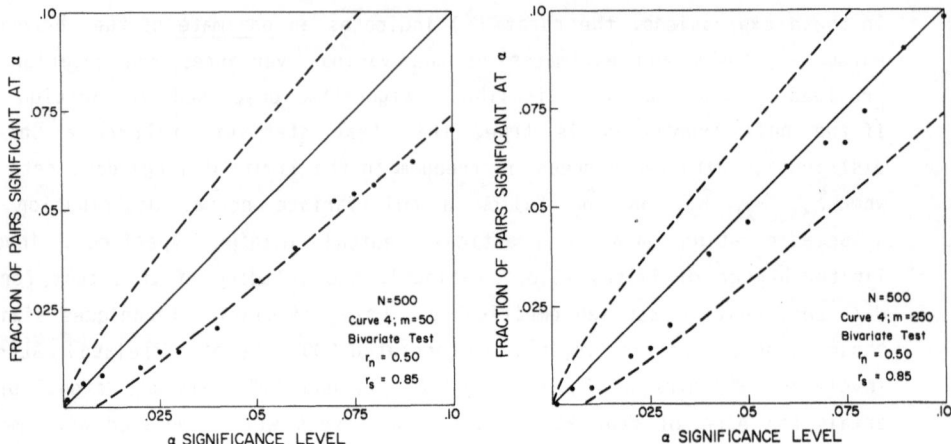

FIGURE 2. "Worst case" agreement between f_s and α for the Chi-square test.

3.2.2. <u>True Positive Fraction test</u>. As an alternative approach, one can test the significance of apparent differences between the True Positive Fractions (TPF's) of the measured ROC curves at some selected value of False Positive Fraction (FPF$_0$). [Null hypothesis: the correlated rating data arose from ROC curves such that TPF$_x$ = TPF$_y$ when FPF$_x$ = FPF$_y$ = FPF$_0$.] One should note that this test is quite distinct from the bivariate parameter test described above, because two binormal ROC curves can cross, allowing the null hypothesis of the TPF test to be true when that of the bivariate test is false.

If the null hypothesis is true, and if $\hat{a}_x$, $\hat{b}_x$, $\hat{a}_y$, and $\hat{b}_y$ are multivariate normal, then (23) the quantity $\underline{v} = (\hat{b}_x - \hat{b}_y)t - (\hat{a}_x - \hat{a}_y)$ should be a normal random variable with zero mean and standard deviation $\sigma_v = [w_{11} - 2tw_{12} + t^2 w_{22}]^{1/2}$, where $t = \Phi^{-1}(1 - FPF_0)$, where Φ^{-1} is the inverse of the cumulative standard normal distribution function, and where the w_{k1} terms are given in Section 3.2.1. Thus the quantity $\underline{v}/\sigma_v$ should follow a standard normal distribution in the limit of large data sets when the null hypothesis is true.

Using the same correlated rating data used to evaluate the bivariate Chi-square test in the previous section, we studied the agreement between f_s and α for this TPF test, employing a "two-tailed" standard-normal analysis at FPF$_0$ values of 0.05, 0.10, and 0.20. In each case, the agreement between f_s and α was at least as good as that shown in Figure 2. As with the bivariate test, agreement was consistently better for larger numbers of trials and for lower ROC curves.

3.2.3. __Area Index test.__ A third possible approach to the difference between measured ROC curves involves the "Area Index", A_Z, which summarizes each binormal ROC curve in terms of the area beneath it (6,7,16). [Null hypothesis: the correlated rating data arose from ROC curves with equal areas beneath them.] One should note that this test is distinct from each of the first two tests described above; since two binormal ROC curves can cross, the null hypothesis of the A_Z test can be true when that of the bivariate test is false and when that of the TPF test is false (except at a particular value of FPF_0).

The Area Index is related to the parameters of an ROC curve by the expression (6,7): $A_Z = \Phi(a/[1+b^2]^{1/2})$, where Φ is the cumulative standard normal distribution function. Thus if the null hypothesis is true and if the data set is large, one can show that the quantity $\underline{v} = \Phi(\hat{a}_x/[1+\hat{b}_x^2]^{1/2}) - \Phi(\hat{a}_y/[1+\hat{b}_y^2]^{1/2})$ should be a normal random variable with zero mean and variance σ_v^2 given by

$$\sigma_v^2 = \sum_{k=1}^{4} \sum_{l=1}^{4} (\partial v/\partial\theta_k)(\partial v/\partial\theta_l) \, \text{Cov}\{\hat{\theta}_k, \hat{\theta}_l\}$$

where $\{\theta_k:k=1,2,3,4\} \equiv \{a_x, b_x, a_y, b_y\}$ represents the set of four parameters of the two ROC curves*.

Monte Carlo simulation of correlated rating data from the four ROC curves specified in Section 3.2.1 showed that the agreement between f_s and α for this test was essentially similar to that found for the bivariate and TPF tests.

3.3 Statistical power

The "power" of a statistical test is the probability that the test will show an __actual__ difference to be statistically significant at a specified significance level (usually at $\alpha = 0.05$). In designing experiments, one usually seeks at least 80% power. Generally, the statistical power of a given test depends on: (i) the magnitude of the difference to be demonstrated; (ii) the number of "trials" in the experiment; and (iii) the amount of correlation between the data sets. In ROC analysis of medical imaging systems, statistical power depends also on: (iv) the balance between "noise only" and "signal present" images used in the experiment; and (v) the number and distribution of "operating points" measured on each ROC curve.

---

*Alternatively, one could use $\underline{v} = \hat{a}_x/(1+\hat{b}_x^2)^{1/2} - \hat{a}_y/(1+\hat{b}_x^2)^{1/2}$ with an analogous expression for σ_v^2. We found empirically that the first formulation of this test gives slightly better results for small data sets.

A fundamental question in the design of ROC experiments for medical image evaluation is: "How many images are required to demonstrate the significance of an assumed difference between two ROC curves?" In other words: "How many images are required to achieve adequate statistical power?"

This question can be addressed by exploring the relationship between the expected sets of confidence rating data that arise from the bivariate binormal model, on one hand, and the variability and correlation of ROC curve parameter estimates obtained from samples of those data sets, on the other. With this approach, the statistical power of the "bivariate Chi-square" parameter test described above can be predicted in terms of a non-central Chi-square distribution with two degrees of freedom (22) for any assumed pair of ROC curves, and the power of the "TPF" and "Area Index" tests can be predicted in terms of a non-central standard-normal distribution. Because the statistical power of each of these tests depends in a complex way on all five factors listed in the first paragraph of this section, no simple "rule of thumb" or table can be formulated to relate statistical power to the set of factors associated with a particular experimental design. A FORTRAN computer program developed in our laboratory (entitled "TESTPWR" and described in the Section 4.2) can be used to predict the power all three tests as a function of the numbers of images of each kind for any assumed set of factors, however.

Monte Carlo simulation studies have shown that this program provides reliable estimates of statistical power for all three tests. Using the four ROC curves employed to evaluate the performance of the three statistical tests in Section 3.2 above, 500 sets of correlated rating data were sampled from pairs of curves with $r_n = 0.5$ and $r_s = 0.85$. Equal numbers of "noise only" and "signal present" trials were assumed. Overall, the fractions of comparisons found significant (f_s) agreed with the predicted power to within a few percent for most pairs of ROC curves and to within 10% for all. Detailed results of these evaluation studies will be reported elsewhere.

4. COMPUTER PROGRAMS FOR ANALYSIS OF CORRELATED RATING DATA.

We have developed two programs in standard FORTRAN that implement the analyses of correlated rating data described here. The initial versions of these programs were designed to run on large-scale computation facilities, but efforts are currently underway to develop versions that can be run on standard 32K systems. Information regarding the availability of these programs can be obtained from the authors.

4.1 "CORROC"

This program computes maximum likelihood estimates of the parameters of the bivariate binormal model from a set of correlated rating data obtained under two conditions (e.g., two imaging systems applied to the same patient sample or two display systems or data processing techniques applied to the same image sample). It then computes the statistical significance ("p-value") of the difference between the two ROC curves using any one of the three statistical tests described in Section 3.2 above.

The program requires that the correlated rating data be tabulated in the form of two IXJ matrices corresponding to "noise only" and "signal present" trials. The (i,j) cell entry of each matrix represents the number of paired observations for which the rating pair (i,j) was obtained, where "i" represents the rating produced under one condition (e.g., imaging system, display, etc.) and "j" represents the rating produced under the other. The numbers of categories used for each condition [I and J] need not be equal, but both must lie in the range ($4 \leq I, J \leq 10$).

4.2 "TESTPWR"

This program predicts the statistical power of all three tests described in Section 3.2 as a function of the number of "noise only" trials. The user is required to specify: (1) the "a" and "b" parameters of each of the two ROC curves to be tested, and the number of rating categories to be used for each measurement; (2) the two correlation coefficients, r_n and r_s, assumed for the underlying "noise only" and "signal present" decision variable distributions [which can be estimated by running the "CORROC" program on pilot study data, if available]; either (3A) the False Positive Fractions to be used as operating points on each of the two ROC curves, or (3B) a code indicating that a variety of operating points should be sampled by Monte Carlo simulation; and (4) the ratio of the number of "signal present" trials to the number of "noise only" trials.

If option (3A) is selected, the program calculates the variances of and covariances among the "a" and "b" parameter estimates of the two ROC curves by using the expected rating data implied by the assumed curve parameters and the specified False Positive Fractions.

If option (3B) is selected, the program generates 400 sets of category boundaries on the decision variables axes [$\{t_i\}$ and $\{u_j\}$] that provide adequate spreads of operating points along each ROC curve relative to the total length of that curve: for K categories, each expected operating point must be in the interval (0.12, 0.8) [measured from the lower left corner], and no two points can be closer than a distance $0.68/(3*(K-1))$ [measured along the curve]. The average variances of and covariances among the "a" and "b" parameters are then computed from the expected rating data associated with each of these sets of category boundaries.

With either option (3A) or (3B), the program then uses the calculated variances and covariances to compute the statistical power of all three tests as a function of the number of "noise only" trials by using the methods sketched in Section 3.3. A key point in this calculation is the fact that the parameter estimate variances and covariances are all simply inversely proportional to the number of "noise only" trials if all other factors are held fixed (21).

5. CONCLUSIONS

A new "bivariate binormal" model provides a basis for evaluating the statistical significance of differences between ROC curves measured from correlated data sets. A new FORTRAN program ("CORROC") can be used to calculate maximum likelihood estimates of the model parameters and to perform any one of three distinct statistical tests of apparent differences. Monte Carlo simulation has demonstrated the reliability of all three tests. Another new program ("TESTPWR") can be used to predict the statistical power of each test as a function of the number of image-pairs used in an ROC experiment.

ACKNOWLEDGEMENT

The work reported here was supported by Contract DE-AC02-82-ER6003 from the U.S. Department of Energy. We are grateful to Evelyn Ruzich for typing the manuscript.

REFERENCES
1. Goodenough, D.J., Rossmann, K., and Lusted, L.B.: Radiographic applications of receiver operating characteristic (ROC) curves. Radiology 110: 89, 1974.
2. Metz, C.E., Starr, S.J., Lusted, L.B., and Rossmann, K.: Progress in evaluation of human observer visual detection performance using the ROC curve approach. In: Information Processing in Scintigraphy (C. Raynaud and A. E. Todd-Pokropek, eds.). Orsay, France: Commissariat a l'Energie Atomique, Departement de Biologie, Service Hospitalier Frederic Joliot, 1975.
3. McNeil, B.J., Keeler, E., and Adelstein, S.J.: Primer on certain elements of medical decision making. N. Engl. J. Med. 293: 211, 1975.

4. Metz, C.E.: Basic principles of ROC analysis. Seminars Nucl. Med. 8: 283, 1978.
5. Turner, D.A.: An intuitive approach to receiver operating characteristic curve analysis. J. Nucl. Med. 19: 213, 1978.
6. Swets, J.A.: ROC analysis applied to the evaluation of medical imaging techniques. Invest. Radiol. 14: 109, 1979.
7. Swets, J.A. and Pickett, R.M.: Evaluation of Diagnostic Systems: Methods from Signal Detection Theory. New York: Academic Press, 1982.
8. Tanner, W.P. Jr. and Swets, J.A.: A decision-making theory of visual detection. Psych. Rev. 61: 401, 1954.
9. Swets, J.A., Tanner W.P. Jr., and Birdsall, T.G.: Decision processes in perception. Psych. Rev. 68: 301, 1961.
10. Swets, J.A. (ed).: Signal Detection and Recognition by Human Observers. New York: Wiley, 1964.
11. Swets, J.A.: The relative operating characteristic in psychology. Science 182: 990, 1973.
12. Green, D.M. and Swets, J.A.: Signal Detection Theory and Psychophysics. (rev. ed.), Huntington NY: Krieger, 1974.
13. Egan, J.P.: Signal Detection Theory and ROC Analysis. New York: Academic Press, 1975.
14. Metz, C.E. and Kronman, H.B.: A test for the statistical significance of differences between ROC curves. In: Information Processing in Medical Imaging (R. DiPaola and E. Kahn, eds.). Paris: INSERM (Vol. 88), 1980.
15. Metz, C.E. and Kronman, H.B.: Statistical significance tests for binormal ROC curves. J. Math. Psych. 22: 218, 1980.
16. Hanley, J.A. and McNeil, B.J.: The meaning and use of the area under a receiver operating characteristic (ROC) curve. Radiology 143: 29, 1982.
17. Hanley, J.A. and McNeil, B.J.: A method of comparing the areas under Receiver operating characteristic curves derived from the same cases. Radiology 148: 839, 1983.
18. Metz, C.E.: Applications of ROC analysis in diagnostic image evaluation. In: The Physics of Medical Imaging: Recording System Measurements and Techniques (A. G. Haus, ed.). New York: Am. Inst. Physics, 1979.
19. Dorfman, D.D. and Alf, E.: Maximum-likelihood estimation of parameters of signal detection theory and determination of confidence intervals -- rating method data. J. Math. Psych. 6: 487, 1969.
20. Grey, D.R. and Morgan, B.J.T.: Some aspects of ROC curve fitting: normal and logistic models. J. Math. Psych. 9: 128, 1972.
21. Kendall, M. and Stuart, A.: The Advanced Theory of Statistics, Vol. 2 (4th ed.). New York: MacMillan, 1979, Chapter 18.
22. Zelen, M. and Severo, N.C.: Probability functions. Chapter 26 in: Handbook of Mathematical Functions (M. Abramowitz and I. A. Stegun, eds.). Washington, D.C.: National Bureau of Standards, 1968.
23. Hanley, J.A. and McNeil, B.J.: Statistical approaches to the analysis of receiver operating characteristic (ROC) curves. Presented at the 4th Annual Meeting of the Society for Medical Decision Making, Boston, October 27, 1982. Abstracted in: Med. Decis. Making 2: 371, 1982.

IMAGING SPATIAL DISTRIBUTIONS OF RESISTIVITY USING APPLIED POTENTIAL
TOMOGRAPHY - APT

D.C. Barber, B.H. Brown and I.L. Freeston
Department of Medical Physics and Clinical Engineering
Royal Hallamshire Hospital, SHEFFIELD S10 2JF, ENGLAND

INTRODUCTION

The measured values of electrical resistance for various tissues cover
a fairly wide range[1]. Table 1 gives some typical values measured using
isolated tissue samples.

TABLE 1

Tissue	Resistivity Ω.m
Bone	150
Fat	15.0
Striated muscle	3.0
Blood	1.6

Images representing the distribution of electrical resistance in the
human body should in principle (assuming these values are maintained in vivo)
exhibit good contrast differences between tissues. These differences should
be rather better than, for example, those found in X-ray tomography where,
with the exception of bone, linear attenuation coefficients for different
tissues differ by only a few percent. Images of resistance should allow good
discrimination of soft tissues.

There has been a small amount of literature published on resistance
imaging[2-10] for both geophysical and medical applications. As far as we
are aware none of this work has resulted in the publication of images from
either laboratory studies or from in-vivo (or in-geo) data. Some computer
simulations have been attempted[5,10] with generally poor results. Some
collection of data from subjects has also been reported[12].

We have developed a new approach to the problem of producing resistance
images which shows some promise. This work is still in a preliminary stage

and much still needs to be done. This paper will describe our progress to date and discuss some of the problems still remaining.

METHODS

All attempts at resistance imaging use a variant of the measurement configuration illustrated in Fig.1. A set of electrodes, 16 in this example, is placed around the boundary of the object being imaged, the aim being to image the distribution of resistance within the slice defined by the common plane of the electrodes.

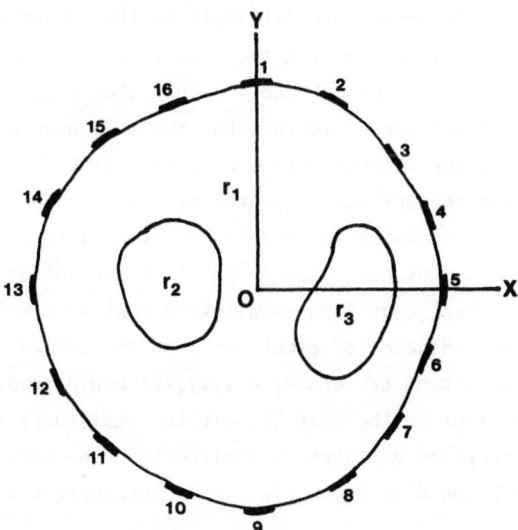

Figure 1: The Measurement Configuration

In order to image the distribution of resistance current is passed between two or more of the electrodes and the voltage difference measured between these or other pairs of electrodes. Which exact set of measurements is made depends on the type of reconstruction being attempted. Consider the simplest case of passing a current between two of the electrodes and measuring the voltage between them. Then from Ohm's Law

$$r = \frac{V}{I} \qquad \qquad \cdots\cdots\cdots (1)$$

the resistance between these two electrodes can be obtained. This resistance must be a function of the distribution of resistance within the region. By making similar measurements between all pairs of electrodes a data set of resistance measurements is obtained and provided a model is available for relating these measurements to the distribution of resistance within the region in principal this distribution of resistance (to a resolution determined by the number of measurements made) can be computed. Typically[10] a discrete resistance network model is used to describe the continuous distribution being measured. Because the relationship between the resistance between two electrodes and the resistance distribution in the network is non-linear a solution can only be obtained by an iterative method. In the description of such a solution by Dines and Lytle[10] they suggest that the solution is likely to prove more difficult as the number of image elements increases (the maximum matrix size they use is 7x7). Their simulated data was obtained directly from a network model rather than a continuous model and it is not clear, on their own admission, how the inaccuracies inherent in this model would affect the reconstruction with real data.

An alternative approach suggested by other authors[3-5] is based on concepts used in computed tomography. If the distribution of the resitance within the region is uniform patterns of electrode voltages can always be found which will produce uniform parallel current flow within the region. For example if the co-ordinates of electrode i in the co-ordinate system of Fig.1 are x_i, y_i then a voltage pattern $V_i = V_1 \cdot y_i / y_1$ would produce such a current flow parallel to the axis OY. If the resistance is no longer uniform but the same pattern of voltages is applied then the voltage between opposing electrodes, say 2 and 8 in Fig.1 divided by the current flowing between them is

$$r = \frac{V_{28}}{I_{28}} \qquad \qquad \cdots\cdots\cdots\cdots (2)$$

which to some approximation represents a line integral of resistance between electrodes 2 and 8. By altering the direction of current flow by activating the electrodes differently enough data may collect to permit a conventional tomographic reconstruction. Since in the case of non-uniform resistance the current flow will no longer be parallel this is only an approximate solution but it might be expected to give useful results. However, Bates et al.[11] have argued that it can lead to serious ambiguities basically because the current flow between two electrodes cannot be simply isolated from current flows between other pairs of electrodes.

A rather serious additional problem with both the above methods is that the contact resistance between the electrodes and the skin is not negligable. Even with careful preparation this contact resistance may well be of the same order of magnitude or larger than the resistance component from the tissue being measured especially with DC or low frequency current. The contact resistance cannot usefully be considered as part of the region being measured (or the resistance network) since it does not contribute to the resistance when current is flowing between other electrodes but only when current is flowing through that electrode. It cannot therefore be estimated using other measurements. This puts in doubt the usefulness of using measurements of voltage from electrodes through which current is flowing. However, the voltage at electrodes other than those through which current is flowing can be measured without taking any current from the electrode and therefore contact resistance is much less important for these measurements. These are the measurements used in the method to be described in this paper.

The impedance value of tissue is dependent on the frequency of the applied current. At the frequencies we have used (50 kHz) the capacitive component of tissue impedance is negligible which is why the term resistance has been used in preference to impedance. The use of higher frequencies, with the determination of both the resistive and capactive terms as a function of frequency may well result in further tissue discrimination but we have not yet attempted this.

The reconstruction algorithm

The distribution of voltage within a region through which current is flowing is given by the solution of the equation.

$$c.\nabla^2 V + \nabla c.\nabla V = 0 \qquad \ldots\ldots\ldots (3)$$

where the conductivity c (the inverse of resistance) is a function of position in the region. If c is replaced by $R = \ln \frac{1}{c}$ this equation becomes

$$\nabla^2 V - \nabla R.\nabla v = 0 \qquad \ldots\ldots\ldots (4)$$

where R is log resistance. The use of log resistance or conductance has the advantage of removing the reciprocal nature of resistance and conductance and converting them into negatives of each other. This paper will reconstruct images of log resistance. The images may be transformed to images of resistance or conductance by a final exponentiation. If R is known throughout a region and the voltage is known at the drive electrodes then solution of Eq.4 (usually numerically) will enable the distribution of voltage on the boundary to be computed. However the inverse problem, that of computing R from boundary measurements, is much more difficult to formulate and to date no general solution is available (apart from the network models). The solution proposed in this paper is based on a tomographic approach. Consider a current I passed between a pair of electrodes. Measurements of the voltage difference between all pairs of adjacent electrodes are made for this configuration of current flow. The electrode pair between which current is passed will be called the drive electrodes. For example, in Fig.2 showing 16 electrodes connected to the boundary of a circular region, current is passed between electrodes 1 and 2 and the voltage differences between all other pairs of adjacent electrodes, e.g. between electrodes 3 and 4, 4 and 5, and so on are measured. Although we would also like to measure the voltage differences between 1 and 2 and 2 and 3 (and 16 and 1) in fact this cannot be done accurately because current is flowing through at least one of these electrode pairs and the voltage measurement is distorted by contact resistance. These values may be approximated by interpolation. The values of voltage differences form a peripheral data profile and therefore suggest the use of a tomographic reconstruction technique.

Most tomographic reconstruction techniques use the concept of a back projection. The back projection of a single profile can often be considered as the simplest distribution of the property being measured (R in the present case) which could give rise to the profile. Suppose for a moment that the resistance throughout the region is uniform. Then for a given drive electrode configuration there exists a set of equipotential lines which end on the electrodes. These are illustrated in Fig.2 for the drive configuration shown.

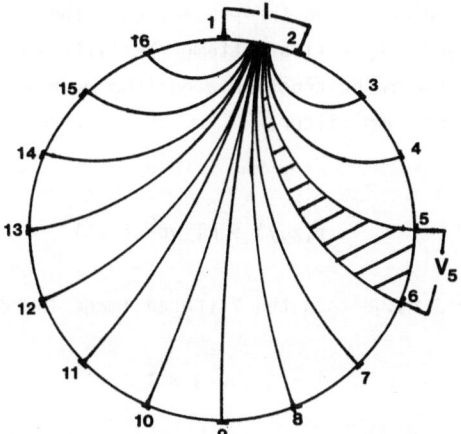

Figure 2: Equipotentials for current passing between electrodes 1 and 2.

For this case of uniform resistance there will exist certain voltage differences between adjacent electrodes. Suppose now that, for a region of identical shape in which the distribution of resistance is no longer uniform we measure an actual set of voltage differences for this drive configuration. This voltage set will in general differ from the uniform case. We assume both sets of measurements are made for the same current passing between the drive electrodes. The voltage V_i is the voltage measured between electrodes i and i+1 in the uniform case and the voltage V'_i is the voltage measured between these electrodes in the non-uniform case. The simplest distribution which explains this difference is that the resistance of the region lying between the equipotentials ending on electrodes i and i+1 is raised in proportion to the ratio of the voltages.

The appropriate region for electrodes 5 and 6 is shown shaded in Figure 2. The log resistance R_i in the region between the equipotentials ending on electrodes i and i+1 is increased to R'_i where

$$R'_i = R_i + \ln V'_i - \ln V_i \qquad \ldots\ldots\ldots\ldots (5)$$

and similarly for the other electrode pairs.

This process is repeated for other drive electrode configurations to produce a set of back projections which are then added together. This result is an unfiltered back projected image. For conventional X-ray tomography the shape of the filter needed to convert this image to the final correct image is well known. However, in the present case the ideal filter is probably not stationary. As a first attempt at filtering prior to a detailed analysis of the reconstruction algorithm we have used a non-stationary modified ramp filter.

Let

$$t(x,y) = FT \; (u^2 + v^2)^{\frac{1}{2}} \qquad \ldots\ldots\ldots \; (6)$$

If g is the unfiltered image then the filtered image in real space is given by

$$f = g + C.g \times t \qquad \ldots\ldots\ldots \; (7)$$

where the factor C is a function of the distance r from the centre of the image. and x represents convolution. C has the form

$$C(r) = 5.0 \; (r_0-r)/r_0 \qquad \ldots\ldots\ldots \; (8)$$

where r_0 is the radius of the image. This filter produces reasonable results across the image (except close to the edge) but can only be considered as a poor approximation to the correct filter.

The reconstruction algorithm assumes we know the V_i i.e. the voltage differences for the uniform case. These will be a function of the drive configuration, the shape of the region and the size of the electrodes and may be obtained from a solution of Laplace's equation

$$\nabla^2 V = 0 \qquad \ldots\ldots\ldots \; (9)$$

in the region. We have not yet attempted this but have been content to use measured values. For general in-vivo work the V_i will have to be computed.

The reconstruction method outlined is simple to implement but is by no means perfect. A possible improvement is to use the reconstructed image as a first approximation and solve Eq.4 to obtain the boundary voltages and their differences. These values will differ from the observed values but these differences may be used to compute an improved image (using possibly a further back projection of the differences). This process can be repeated until the recomputed data matches the measured data. It is not known however, whether this process will converge.

Data collection

Although by no means a trivial electronic problem the concept of data collection in our system is fairly straightforward. Each pair of drive electrodes is driven in turn by a constant current generator and the values of voltage differences between adjacent pairs of electrodes measured. Our system uses 16 electrodes. Voltage differences from electrode pairs for which one electrode is a drive electrode are not measured. The voltage differences are digitised and stored in a Data General Eclipse computer. 0.04 mS is allocated for the collection and digitisation of each voltage difference; therefore as will be seen below data collection is possible for a complete data set within 5 mS. Generally, several sets of data are averaged within the computer to reduce noise. If higher collection speeds were required data could be collected in parallel. Because the dynamic range of the voltage differences is large the data is scaled in a systematic way before digitisation. We shall not be concerned with these details here. For the algorithm described here the Eclipse computer is more than powerful enough. However, for a more accurate algorithm the full power of this or a similar machine may be needed.

Most of our experimental work has been done using a phantom consisting of a 15 cm internal diameter dish with 16 equispaced electrodes set into the edge of the dish. The dish is filled with physiological saline to a depth sufficient to cover the electrodes (~4 mm) and carefully levelled to ensure a uniform depth of saline. Circular brass or perspex objects may be placed in the dish for imaging.

This phantom therefore closely approximates to a two dimensional distribution of resistance. We also have a three dimensional phantom consisting of a long (30 cm) hollow cylinder of perspex of 8 cm internal diameter blanked off at one end. This cylinder may be filled with saline and objects inserted for imaging through its open upper end. The electrodes are placed in a ring 15 cm from either end.

The number of independent measurements

If there are n electrodes then there are apparently n(n-1) possible drive electrode configurations and therefore $n^2(n-1)$ measurements available. Not all these measurements are independent. Consider the two cases of applying the same current between electrodes i and i+1 and between i+1 and i+2. Each of these operations will produce a set of n voltage values which we can represent as two vectors $\vec{V}_i$ and $\vec{V}_{i+1}$.

Because the resistance system being measured is linear, if we apply current between i and i+1 and i+1 and i+2 simultaneously the voltages produced are the same as $\vec{V}_i + \vec{V}_{i+1}$. But because current is flowing both in and out of electrode i+1 no net current flows in this electrode and the voltage sum $\vec{V}_i + \vec{V}_{i+2}$ represents the voltage which would be obtained by directly passing current between i and i+2. In other words the voltage distribution from any drive combination in which the drive electrodes are not adjacent can be produced by summing the voltages produced from a set of adjacent pairs. There are n such adjacent pairs and each produces n measurements which reduces the total number of measurements to n^2. In fact we can only collect n-3 measurements because we cannot use voltage differences which include a drive electrode. In addition the principal of reciprocity states that if we apply a current between two of the electrodes, say A and B and measure the voltage between another pair, say C and D to obtain V_{CD}, and then pass the same current between C and D and measure the voltage between A and B then $V_{AB} = V_{CD}$. This reduces the number of independent measurements by half. The number of independent measurements is therefore n(n-3)/2.

For drive configurations other than the adjacent set the number of measurements is n(n-4)/2. If we could use the voltages on the drive electrodes a rather more rigorous analysis than given here shows that there are n(n-1)/2 independent measurements. Clearly the fraction of 'lost' measurements decreases with increasing n.

Assuming that a circular region is being imaged then the number of independent image points which can be obtained for this area is given by n(n-3)/2. If we assume these data points are uniformly distributed over the circular region this leads to an image sample spacing of

$$ a \qquad \left[\frac{\pi}{2} \cdot \frac{1}{n(n-3)} \right]^{\frac{1}{2}} D \qquad\qquad \cdots\cdots\cdots (10) $$

where D is the diameter of the region. For a unit diameter and a value of
n = 16 this gives a data point spacing of 0.087 which corresponds to a
resolution of 0.174.

Choice of drive set

A drive set is a set of drive electrode configurations all of the same
spacing. One important set is the adjacent electrode set in which the drive
electrode pairs are 1-2, 2-3 ... etc. Another important set might be that in
which the drive electrode are diametrically opposite, e.g. for a 16 electrode
system 1-9, 2-10 ... etc. The notation S_n will be used to indicate the
drive set in which the drive electrodes are n spaces apart. S_1 is the
adjacent drive electrode set. Since we can derive any drive set from the
adjacent set it would seem that all drive sets are equivalent. S_1 can only
be derived from sets for which n is odd but these odd set would all appear to
be equivalent and only measurements from one drive set need to be considered
in the reconstruction. The problem of choice of drive set is complicated by
the fact that the pattern of back projection is different for each drive
configuration. The drive set chosen for the images shown in this paper is
S_1. The reason for this choice is that it gave the reconstruction of
highest resolution over all other odd sets tested, the highest sensitivity in
terms of image amplitude and the most artefact free reconstruction for a
variety of object positions. Figure 3 shows the Fourier transform of a 1.5 cm
perspex object (i.e. 10% of the image diameter) reconstructed using drive sets
S_1, S_3, S_5 and S_7. Clearly the differences are not great although they
become relatively larger at higher frequencies and are complicated by the fact
that the signal to noise ratio improves from S_1 to S_7. Relative values of
signal to noise ratio for a 1.5 cm object are given in Table II and it is
possible that a better image than S_1 could be produced by suitable
processing of one of the other drive set images. However, S_1 does have the
advantage of a full set of 104 measurements compared to 96 for S_3, S_5 and
S_7. It is likely that choice of the best drive set may be changed in
future, especially as more electrodes are added.

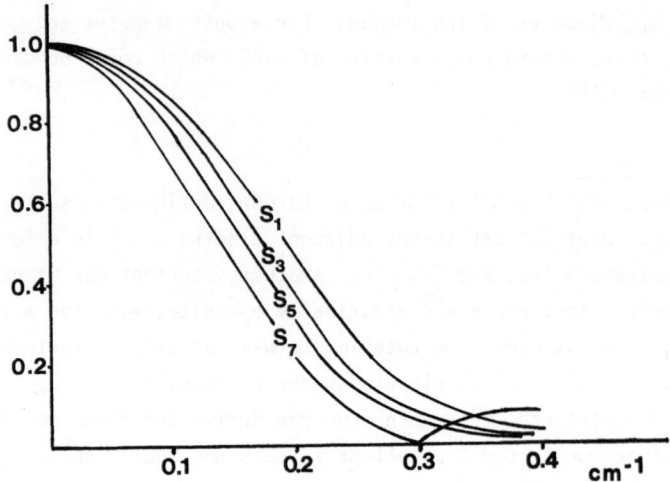

Figure 3: Modulus of the Fourier Transform of a 1.5 cm object at the centre of the image for drive configurations S_1, S_3, S_5 and S_7.

TABLE II

Drive Set	Relative S/N ratio object at centre	Relative S/N ratio object at 3.5 cm from centre
S1	1.0	1.4
S3	2.1	3.3
S5	2.5	4.1
S7	2.7	4.1

RESULTS

Figures 4 to 7 are images of a 1.5 cm circular perspex object at different positions in the 15 cm dish surrounded by saline. The images were reconstructed from measurements from 16 electrodes. Measurements of the full width at half maximum height (FWHM) are given relative to the image diameter of 15 cm for these images in Table III. The average value is 0.17 which agrees well with the theoretical value given above. The reconstruction is producing images as good as could be expected given the number of data points. Fig.8 shows the image of two 1.0 cm perspex objects and a 1.0 cm brass object and shows that multiple objects can be imaged clearly.

Images of a 1.5 cm. diameter perspex object at various distances r
from the center of the 15 cm, dish phantom.

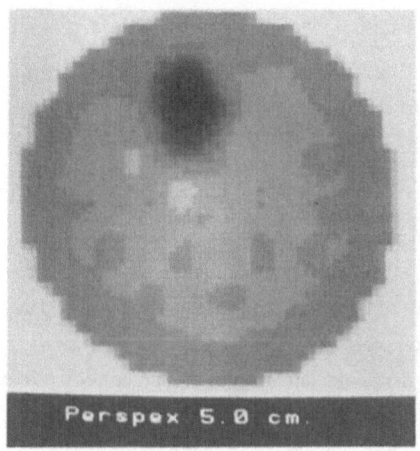

Figure 4: r = 5.0 cm.

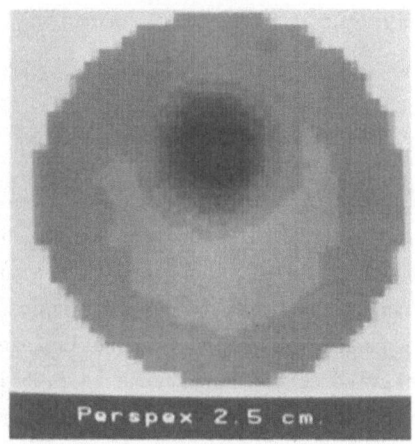

Figure 5: r = 2.5 cm.

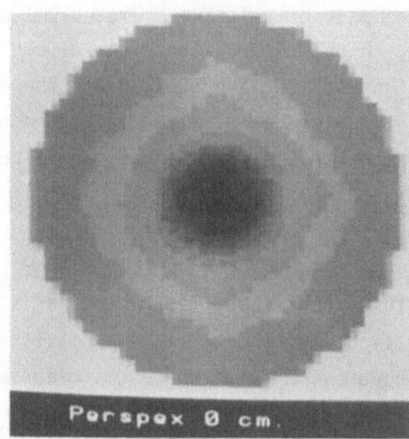

Figure 6: r = 0.0 cm.

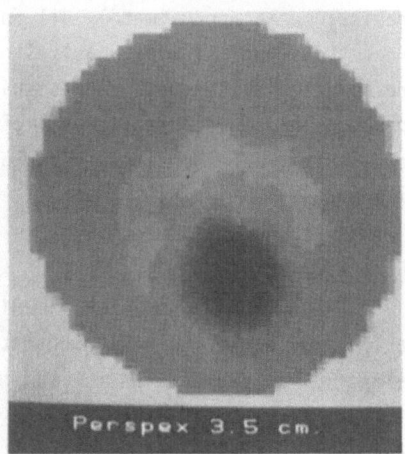

Figure 7: r = 3.5 cm.

TABLE III

Relative Distance from centre	Relative FWHM
0	0.19
0.17	0.18
0.23	0.16
0.33	0.14

Sensitivity

Ultimately the sensitivity of an imaging procedure is dependent on the noise level. However, in practice an image must achieve a reasonable absolute contrast if only to reduce the effect of rounding errors in its reconstruction. The peak resistance contrast of the object in Fig.6 relative to the background is 2.05:1. This is an image of an object which effectively has an infinite resistance and therefore the contrast would appear to be poor. However, Seagar[13] has shown that once a certain ratio of object to background resistance is exceeded further changes in resistance produce little change in the measured values because the pattern of current flow remains the same. He has also shown that the resistance ratio needed to produce half the contrast of an object of infinite resistance is approximately 4:1 for an object of relative diameter 0.1 and that the signal size is nearly linear with the natural logarithm of contrast ratio below this point. A resistance contrast ratio of 2:1 should therefore produce an image contrast ratio of 1.25:1 which can easily be detected with our system. The sensitivity for objects of this size would appear to be adequate.

Linearity

Equation 4 shows that imaging of log resistance distributions is not a linear process in the sense that the image of two log resistance distributions is not the same as the sum of separate images of these distributions. It is this property of Eq.4 which is likely to pose the most serious problems in resistance imaging. Consider that a solution to Eq.4 is V where $V = V_p + V_u$, V_p being a perturbation of the uniform voltage distribution V_u. Inserting V in Eq.4 gives

$$\nabla^2 Vp - \nabla Vp.\nabla R - \nabla Vu .\nabla R = 0 \qquad \cdots\cdots\cdots(11)$$

since $\nabla^2 Vu = 0$

If ∇Vp is small compared to ∇Vu this becomes

$$\nabla^2 Vp - \nabla Vu.\nabla R = 0 \qquad \cdots\cdots\cdots(12)$$

This is now linear since if Vp_1 and Vp_2 are solutions of this equation for R_1 and R_2

$$\nabla^2 (Vp_1 + Vp_2) - \nabla Vu(\nabla R_1 + \nabla R_2) = 0 \qquad \cdots\cdots\cdots(13)$$

Eq.12 implies that to a first order the equipotentials are not disturbed from the uniform resistance positons, a condition required by the reconstruction algorithm. This condition is only achieved for small values of resistance gradient, a condition not present in our phantom experiments. Figure 8 possibly shows some distortions due to non-linearities.

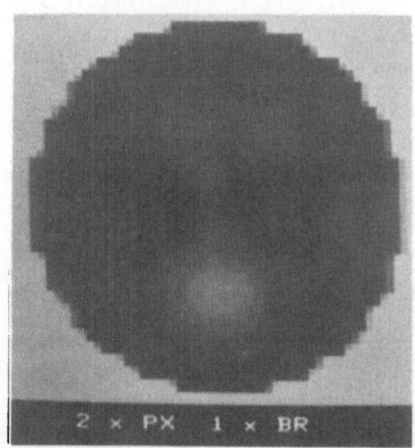

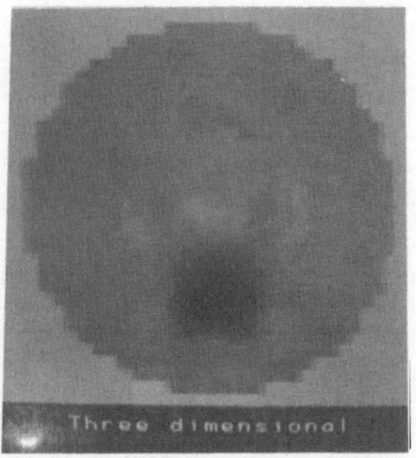

Figure 8

An image of two 1.0 cm perspex objects and a 1.0 cm brass object.

Figure 9

An image of a 0.8 cm diameter object in the 3-D phantom.

Three dimensions

Resistance imaging, if it is to be clinically useful must produce tomographic images from a three dimensional distribution. In the three dimensional situation electrodes would be placed around a generally cylindrical object. When current is passed between the drive electrodes current flow is no longer confined to the plane of the electrodes and clearly any measurements will include information from either side of the electrode plane. Several possible ways of dealing with this problem can be suggested. One possible way is, at the expense of extra electrodes, to mount guard electrodes above and below the electrode plane in the hope that the current flow in the plane of interest cn be confined to that plane. This has two problems. Firstly Plonse and Collin[14] have shown that the use of guard electrodes on an inhomogeneous medium can lead to serious errors of measurement, basically because current flow cannot be reliably confined to a plane. Secondly because of variations in contact resistance it would be very difficult to ensure that the voltages under the guard electrodes matched the electrodes being guarded. Use of strip electrodes is another possibility but there are difficulties of ensuring uniform contact. A more theoretical approach is to assume that the resistance does not vary in the direction at right angles to the collection plane. For a given distribution of resistance in the plane of the electrodes it may be shown that there exists a transformation which converts the observed voltage differences measured for a given drive configuration into the voltage differences which would be observed if the distribution of resistance was being measured as a two dimensional problem. In other words provided the resistance is uniform at right angles to the plane of the electrodes a three dimensional problem can be converted into a two dimensional problem.

$$V_{2D} = T(V_{3D}) \qquad \dots\dots\dots(14)$$

In practice we would initially only have the transform T for the uniform case. Figure 9 shows an image reconstructed from data using this transform taken from our three dimensional phantom. The insulating object is well reconstructed. In practice such axially uniform distributions will only be approximated. However, preliminary experimental work suggests that the axial uniformity has only to be maintained over a limited distance about the measuring plane for this to work. Once an approximate image has been

produced it is possible to consider recomputing the transform T based on
this new data. Further refinements may possibly be achieved by collecting
more data from sets of electrodes on either side of the plane of interest.

Conclusions

This paper has described a method of collecting and processing data
to produce images of electrical resistance in a region. The method has been
shown to produce images of resolution consistent with the amount of data
collected and have sensitivity sufficient to image the resistance
differences found in vivo. Many problems still exist with this technique
but we have begun to collect some in vivo data and hope to produce some
useful images in the not too distant future.

REFERENCES

1. Geddes, L.A. and Baker, L.E. The specific resistance of biological material - A compendium of data for the biomedical engineer and physicist. Med. and Biol. Eng., Vol.3, p 271-293, 1967

2. Henderson, R.P. and Webster, J.B. An impedance camera for spatially specific measurements of the thorax. IEEE Trans. Biomed. Eng., Vol.25, p 250-254, 19

3. Price, L.R. Electrical impedance computed tomography (ICT). A new CT imaging technique. IEEE Trans. Nucl. Sci., Vol. NS-26, p 2736-2739, 1979

4. Lytle, R.J. and Dines, K.A. An impedance camera: A system for determining the spatial variation of electrical conductivity. Lawrence Livermore Lab. Rep. UCRL, 52413, 1978

5. Schomberg, H. Reconstruction of spatial resistivity distribution of conduction objects from external resistance measurements. Phillips GmbH, Hamburg, Man. MS-H, 1908V/78, 1978

6. Yamashita, Y. and Takahashi, T. Methods and feasibility of estimating impedance distribution in the human torso. Proc. of the Vth ICEBI, Tokyo, 87-90, (1981)

7. Mochizuki, A., Takado, H and Saito, M. Impedance computed tomography and the design of hyperthermia. Proc. of the Vth ICEBI, Tokyo, 95-98, (1981)

8. Nakayama, K., Yagi, W and Yagi, S. Fundamental study on electrical impedance CT algorithm utilising sensitivity theorem on impedance plethysmography: Proc. of the Vth ICEBI, Tokyo, 99-102, (1981)

9. Dines, K.A. and Lytle, R.J. Computerised geophysical tomography. Proc. IEEE, Vol.67, p1065-1073, 1979

10. Dines, K.A. and Lytle, R.J. Analysis of electrical conductivity imaging. Geophysics, Vol.46, No.7, p1025-1036

11. Bates, R.H., McKinnon, G.C. and Seager, A.D. A limitation of systems for imaging electrical conductivity distributions. IEEE Trans. on Biomed. Eng., Vol.27, No.7, p 418-420, 1980

12. Jossinet, J., Fourcade, C. and Schmitt, M. A study for breast imaging with a circular array of impedance electrodes. Proc. of the Vth ICEBI, Tokyo, 83-86, (1981)

13. Seagar, A.D. Ph.D. Thesis, University of Canterbury, Christchurch, New Zealand 1983

14. Plonse, R. and Collin, R. Electrode guarding in electrical impedance measurements of physiological systems - a critique. Med. and Biol. Eng. and Comput., Vol.15, p519-527, 1977

AN UNCOLLIMATED COMPTON PROFILE METHOD FOR DETERMINATION OF
OSTEOPOROTIC CHANGES IN VERTEBRAL BONE DENSITY AND COMPOSITION

SHARON K. CLAYTON*, SAMIM ANGHAIE, ALAN M. JACOBS
Department of Nuclear Engineering Sciences
University of Florida
Gainesville,Florida 32611, USA

ABSTRACT. An approach to determine both the density and composition of the
human vertebra based on Uncollimated Compton Scattering is presented. The
proposed method uses the photon energy-history and its relationship to the
transit path of the photon rather than the current practice of rigorous
collimation. The results using a proposed model of the human vertebra
indicate that the method can be used to determine the small density
changes in the trabecular region. It is the density of this region that
will allow the detection at an earlier stage than is currently attainable
and allow the possibility of prophylactic treatment.

1. INTRODUCTION

One of the first x-ray images reported was of the bones of the hand.
Since that time, many other methods using radiation have non-invasively
interrogated internal structures. However, no low-cost method of effectively detecting small changes in the loss of bone with aging has been developed.
Early efforts concentrated on film densitometry.(1,2) These methods were
relatively unsuccessful since a thirty percent change in bone density must
occur before a significant change can be detected on a radiograph.(3)
Radiogrammetric parameters such as the width of the cortex have been
investigated, but no conclusive evidence at an early stage could be
determined by these methods.(4,5)

The development of radioisotopes opened a new path for bone studies.
Photon absorptiometry using a gamma-ray source to make transmission measurements through a bone was thought to be the answer to the problem.(6-11)
This method was directed toward the appendicular skeleton and it has since
been shown that the axial skeleton is the critical region for the early
loss of bone.(12,13) The use of dual-photon absorptiometry allowed the
axial skeleton to be measured by the removal of the restriction on a
constant thickness of tissue-like material surrounding the bone.(14,15) The
major failure of this method as well as the Neutron Activation method was
described by Ruegsegger when he said that trabecular bone shows a more
rapid change in mineralization than does compact bone, so a method for
detection of minute alterations in mineralization must allow for separate
quantification of compact and spongy bone.(16) Both methods sense an average
vertebral measurement.

* Currently employed at Orlando Regional Medical Center,Orlando, Florida

It is the ability to detect the density changes of both the cortical and trabecular regions that will allow the early detection and screening for osteoporosis. Currently, only CT allows this quantification(17-23) but the cost inhibits its use as a screening modality. The method using a variation of Compton scattering techniques to include the compositional dependence of the photoelectric effect will allow this separate quantification at a reasonable cost. Compton scattering was first described in medical applications by Odeblad and Norhagen.(24) It has since been described for in vivo diagnostic tests for both lung and bone studies.(25-44) Attenuation and multiple-scatter problems have thus far limited the clinical application of the previous Compton scattering techniques. This paper will describe the Uncollimated Compton Profile Method which will allow these problems to be overcome and a separate quantification of the densities of the trabecular and cortical regions to be determined.

2. THEORY

The basic principles of the uncollimated detector approach will be summarized with reference to Figure 1. The following development and notation closely follow that described by Jacobs.(45) As illustrated, a gamma-ray source (S) illuminates a chord of the object. The scattered radiation is sensed by a detector (D). Points A and B are the entrance and exit points of the object. Point B is shown for an arbitrary scattering point (P), but the uncollimated detector actually senses all points along the illuminated chord. The energy resolution of the detector provides the collimation "electronically", allowing the determination of the point of scatter by the following Compton kinematics relationship:

$$E' = \frac{E_0}{1 + 0.00196E_0(1 - \cos\theta)} \qquad (1)$$

where E_0 is the initial energy(keV), θ is the polar angle of scatter, and E' is the scattered energy(keV). This relationship provides a one-to-one correspondence between the angle of scatter and the scattered energy for each initial energy.

Although the above discussion and illustration describe P as a point, it is actually a volume defined by the size of the source collimators and the energy resolution of the detector. To further quantify scattered-ray densitometry, it will be useful to define some parameters. Source-to-object interactions and the source collimation system beam shaping characteristics are included by defining:

F_S = fraction of source photons which reach point A.

Detector efficiency and any object to detector interactions are included in

F_D = fraction of photons reaching point B which are detected at D.

The dimensions of the scattering volume, the solid angle limitations, and
the differential scattering cross section are included in the following
expression:

$\rho\sigma(\Theta)F_V$ = fraction of photons which reach point P and are sensed at D

where ρ is the volume-averaged density at point P and $\sigma(\Theta)$ is the differential
scattering coefficient at the requisite polar angle Θ.

Using the above definitions, the detected photon rate (D) for a given
source strength (S) can be written as

$$D = SF_S e^{-\ell(A,P)} \rho\sigma(\Theta)F_V e^{-\ell(P,B)} F_D \qquad (2)$$

where the factors are written in the order of the time-history of the
photon. The exponential terms are the attenuation from A to P and P
to B. It is the information included by these terms that will allow the
determination of the densities and composition. This equation assumes that
only once-scattered radiation is detected. If a constant F is defined as
the natural logarithm of $SF_S F_V \sigma(\Theta) F_D$, equation 2 can be rewritten as

$$\ln D = F + \ln\rho - \ell(A,P) - \ell(P,B) . \qquad (3)$$

This is the general form of the equations used to solve all
scattered densitometry problems using this approach. Several schemes
have been suggested for applying this to imaging and the details are found
in the literature.(46,47)

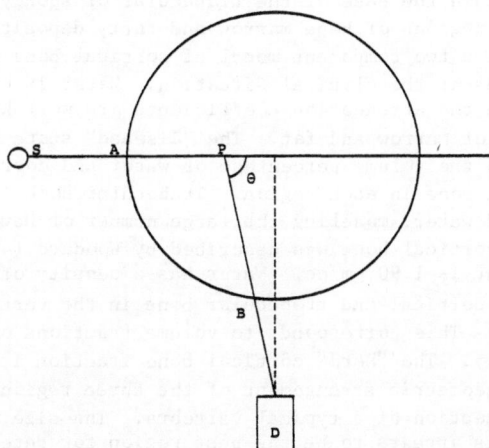

FIGURE 1. Basic configuration of Uncollimated Compton Profile Imaging. S
is the position of a collimated gamma-ray source. D is an uncollimated detector. Points A and B are the entrance and exit
points of the incident and scattered photons. P is the arbitrary
scattering point with scattering angle Θ.

Equation 3 can be rewritten more explicitly in the following form to include the determination of n-components,

$$\ln D_{ij} = F_{ij} + \ln\rho_i - d \sum_{k=1}^{i-1} \mu_{oj}\rho_k \quad -\bar{\rho}_i L_i \mu_{ij} \quad . \qquad (4)$$

The densities and attenuation coefficients are represented by ρ and μ. Subscript i represents the discrete pixel number in the approximation of the line integrals of the exponential attenuation terms. The pixel width is d. The exit pathlength for each pixel is L_i. Using the method of multiple energies to discriminate between various materials so common in many imaging modalities, the subscript j represents the energy of the source. Therefore, if n energies are used, n components may be determined if the set of equations are independent.

3. APPLICATION OF COMPTON PROFILE IMAGING TO OSTEOPOROSIS
3.1 Vertebra Model

The human vertebra consists of a thin shell of cortical bone surrounding a much larger region of trabecular bone. The vertebral model chosen for the evaluation of Compton Profile Imaging is based on the desire to determine a clinically significant parameter at the lowest possible expense. As stated previously, the method can determine n components with n energies. In general, the lowest expense can be realized by using the least number of sources. This dictates the necessity of describing the vertebra by the fewest components that can adequately describe the vertebrae.

A two component model is believed to provide the necessary information. In osteoporosis, the composition of the two types of bone do not appear to change significantly but in the case of the trabecular or spongy bone, areas of bone are replaced by regions of bone marrow and fatty deposits.(48) It is for this reason, that a two component model of cortical bone and water appears to closely represent the clinical situation. Water is used for the non-bone component since the attenuation coefficients are well known and the density is between that of marrow and fat. The "disease" state is approximated by an increase in the volume percentage of water and corresponding decrease in the cortical bone in each region. Trabecular bone is represented by a large percentage of water, modeling the large number of Haversian canals.

The composition of cortical bone was described by Woodard.(49) The density of this component is 1.90 gm/cc. Water has a density of 1.0 gm/cc. The densities of normal cortical and trabecular bone in the vertebrae are 1.85 and 1.08 gm/cc.(50) This corresponds to volume fractions of water of 0.6 and 0.91 respectively. The "hard" cortical bone fraction is 0.00.

Figure 2 shows the geometric arrangement of the three regions of bone densities in the cross section of a typical vertebra. The size represents an L3 vertebra since this appears to be the best region for detecting early osteoporotic changes.

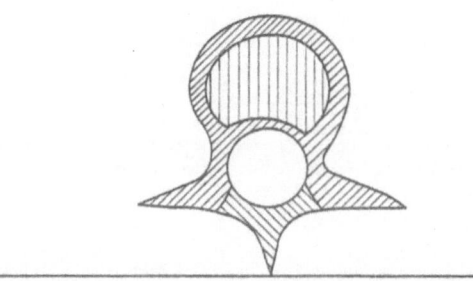

FIGURE 2. Geometric arrangement of the three bone regions of a typical
L3 vertebra.

3.2 Energy Selection

The first consideration in the selection of the two energies is the
necessary condition of sufficiently different attenuation coefficients so
that the equations will be independent. This is a result of the densities
and pathlengths being independent of energy. The Compton, photoelectric,
and total attenuation coefficients for each component are shown in Figure 3.
As shown, the photoelectric interaction is very large at low energies in the
cortical bone and this should be minimized to reduce attenuation which leads
to a higher patient dose. The optimum energy for bone mineral determination
has been reported to be about 90 keV.(51)

Since the energies must be available in radionuclides, the half-life,
specific activity, cost, availability, and other emissions must be considered.
Allowing for the maximization of as many of the above considerations as
possible, ^{241}Am and ^{153}Gd are chosen as the sources with primary energies of
60 and 100 keV, respectively.

3.3 Other Parameters

The location of the source and detector on the plane of interest is an
important consideration. It has been shown that the earliest changes occur
in the central part of the trabecular region.(52) Therefore, the line of
illumination should pass through this region. The differential scattering
cross section depends on the angles of scatter and is considered in the
determination of the placement. Ninety degrees is chosen to provide a good
range of scattered energies for the incident energies and geometry, and to
provide the best illumination of the vertebra. Figure 4 shows the geometric
arrangement for the discrete calculations.

468

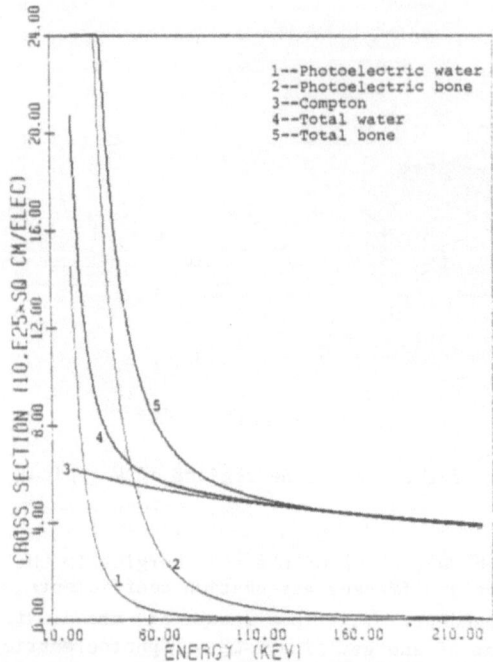

FIGURE 3. Cross sections for water and cortical bone.

For a discrete formulation, the line of illumination must be divided
into pixels. The choice of the width of the pixel is determined by the
energy resolution of the detector system. A resolution of 0.35 to 0.5 keV
is the limit on current commercial systems in the energy range of interest.
This dictates a pixel width of 0.8 cm for the geometrical arrangement of
Figure 4.

A source illumination area of 1cm by 1cm was used in the calculations.
The detector was assumed to have a diameter of 0.5cm and an efficiency of
0.15. The only other parameter of interest is the volume fraction of water
in each region. The results of varying this parameter, simulating bone loss,
will be discussed later.

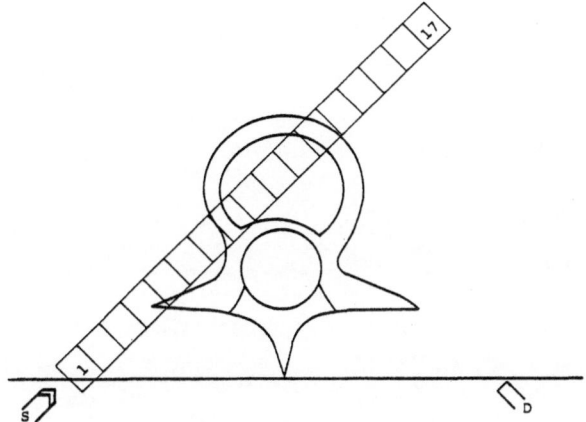

FIGURE 4.   Geometric arrangement for the discrete solution.

4.   RESULTS

The spectrum generated for the case of the normal bone by the
FORTRAN program in reference 53 is shown in Figure 5. The spectra for
several cases of loss of bone were calculated and the results indicate that
the requirements on the reverse problem, of calculating the densities from
the calculated detection rates, are reduced to observing a count rate high
enough to overcome the statistical uncertainty in the detection rate. It
shows a magnification effect in that the larger losses of bone show an
increasing effect as the loss of bone increases.   The effects of the
multiple-scatter will be shown in the following section.

4.1 Multiple-Scatter Considerations

Densitometry of two-phase fluid flow in optically opaque systems is an
application of the Compton Profile technique which includes many of the
features found in the present composition measurement problem. Of most
direct and relevant significance is the complication of determining the
detector response to orders of photon scattering greater than the once-
scattered component. The single-scatter spectrum provides the basis for the
composition determination presented earlier. The actual detector spectrum
response to the scattered photon field must be reduced to that due to only
the once-scattered component. Anghaie and Jacobs have considered in detail
the effects of multiply-scattered detected photons on two-phase density
distribution measurements.(54,55) The methods and calculation schemes
employed in these applications are directly applicable to the vertebral
composition situation.

470

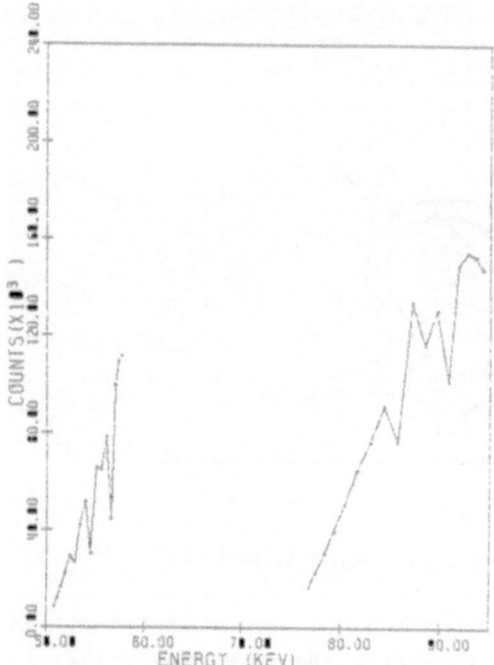

FIGURE 5. Detected spectrum for the model of normal vertebral bone.

A multiple-scatter factor, B(E), is defined to be the ratio of the detector spectrum response rate due to all photon scattering-orders to the spectrum response rate due to only once-scattered photons. Denoting the actual detector response rate by $D_{meas}(E)$, the detector response rate due to once-scattered photons,D(E), is given by

$$D(E) = \frac{D_{meas}(E)}{B(E)} \tag{5}$$

The response,D(E),is then used to determine the vertebral composition distribution by the deductive route developed earlier. Clearly, B(E) has a minimum value of unity which indicates that only once-scattered photons of energy E are actually detected.

Monte Carlo numerical experiments of 100,000 photon histories each are employed to estimate the factor B(E). The object illustrated in Figure 6 is chosen to resemble the vertebral model and to be geometrically consistent with the required inputs to Monte Carlo codes implemented on readily available computers. Also indicated in Figure 6 is the relative orientation of the incident photon beam, object, and detector. Based on the study in reference 55, a detector position at 150° from the incident beam is examined as well as the 90° position previously presented.

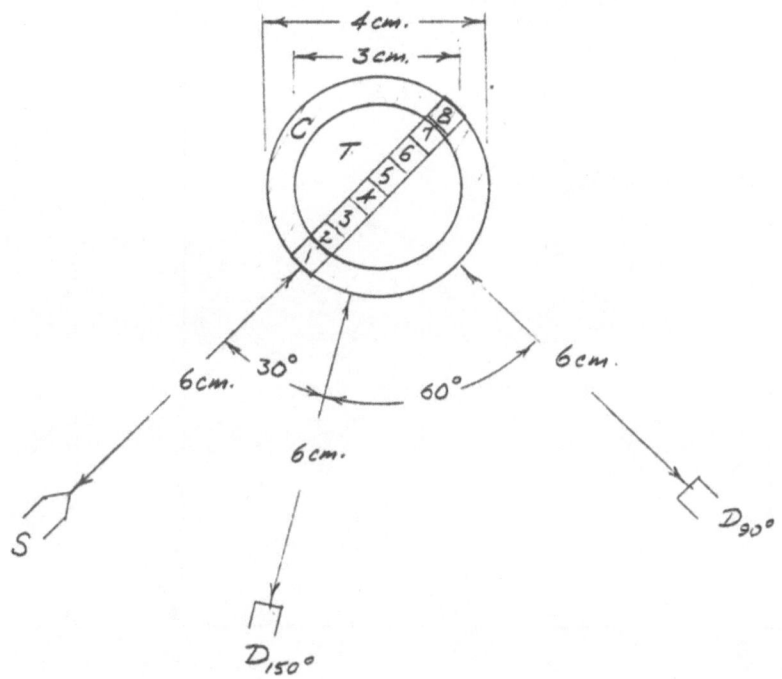

FIGURE 6. Object, incident beam and detector orientations used for
determination of B(E). Region C represents cortical bone(ρ =
1.9 gm/cc). Region T represents trabecular bone(ρ = 1.1 gm/cc)
presumed to be a homogeneous mixture of bone and water.

The results of the calculation of B(E) for incident photon energies
of 60 and 100 keV are presented in Figure 7 for the detector at the 90°
position from the incident beam.   Rather than expressing the abscissa
as detected photon energy, E, it is presented as the pixel index for the
eight (0.5 cm) diameter elements. The pixel index (or illuminated chord
position) is a function of the once-scattered photon energy through equation
1. The maximum value of B(i.e., the worst case) occurs for an incident
beam energy of 100 keV and is approximately 1.14. Thus, at worst, only
14 percent of the detected photon signal is due to multiply-scattered
photons. Of equal interest is the rather small and unstructured variation
of B(E) which indicates that an iterative approach to including a progres-
sive(rather than sharp) bone composition variation would converge rapidly.

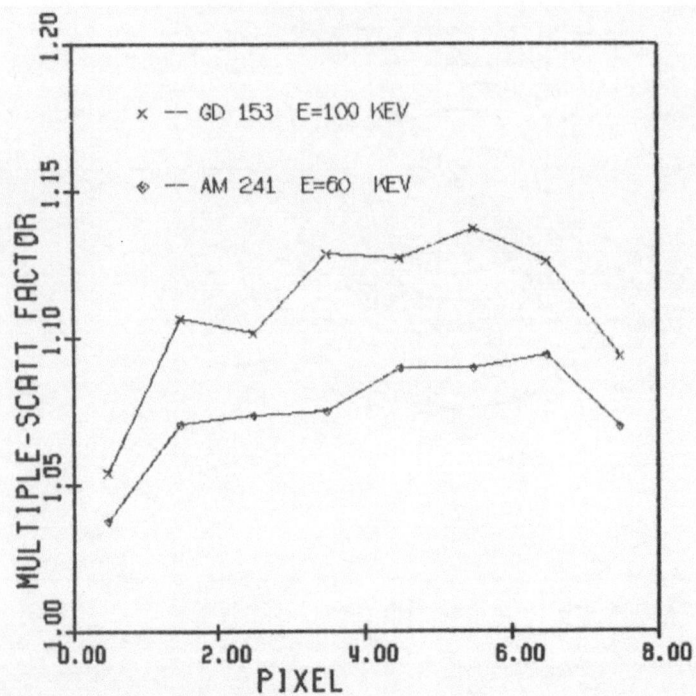

FIGURE 7.   The multiple-scatter factor,B, as a function of object pixel
index for 90° detector orientation relative to incident beam
for E_0= 60 and 100 keV.

Figure 8 presents the results of the calculation of B for the
same incident energies but for the 150° orientation of the detector from the
incident beam.   The advantage of this orientation is clear from the results.
A disadvantage is that the position resolution is degraded(esp., for deep
pixels).   In the region of greatest interest(i.e. pixels 1 through 4),the
maximum value of B is about 1.05 indicating only a 5 percent signal contribution by multiply-scattered photons.   The variation of B is smooth and
again iterative approaches(if, indeed, necessary) could be easily employed
to obtain B for actual bone composition variation.

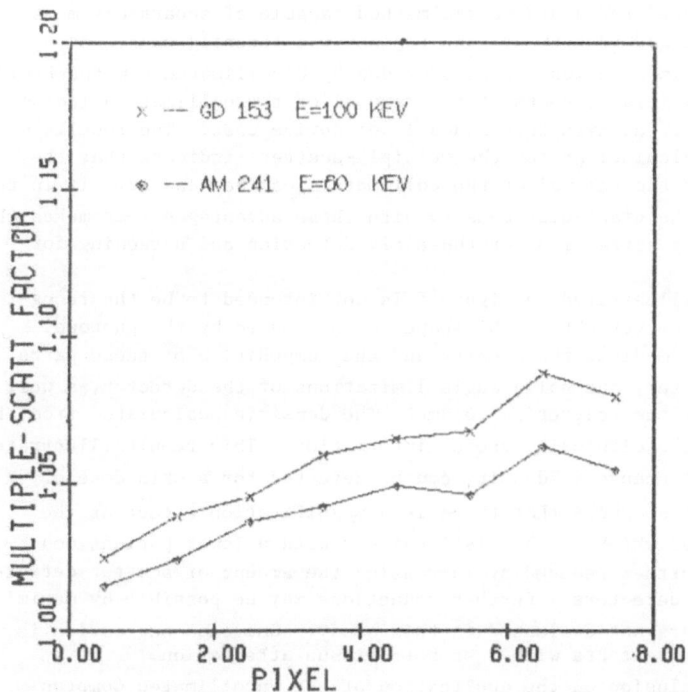

FIGURE 8.   The multiple-scatter factor,B, as a function of object pixel
index for 150 detector orientation relative to incident beam
for E_0= 60 and 100 keV.

Relevance of the multiple-scatter correction is evident only in actual
measurements (which are not the subject of this paper). The above
results of the B calculation for an object resembling the calculational
model of the human vertebra, imply two important points: 1. The maximum
contribution of multiple-scatter to the detected spectrum should be low.
2. The variation of B with photon energy (or scatter location) is
unstructured,indicating a relatively easy-to-apply iterative process for an
actual composition variation. This variation is more quickly converging
than the two-phase flow application which is highly successful.

5. CONCLUSIONS

The clinical need for a diagnostic method capable of separately measuring the cortical and trabecular bone regions was recently expressed by Wahner(56). This information can be provided by Uncollimated Compton Profile Imaging. The beneficial effects of the removal of the collimation include more information for a given dose and a lower device cost. The results of the Monte Carlo calculations for the multiple-scatter indicate that the negative effect of the removal of the collimators can be handled. It is the ability to sense the trabecular density with these advantages that makes the method particularly attractive for the early detection and screening for osteoporosis.

The spectrum illustrated in Figure 5 is not intended to be the recognizable image of the vertebra. The shape is influenced by the photons' pathlengths in the medium, the density and the composition of these paths, the angles of scatter, the solid angle limitations of the detector, as well as, the density of the scattering volume. The densities calculated from this spectrum will be the clinically useful information. This result illustrates that a one percent change in density can be detected for a skin dose of about 7 rem. It also shows that there is a magnification effect at the greater bone losses which can be distinguished with a lower patient dose. The dose can be further reduced by increasing the amount of scatter detected by using multiple detectors. Further reductions may be possible by maximizing other parameters not evaluated in this study. One such suggestion is to examine another vertebra with less soft tissue attenuation.

The final conclusion on the application of the Uncollimated Compton Profile Method, which has been shown to be successful in two-phase flow in pipes, to osteoporosis awaits experimental development. The results of this study indicate that the method is capable of detecting the early trabecular bone losses, that no other available screening method can obtain, for a device cost of less than $ 50,000. This modest cost makes the method feasible for screening. The early detection would allow preventative measures such as estrogen treatments to be initiated and the painful and debilitating effects of osteoporosis to be avoided for some of the more than 6 million persons in the U.S. alone.

REFERENCES

1. Vose, G.P., 1969, Radiology, 93:841-844.
2. Colbert,C., and Bachtell,R.S., Non-Invasive Measurements of Bone Mass and Their Clinical Application, CRC Press, 1981.
3. Ardran, G.M., 1947, Br. J. Radiol., 27:107-109.
4. Meema, H.E., and Meema, S., Non- Invasive Measurements of Bone Mass and Their Clinical Application, CRC Press, 1981.
5. Goldsmith, N.F., Johnston, J.O., Ury,H., Vose, G.P., and Colbert, C., 1971, J. Bone Joint Surg., 53A(1):83-100.
6. Gershon-Cohen,J., Cherry, N.H., and Boehnke, M., 1958, Radiat. Res., 8:509-515.

7. Cameron, J.R., and Sorenson,J. , 1963, Science, 142:230-232.
8. Cameron, J.R., Grant,R., and MacGregor, R., 1962, Radiology, 78:117.
9. Sorenson, J.A., and Cameron, J.R.,1970, Symposium Ossium, Churchill Livingston.
10. Smith, D.M., Johnston, C.C., and Yu, P., 1972, JAMA, 219(3):325-329.
11. Dequeker, J., Roh,Y.S., Dessel, D.V., Gautama, K. and Burssens,1973, J. Belge Rhum. Med. Phys., 28:293-301 .
12. Riggs, B.L., Wahner, H.W., Dunn, W.L., Mazess, .R.B., Offord, K.P., and Melton, L.J., 1981, J. Clin. Invest., 67:328-335.
13. Mazess, R.B., 1979, Calcif. Tissue Int., 28:89-92.
14. Peppler, W.W., and Mazess, R.B., 1981, Calcif. Tissue Int., 33:353-359 .
15. Krolner, B., and Pors Nielsen, S.,1982, Clin. Sci., 62:329-336 .
16. Ruesegger, P., Elsasser, U., Anliker, M., Gnehm, H., Kind, H., and Prader, A., 1976, Radiology, 121:93-97.
17. Genant, H., Boyd, D., Rosenfeld, D., Abols, Y., and Cann, C.E.,1981, Non-Invasive Measurements of Bone Mass and Their Clinical Application, CRC Press.
18. Cann, C.E., Genant, H.K., Ettinger, B., and Gordan, G.S., 1980, JAMA, 244(18):2056-2059.
19. International Workshop on Bone and Soft Tissue Densitometry Using Computed Tomography, J Comput. Assist. Tomogr., 3(6):847-862,1979.
20. Bradley, J.G., Huang H.K., and Ledley, R.S., 1978, Radiology, 128:103-107 .
21. Lee, B.C.P, Kazam, E., and Newman, A.D., 1978, Radiology, 128:95-102.
22. Grossman,Z.D., Wistow, B.W., Wallinga, H.A., and Heitzman, E.R., 1976, Radiology, 121:369-373.
23. Reich, N.E., Seidelmann, F.E., Tubbs, R.R., MacIntyre,W.J., Meaney,T.F., Alfidi, R.J. and Pepe, R.G., 1976, Am. J. Roentgenol., 127:593-594.
24. Odeblad, E., and Norhagen, A.,1956, ACTA Radiol., 45:161-167.
25. Guzzardi,R., and Mey, M.,1981, Phys. Med. Biol., 26(1):155-161.
26. Stalp,J.T, and Mazess, R.B., 1980, Med. Phys., 7(6):723-726.
27. Kerr, S.A., Kouris, K., Webber, C.E., and Kennett,T.J., 1980, Phys. Med. Biol., 25(6):1037-1047.
28. Huddleston, A.L., Agarwal,S.K., Friesen, E.J., and Bhaduri, D.,1978, Appl. Radiol., 7:232-237.
29. Hazan, G., Leichter, I., Loewinger, E., and Weinreb, A., 1977, Phys. Med. Biol., 22(6):1073-1084.
30. Webber,C.E., and Kennett, T.J, Phys. Med. Biol., 21(5):760-769,1976.
31. Kennett, T.J., and Webber, C.E., 1976, Phys. Med. Biol., 21(5):770-780.
32. Ullman, J., IEEE Trans. Nucl. Sci., NS-23(1):599-605,1976.
33. Clark, R.L., and Van Dyk, G., 1973, Phys. Med. Biol., 18(4):532-539.
34. Garnett, E.S., Kennett, T.J., Kenyon, D.B., and Webber, C.E.,1973, Radiology, 106:209-212.
35. Kennett,T.J., Garnett, E.S., and Webber, C.E., Journal De L'Assoc. Canadienne Des Radiologistes, 23:168-170, 1972.
36. Reiss, K., and Schuster, W., 1972, Radiology, 102:613-617.
37. Jacobs, A.M., Towe,B.C., and Harkess, J.E., 1979, Proc. SPIE Med. Imaging II, 206.
38. Battista, J.J., and Bronskill, M.J.,1978, Phys. Med. Biol.,23:1-23.

39. Battista,J.J., Santon,L.W., and Bronskill, M.J., 1977, Phys. Med. Biol., 22(2):229-244.
40. Walford,G.V.,and Fenton, T.R., 1975, IEEE Trans. Nuc. Sci., NS-22:428-436 .
41. Farmer,F.T., and Collins,M.P., 1974, Phys. Med. Biol., 19(6):808-818.
42. Farmer,F.T., and Collins,M.P., 1971, Phys. Med. Biol., 16(4):577-586.
43. Lale, P.G., 1968, Radiology, 90:510-517.
44. Lale, P.G., 1959, Phys. Med. Biol., 4:159-167.
45. Jacobs, A.M., 1979, First Report on the Evaluation of Gamma-ray Scattering Techniques for the Tomographic Evaluation of Water Two-Phase Density Distributions, EG&G Consultant Agreement No. K-8118-TKP-70 -79, State College, Pennsylvania.
46. Jacobs,A.M., "Research Proposal Submitted to EG&G Idaho, Inc.",1980.
47. Jacobs,A.M., Non-Invasive Studies of Body Chemistry, Raven Press(in press).
48. Urist,M.R.,Gurvey,M.S., and Fareed,D.O., Osteoporosis, Grune & Stratton, 1970.
49. Woodard,H.Q., 1962, Health Physics,8:513-517.
50. Blanton,P.L., and Biggs, N.L., 1968, Am. J. Phys. Anthrop., 29:39-44.
51. Watt, D.E., 1975, Br. J. Radiol., 48:265-274.
52. Atkinson, P.J., 1967, Calc. Tiss. Res., 1:24-32.
53. Clayton, S.K., 1983, Master's Thesis, University of Florida.
54. Anghaie, S., Ph.D. dissertation, The Pennsylvania State Univ, 1982.
55. Anghaie, S., Finlon,K., and Jacobs, A.M.,1983, Proceedings of the Third Multi-Phase Flow Heat Transfer Symposium, Miami(in press).
56. Wahner, H.W., 1982, Appl. Radiol, 9:154-159.

AUTOMATED TISSUE CHARACTERIZATION WITH NMR IMAGING

DOUGLAS A. ORTENDAHL, NOLA M. HYLTON, LEON KAUFMAN, LAWRENCE E. CROOKS

Radiologic Imaging Laboratory, University of California, San Francisco
400 Grandview Drive, South San Francisco, CA 94080

INTRODUCTION

Nuclear magnetic resonance imaging is a rapidly evolving modality which has aroused great excitement in the medical community (1,2). NMR has shown excellent soft tissue contrast without the necessity of intravenous contrast agents. It also has the advantage of using no ionizing radiation.

Unlike CT which images electron density only, NMR images are a function of 4 different parameters: hydrogen density (since we limit this discussion to proton NMR), relaxation times T1 and T2 and flow. In our spin echo technique the signal intensity is given by

$$I = N(H) f(v) \exp(-TE/T2) [1-\exp(-TR/T1)] \qquad (1)$$

where N(H) is the spin density which we will call hydrogen density, H; f(v) is a function of flow; TE and TR are acquisition parameters, echo delay and repetition interval, respectively. It is this multiparametric feature which provides the high soft-tissue contrast. Changes in contrast are a reflection of change in one or more of these four parameters. In addition contrast can be altered by changing the acquisition parameters as clearly shown in Figure 1. In particular note the better contrast for resolving the multiple sclerosis lesions at longer TE and TR values. Routinely several images of the same section are acquired with different settings of TE and TR. This in combination with the multiple sections which are obtained provides the physician with a large number of images (50-100 per patient) (3). Properly utilizing that much information will be a significant challenge to the radiologist. In particular it is important that the multi-parametric nature is fully utilized, requiring the use of new techniques to present the data. Some of the advantages of NMR will be lost if images are interpreted strictly as in CT.

As NMR moves into clinical utilization, it is important to begin exploring these techniques. At our institution the thrust of the research program is to fully explore the potential of NMR imaging by examining such areas as acquisition techniques, clinical protocols and computer processing. The superb contrast available with NMR is due primarily to the difference in relaxation times of tissue. This suggests that techniques to extract additional information from the relaxation times may prove fruitful.

One such area is the use of the NMR parameters, primarily the relaxation times, to characterize tissue. Since the first discussion of NMR as an imaging tool there has been speculation on the use of T1 and T2 for pathologic examination (4). In this paper we present early results on the use of the NMR image parameters to produce computer generated maps of the various tissues in the section.

Such a task would be extremely difficult with x-ray CT where only electron density is available to characterize the tissue. With NMR there are four parameters available which makes the task more manageable. Throughout this work the emphasis is on learning what NMR's capabilities are in this area. For this reason techniques of pattern recognition which will be essential in a final version of the program have not yet been emphasized.

The goal of such research is not to replace the radiologist with a computer operator, nor the original images with a computer printout containing the diagnosis, but to provide the physician with the maximum amount of information. This does not necessarily make his job easier, but hopefully the diagnosis will reflect all the available information.

RELAXATION TIMES

The T1 or spin-lattice relaxation time is the time for the spin system to return to equilibrium after being disturbed. This time is highly dependent on local magnetic environment. Typical T1 values in tissue range from 0.2 - 3.0 seconds. The T2 or spin-spin relaxation time is the time for transverse magnetization to decay due to loss of phase coherence after the 90° RF pulse. T2 is always less than T1 and for tissue is 20 - 150 msec.

The considerable interest in tissue characterization by NMR imaging is in part due to early in vitro research which suggested that NMR imaging might differentiate malignant from benign processes. In vitro measurements in rats (4) and humans (5-7) showed differences in T1 and T2 between malignant and benign tissues. Extensive animal work at our institution has studied the NMR characteristics of normal and abnormal tissue in vivo (8-12). This work has shown substantial differences among normal and abnormal tissues. A sample of this work is shown in Figure 2. Substantial differences are observed in the T1 and T2 values. This gives NMR its excellent soft-tissue contrast since hydrogen concentration differences among these tissues account for less than 15%. Neither T1 nor T2 would by itself be able to differentiate each of the tissues but by using both T1 and T2 information all the tissues are distinguishable. It has been found that the primary determinant of the relaxation time is the water content. Investigators in our laboratory have found a rough inverse relationship between water content and the relaxation time for both T1 and T2. In Figure 2 we note considerable scatter among the tumors. This is due to the variation in water content among tumors of different stages of development. Such variation will of course make the determination of malignancy by NMR a very elusive goal. Although there is much scatter in the T1 and T2 values of the tumors, the knowledge of both the T1 and T2 is usually enough to separate them from normal host tissue and other types of lesions such as abcesses and hematomas.

The relaxation times T1 and T2 may be calculated by acquiring images at different values of TE and TR and fitting the data to equation 1. A minimum of 2 images obtained at the same TR and different TE values are needed to determine T2, while two images at different TR values and constant TE are required for T1. Three images would be enough for obtaining both T1 and T2, but four are acquired since first and second echo images are obtained at the same time. The echo delays, TE, are 28 and 56 msec. in our imager. Standard protocols for our system use TR values of .5, 1.0, 1.5 or 2.0 sec.

The accuracy of any tissue mapping system will be determined by the signal/noise of the input parameters. There are two components to this signal/noise: electronic and biologic. In a well designed and

shielded system, the electronic noise is almost entirely due to random
thermal currents in the patient which induce noise in the RF coil.
This noise is independent of the signal and is the same for intensity
images acquired with different TE and TR values but equal averages.
This noise will be propagated into the calculated relaxation time
images. The T1 or T2 signal/noise (T/ΔT) will depend on the value of
the relaxation time and the parameters used in the calculation.

Any viable technique to increase the utility of NMR images must
in general be able to use images obtained for routine clinical purposes. For this reason we have avoided special acquisitions to obtain
images with unusually high signal/noise. An example of the T1 and T2
images obtained routinely in our laboratory is shown in Figure 3. T2
signal/noise is acceptable using spin echos at 28 and 56 msec.
Accuracy could be improved by as much as a factor of two by using a
third echo at 84 msec. (13) This could be done with no increase in
acquisition time, but with the added expense of archiving and reconstructing an additional image for each section. With the multi-
section acquisition technique used, RF irradiations are performed
every 100 msec at a different section before returning to the same
section after time TR. Thus accumulating more than 3 echos would
decrease the number of simultaneous slices.

The T1 image quality in Figure 3 is excellent. Excellent gray-
white contrast is observed. Improving signal/noise beyond what is
shown here would require more averaging and longer imaging time. Our
typical protocols call for TR values of 1.5 or 2.0 sec. which provide the most diagnostically useful images. Multi-section imaging
makes time per section independent of TR. The addition of an acquisition with TR = 0.5 sec allows for the T1 calculation.

A more difficult problem is faced when a biologic variability is
considered. It has already been shown that tumors exhibit significant
variability in T1 and T2 values. While the other types of tissues
shown are more consistent in their T1 and T2 values the size of the
one standard deviation rectangle still demonstrates considerable
variation among different subjects. This is most likely due to
natural differences in hydration. In addition to variation among
subjects there will also be variations in relaxation times over the

image due to natural differences in tissues and partial volume effects for mixtures of tissues. At an organ boundary the intensity will represent the sum of the intensities from each side of the boundary. The resultant calculated relaxation times at that point may well not agree with either type of tissue.

The diagnostic usefulness of the T1 and T2 images in interpreting the NMR images is illustrated in Figure 4. In this case there is no problem identifying the lesion in the left side of the brain. But clinically it is important to determine whether it is edema or hemorrhage. The long T2 is consistent with either diagnosis, the short T1 indicates hemorrhage.

Once T1 and T2 have been determined it is then easy to use equation 1 to solve for hydrogen density. An example of a hydrogen density image is shown in Figure 3. Strictly speaking this is a free hydrogen image since hydrogen bound in proteins and other large molecules will give very weak NMR signals.

TISSUE TYPING ALGORITHM

Ignoring flow for the moment, three parameters, T1, T2, and H, are required to completely determine equation 1. We assume that intensity images are acquired at four settings of TE and TR: I1(TE1, TR1), I2(TE2, TR1), I3(TE1, TR2) and I4(TE2, TR2). If T1, T2 and H are taken as orthogonal basis vectors for a three-dimensional space, then this space is also spanned by I1, I2, I3 and I4. The latter are not orthogonal and are redundant in the sense that three of the intensity images are sufficient to determine T1, T2 and H. In the ideal noiseless case each type of tissue would represent a point in this space. The potential advantage of NMR is apparent when this is compared to x-ray CT where a tissue would be assigned a CT number, just a point in the one-dimensional electron density space.

When noise is introduced, tissues are no longer represented by points, but by three-dimensional probability distribution functions. At this point several simplifying assumptions are made. First this probability function is assumed to be separable. That is the probability density for the ith tissue type is given by:

$$P_i(T_1, T_2, H) = Q_i(T_1)R_i(T_2)S_i(H). \qquad (2)$$

Second, we assume that the probability distribution functions are gaussian. These three-dimensional probability functions P_i will overlap; the major task will be identifying tissue with this overlap.

Most of the contrast that is found with NMR is due to the differences in T1 and T2. Our experience has been that the H image is not particularly useful for tissue discrimination. Since it is a derived image it tends to be much noisier than the intensity images. For that reason instead of using T1, T2 and H as the basis we choose to use T1, T2 and I, one of the intensity images which we typically choose to be either I1 or I3. This basis will span the space but is not orthogonal.

For each tissue type that is to be mapped a template is created consisting of the means and standard deviations of T1, T2 and I: $\mu_i(T1), \sigma_i(T1)$; $\mu_i(T2), \sigma_i(T2)$; $\mu_i(I), \sigma_i(I)$. A unique color is assigned to each tissue type. In principle the template is determined a priori, in practice we have found it necessary to adjust the template to fit the individual case.

In the first pass through the algorithm the T1, T2 and I for each pixel in the image is compared with the template. A match is declared if each of the three parameters is within N standard deviations of the expected mean. N is usually chosen to be 2-4. It is quite likely that more than one tissue will be selected. If this occurs the most likely candidate is selected assuming gaussian distributions by using the expression:

$$[(\mu_i(T1)-T1_j)/\sigma_i(T1)]^2 + [(\mu_i(T2)-T2_j)/\sigma_i(T2)]^2 + [(\mu_i(I)-I_j)/\sigma_i(I)]^2 \qquad (3)$$

where the subscript i refers to the ith tissue type and j refers to the parameter values for the jth pixel. The template which minimizes this expression will maximize the probability density in equation 2.

As a second pass over the image an attempt is made to type pixels which failed to match any of the templates. For each undefined pixel the eight nearest neighbors are polled. If a specified plurality of these are of one tissue then this isolated pixel is also defined to be of that type.

FLOW CHARACTERIZATION

Flow is manifest by NMR in several ways. If the velocity of the

protons is fast (V >20 cm/sec), the excited protons can move out of
the imaging plane before readout will occur. Areas of flow will have
very low intensity. This is shown in Figure 5. At slower velocities
there is not a significant loss of excited nuclei due to exit from the
imaging plane. In this velocity regime it has been shown that NMR
intensity is changed by flow (14-16). At the time of the 90° RF pulse
which rotates the magnetization into the x-y or readout plane, all of
the spins will be in phase with each other. Variations in local
magnetic field due to external sources such as the inhomogeneity of
the main field or internal sources such as the molecular environment
will cause variations in precession frequency which will quickly cause
the precessing protons to become out of phase. Signal intensity
depends on the degree of phase coherence. In the spin echo technique
a 180° pulse at time τ after the 90° pulse will invert the
magnetization and cause refocussing of the phase at time τ after the
180° pulse. This applies to stationary objects. If there is flow
then the Carr-Purcell pulse sequence predicts that complete refocusing
will not occur at the expected time for odd spin echoes, however these
flow effects will cancel for even echoes (17,18). This means that
signal attenuation would be expected for the first echo but not for
the second echo. This has important consequences in terms of
characterizing flow with NMR images. If the first echo signal is
attenuated relative to the second echo then the apparent T2 will be
longer than for the no flow state. If the first echo is depressed so
that its magnitude is less than the second echo, T2 will become
negative, a clearly unphysical state for stationary tissue. This
negative T2 can be used as a signature for flow.

The amount of recovery of the magnetization before the next pulse
repetition is given by $(1-e^{-TR/T1})$. In general full recovery is not
achieved, and therefore the amount of signal obtained will be less
than if the sample were at complete equilibrium. If flow is slow then
protons with full magnetization can move into the imaging volume,
producing more signal than the ones they replace. This has been
called paradoxical enhancement (14). It can provide information about
the direction of flow as shown in Figure 6. In the cephalic and
caudal slice both the aorta and inferior vena cavae (IVC) are dark in
the first echo image as explained above. In the cephalic section the

aorta is greatly enhanced due to the entrance of fully magnetized protons into the imaging volume. Similarly in the caudal slice the IVC is enhanced showing the return flow into the imaging volume.

RESULTS

Tissue Type Maps

As a first example of tissue type maps we show in Figure 7, a patient with a glioma of the brain stem. In this case we are able to map gray and white matter, CSF and the tumor. The gray-white differentiation is quite good. Note the areas of CSF. These maps would normally be displayed in color, but are presented here in black and white.

In Figure 8 is an example of a patient with prostate cancer. The mapping program is able to identify muscle, bladder, fat, marrow in the illium and the tumor. Because of the similarity of marrow and fat we find some marrow in areas of known fat. Because of noise, tumor is seen in areas which are known not to be cancerous. This type of noise is observed in many of the examples shown here.

A multi-slice example is presented in Figure 9. The lower slice was used to develop the signature, labeling gray and white matter along with CSF. This same signature when used two sections higher shows excellent mapping of the gray and white matter. The areas of CSF are also clearly defined. The relatively small amount of CSF present in this section would make it difficult to develop an accurate CSF signature using this section alone.

As a final example of tissue mapping we show in Figure 10 a section through an adult male pelvis. In this case muscle, fat, and bladder are labeled. It was not possible to differentiate signatures between fat and marrow for this patient. A priori knowledge of the location is used in this case to define the fat-like substance in the illium and pelvis as marrow. Below the bladder we are able to identify the seminal vesicles with a unique signature. Again noise causes a scattering of pixels throughout the image to be labeled as a seminal vesicles. Moving down two sections we find that the bladder is no longer easily discerned in the intensity images, but the tissue map is able to pick up a small amount of bladder. Also note that a small amount of seminal vesicle type tissue is identified below the bladder where it would be expected.

Flow Maps

An example of a flow map is presented in Figure 11. In this abdominal section a negative T2 signature is used to label areas of flow in white. Good delineation is seen in the aorta, IVC and hepatic vessels. Some areas of the IVC are missed because the intensity was to low to get a negative T2 signature. For this image the second echo intensity was required to be more than 50 intensity units above that of the first echo before flow was assigned. For a pixel to be a candidate for flow the intensity must be greater than 8% of the maximum intensity in the image. At this threshold noise may mimic flow as is seen in the bowel where random fluctuations produce a second echo intensity larger than the first.

CONCLUSION

These results indicate promise for tissue characterization with NMR imaging. However, significant problems remain. The spread in T1 and T2 values makes patient independent signatures difficult. Pattern recognition techniques may prove useful in adjusting the tissue type templates for the individual patient. Readily identified tissue such as muscle or fat might be used as standards in this adjustment process. Pattern recognition could be employed to reduce the extraneous noise in the maps due to isolated pixels. Pattern recognition was not emphasized in this work because it was desired to see what could be done on the basis of NMR alone.

The flow maps also are in need of additional research. Software could be written to trace vessels from one section to another. By following the vessel to the outer section paradoxical enhancement would allow direction of flow to be determined.

ACKNOWLEDGEMENTS

This work is supported in part by Diasonics (NMR), Inc. and by USPHS Research Career Development Award GM00493 from the NIGMS.

REFERENCES
1. Nuclear Magnetic Resonance Imaging in Medicine. Edited by L Kaufman, LE Crooks and AR Margulis. Igaku-Shoin, New York, 1981.
2. Clinical Magnetic Resonance Imaging. Edited by AR Margulis CB Higgins, L Kaufman and LE Crooks. Radiology Reseach and Education Foundation, San Francisco, 1983.
3. Crooks LE, Ortendahl DA, Kaufman L, et al. Clinical Efficiency of Nuclear Magnetic Resonance Imaging. Radiology 146:123, 1983.
4. Damadian R. Tumor detection by NMR. Science 161:1151, 1971.
5. Damadian R, Zaner K, Hor D, et al. Human tumors detected by NMR. Proc Nat Acad Sci USA 71:1471, 1974.
6. Medina D, Hazlewood CJ, Cleveland, et al. NMR studies on human dysplasias and neoplasms. J Nat Cancer Inst 54:813, 1975.
7. Eggleston JC, Saryan LA, Cxeisler JL, et al. NMR studies of several experimental and human malignant tumors. Cancer Res 33:2156, 1973.
8. Hansen G, Crooks LE, Davis PL, et al. In Vivo Imaging of the Rat Anatomy with Nuclear Magnetic Resonance. Radiology 136:695, 1980.
9. Herfkens R, Davis PL, Crooks LE, et al. NMR Imaging of the Abnormal Life Rat and Correclation with Tissue Characteristics. Radiology 141:211, 1981.
10. Davis PL, Kaufman L, Crooks LE, et al. Detectability of Hepatomas in Rat Livers by Nuclear Magnetic Resonance. Investigative Radiology 16:354, 1981.
11. In Nuclear Magnetic Resonance Imaging in Medicine, Edited by L Kaufman, LE Crooks and AR Margulis, Igaku Shoin, New York, New York, 1981: Pl Davis, L Kaufman, LE Crooks and AR Margulis: NMR Characteristics of Normal and Abnormal Rat Tissues, Chapter 5.
12. Davis PL, Sheldon PE, Kaufman L, et al. Nuclear Magnetic Resonance Imaging of Mammary Adenocarcinomas in the Rat. Cancer 51:433, 1983.
13. Ortendahl DA et al. Signal to Noise in Derived NMR Images. Submitted for publication.
14. Crooks LE, Sheldon PE, Kaufman L, et al. Quantification of Obstructions in Vessels by Nuclear Magnetic Resonance. IEEE Trans. Nucl. Sci. NS-29:1181, 1982.
15. Kaufman L, Crooks LE, Sheldon PE, et al. Evaluation of NMR Imaging for Detection and Quantification of Obstructions in Vessels. Investigative Radiology 17:554, 1983.
16. Kaufman L, Crooks LE, Sheldon PE, et al. The Potential Impact of Nuclear Magnetic Resonance Imaging on Cardiovascular Diagnosis. Circulation 67:251, 1983.
17. Carr HY, Purcell EM. Effects of diffusion on free precession in nuclear magnetic resonance experiments. Phys Rev 94:630, 1954.
18. Singer JR. NMR diffusion and flow measurements and an introduction to spin phase graphing. J Phys E (Sci Instrum) 11:281, 1978.

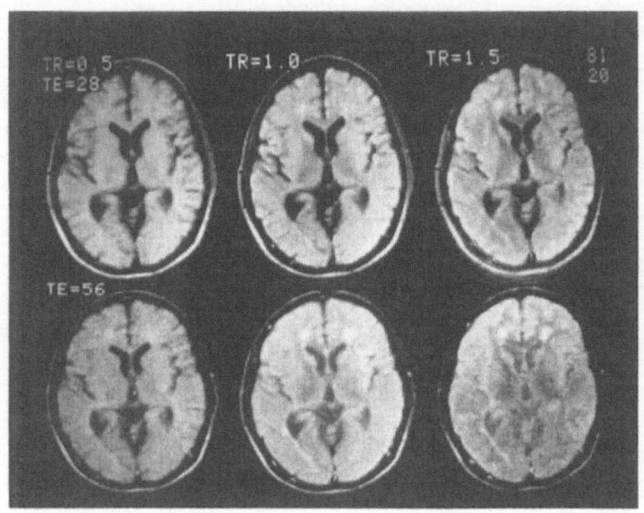

FIGURE 1. Images acquire at different values of TE and TR for a patient with multiple sclerosis. Lesion contrast is best at long TR and TE.   Note how contrast between CSF and brain is lost at TR = 1.5 sec, TE = 56 ms.

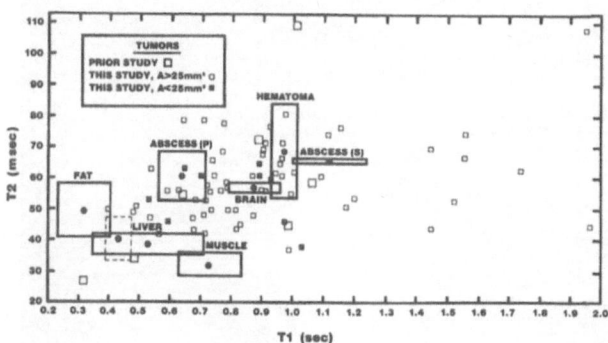

FIGURE 2. A plot of T1 vs. T2 for various normal and abnormal tissue. By using both T1 and T2 information, most tissues become separable. The rectangles represent one standard deviation.

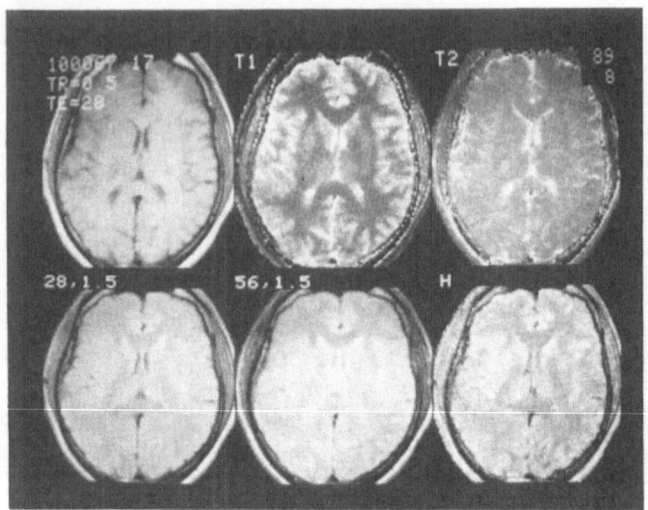

FIGURE 3. Spin echo, T1, T2 and hydrogen images for a normal
volunteer. Excellent gray-white contrast is seen in spin echo and T1
images. T2 shows no gray-white differentiation while hydrogen density
shows some contrast.

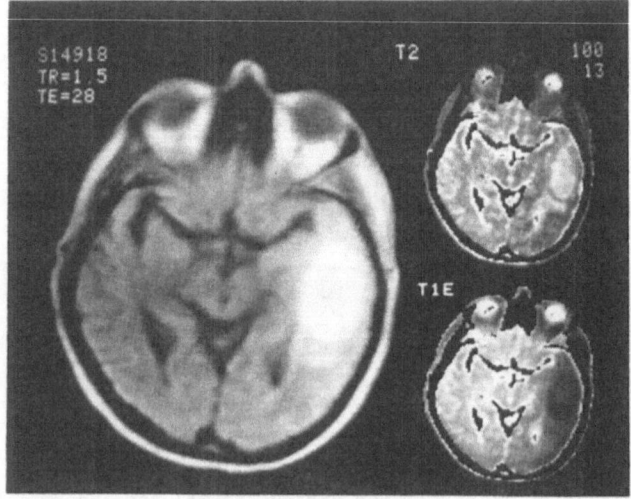

FIGURE 4. A patient with a cerebral infarction of the left temporal
lobe. The long T2 and shortened T1 are consistent with a diagnosis of
hemorrhage.

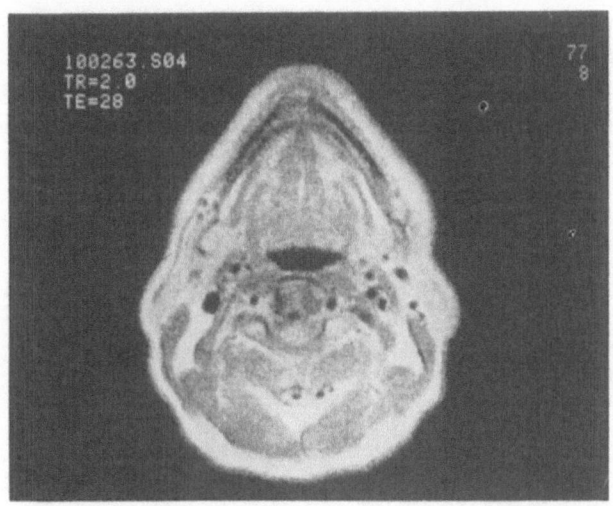

FIGURE 5. In this high resolution image of the neck the vessels are
clearly shown as areas of low intensity. Occlusion of the internal
carotid artery is seen on the left side.

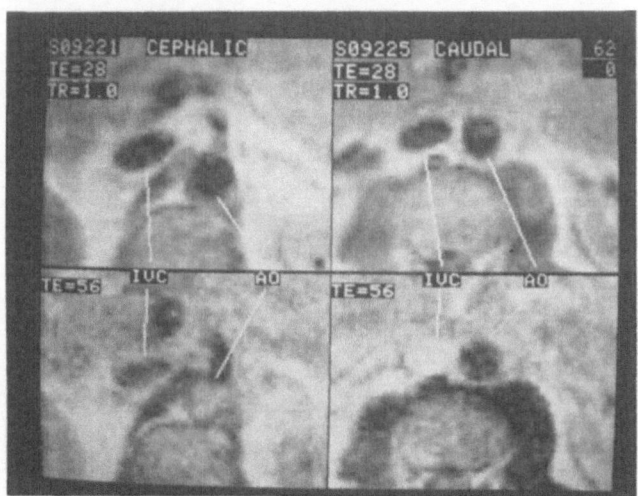

FIGURE 6. Flow direction sensitivity is demonstrated in these
abdominal sections. Enhancement of the aorta in the second echo of
the uppermost section shows blood flow into the imaging volume. The
IVC enhances in the lower section showing return flow.

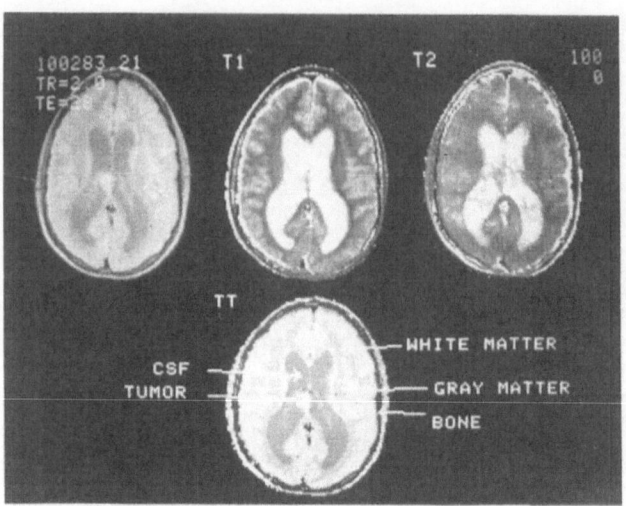

FIGURE 7. Tissue type map of a patient with glioma of the brain stem. The tumor is well differentiated in the map, as is the gray and white matter.

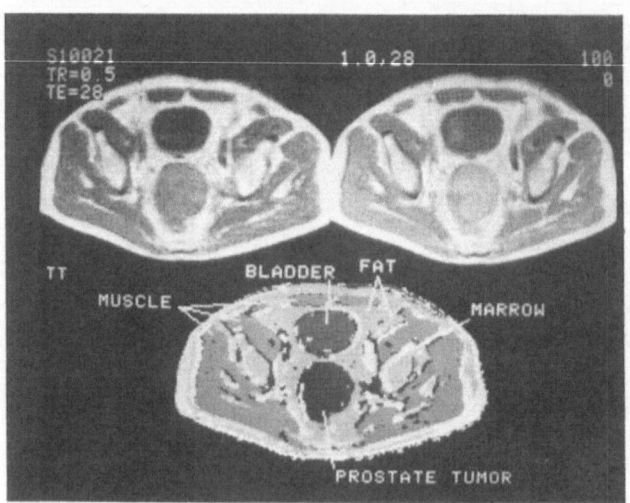

FIGURE 8. Tissue type map of a patient with prostate cancer. Muscle, fat, and marrow in the illium are well defined. Bladder and tumor are also well defined.

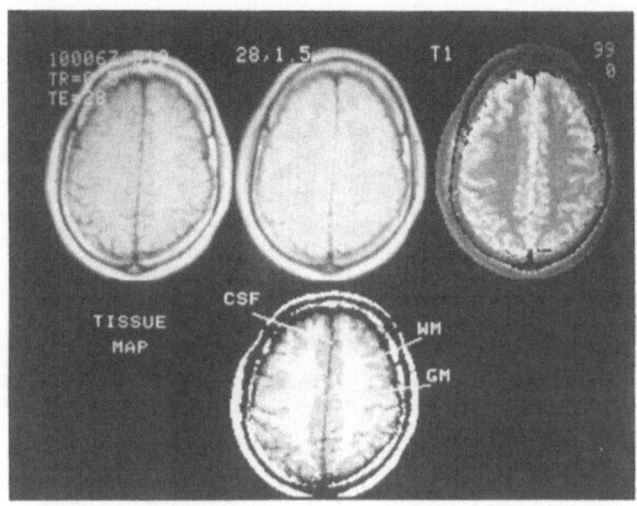

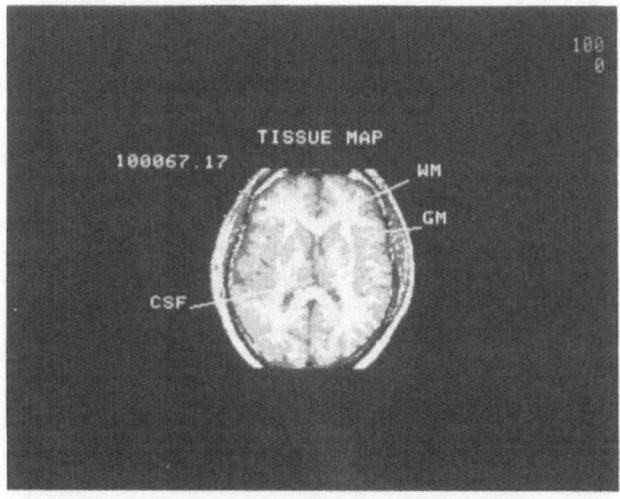

FIGURE 9. Two sections through the brain separated by 1.6 cm. The lower slice is the same section as Figure 3. Gray and white matter are well seen in both slices. Note the excellent definition of CSF in the upper slice using a signature developed for the lower section.

492

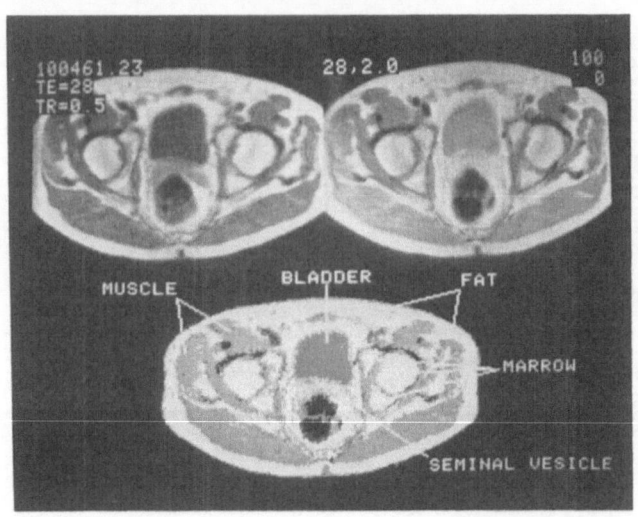

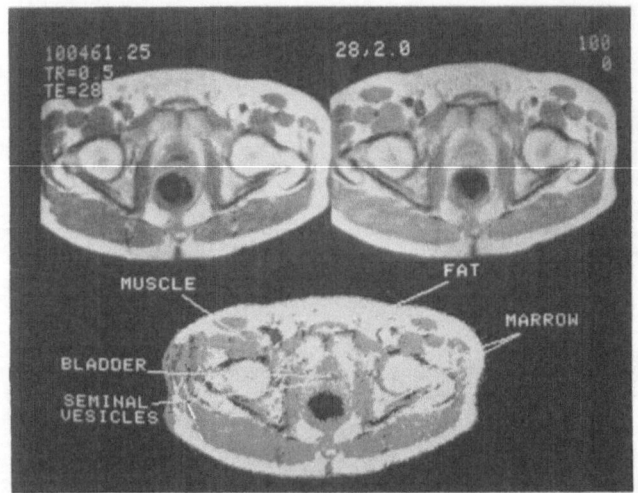

FIGURE 10. Two sections through the male pelvis separated by 1.6 cm. Bladder and seminal vesicles are well defined in the map. The similarity of marrow and fat made them indistinguishable. Marrow is shown by location of fatty tissue in the illium and pelvis. In the lower section, the mapping program is able to show both bladder and seminal vesicles even though they are more difficult to appreciate in the intensity images.

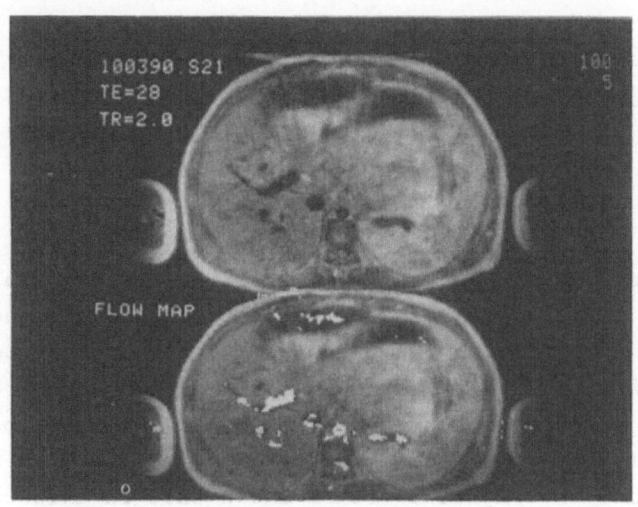

FIGURE 11. A negative T2 signature for flow is used to map the areas of flow. Good definition of the IVC, aorta and hepatic vessels is observed.

ZONAL PARAMETRIC IMAGING

T. SANDOR, L.M. BOXT, D.P. HARRINGTON, ·W.B. HANLON

ABSTRACT

A new method is described that modifies the original concept of parametric or functional imaging. While the conventional parametric image replaces a temporal sequence of images with a single static image based upon a selected parameter, in the new approach fixed zonal areas and bands are established within the imaged organ, and the mean value for each zone is computed. It is shown that in this way parametric images can be quantified and objectively compared. Examples for various organs are given.

1. INTRODUCTION

Examinations utilizing sequential images are increasing in number in radiology. Most of them are originated by nuclear medicine, angiography, ultrasonography and computerized tomography. The studies may be classified arbitrarily into three major categories:

1. Perfusion analyses that follow the time sequence of the injected contrast medium into a selected organ, in order to assess the extent, degree or rate of contrast propagation and in turn blood flow characteristics,

2. Image processing related to the determination of shape and function of selected organs and their changes with time,

3. Image principal component analysis; this is an experimental technique in medical image analysis that computes enhanced images or features from the original image sequence via the Karhunen Loeve transformation [1]. The principal components correspond to the eigen vectors of the image covariance matrix. As a result of this transformation the information content of the images is redistributed among the principal components in such a way that

the first few components corresponding to the highest eigenvalues contain most of the information, and the remaining components consist mainly of noise.

Due to technical developments of the past few years, real time angiographic imaging, in which the end product is a time series of digital images, has become common in radiology departments. Since the second generation of digital subtraction equipment includes a dedicated computer, an effort to quantify perceptual observations, which describe diagnostic properties of the visualized organ or vasculature has become obvious. This could be achieved if the quality of the images would be equivalent to that of the cine angiographic images. The commercially available digital subtraction equipment, however, at least until now, has not exceeded the 512x512 image matrix size, a resolution that corresponds in the case of a 25 cm image intensifier with a 1.25 magnification factor to approximately 0.4 mm in the object space. This shows clearly that in the image intensifier-video camera combination, in which a high quality image intensifier's resolution is 4 line pairs per millimeter, the video system represents the resolution bottle neck. Consequently, the studies requiring the assessment of fine image detail, such as blood vessel analysis in terms of percent stenosis or small changes in vessel diameter, are not suitable for most of the currently available digital subtraction equipment. This type of sequential image analysis, that can be assigned to the second category in the above classification, is best performed with cinedensitometry, where the scanning resolution compared to a video system can be increased by about a factor of four considering 35 mm cinefilm as image recording medium.

Low resolution, however, is much less of a hindrance for perfusion studies as demonstrated by the analyses performed in nuclear medicine [2].

Quantification of perfusion can be important for various organs. The most commonly investigated organs are the kidney, the brain, the heart, the spleen, as wellas tumors at various locations. Perhaps, the simplest approach to quantify perfusion is to position an analyzing window over the area to be studied, for instance, over a region of a CT scan of the brain, integrate the CT numbers over the window and follow this procedure through the time sequence of the images. The result of such a computation is a dye dilution curve. While these curves can be shown to be different for different organs, or even within the same organ, it is very hard to extract diagnostically significant information from them. Furthermore, using only a few analyzing windows over an organ, will leave a vast amount of information imbedded in the imagery untapped.

To obviate this, the concept of functional or parametric images was introduced into nuclear medicine by Kaikara et al in 1969 [3], and the technique was later implemented to radiographic images by Tasto, Hoehne and others [4-7]. Such images are, in general, two dimensional pictorial representations of three dimensional data sets, where the third dimension is usually time. In other words, the end result of this picture processing method is a new static image that condenses information from a time sequence as a function of a single parameter, that can be the arrival time of the contrast, the maximum opacification, the area under the washout curve, the variance within the pixel sequence, etc. This information is computed for each pixel of the image sequence, thus the parametric image utilizes the whole image area. A schematic presentation of the principle is shown in Figure 1.

This concept has, however, one shortcoming: the substrate for analysis is digitized imagery, but the product is an analog image. Therefore, the physician when making his diagnosis must again subjectively interpret an analog image. This method should work very well in the case of gross abnormalities, but cannot be relied upon for identification of subtle changes. (At present we do not even know what the "normal" pattern is for the parametric imagery of various organs.)

Extracting quantifiable diagnostic information from radiologic images requires a feature extractor, whose purpose is to reduce the images by measuring certain characteristic

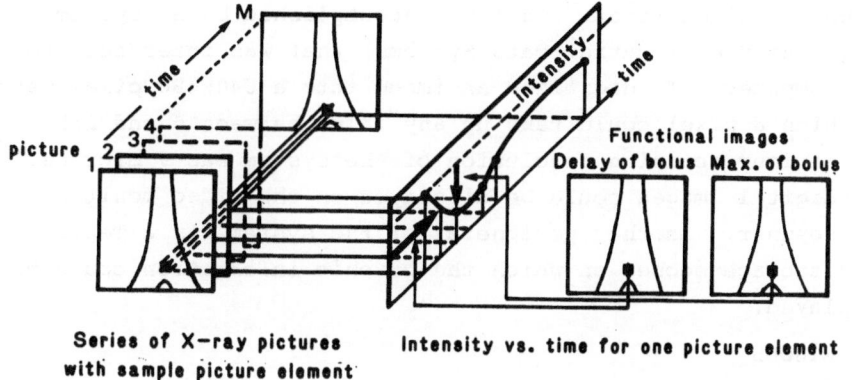

Series of X-ray pictures
with sample picture element

Intensity vs. time for one picture element

FIGURE 1. The principle of parametric imaging.

features in them. These features should then be passed to a
classifier, in order to evaluate the features and classify the
cases into normal or abnormal categories.

Since the conventional parametric images are analog, the
above procedures cannot be applied to them. To obviate this
shortcoming, we have expanded the concept of functional images:
Our method generates a new representation, in which fixed size
zonal areas are established within the boundaries of the
selected organ's image and the mean values of the respective
zones are computed. From these data new parametric images
("zonal parametric images") are computed. Features from these
images in terms of different parameters can be represented in
graphic form that can be used for further computations.

2. EQUIPMENT

Image sequences used in this study have been generated with
different imaging modalities, such as standard digital subtraction
angiography (Philips DVI), CT headscanning (Siemens Somatom-2),
conventional 35 mm cineangiocardiography and fundus photography
(Zeiss). Those images, which were obtained in digital form,
were fed into a VAX 11/780 computer for further analysis. The
imagery obtained with cineangiography and the fundus camera had

to be digitized first.   This was accomplished by an EyeCom
image analyzer (Spatial Data Systems) that was interfaced to
the computer.   It digitized an image into a 640x480 pixel matrix,
in which a pixel could take up any value between 0 and 255.
The maximum scanning resolution of the system was 9 microns.
The digital images could be displayed on the video monitor of
the scanner.   Another peripheral of the system was a Tektronix
4014 storage scope, on which the graphic information could be
displayed.

3. METHODS

In order to implement the method, a grid system specific to
the particular organ to be studied was designed in order to
overlay it on the organ's image.   In the case of the kidney,
for instance, where the cortical area may be judged more
significant than the medulla, the grid system shown in Figure
2 has been developed.   This grid contains 6 bands with 20
subdivisions each.   The three outermost bands have the same
total width as any one of the inner bands.   At present, the
operator traces the outer contour of the organ, marks the
cephalic and caudal poles of the pattern, and the computer then
plots the grid superimposed on the organ's image displayed on
the screen of the EyeCom image analyzer.

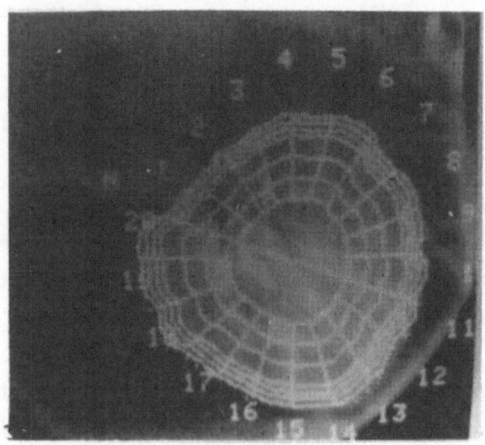

FIGURE 2. Grid designed for renal studies.

The program then computes zonal parametric images, with the following parameters: the maximum contrast density of the zone, the arrival time of the maximum contrast for each zone, the area under the zonal dilution curve and finally the variance for each zone. The computations can be done with or without subtraction, that is, a masked image without contrast may be subtracted from the rest of the sequence.

The results of the computations for each parameter are presented in graphic form (Fig. 3) on the screen of a Tektronix 4014 storage scope. In addition to the four parameters, the mean washout curve of the whole organ plus and minus one standard deviation are computed for all the zones and plotted.

Inspection of the display clearly indicates that the graphic representation of the data in the present form is too congested. There are six curves for each parameter and their assessment would not be straightforward even if the congestion of the display would be obviated. Two further procedures have been developed in order to make the diagnostic significance of these curves more appreciable and more quantitative. One is for the individual assessment of the case to be studied, the other is for group comparison. The former is an added pictorial representation of the results: from the trend shown by the curves or from some unusual sudden changes that can be either noticed or extracted by statistical methods, some abnormal functioning of the organ can be suspected. To correlate graphic and pictorial information and to verify the results visually, the graphic data (feature vector) (Fig. 3), the zonal parametric images as well as a selected contrast-filled image from the sequence can be displayed simultaneously (Fig. 4). This approach has been found very efficient, and is expected to improve the physician's ability to correlate qualitative and quantitative diagnostic information.

In the second procedure, which is currently developed, the shape and similarity of zonal parametric images are assessed for a normal patient group. If such zonal patterns are persistent, that is, if a feature vector can be established, then the method can be used as an objective diagnostic tool

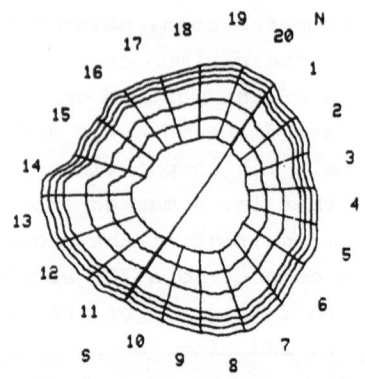

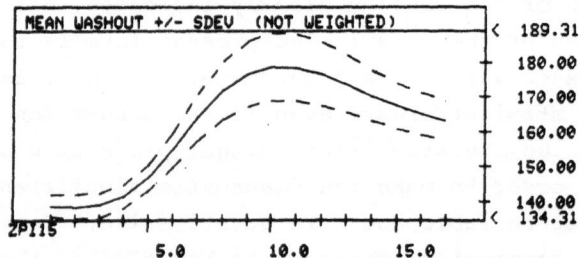

FIGURE 3. a) Zonal graphic information obtained from a renal
study. Top: grid overlaid on renal image; bottom: mean
washout curve computed for the whole organ versus time.

to delineate normal and abnormal populations.

To facilitate the comparison of diagnostic cases with the
normal group, the following model has been designed: Let the
number of patients in the control group be N, and let the zonal
parametric image be divided into RxC subdivisions, where R and
C denote the number of subdivisions and bands, respectively.
Then for each patient a matrix, {M(P)}' can be defined, so that
the general element of the matrix, $M(P)'_{ij}$ represents the
computed value of the zonal parametric image of parameter P,
for the ith subdivision within the jth band (i=1,2,...,R and
j=1,2,...,C).

To combine the parametric images into a homogenous group,

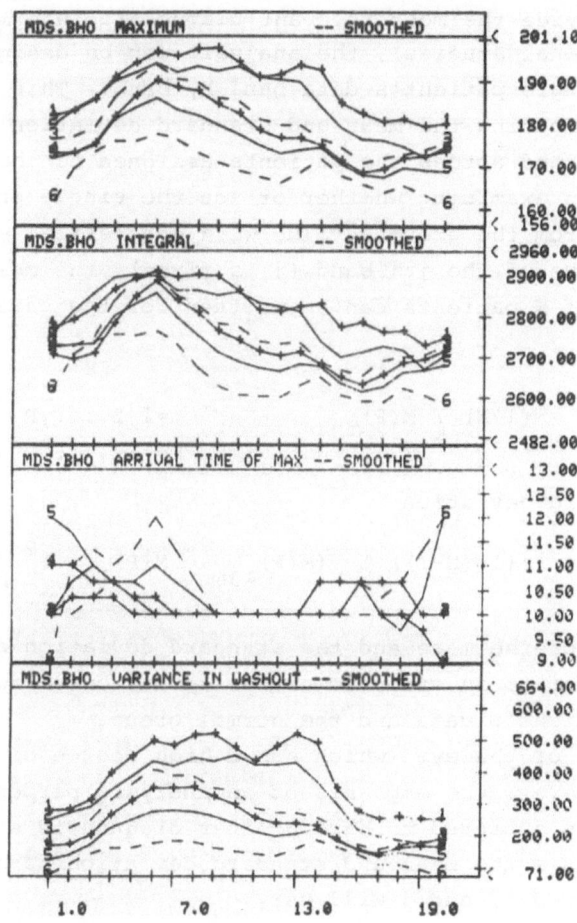

FIGURE 3. b) Zonal graphic information obtained from a renal
study. Plot of zonal parametric means against zone number.
The curves are labelled according to band numbers.

they have to be normalized, first. The normalization is performed
by dividing all elements of the matrix by $\sum_{i}\sum_{j} M(P)'_{ij}$; for the
new matrix, $\{M(P)\}$ that results from this procedure, $\sum_{i}\sum_{j} M(P)_{ij}=1$.

If it is assumed that the band structure of a zonal grid

system may provide the most relevant diagnostic information
(such as for renal studies), the analysis can be designed by
comparing a single patient's data band by band. This can be
achieved by computing the mean and standard deviation of the
data for each band across the patients assigned to the normal
group, and then examining whether or not the single patient's
data differs from the group's value with statistical significance.
Thus in the case of the jth band (j is fixed), the mean of the
normal group of N patients can be written for the parameter
P as

$$M(P)_{ij.} = (1/N) \sum_{k} M(P)_{ijk} \qquad \begin{aligned} &i=1,2,\ldots,R \\ &k=1,2,\ldots,N \end{aligned}$$

and the standard deviation

$$(SD)_{ij} = \left[(1/(N-1)) \sum_{k} (M(P)_{ijk} - M(P)_{ij.})^2 \right]^{\frac{1}{2}}$$

The values of the mean and the standard deviation are plotted
as a function of i, in order to assess deviations between the
individual patient's data and the normal group.

In the case of the eye (which has a high degree of circular
symmetry), however, the emphasis of an analysis perpendicular
to the bands is expected to have greater diagnostic significance.
For such analysis the mean and standard deviation have to be
defined for fixed i, and j will vary.

Such dichotomy in the analysis may be required not only across
different organs, but across different zonal parametric images.
For instance, the analysis of zonal parametric images referring
to maximum contrast may be considered optimal by using the band
mode, and for the zonal parametric imaging associated with
the arrival time, the radial mode may be needed.

4. RESULTS

In the case of intravenous subtraction angiography, nine
intravenous renal subtraction studies were selected, and
subjected to normalized grouping. The results of the analysis
for the four parameters can be seen in Figs. 5(a,b,c,d). The

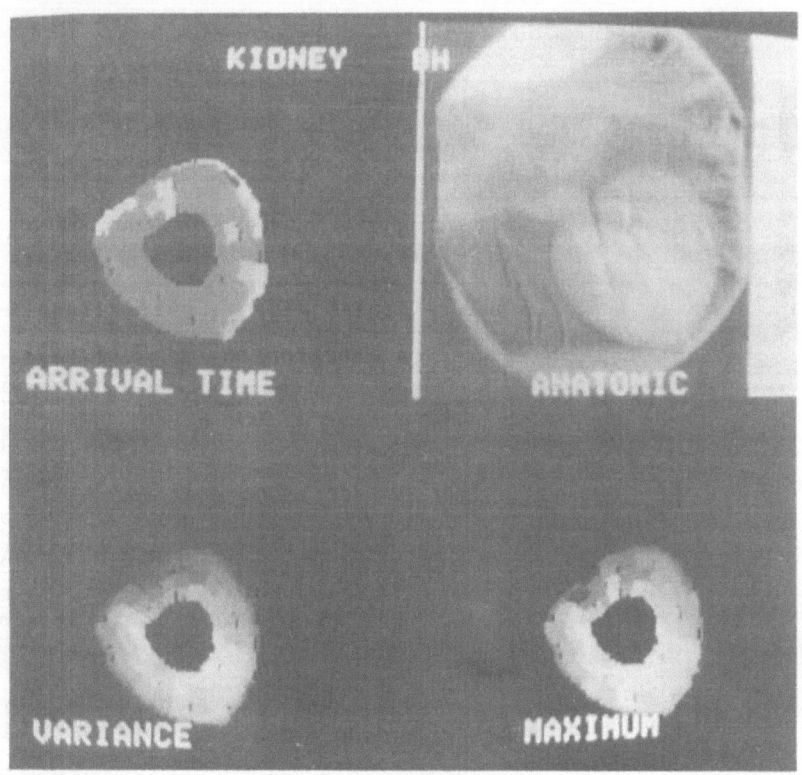

FIGURE 4. Pictorial representation of zonal graphic results shown in Fig. 3 for three parameters accompanied by a selected contrast-filled image labelled anatomic, as seen on the video display.

bands are numbered from the cortical area inward, and the subdivision numbers start at the caudal position and proceed clockwise (see Fig. 3). Each of these zonal parametric images appear to have a pattern, but these patterns differ from each other.

An example of the graphic and pictorial zonal parametric information in an intravenous renal study selected from the above group has already been shown in Figs. 3 and 4. The latter contains only three zonal parametric images, the

504

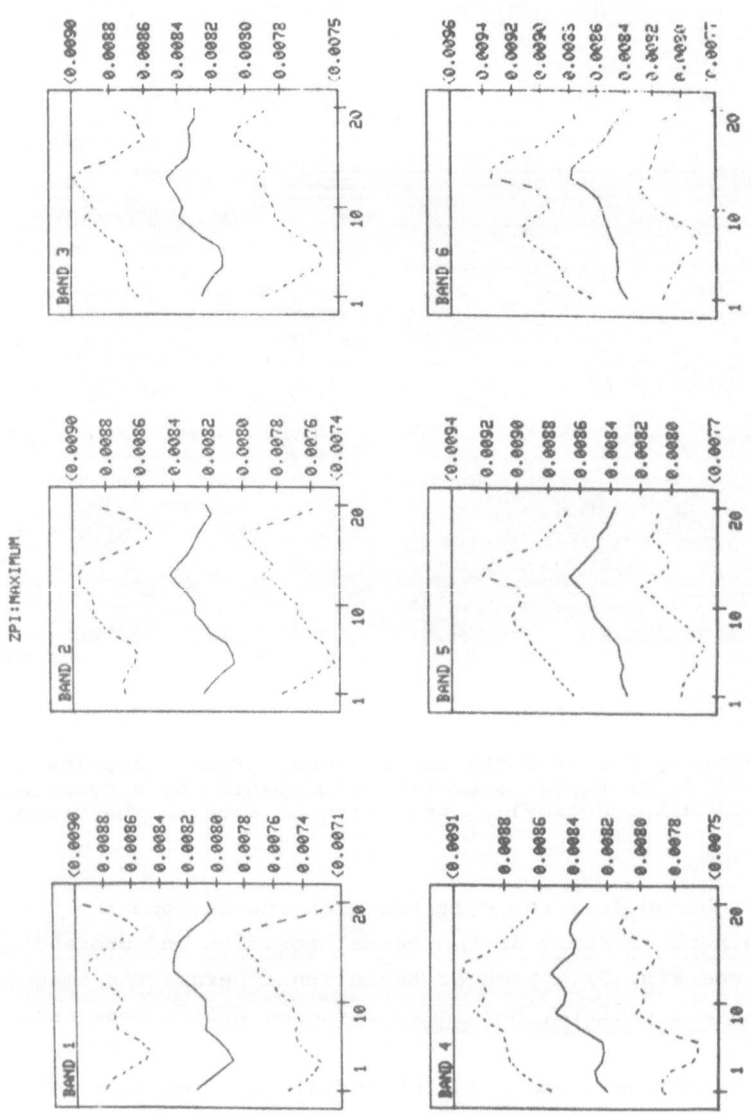

Figure 5. a) Combined data for nine normal renal studies. Parameter: maximum of zones. Abscissa: zone number. Ordinate: arbitrary units. Solid line indicates mean value, dotted lines represent mean +/- one standard deviation.

505

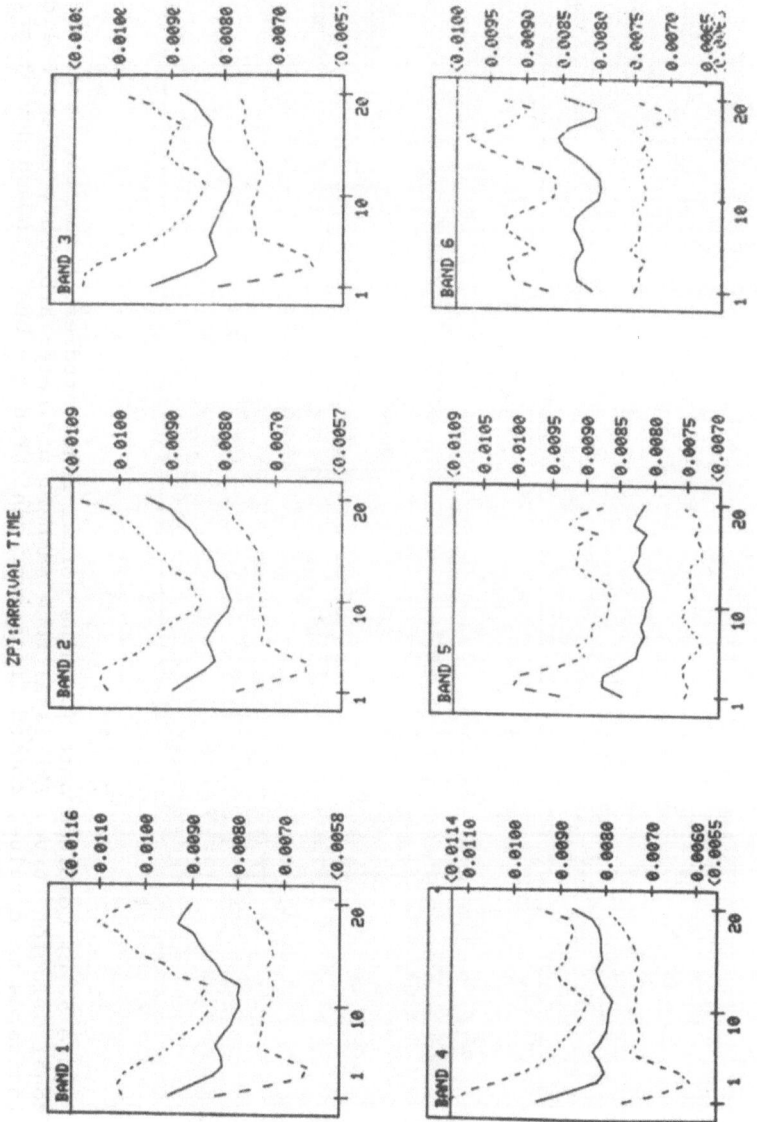

Figure 5. b) Combined data for nine normal renal studies. Parameter: arrival time of zonal washout maximum. Abscissa: zone number. Ordinate: arbitrary units. Solid line indicates mean value, dotted lines represent mean +/- one standard deviation.

506

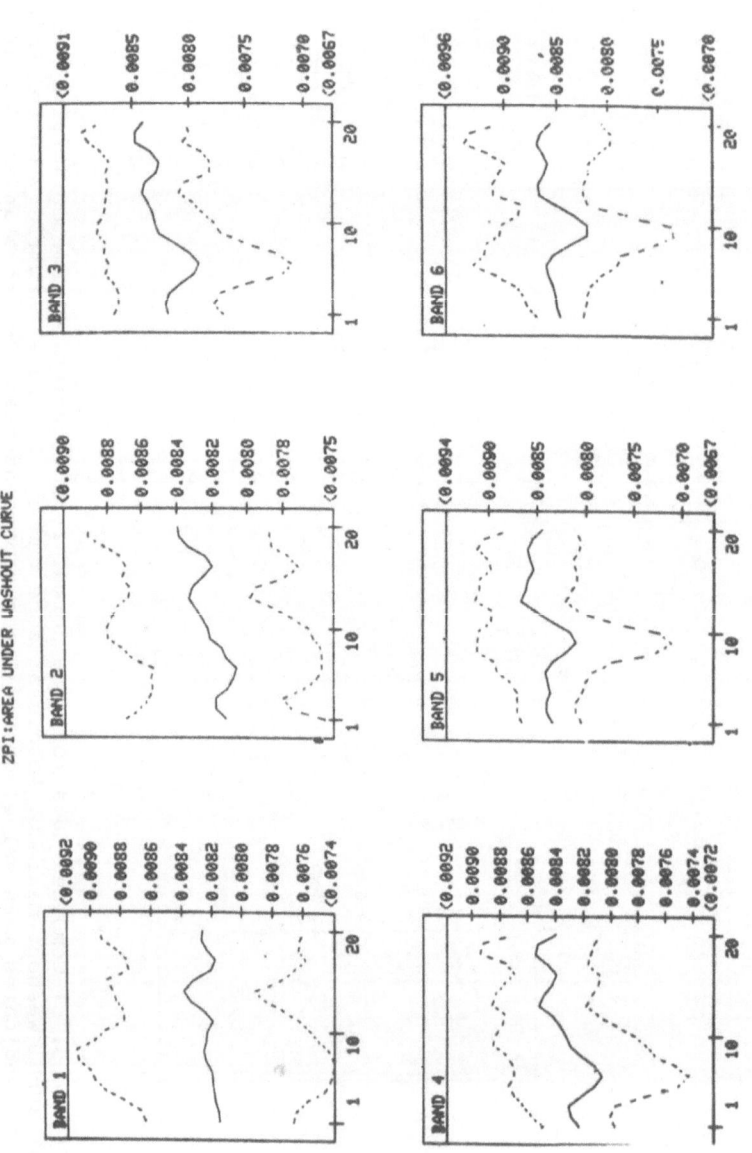

Figure 5. c) Combined data for nine normal renal studies. Parameter: area under zonal dilution curve. Abscissa: zone number. Ordinate: arbitrary units. Solid line indicates mean value, dotted lines represent mean +/- one standard deviation.

507

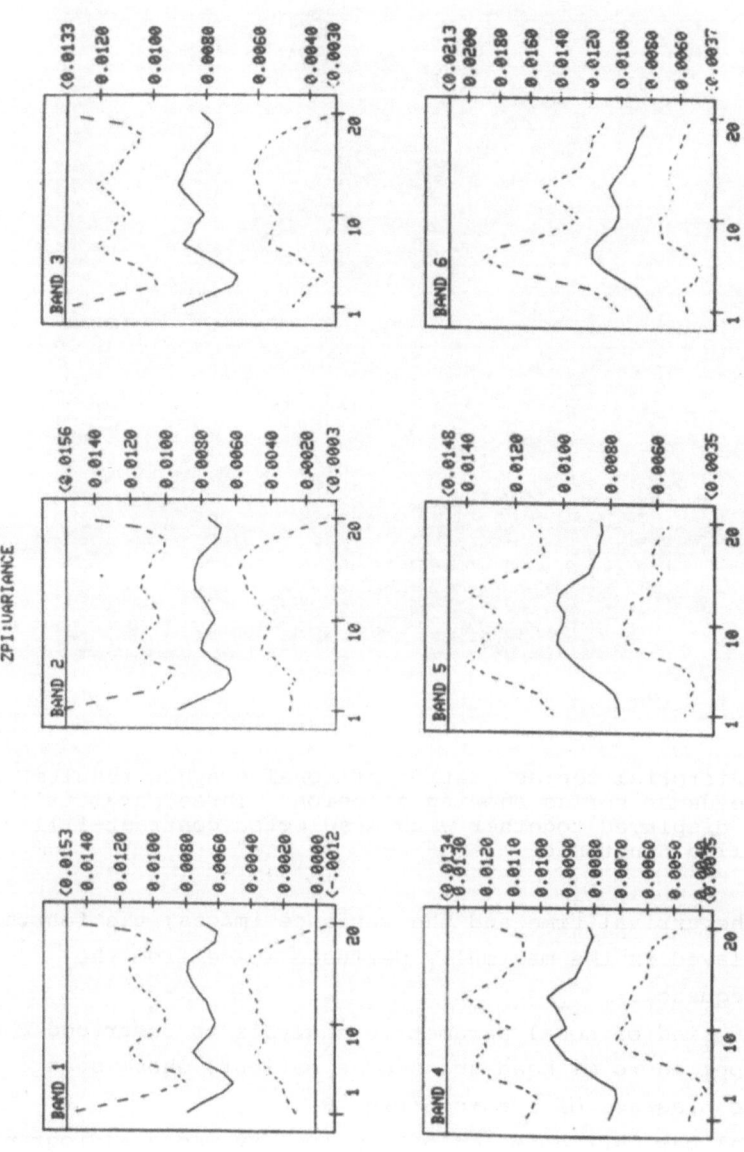

Figure 5. d) Combined data for nine normal renal studies. Parameter: zonal variance. Abscissa: zone number. Ordinate: arbitrary units. Solid line indicates mean value, dotted lines represent mean +/- one standard deviation.

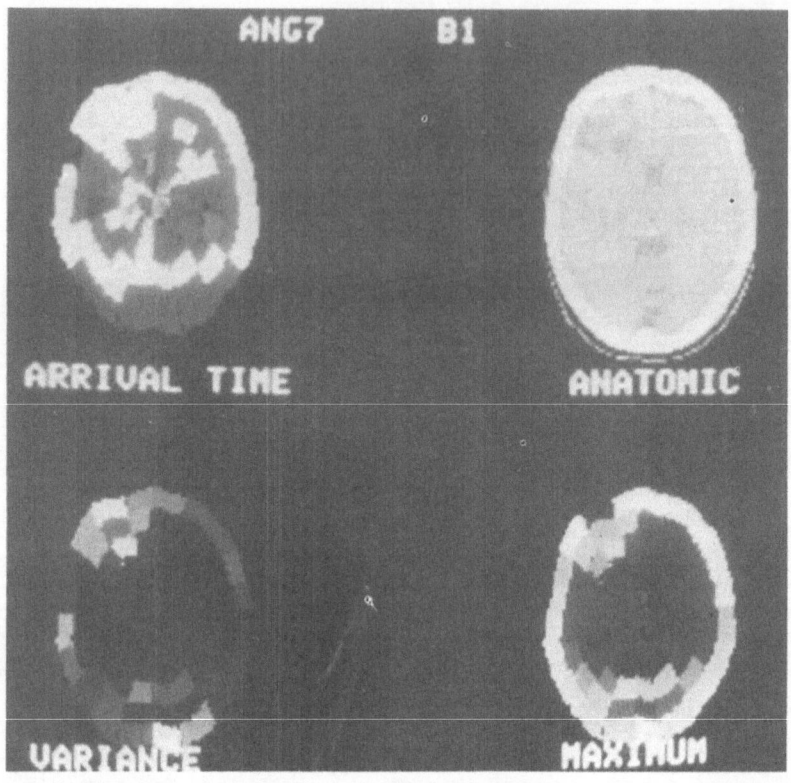

FIGURE 6. Pictorial representation of zonal graphic results for a CT headscan series showing a lesion. Three parametric images are displayed together with a selected contrast-filled image labelled: anatomic.

maximum, the arrival time and the variance images; the fourth image displayed is the maximally perfused image from the original sequence.

The same kind of zonal parametric analysis as described above has been applied to CT head scans of a patient, whose scan reveals the presence of a tumor (Fig. 6).

The zonal parametric images of a pulmonary wedge angiographic study is shown in Fig. 7 for a pediatric patient with congenital heart disease. The variance image demonstrates excellent

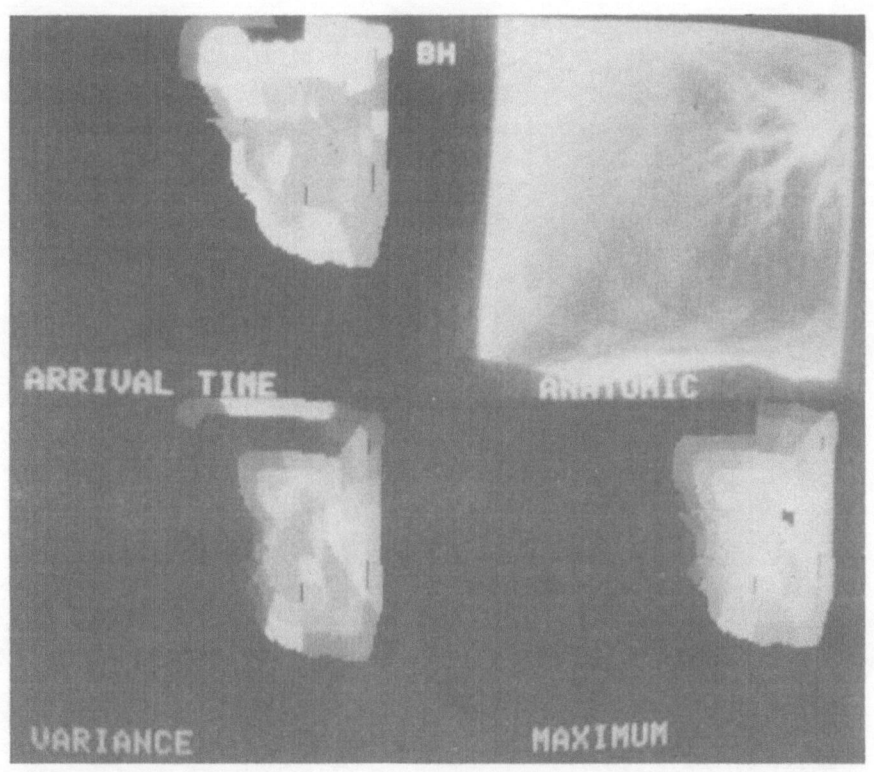

FIGURE 7. Pictorial representation of zonal graphic results for a pulmonary wedge angiographic series. Three parametric images are displayed together with a selected contrast-filled image labelled: anatomic.

quality as suppressing non perfused background compared to the perfused area.

Zonal parametric images from a fluorescein angiographic study are shown for a diabetic patient, who has leakage of contrast in the retinal vasculature (Fig. 8).

5. DISCUSSION AND CONCLUSIONS

This paper describes a means of extracting quantifiable diagnostic features with regard to perfusion and radiologic image sequences. It intends to go beyond the original concept

510

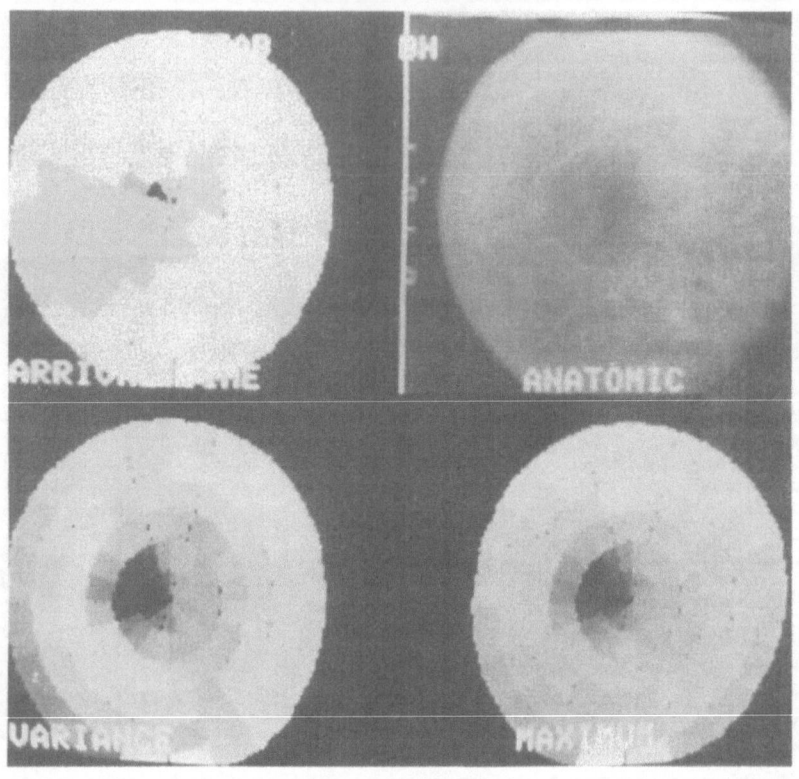

FIGURE 8. Pictorial representation of zonal graphic results
for a fluorescein retinal angiographic series. Three parametric
images are displayed together with a selected contrast-filled
image labelled: anatomic.

of standard parametric imaging that leaves the classification
of the image sequence to the subjective judgement of the
radiologist. For the radiologist to make a meaningful
judgement, the normal diagnostic pattern should be known
separately for each parameter, and they have to be evaluated
and combined for his diagnosis. This is clearly a difficult
pattern recognition and classification task, that can hardly
be done with great precision in a subjective manner.

We expect that zonal parametric imaging facilitates automated

feature extraction in sequential radiologic image studies,
which in turn, advances computer-aided diagnosis.

Although the investigations are clearly at a very early
stage, we can already make some observations on the method:

1. The apparent significance of the various zonal parametric
images may vary depending on the modality in the organs studied.
For low rate image sequences, such as CT, pulsed images in
subtraction angiography or fundus camera images of the eye,
the quality of information provided by the time arrival study,
is low. This is due to the fact that these image sequences
contain few images (15-30) so that the resolution of the
resultant feature curve is coarse. In the case of high
exposure rate, however, that can be achieved in digital
subtraction or with the most advanced fundus camera systems,
the arrival time has tremendous potential. For diabetic
patients, for instance, the severity of leakage from the
damaged vasculature of the eye could be easily assessed.

2. The integral under the absolute zonal washout curve
depends upon the amount of contrast medium injected, the
length of injection, the cardiac function of the patient.
The usefulness of the technique without normalization is,
however, severely impeded.

3. The pattern in the zonal image of maximum contrast is,
in principle, not affected by injection technique and this
image is perhaps the easiest to interpret for radiologists.
Good quality zonal images are obtainable with this parameter
for all modalities tested.

4. The zonal variance image has, perhaps, the greatest
potential. Since the image area, which is not perfused, has
very low variance, the perfused region undergoes a very
efficient enhancement, which could be almost equivalent to
subtraction. Pictorially, this enhancement is most visible
for vascular images (renal and pulmonary studies), and in the
graphic representation is significant for CT.

The preliminary studies obtained with different organs
indicate both promise and difficulties of the method.

Renal angiography appears to be excellently suited for

zonal parametric imaging. The organ usually undergoes little motion, and the case shown, in this regard, is fairly typical. The limited statistics that has been collected so far indicates a promise for a general pattern, but more data are required to obtain statistically significant results.

There is one kind of difficulty associated with renal zonal parametric images; superimposed structural artifacts, such as undesirable overlapping vasculature, bowel gas, etc., can frequently interfere with the assessment of the image sequence. Hence, the accumulation of cases for the control group is rather slow. The amount of computation required is substantial, and while the state of the art computer hardware can handle it, it certainly imposes enhanced needs for massive data processing of the image sequences.

REFERENCES

1. Santisteban A, Munoz L. 1978. Principal components of a multispectral image: application to a geological problem. IBM Journal of Res. and Devel. 22:444-454.
2. Jones RH, Goodrich JK, Harris CC, Sabiston DC. 1972. Evaluation of the accuracy of radionuclide measurement of regional pulmonary perfusion. Inv. Rad. 7:357-364.
3. Kaikara S, Natarajan TK, Maynard CD, Wagner HN, Jr. 1969. Construction of a functional image from spatially localized rate constants obtained from serial camera and rectilinear scanner data. Radiology. 93:1345-1348.
4. Tasto M, Felgandreher M. 1974. Verfahren zur Darstellung des zeitlichen Verlaufes einer Bewegungsgrosse und Anordnung zur Durchfuhrung des Verfahrens. German Patent P2447396.9.
5. Hoehne KH, Bohm M, Erbe W, Nicolae GC, Pfeiffer G, Sonne B, Buecheler E. 1978. Die Messung und differenzierte bildliche Darstellung der Nierendurchblutung mit der Computerangiographie. Fortschr. Roentgenstr. 129:667-672.
6. Hoehne KH, Bohm M, Nicolae GC. 1980. The processing of X-ray image sequences. P. Stucki ed. Advances in Digital Image Processing. Plenum Press. pp. 147-163.
7. Gallagher JH, Meaney TF, Flechner SM, Novick AC, Buonocore E. 1981. Parametric imaging of digital subtraction angiography studies for renal transplant evaluation. SPIE. Digital Radiography. 314:229-234.
8. Bursch JH, Hahne HJ, Brennecke R, Gronemeier D, Heintzen PH. 1981. Assessment of arterial flow measurements by digital angiography. Radiology. 141:39-47.
9. Sandor T, Harrington DP, Boxt LM, Murray PD, Hanlon WB. 1982. Quantitation of zonal parametric images. Proc. SPIE. 347:302-306.

INTERACTIVE 3D DISPLAY OF MEDICAL IMAGES

Stephen M. Pizer, Henry Fuchs,
E. Ralph Heinz, Edward V. Staab, Edward L. Chaney, Julian G. Rosenman,
John D. Austin, Sandra H. Bloomberg, Earle T. MacHardy,
Peter H. Mills, Dorothy C. Strickland
University of North Carolina, Chapel Hill, NC, USA

1. INTRODUCTION

3D display has the potential for increasing the information from medical images that can be used for diagnosis or treatment. It can be accomplished both by displays which present reflections from computed surfaces and by translucent, projective displays. Taking into account both types of display, this paper will

(1) discuss the strengths and weaknesses of 3D display and indicate areas of medical imaging where it seems that these strengths can be capitalized upon.

(2) survey the kinds of preprocessing necessary to prepare an image for 3D display from a series of 2D grey-scale slice images.

(3) present types of interaction and display features that are important as part of 3D display, in particular for projective, translucent 3D display.

(4) summarize the features of system software at UNC that supports the required interaction and display on a particular projective 3D display, a varifocal mirror system designed as an add-on to a color raster graphics system [Fuchs, Pizer, et al, 1982a,b].

We will focus on the varifocal mirror display, but also discuss shaded graphics display. Figures showing the results of shaded graphics reflective surface display will be included, as will stereo pairs taken by photographing the results of projective display by the varifocal mirror from two different angles. Of course, none of these images will be able to capture the effectiveness of interactive display or of the true 3D effect that the varifocal mirror provides.

2. STRENGTHS AND WEAKNESSES OF 3D DISPLAY

As compared to information from a pile of grey-scale slice images, 3D display seems to have a major strength where the comprehension of global 3D structure is important but seems not to be helpful where local issues are the major concern, even if these local issues must be addressed in many of the original image slices. The comprehension of the amount of plaque on the carotid artery wall and the degree of ulceration of the plaque is a local matter, and we have found that in this case 3D display adds little to the information that can be comprehended from grey-scale CT slices from which the 3D display derives.

On the other hand, we have found frequently that radiologists are not able to comprehend 3D structure from the 2D grey-scale slices. For example, we have made 3D images showing artery structure and the relation of clot or plaque to artery (figures 1-3) which allow the viewer to view aspects of global artery structure that are not apparent from the original images. For situations in which such comprehension is diagnostically important, 3D display should be helpful. In particular, such comprehension seems important in cases where

514

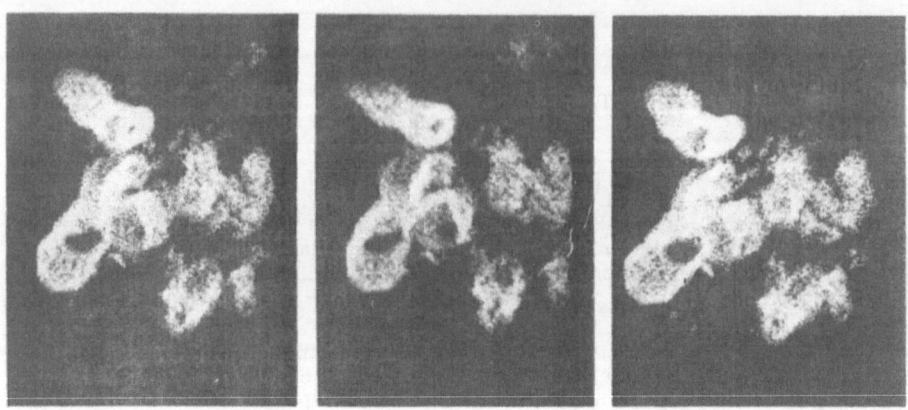

Figure 1
View from three nearby angles of varifocal mirror display of edge strength of blood from CT scans; either adjacent pair may be viewed in stereo.

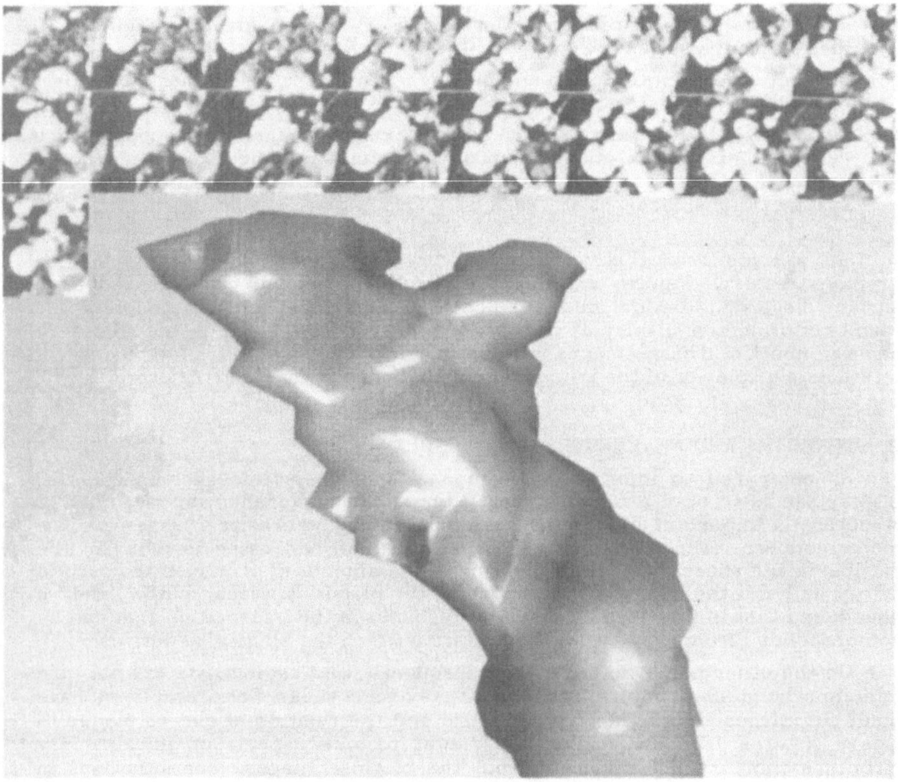

Figure 2
Shaded graphics presentation of carotid artery blood surface from CT scan. Surface indicates ulcer in plaque on vessel wall.

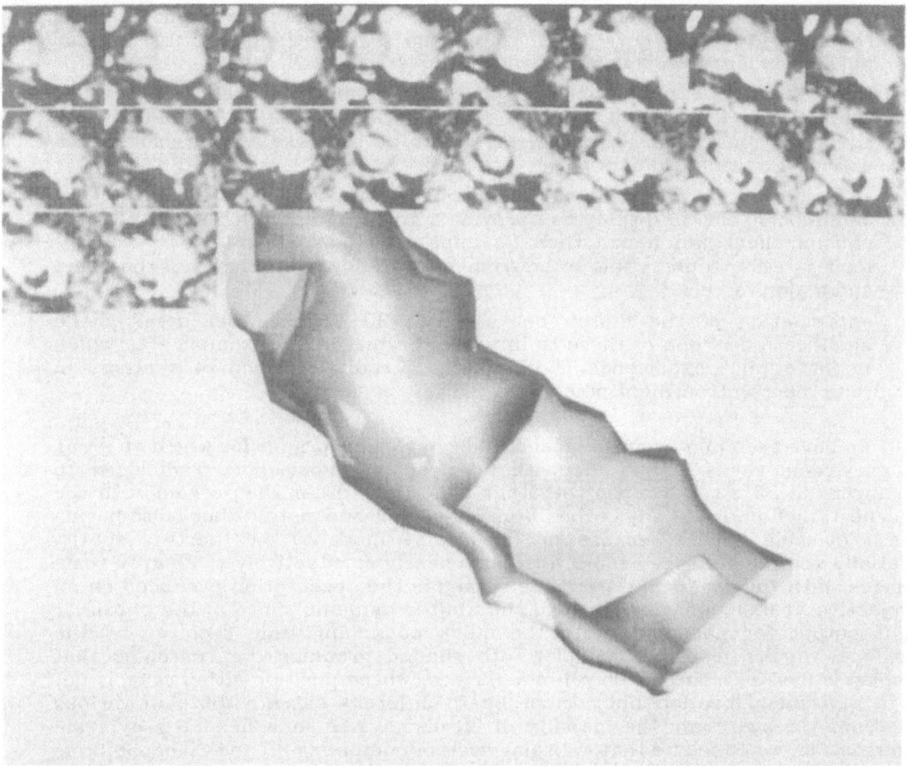

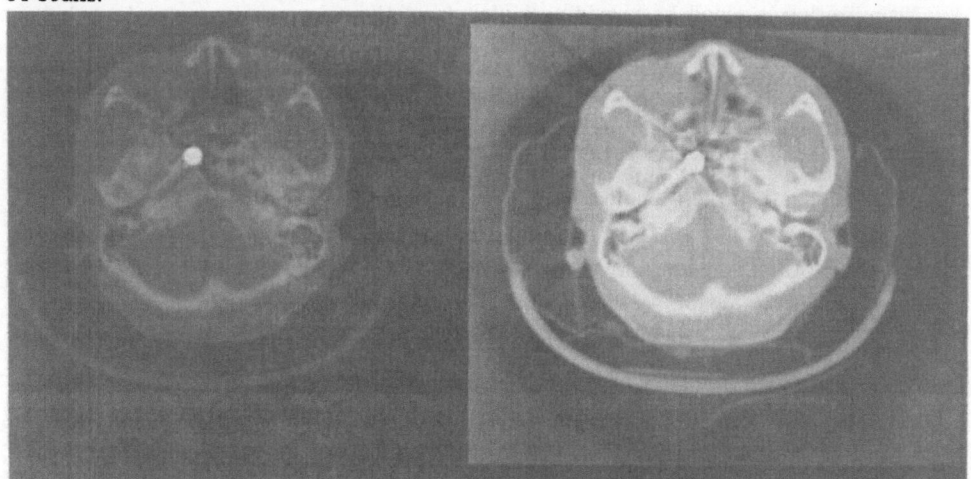

Figure 3
Shaded graphics presentation of clot inside (transparent) carotid artery from
CT scans.

Figure 4
CT scan of bullet in brain
a) before any contrast enhancement
b) after range limited histogram equalization using range of body intensities.

(1) the 3D structure is itself the basic goal, as when directing a surgeon. Others [Herman, Vannier] have commonly found 3D display important for this purpose in surface displays of bone surfaces.

(2) the extent of a complex object is the goal, as when one wishes to measure volume or shape. Examples are in measuring heart chamber volume or wall shape or tumor size. We have seen this to be the case in appreciating the extent of a brain tumor.

(3) appreciation of grey scale variations is the goal but the structure is very complex, so the 3D display can provide a guide for the selection of possibly oblique slices which can then be appreciated as 2D grey-scale images. Harris [1982] reports this to be frequently the case in images of the heart and major vessels.

(4) appreciation of the match between two 3D objects, and possibly the modification of one of these to improve the match. An example with which we have pilot experience is in matching radiation dose to anatomy in radiotherapy treatment planning.

We have seen numerous clinical studies of various organs for which an array of grey-scale slices is not adequate for even an experienced radiologist to comprehend 3D structure. On the other hand, with other than organs with the sharpest, high-contrast edges the 3D display is not adequate without also having the grey-scale slices, because no 3D display modality can portray subtle, spatially complicated grey-scale variations nearly as effectively as 2D grey-scale images. With the varifocal mirror the reason is the obscuration produced on all projective, translucent displays and the limited dynamic range of the phosphor light output for phosphors with the quick quenching time required by the varifocal mirror display principle. With shaded graphics the reason is that display is based on the portrayal of a surface, whose position either is or is not at a particular location but cannot be to different extents there in various locations. To overcome the inability of 3D displays to show needed grey scale information, we conclude that a display system combining 2D and 3D capabilities is required. Pilot studies support this conclusion.

Furthermore, interaction is most important with 3D display. It is important both to aid visualization of the 3D objects being displayed and to allow convenient manipulation and measurement of the objects in the image. Visualization is aided by providing a view from the appropriate orientation, by the kinetic depth effect, and by removal of obscuration by dimming or removal of objects or regions not presently of interest. Manipulation and measurement is provided by allowing translation and rotation of image objects including cursors and by providing a means of specifying irregular volumes of interest. Both of these interactive objectives are severely compromised if response is not provided in a fraction of a second. Motion-related perception of 3D is distinctly lessened and poor feedback harms interactive control. Ways of providing responsive interaction are discussed in section 4 below.

3. PREPROCESSING FOR 3D DISPLAY

Preprocessing for varifocal mirror display has three major objectives: 1) transformation of the image data from a 3D array of intensities in which it normally arrives as a pile of slices to the format required by the varifocal mirror display system, 2) accomplishment of contrast-enhancing and edge strength transformations that improve the perceptibility of image features on the 3D display, and 3) selection of regions or image objects that one wishes to have the option of displaying separately on the 3D display. The first step simply involves transformation of the original pixels into the form of a set of (x,y,z,i) 4-tuples, where i is intensity. Among the options in accomplishing this transformation are scaling and interpolation. While interpolation in all three dimensions is often desirable to remove pixel artifacts, the most important is that in the depth (z) dimension, since without this the view from the side shows the slices from which the image was produced, severely limiting any other perception. We have found that slice artifacts are largely removed if as few as two pixel values are interpolated between each pair of pixels in the same (x,y) positions on adjacent slices, interpolating not at fixed depths between the slices but rather at random depths (different for each pixel pair) uniformly distributed between the slices. It seems that this idea can usefully be extended to interpolation in the x and y dimensions.

As will be explained in section 4, it is useful to randomly shuffle the resulting 3D points before they are used to define objects for 3D display.

A major advantage of varifocal mirror display over shaded graphics display is that it can be used as an exploratory modalilty. Shaded graphics' strength seems to be as a means of showing someone 3D views of objects that have already been perceived as objects, though not necessarily in 3D, for example in guiding surgeons. Especially with the noisy, blurred, low contrast objects in medical images, this perception requires human involvement in defining the object surfaces that shaded graphics requires. On the other hand, if a display is to be used to explore images for the information they contain, only automatic preprocessing involving little or no loss of image information should be used. The major objectives of this preprocessing is contrast enhancement and limiting the obscuration that all projective, translucent, true 3D displays produce when one object is in front of or behind another.

The most effective contrast enhancement method for 2D medical images that we know of is our method of adaptive histogram equalization [Pizer, 1981, 1983]. We have sometimes used it with good effect in 3D varifocal mirror display, but there it has two major weaknesses. The first is that it enhances contrast which is not of interest as well as that which is. In 2D this is no problem, but in 3D the uninteresting objects can obscure the interesting ones. The second weakness is that it destroys the intensity ordering relationships within the image, so that windowing can no longer be used to pick out objects of interest and remove others from obscuring the objects of interest. As a result we recommend global histogram equalization, with the histogram coming only from the range of intensities in the body (see figure 4) or a smaller range selectable based on the organ system of interest. After this transformation, the image objects become far more apparent than if no contrast enhancement were done, and also intensity windowing, as described in section 3, can be applied to reduce obscuration.

Obscuration is also lessened by displaying edge strength to show surfaces rather than the original or contrast-enhanced grey-scale values, which result in the inside of objects obscuring their surfaces. Edge strength transformations, such as that due to Sobel and its 3D extension, both of which are used by us (see figure 5), are effective only after appropriate contrast enhancement. The same contrast enhancements discussed in the previous paragraph are applicable, except that adaptive histogram equalization can indeed be attractive for this application. Edge strength display is often very effective, since it allows the viewer to put points in the contrast-enhanced image with a high intensity gradient to be coalesced into a surface by the viewer while allowing him to ignore the scattered non-surface high-gradient points that come from image noise. However, when the noise level in one part of the image is comparable to

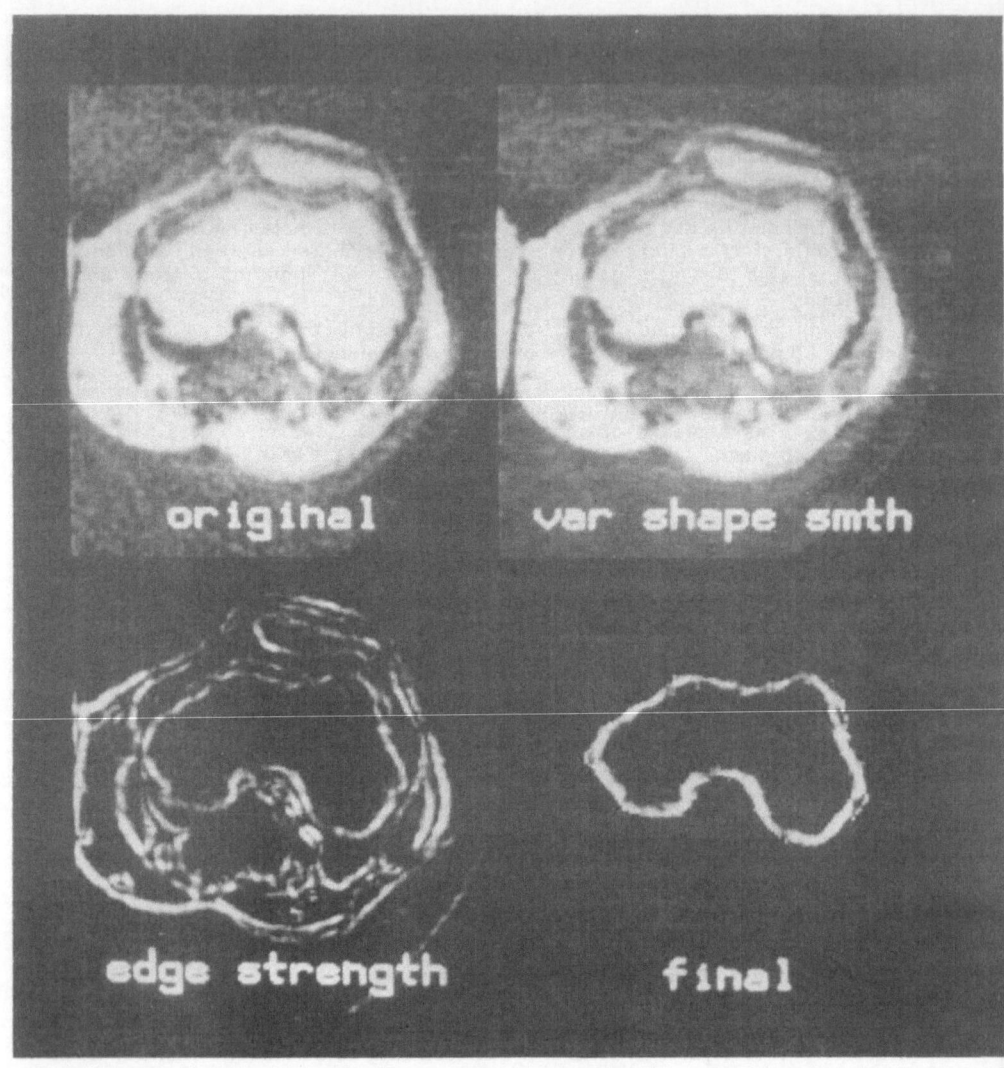

Figure 5
Preprocessing for varifocal mirror display of NMR images of the knee.

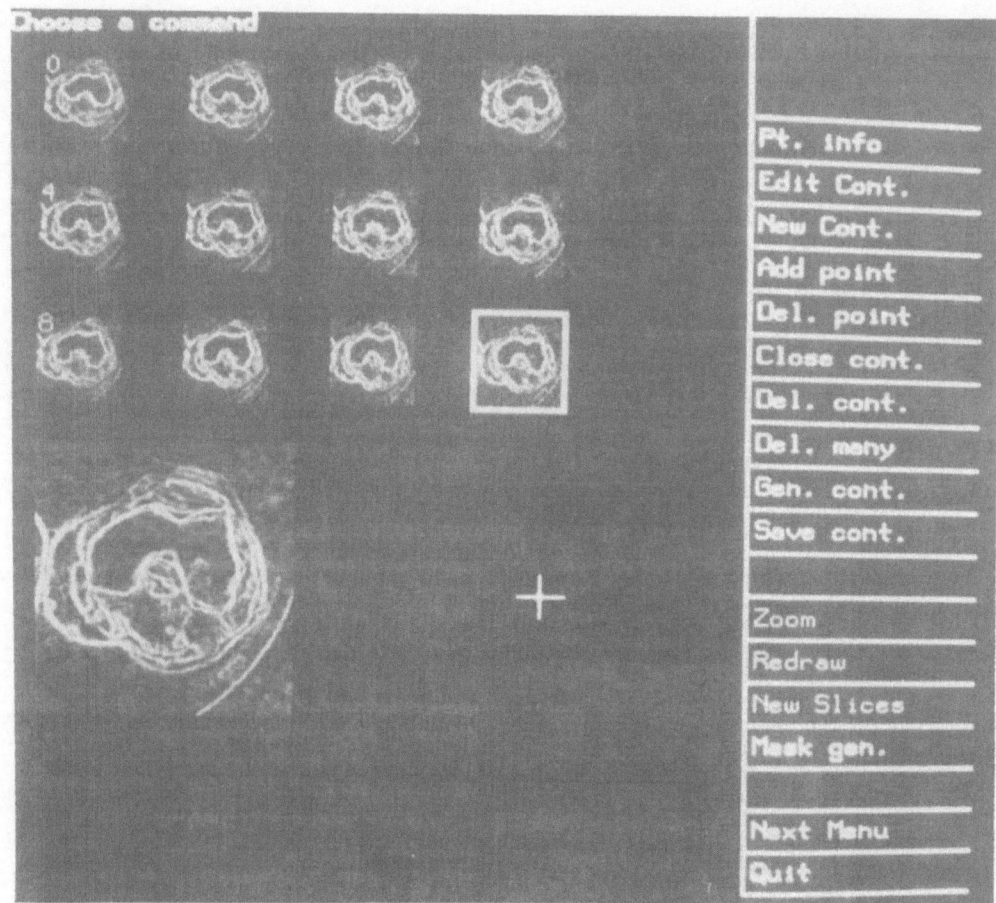

Figure 6
Result of Hough-transform-based slice-to-slice edge following of femur
marrow surface on NMR images of knee.

edge intensity difference in another, the high-gradient points due to noise can swamp the image and no windowing can remove the noise points without also removing important object edge points. This high relative noise can occur when adaptive histogram equalization is used in a image where noise appears in a region with a low contrast range and is thus enhanced by the processing. In this kind of a situation a global contrast enhancement that is not locally adaptive such as the range-limited histogram equalization method described above should precede edge strength measurement. Alternatively, the image can be pre-smoothed by a method that preserves edges (see figure 5), such as one we have developed based on accepting pixels into a local average only if they are appropriately close in intensity to that of the pixel whose smoothed value is being computed [Austin, 1982].

Object or region specification can also be important as a step towards limiting obscuration by allowing the objects or regions thus defined to be selected among or displayed using differing relative intensities or display modes such as color or blink. The specification to which we refer is of regions which are not simply a range in each of x, y, and z, as can be defined in real time on line by the display device, as described in section 4. Ideally the specification of general objects or regions should be done based on simultaneous 2D and 3D display, as discussed in section 2. However, at present we have developed a program for specifying objects using a sequence of slices, displayed as an array of 2D images. In this program the user specifies a closed contour on one slice, and the program determines the corresponding contour on succeeding slices, using edge strength and direction values computed for these slices (see figure 6). The user can edit contours where the edge that is found is in some part not the one desired, and then the edited edge forms the basis for the edge on the next slice.

The method for finding a contour on one slice given a prototype contour on the previous slice and the edge strength and direction values on the new slice is based on the Hough Transform [Ballard & Brown, 1982]. The contour on each slice is represented as a cyclic series of points connected by line segments. Each point on one slice is replaced by another on the next slice by fitting the line segments connecting the points to the edge information in the new slice. For each line segment in the prototype, a rectangular box is centered about the line (see figure 7). The width of the box is a parameter of the program specifying the distance from the prototype to search for the new edge. All pixels in the box whose edge strength is above a given threshold are given votes as to the identity of the new line segment. Each such pixel votes most strongly for the line through it with its edge direction value, and less strongly for lines with nearby slopes and intercepts. The line segment chosen is the one with the most votes, if this number of votes is above some threshold. If not, the prototype segment is used.

The new edge points are determined by intersecting the new line segments. For a pair of line segments sharing a point in the prototype, the intersection of the new line segments with the ends of their boxes near the point are each calculated, as well as the intersection of the two line segments. If this intersection of the lines is near enough to the box intersections, the intersection of the lines is used as the new point. If not, the new point is a weighted average of the two box intersections, with the weights being the number of votes received by the respective line segments.

The success of the object specification method just described depends on the contrast of the edges in the underlying image and on separation of edges relative to the distance moved by an edge from slice to slice. The edges thus produced can be used as the basis of a region definition for varifocal mirror display by selecting an annulus about the edge, the region inside the edge, the

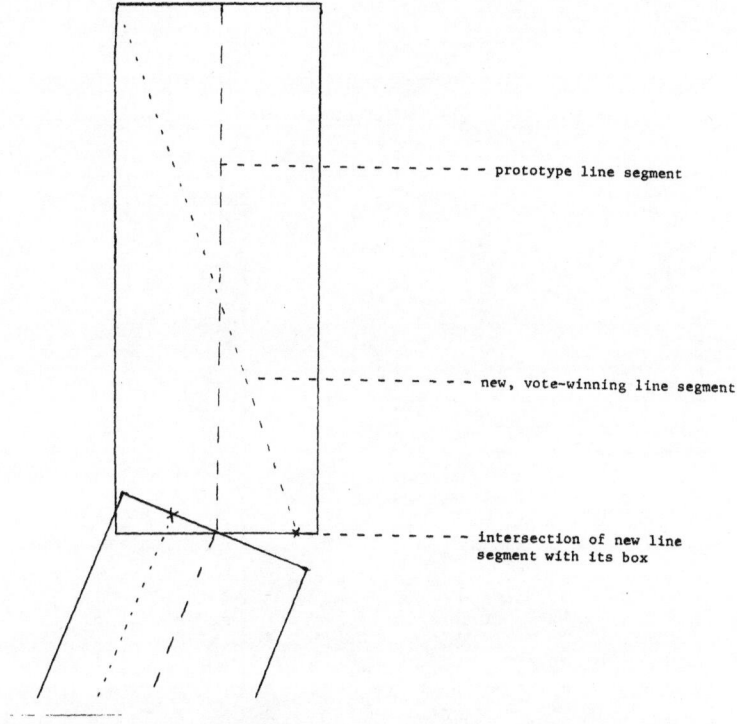

Figure 7
Boxes and linear segments of edges in Hough-transform-based slice-to-slice
edge following method.

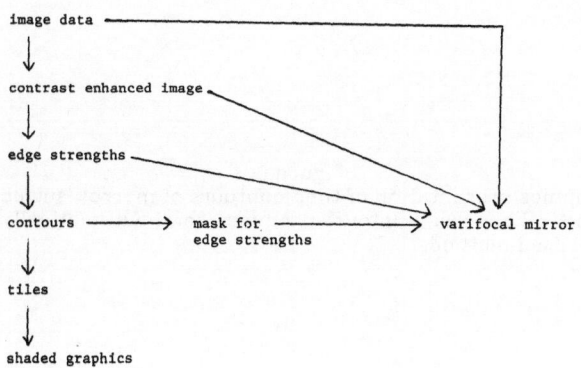

Figure 9
Preprocessing for varifocal mirror and shaded graphics display.

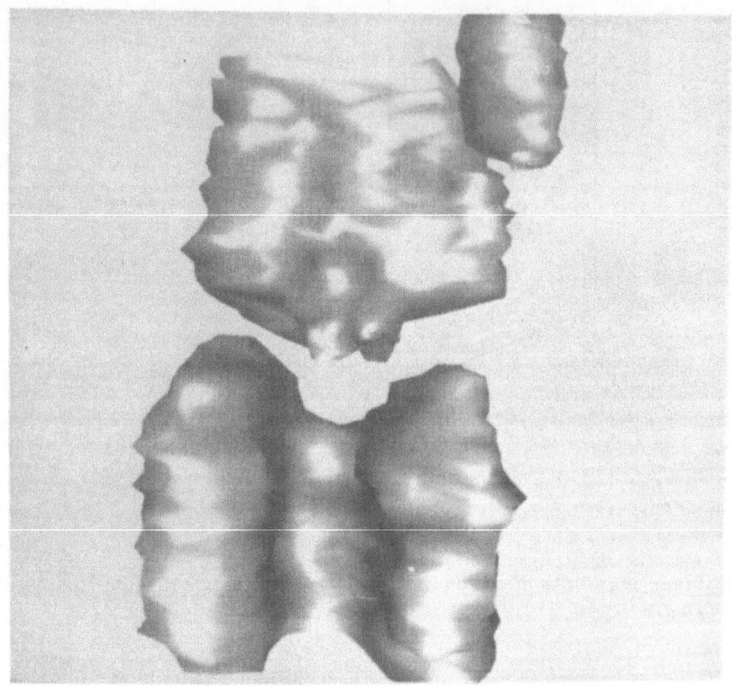

Figure 8
Shaded graphics presentation of tiled contours of marrow surfaces in knee
bones from NMR images. Contours produced semi-automatically using Hough-
transform-based method.

region outside the edge, or some union of these,. In this case the edge need not be exact. It is also possible to use these results to define contours for tiling and subsequent shaded graphics display (see figure 8), but the accuracy requirements there are much more stringent.

The preprocessing necessary for varifocal mirror and shaded graphics display is summarized in figure 9.

4. INTERACTION AND DISPLAY FEATURES FOR VARIFOCAL MIRROR 3D DISPLAY

For visualization it is important for a projective, translucent 3D display to provide the ability to select among objects, to allow, for each object, selection of orientation, relative intensity, and other intensity properties such as blink, and to allow spatial and intensity windowing. For manipulation of image objects it is also important to allow object translation, pointing, region specification, and plane selection to indicate slices of interest that can be displayed on the 2D display component of the display system that presents grey-scale information most effectively. In the following we describe how our raster-graphics-system based varifocal mirror display system described in Fuchs and Pizer [1982a,b] provides these capabilities.

The object descriptions produced by the preprocessing each consist of a set of (x,y,z,i) 4-tuples. Each object needs to be rotated and translated and have its intensities transformed to a set of (x',y',z',i') 4-tuples. This is accomplished by the display processor in the raster graphics system on which our varifocal mirror display system is based, using standard graphics techniques. Then as described in Fuchs and Pizer [1982a], each z' is used to select a depth bucket of the refresh buffer, into whose first free location the corresponding (x',y',i') is placed. More precisely, the triple $(x',y',0)$, i.e. the new location but with zero intensity followed by the triple (x',y',i') is placed into the refresh buffer. The first triple is required to allow the CRT beam to move to (x',y') without leaving a trail or a smear before the beam is appropriately intensified.

In order to allow the viewer to receive immediate feedback from his interaction we wish to display whatever points have been transformed into the refresh buffer after 1/30 sec. Because the object descriptions have their points in random order, a full but coarse coverage of the object will provided by this initial display. If at that time further modification of the interactive parameters has been done, a new refresh buffer will be computed based on the new transformation. However, if the user has not changed the orientation, translation, or other interactive parameter, the processor can continue filling the original refresh buffer with further points from the object descriptions. We call this approach successive refinement, and have found it quite successful. Furthermore, after the refresh buffer or one of its depth buckets becomes full, one can make space for additional points from the object description to be transformed by reordering the points so that almost all successive points in a depth bucket are near enough in (x',y') so that little CRT beam movement is required and thus intervening zero-intensity points need be inserted only where the nearness required cannot be achieved.

Pointing is achieved by having an object describing a cursor and logically attaching it to an interactive device. Region specification can be accomplished by painting using such a cursor and creating a new object description on the fly from the region that is painted or its surface (computing this surface quickly is a problem yet to be solved). Alternatively the cursor can be used as an eraser by recording the region painted and not loading into the refresh buffer any point whose transformed value is in the erased region.

Spatial and intensity windowing, which are global to the whole image, can be accomplished in real time using the color lookup tables and viewport registers of the raster graphics system. Since the x,y,i values in the refresh buffers are stored in the frame buffer in the locations used for red, green, and blue for color video display, the red and green lookup tables can be used to do windowing in the x and y directions, respectively, on the varifocal mirror. All table entries for x (or y) values less than an interactively specified minimum and greater than an interactively specified maximum are set to zero, with the result that all such points appear at an edge of the picture. Similarly, intensity windowing can be done by loading an appropriate blue lookup table. Note that on the varifocal mirror intensities above as well as below the window should be mapped to zero intensity to avoid obscuration.

Depth windowing is more important than x and y spatial windowing, since it relieves more obscuration. Here we take advantage of the fact that distance along the frame buffer, i.e. successive lines when the buffer is used for video display, correspond to successive levels of depth on the varifocal mirror display. Thus, restricting display to a certain range of video lines is equivalent on the varifocal mirror to restricting display to a certain range of depths. This is just the function of the video-y viewport registers in many raster graphics systems. Thus, settings of interactive controls determining a desired depth window are used to load the video-y viewport registers and thus restrict display to the desired depth window.

A factor worthy of discussion is the number of points required for 3D varifocal mirror display. Because obscuration needs to be avoided, it is frequently the case that the number of points desired is proportional to the square of the number of points in a linear dimension rather than the cube. This limitation is acheived, for example, by the edge strength transformation followed by accepting points above some edge strength threshold, or spatial or intensity windowing. Our experience indicates that a 256 x 256 x 64 depth bucket x 16 intensity system is adequate and a 512 x 512 x 128 x 32 system can be justified. Furthermore 32K points is clearly inadequate and 64K is still not enough. Based on our experience with our system and that of others, we suspect that perhaps 200,000 points will be satisfactory to display multiple objects, each with appropriate point density.

These numbers can be used to compare raster-based systems to point-based systems, such as ours. A raster-based system must store only i but do so at many unused points. A point-oriented system must store (x,y,i) for each point. Even at the lower resolution a raster system would require a refresh buffer of 20 million bits, whereas a point-based system would require 4.4 million bits, or 8.8 million if space is allocated so that every point can include a zero intensity entry. Furthermore, many of the interactions are difficult with a raster-based system.

5. SOFTWARE TO SUPPORT VARIFOCAL MIRROR DISPLAY

Varifocal mirror display is simply a graphics display, and the software to support it is no different in principle than that to support other graphics displays, such as vector graphics and raster graphics systems. The only exception is that varifocal mirror software must include software appropriate for the special preprocessing required, and certain of the transformations are specialized to the varifocal mirror display. Thus, the software used after preprocessing consists of programs to transform object descriptions for multiple objects into refresh buffers and software to load the display device registers and tables.

Our varifocal mirror display is implemented as an add-on to an Ikonas RDS-3000 raster graphics system that contains an AMD 2900-based parallel bit-sliced microprocessor as the display processor and also a fast multiply/accumulate chip. Our software operates by loading object descriptions, at user command, into part of the frame buffer. Then interactive devices are logically attached to objects specified by the user, so that transformations specified by the position of the devices are loaded from the host computer to the raster graphics system. These transformations are applied to the appropriate objects via the display processor and multiply/accumulate chip and stored in the refresh buffer.

The refresh buffer is organized by the level of dynamism of the objects, these levels being determined by the user. We normally use two levels, dynamic and static, or three, busily dynamic, dynamic from time to time, and static. The loading of a refresh buffer is done in increasing order of dynamism, while assuring that enough space is left to hold the more dynamic objects. The result is that when a dynamic object is moved, only the part of the buffer at its level of dynamism or above need be erased and refilled, considerably speeding the effect of interactions.

The software we have developed supports both single and double refresh buffers. The successful idea of successive refinement has been extended to using a single buffer (of double the size of a double buffer) if interaction is not occurring after the double buffer is full, and switching back to double buffering when interaction recommences.

6. CONCLUSIONS

Interaction has been seen to be crucial in 3D display of medical images. For exploratory display projective, translucent 3D display seems neccessary. We have therefore developed a varifocal mirror display system that supports interactive use, using a design as an add-on to a raster graphics system that keeps the additional cost of 3D display relatively low. Further developments are needed to make such a display clinically useful, especially in the area of simultaneous 2D and 3D display, interaction based on successive refinement, and improved 3D interactive devices. However, our studies suggest that such a system will be clinically important in areas where global structure properties or relationships are clinically relevant. Finally, we have designs which will allow 3D dynamic display and envision this also being of clinical importance, for example for studying the heart.

ACKNOWLEDGEMENTS

The work reported above is partially supported by NIH Grant # NS/HL 16759-01 and partially by funds provided by Technicare, Inc. and Atari, Inc. We thank Greg Abram for the shaded graphics display software used to create figures 2, 3 and 8 and Brad Hemminger for assistance with the surface reconstruction software used to define the objects in these figures. We thank Bo Strain and Karen Curran for photography.

REFERENCES

Austin, J.D., B.M.W. Tsui, S.M. Pizer (1982), "Processing of NMR Images", Southeastern Chapter Meeting of the Society of Nuclear Medicine, Charlotte, North Carolina, October 1982.

Ballard, D.H., C.M. Brown (1982), *Computer Vision*, Prentice-Hall, Inc., Englewood Cliffs, New Jersey.

Fuchs, H., S.M. Pizer, E.R. Heinz, S.H. Bloomberg, L.C. Tsai, D.C. Strickland (1982a), "Design of and Image Editing with a Space-filling 3-D Display Based on a Standard Raster Graphics System", *Processing and Display of 3-D Data*, SPIE, Vol. 367, pp. 117-127.

Fuchs, H., S.M. Pizer, L.C. Tsai, S.H. Bloomberg, E.R. Heinz (1982b), "Adding a True 3-D Display to a Raster Graphics System", *Computer Graphics and Applications*, IEEE, Vol. 2, No. 7, pp. 73-78.

Harris, L.D. (1982), "Display and Analysis of Medical Volume Images", *Nuclear Medicine and Biology*, Pergamon Press, Vol. II, pp. 2181-2184.

Herman, G.T., J.K. Udupa (1981), "Display of 3D Discrete Surfaces", *Proc. SPIE*, Vol. 283, pp. 90-97.

Pizer, S.M., "Adaptive Grey Level Assignment in CT Scan Display", submitted for publication.

Pizer, S.M. (1981), "An Automatic Intensity Mapping for the Display of CT Scans and Other Images", *Information Processing in Medical Imaging* Proc. VII International Conference on Information Processing in Medical Imaging, Stanford, California, in press.

Vannier, M.W., J.L. Marsh (1983), "Craniofacial Disorders", *Diagnostic Imaging*, Miller Freeman Publ., Vol. 5, No. 3, pp. 36-43.

CAN WE PREDICT VISUAL PERFORMANCE
USING A MODEL OF THE HUMAN EYE?

Brent Baxter * Celia Blackburn # Richard Normann @

Departments of: Radiology and Computer Science *, Electrical Engineering
, and Bioengineering @ University of Utah, Salt Lake City, Utah

ABSTRACT

This paper describes an approach for analyzing radiographic
tumor detection which is based on the light adaptation properties of
photoreceptor cells (the cones) in the retina. Factors which affect the
sensitivity of these cells will be discussed, changes in sensitivity due
to light adaptation will be demonstrated and preliminary results from
experiments dealing with the effect of age and radiologic training will
be presented. A computer model of these processes has been constructed
that appears to be useful for predicting the sensitivity of the visual
system for detecting low contrast patches on a variety of background
intensity distributions. Predictions of observer performance based on
calculations from this model will provide a means for evaluating the
clinical usefulness of image processing/enhancement schemes.

1.0 INTRODUCTION

Detection of low contrast lung nodules shadows is an important function of chest radiography that is often difficult to accomplish in a reliable fashion. When a marginally visible tumor is missed there is a possibility of delayed diagnosis and treatment, or where more than one abnormality is present, inappropriate treatment may be undertaken. The problem of missed nodules is further complicated by the variety of densities and textures on which tumor shadows may appear. Our objective in this research is to develop an accurate model of the visual system that may be used to predict the contrast necessary for reliable tumor detection.

Visual sensitivity depends on a variety of factors including the average light intensity present in the viewable image. The well known Weber-Fechner relation states that for photopic light levels (*) the intensity increment required for detection of a test patch is approximately proportional to background intensity. Factors other than changes in area of the pupil are required to account for this large change in visual sensitivity, since pupillary area can only change by about a factor of 10:1.

The distribution of light within the background can also affect visual sensitivity. It is more difficult to detect a test patch placed in a dark part of the background when there are nearby bright areas. Our approach to analyzing these changes in visual sensitivity is based on a model of the photoreceptor cells that converts a pattern of light intensities in the image into a pattern of photoreceptor hyperpolarization (output voltages). Basic to this approach is the hypothesis that test patch detectability is dependent on the photoreceptor output voltages produced by viewing the test patches. We assume that when a test patch causes a large enough change in photoreceptor output, the patch will be seen. Further, we assume there is a single fixed voltage threshold for each observer.

----

* Photopic light levels are those required for color vision. Color vision is active over at least-eight orders of magnitude in light intensity.

2.0 BACKGROUND: A Model of Retinal Photoreceptors (The cones)

Images viewed by an observer are not projected onto the retina with complete radiometric fidelity, but are modified by the optical components of the eye (lens, cornea, vitreous and retinal tissue layer). Focusing is imperfect because of optical aberrations and diffraction effects, and because light is scattered at the interfaces of each optical structure in the eye, introducing a low intensity veiling glare over the entire retina. For this reason the retinal image of a point of light consists of a slightly blurred point with a dim halo surrounding it.

Optical Scatter: In an image containing both bright and dark regions, light from the bright region is scattered into darker regions, increasing the average light level and reducing contrast in the darker regions. In the same manner, optical scatter also reduces the visibility of low contrast tumor shadows when they appear in dark parts of a radiograph. The effect of optical scatter on visual sensitivity may be illustrated by viewing a color slide while placing a scattering device (a section of nylon stocking) in front of the projector lens.

The optical point spread function used in our model is based on data from studies by other workers (1,2,3,4) using young adult observers. We have made adjustments to this optical point spread function data for angles greater than about 5 minutes of visual angle for the purpose of simulating increased optical scatter in older observers. Our experiments suggest that the amount of optical scatter in the eye increases with age. (See section 3.4)

Light Adaptation: Photoreceptor cells in the retina produce a graded voltage response to graded light stimulation. The strength of this electrical signal depends on the sensitivity of the cell as well as on the absolute light intensity falling on the cell (5,6). Changes in photosensitivity (also called light adaptation) occur as the average light intensity falling on the cell changes. This may be due to an actual change in illumination or to the scanning effect of the involuntary eye movements. (See next paragraph) The response of a cone type photoreceptor cell to light, including light adaptation effects, is closely approximated by,

$$V = V_{max} I/(I + S) \tag{1}$$

where I is the instantaneous light intensity incident on the cell, S is an adaptation parameter which depends on a local average of the light intensity (7), V is the output voltage from the cell, and Vmax is the maximum voltage the photoreceptor cell can produce. The adaptation parameter, S, partially tracks changes in illumination level, thus allowing the photoreceptor cell output to be relatively independent of absolute light level.

Eye Movements: Small involuntary eye movements (microsaccades) consist of abrupt changes in location of the visual axis of the eye with intervening periods of slow drift, and high frequency tremor. These eye movements cause a photoreceptor to scan the light pattern in a small region of the image. Ditchburn and others (8,9,10,11) have measured the amount of time the visual axis spends away from a sharp fixation target and have estimated the distribution function which represents the probability the eye will be at some distance from the fixation target. We have modified their distribution function to account for viewing conditions typical of diagnostic x-ray image interpretation. For a given image, eye movements determine the average light level to which a photoreceptor cell is exposed, thereby controlling its state of light adaptation.

The Detector: A binary threshold operation is included in the model because we hypothesize that a fixed increment in retinal output voltage is produced by viewing a test patch that is just visible. We refer to this signal level as the photoreceptor voltage increment. A more sophisticated detector process has been developed for future work that should permit the detector to accurately test the visual system's sensitivity to test patches of various sizes, patches with varying amounts of edge sharpness and backgrounds with varying amounts of noise. This detector should respond to the presence or absence of a test patch in a manner statistically similar to the human visual system.

3.0 PREDICTING VISUAL SENSITIVITY: Calculations based on the model

A series of experiments was carried out using image backgrounds and test objects relevant to the problem of detecting low contrast tumor shadows on radiographic images. These experiments were performed to assess our hypothesis that detection of test patches could be associated with photoreceptor voltage increments which exceeded a fixed threshold.

Measurement of Observer Contrast Sensitivity: Observers from 14 to 70 years of age viewed a stimulus pattern containing a variable intensity test patch projected on either a uniform background or on a nonuniform background having a dark central test area. Patches were projected onto locations selected at random by the experimenter. At each trial the observer was asked if the patch was visible. If not, the intensity of the patch was increased and the process repeated until the observer detected the test patch. Before and after each trial the observer's gaze was directed away from the projection screen to eliminate temporal cues that would have increased the measured visual sensitivity. While this method (method of ascending limits) is known to be adversely affected by inter-observer variations in criterion level and to errors of anticipation, it was selected because these effects are small and because the protocol allowed us to collect observer data rapidly.

Images judged by each observer to have just visible test patches were processed using the model to calculate the pattern of photoreceptor output voltages produced within the observers' eyes. Photoreceptor voltage increments for each observer were obtained by calculating the difference in photoreceptor output across the boundary of the test patch.

Experimental Results: The intensity differences shown in Figure 2 are the ratio of test patch intensity, $\triangle$ I, to the light intensity of the immediate background, I. Note how the intensity difference varies as a function of observer age for both uniform and nonuniform backgrounds. Despite limitations in the observer testing procedure noted above, the experiment shows an increase in contrast required for detection of test patches on nonuniform backgrounds. We ascribe this result to light scattered from the bright periphery onto the darker central region containing the test patch.

Determination of Optical Scatter: By our hypothesis, the calculated output voltage difference for a given observer should be the same for just detectable patches on both uniform and nonuniform backgrounds. For young observers, output voltages were nearly the same for both uniform and nonuniform backgrounds and they could be made equal by small adjustments to the scatter component of the model. We adjusted the light scatter part of the model for each observer until the photoreceptor voltage increments were the same for both the uniform and nonuniform backgrounds. Figure 3 shows the magnitude of these adjustments as a function of the age of the observer. We found similar amounts of light scatter in observers age 30 and younger, but light scatter increased by a factor of two by age 50 and a factor of three by age 65. There were no significant differences between radiologists and nonradiologists. Note how the separation between intensity difference data for uniform and nonuniform backgrounds in Figure 2 is generally greater for older observers. This trend corresponds to the increased light scatter with age shown in Figure 3.

Changes In Photoreceptor Voltage Increments: Figure 4 shows the variation of photoreceptor voltage increment with observer age. Voltage increments were smallest (highest visual sensitivity) for teenage observers, with approximately a twofold increase by age 65. It is interesting to note that observers with radiologic training exhibited lower voltage increments than untrained observers. Trained observers also showed a more gradual increase in photoreceptor increment with age and there was less interobserver variation. These results suggest that radiologists may be slightly better than untrained observers at detecting low contrast structures, perhaps because of skills developed through clinical practice in operating near the visual system's inherent noise level.

Evaluating Image Processing Techniques: Several techniques might be devised for evaluating imaging system utility on the basis of our photoreceptor model. Suppose a test image were to be processed using two image enhancement schemes. The enhancement algorithm for which the calculated photoreceptor voltage increment is largest should produce images where the patch would be easiest to see. Alternatively, one could iteratively adjust the test patch contrast until the enhanced image gave a photoreceptor voltage increment equal to a standard

comparison value. The enhancement algorithm able to accomodate lowest
contrast patches would be preferable.

4.0 CONCLUSION

What may we conclude about predicting test patch detection on
the basis of calculated patterns of retinal photoreceptor output
voltage? Test images used in our study contained both uniform and
nonuniform backgrounds which varied over a 300 to 1 range in light
intensity, yet calculated voltage increments for a given observer ranged
over only about 15% of the total range . Further, estimates of optical
scatter in the eyes of our observer are consistent with gradual
opacification of the lens known to occur in older observers [13].

Limitations in the visual model used in these experiments
include its inability to deal with noisy image backgrounds or
backgrounds containing large amounts of anatomical structure. Also we
have yet to systematically explore the effect of edge sharpness on
detection performance. Despite these deficiencies, the photoreceptor
model appears capable of accounting accurately for changes in visual
sensitivity caused by light adaptation where there are large intensity
differences in the image. Improvements to the model planned for future
work should remove these restrictions.

FIGURES

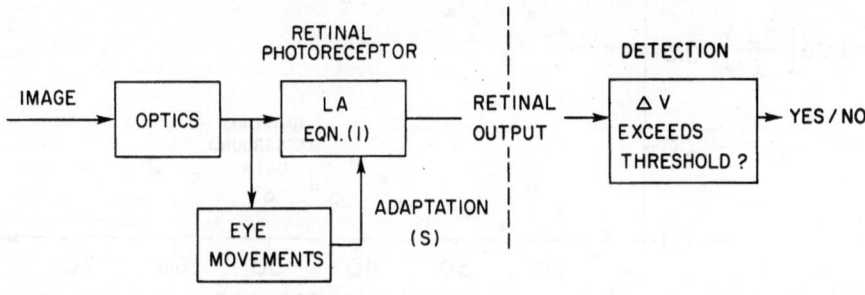

Figure 1 - This functional model of the eye converts patterns of light
            in a viewable image into patterns of photoreceptor output
            voltages.

538

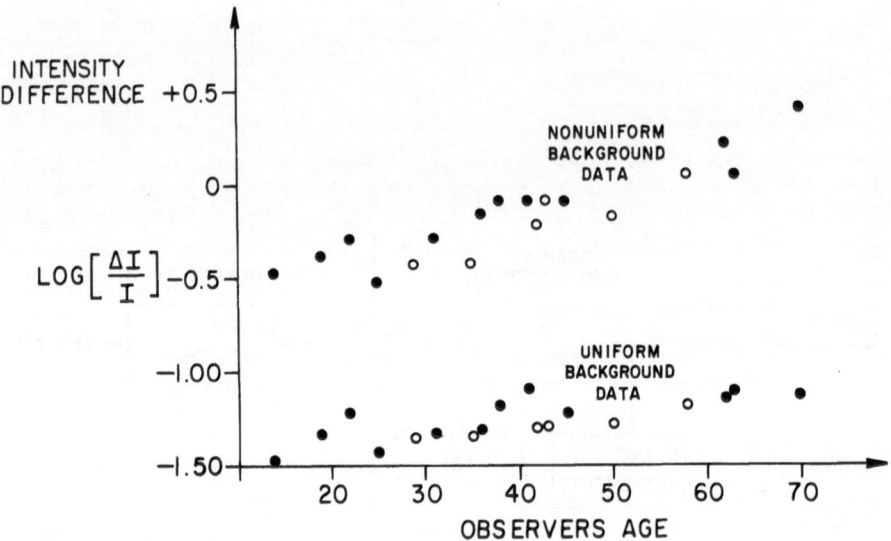

Figure 2 - Intensity difference data from psychophysical experiments. Open circles are for radiologists.

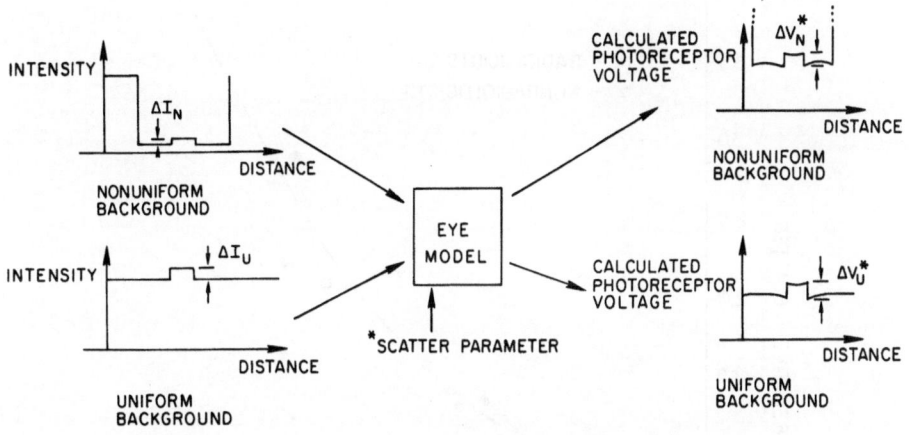

Figure 3 -Eye model was adjusted to estimate optical scatter in observers' eyes (A).

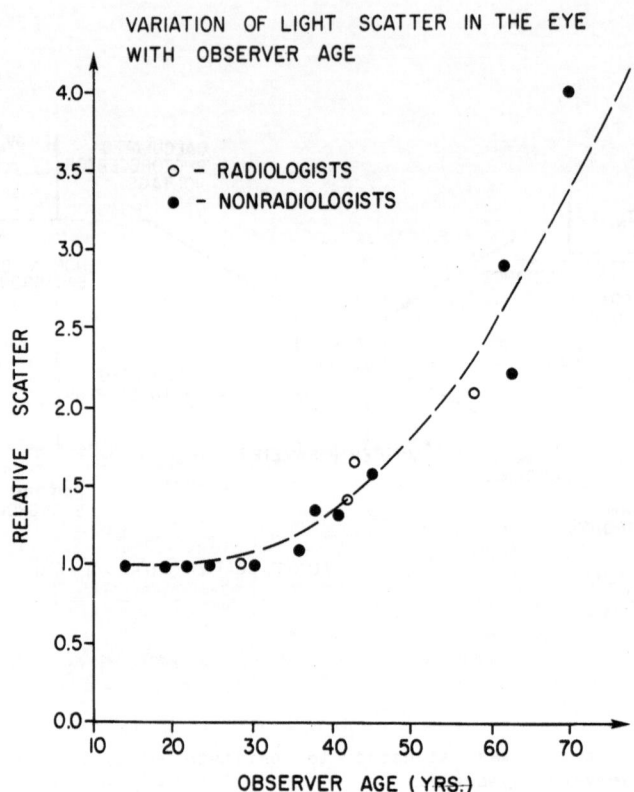

VARIATION OF LIGHT SCATTER IN THE EYE
WITH OBSERVER AGE

Figure 3 -   Optical scatter was found to increase
with age for both trained and untrained observers (B).

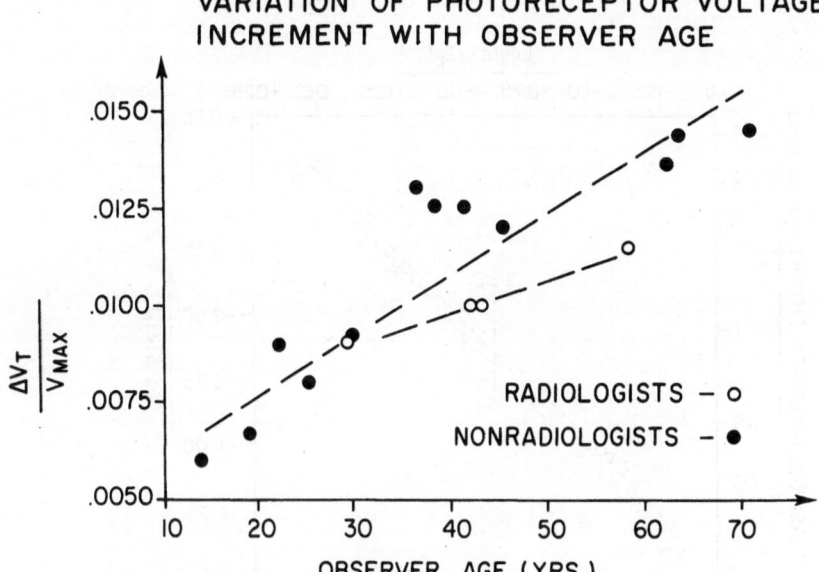

Figure 4 - Photoreceptor voltage increment also was found to increase with age, but the increase was less pronounced for radiologists.

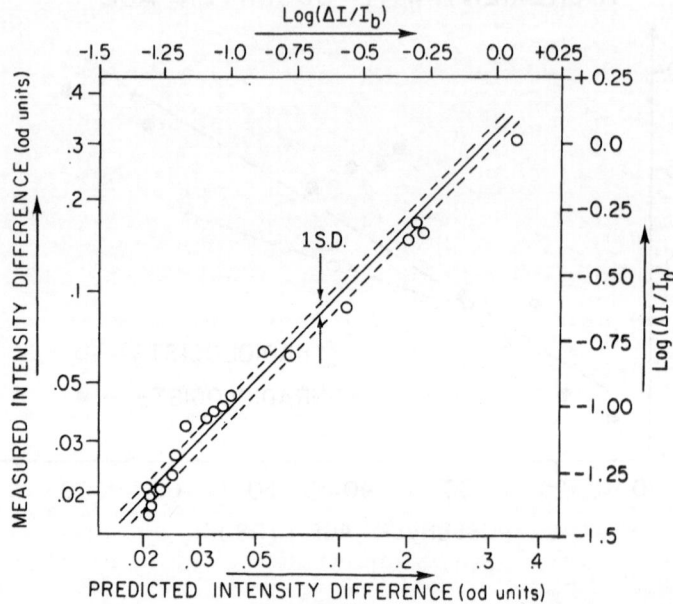

Figure 5 - Scatter diagram showing intensity differences predicted using photoreceptor model vs. intensity differences measured for the observers used in our study.

REFERENCES

1. Campbell FW and Gubisch RW: Optical Quality of the Human Eye. J. Gen. Physiol. 186:558-578, 1966.

2. Gubisch RW: Optical Performance of the Human Eye. J. Opt. Soc. Am. 57(3), 1967.

3. Vos JJ, Walraven J, and Van Meeteren A: Light Profiles of the Foveal Image of a Point Source. Vision Research 16:215-219, 1976.

4. Ravindra H: Diagnostic X-ray Interpretation and Retinal Photoreceptor Properties. PhD Dissertation, University of Utah, 1982.

5. Normann RA and Perlman I: The Effects of Background Illumination on the Photoresponses of Red and Green Cones. J. Physiol. 286:491-507, 1979.

6. Normann RA and Werblin FS: Control of Retinal Sensitivity, I. Light and Dark Adaptation of Vertebrate Rods and Cones. J. Gen. Physiol. 63:37-61, 1974.

7. Baxter B, Ravindra H, and Normann RA: Changes in Lesion Detectability Caused by Light Adaptation in Retinal Photoreceptors. Invest. Radiol. 17:394-401 Jul/Aug 82.

8. Ditchburn RW: Eye Movements and Visual Perception, Clarendon Press. Oxford, 1973.

9. Ditchburn RW and Ginsborg BL: Involuntary Eye Movements During Fixation, J. Physiol. 119:1-17, 1953.

10. Higgins GC and Stultz KF: Frequency and Amplitude of Occular Tremors. J. Opt. Soc. Am. 43(12):1136-1140, December 1953.

11. Barlow HB: Eye Movements During Fixation. J. Physiol. 116:290-306, 1952.

12. Miller D and Miller R: Glare Sensitivity in Simulated Radial Keratotomy. Arch. Ophthalmol. 99:1961-1962, 1981.

13. Weale RA: The eye and aging. Interdiscipl. Topics Geront. 13:1-13, Darger, Basel 1978). See especially figure 5, page 7.

UNIFIED ANALYSIS

OF MEDICAL IMAGING SYSTEM SNR CHARACTERISTICS

Robert F. Wagner and David G. Brown

Office of Science and Technology

National Center for Devices and Radiological Health

ABSTRACT

The ideal observer signal-to-noise ratio has been derived from statistical decision theory for all of the major medical imaging modalities. This yields a context for image performance assessment and instrumentation design and optimization. Measurements on human observers show that they can come close to ideal performance, except when the noise has negative correlations as in images reconstructed from projections. In this latter case they suffer a small but significant penalty.

INTRODUCTION

In the analysis of the sensitivity of medical imaging systems there are a number of structures that are as common to all of the systems as the harmonic oscillator is to so many problems in physics. The purpose of this paper is to sketch our general signal-to-noise ratio (SNR) analysis of the sensitivity of these imaging systems, emphasizing the common elements, and to give some applications of this general approach to particular systems.

THE IDEAL OBSERVER SNR

The concept of the ideal observer is central to all of our analysis. The ideal observer is one who has access to the raw image data at the first stage of detection, and is able to extract all of the information in this data without its display as an image. The image evaluation problems which we know how to solve involve presenting an ideal observer with a well defined decision task and keeping score on his performance. For example, we might show noisy image data to the ideal observer and ask him to tell us whether it corresponds to a single lesion in the object or two lesions near coalescence, as in Figure (1a). This is the generalization of the Rayleigh resolution task to a binary discrimination task for noisy images. It can also be thought of as the simple extension of the signal detection task of Figure (1b) where the observer is asked whether the noisy image data corresponds to a signal upon a background, or simply a uniform background. In the analysis of these tasks we shall speak of the difference signal ΔS, which is the result of subtracting the two alternatives of the binary task.

The performance of the ideal observer as summarized, for example, by his per cent correct score in a two alternative forced choice (2AFC) experiment, is determined by the signal and noise characteristics of the image data at the first stage of detection. In the limit of low contrast images the following expression for the ideal observer signal-to-noise ratio uniquely determines his score (1), (2):

$$SNR_I^2 = \int \frac{[\Delta S]^2 \, MTF^2 \, G^2}{NPS} \, df \qquad (1)$$

This requires knowledge of the difference signal, the slope of the large-area or macro-transfer characteristic G, the micro- or modulation transfer function (MTF), and the noise power spectrum (NPS)--all in absolute commensurate units. These functions of spatial frequency are integrated over a number of dimensions appropriate to the problem to give what is recognized as the matched filter SNR.

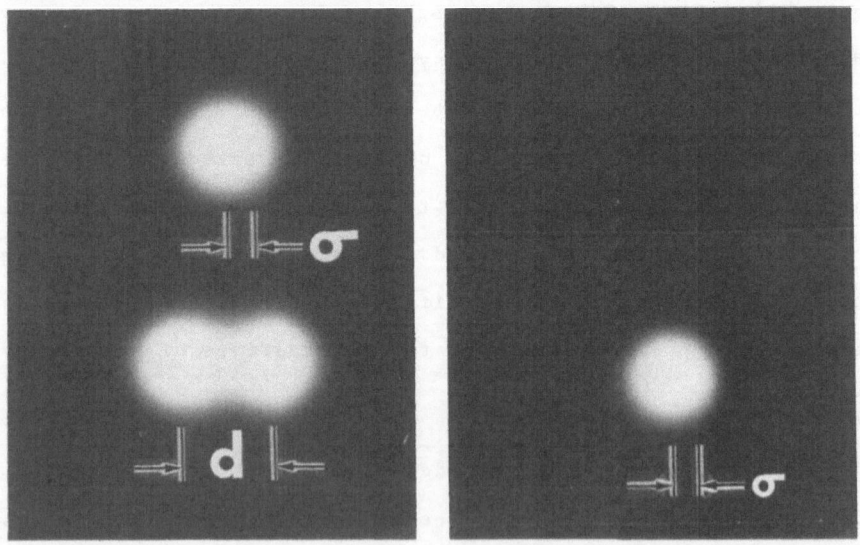

Fig. 1.   Discrimination (a, left) and Detection (b, right) binary tasks.

For photon noise limited images the quotient of the properly normalized $G^2 MTF^2$ and the NPS is identified as the equivalent number of input quanta, or noise equivalent quanta (NEQ), per unit area that for an ideal imaging system would give the same SNR as the real exposure quanta degraded in information content by the actual imaging system (1), (2), (3):

$$SNR_I^2 = \int [\Delta S]^2 \; NEQ(f) \quad df \qquad (2)$$

Most of the interesting radiation physics is contained in Δ S; however, we shall concentrate here on the function describing the detected radiation that is effective in carrying information, namely, NEQ. NEQ is a function of spatial frequency, indicating that the number of quanta available to image low frequencies is not available to the high frequencies. We refer to the NEQ bandwidth as the system aperture in frequency space. Some examples of the NEQ spectrum for conventional radiography (1) and for CT (2) at typical operating points are given in Fig.(2) and Fig. (3). We see that conventional radiographic systems operate with large area NEQ values of about $4\times10^4/mm^2$ and with an average bandwidth equivalent to an aperture of about 0.25 mm. The first and second generation CT head scanners operated with about 10^8 counts/cm along the periphery of the cut, with a bandwidth corresponding to an aperture of about 1 to 2 mm.

The system aperture is an essential concept in the unified view. It corresponds to a distance over which signal counts are irretrievably coupled to background noise counts by those contributors to system blur which do not also blur the noise. A list of system apertures for various modalities is given in Table I. We often refer to the system aperture as the terminal blur since it cannot be processed away by image processing, except in the non-physical limit of a noise free image source and detector.

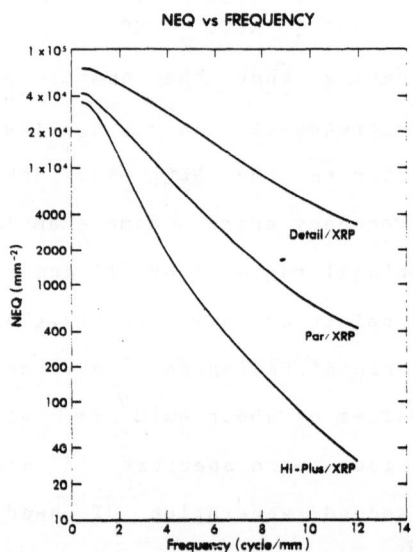

Fig. 2. NEQ spectrum for three conventional radiographic systems
at typical operating levels.

For thermal noise limited images a concept of a spatial frequency dependent noise equivalent temperature can be defined by analogy with the noise equivalent quanta concept. We do not at present have measurements of NMR systems to demonstrate this concept.

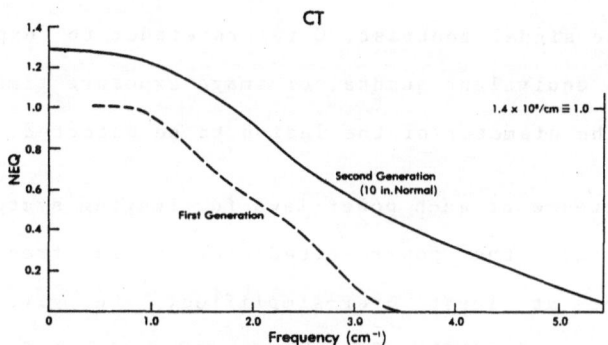

Fig. 3.   NEQ spectrum for first and second generation CT scanners in head mode.

Discrimination tasks such as that of Fig. (1a) have been used by Wagner, Brown, and Metz (4) to obtain new information on the coded aperture problem, where a more general SNR for high and low contrasts is required. They also have been found by Hanson (5) to have a sensitive dependence on the high frequency region of the NEQ spectrum. This emphasizes the need to make accurate image performance measurements such as MTF and NPS out to frequencies expected to be significant in the imaging task.

When the integral for SNR_I^2 of Equation (1) is carried out for the elementary signal detection task, the result has the form:

$$SNR_I^2 = C^2 \, Q \, d^n$$

where C is the signal contrast, Q refers either to exposure quanta, noise equivalent quanta, or image exposure time, and d refers to the diameter of the lesion to be detected.

The existence of such power laws for imaging systems is well-known but the power cited for n is frequently incorrect, or at least over-simplified. We give our rigorously derived results for the exponent n as a function of imaging modality and lesion size in Table II; "large diameter" and "small diameter" regimes are defined with respect to the size of the system aperture, e.g. large means much greater than the system aperture, etc.

TABLE I -

THE APERTURE or

THE TERMINAL BLUR

RADIOLOGY: Focal spot & portion of screen (NEQ bandwidth)

CT, DR: { Focal spot & detector aperture (sampling greatly complicates)

RN: Collimator, detector

NMR: { $1/T_2$
Field inhomogeneity
Chemical shift

We see first of all the general result that for imaging in two dimensions the exposure or imaging time t depends on the inverse 4th power of lesion diameter, and in three dimensions on the inverse 6th power of lesion diameter (6)-- for small diameter lesions. There is always a large diameter regime in which the dependence is not so severe. One application of this distinction is to the problem of "resolution" in conventional and tomographic radiography.

Table II

IDEAL POWER LAW: $c^2 Q d^n$ = const

MODALITY	Large d	Small d
Photog/Proj Imaging	$2 \leftarrow n \rightarrow 4$	
2D CT - line $\int s$	3	4
2D FT	2	4
3D CT -planar $\int s$	5	6
3D FT	3	6

At any given state of technology it is always possible to move from the 4th or 6th power dependence to, say, a 3rd or 5th power dependence merely (!) for the cost of smaller sources and detector apertures--with noticeable improvement in detail resolution without an exposure cost. This has been taking place over the last five years in x-ray CT. It is also possible to achieve this in positron emission tomography. The situation is somewhat more complicated, however, for radionuclide imaging and single photon emission

CT which are intrinsically dependent on hardware
collimation. Analysis of the dose/ or exposure/resolution
function for these systems requires the detailed analysis of
ref. 4.

Our analysis generates the exact form of the SNR as a
function of lesion and aperture size for Gaussian lesions
and apertures. We find the form of the SNR not only in the
limiting cases but over the transition region. One
interesting result we find is that CT methods for NMR
(referred to as projection reconstruction, or PR methods)
using m views have an m-fold advantage over non-PR
techniques for estimating large area or low frequency
information due to their use of m times as many estimates of
the information in the low frequency regime. This advantage
gradually diminishes to unity in the limit of pixel size
lesions. It must be balanced, however, against the
considerations of the next section.

PERFORMANCE OF REAL OBSERVERS

The performance of real observers can be measured by the true positive and false positive scores in yes/no type experiments or by their percent correct scores in 2AFC experiments. These scores can be transformed into SNRs by the use of appropriate inverse error functions (7). The performance of the ideal observer in the same experiment can either be measured with a computer simulation or by calculating the SNR from the imaging parameters. The ratio

$$\text{OBS EFF} = \frac{\text{SNR}^2_{\text{Real}}}{\text{SNR}^2_{\text{I(deal)}}} \tag{3}$$

then expresses a statistical efficiency for the real observer and represents the fraction of the information in the image that he extracts in performing it.

Before proceeding with this discussion, it is necessary to introduce the SNR of an almost- or quasi-ideal observer. This observer ignores the true character of the noise correlations in the image, treating the noise as if it were white. For images whose noise is colored in the frequency domain, or correlated in the spatial domain, the performance of this quasi-ideal observer is not optimal since he

554

effectively makes an incorrect assumption about the
independence of the noise samples. This quasi-ideal
observer SNR is given by

$$SNR_{II}^2 = \frac{G^2[\int [\Delta S]^2 \ MTF^2 \ df]^2}{\int NPS \ [\Delta S]^2 \ MTF^2 \ df} \qquad (4)$$

This SNR has been used by Otto Schade (8), Wagner, Brown,
and Pastel (2), and P.F. Judy (9). Its denominator may be
identified as the unnormalized noise granularity function
(10).

Now we may rewrite the definition of observer
efficiency

$$OBS \ EFF = \frac{SNR_{Real}^2}{SNR_{I(deal)}^2} \left(x \ \frac{SNR_{II}^2}{SNR_{II}^2} \right)$$

$$= \frac{SNR_{Real}^2}{SNR_{II}^2} \ x \ \frac{SNR_{II}^2}{SNR_{I}^2}$$

$$= 0.5 \pm 0.2 \ x \ \begin{pmatrix} Observer \\ Reconstruction \\ Efficiency \end{pmatrix} \qquad (5)$$

The first factor in this expression has been found by
Burgess and collaborators to cluster about 50% for a wide
range of observer detection and discrimination tasks as long
as there is enough contrast in the image (7), (11), (12).
We shall define the second factor as the
"reconstruction/observer efficiency" since, in practice, it

is generally only appreciably different from unity for images that have been reconstructed from projections. In these images the negative correlations are not used optimally by the observer, leading to this reconstruction/observer efficiency loss. (The inverse of the reconstruction/observer efficiency is referred to as the reconstruction/observer penalty (13).) A list of these efficiencies is given in Table III. The values follow from using the appropriate noise power spectra in Eqs. (1) and (4).

TABLE III

RECONSTRUCTION/OBSERVER EFFICIENCY

2D PR (CT)	---	2/pi
3D PR		
LINE INTEGRALS -	pi/4	
PLANAR INTEGRALS -	1/3	

The ideal observer beats this penalty by either using a complicated averaging scheme in testing the image for the presence of a lesion, or equivalently by (p)re-whitening or uncorrelating the image noise before testing for the lesion. A poor (but practical) man's version of a pre-whitening filter—with respect to the CT negative noise correlations—can be achieved by means of gross image smoothing. Joseph has found that in CT this requires first expanding the data scale to maintain numerical precision and then using a filter function with a very poor high frequency response (14).

The smallest value in Table III occurs for 3D reconstruction from planar integrals. We therefore expect to see a re-opening of the question of image smoothing for data acquired by that technique. Our analysis shows that optimal smoothing can raise this factor from 1/3 to about 2/3; the corresponding optimal smoothing for 2 dimensional CT raised the factor from 2/pi = 0.6 to about 0.8 (2). That is, the relative effect is much greater in the 3 dimensional case.

NON-GAUSSIAN STATISTICS

In principle, the above analysis is only rigorous for additive Gaussian noise. However, for photon images the multiplicative Poisson noise becomes additive Gaussian noise in the limit of low contrast imaging, and so the above analysis applies in that limit. In ref. (4) the high contrast case was considered, including the Poisson statistics of x and gamma rays, in a study of the multiplex advantage of coded aperture imaging.

In ref. (15) amd (16) the fundamentals of statistical decision theory from which the above analysis derives were applied to the Rayleigh statistics that result from envelope detection of signals returned from ultrasound scattering phantoms. In ref. (17) this work was extended to the more general case of Rician statistics. The results fall within the general framework given here, but additional considerations are required. These will not be treated here.

EXPOSURE EFFICIENCY

Finally, some considerations of system efficiency and exposure optimization are given in refs. (1), (2), (18) including effects of scatter and beam energy (19), (20). There, the generalization of some of the above concepts to detective quantum efficiency, and the generalization of this to exposure and dose efficiency are given. These concepts involve normalization of the above SNR quantities (squared) by exposure quanta or dose. At that point the distance between the performance of the actual system being evaluated and the physically ideal system can be determined.

CONCLUSIONS

The ideal observer SNR derived from statistical decision theory leads to an absolute scale of image system performance evaluation: it requires measurement of the large area and micro-area transfer characteristics and the noise power spectrum at a given operating point as a function of spatial frequency. (The commonly measured "pixel variance" does not appear in this analysis.) This information can then be used to see how far a given system falls short of the optimal design, to project possible improvements, and to chart the optimization procedure.

ACKNOWLEDGEMENT

558

We gratefully acknowledge the valuable assistance of Mary Pastel Anderson.

REFERENCES

1. Sandrik JM, Wagner RF. Absolute measures of physical image quality. Measurement and application to radiographic magnification. Med. Phys. 9, 540 (1982).

2. Wagner RF, Brown DG, and Pastel MS. The application of information theory to the assessment of computed tomography. Med. Phys. 6, 83 (1979).

3. Shaw R. Evaluating the efficiency of imaging processes. Rep. Prog. Phys. 41, 1103 (U.K. 1978).

4. Wagner RF, Brown DG, and Metz CE. On the multiplex advantage of coded source/aperture photon imaging. Proc. of the Soc. of Photo-Opt. Instr. Engr. (SPIE, Bellingham WA) 314, 72 (1981).

5. Hanson KM. Variations in task and the ideal observer. Proc. of the SPIE 419, (1983).

6. Barrett HH, and Swindell W. Radiological Imaging: The theory of image formation, detection and processing. Two Vols. (New York: Academic Press 1981).

7. Burgess AE, Wagner RF, Jennings RJ, and Barlow HB. Efficiency of human visual discrimination. Science 214, 93 (1981).

8. Wagner RF. Decision theory and the detail SNR of Otto Schade. Photog. Sci. Eng. 22, 41 (1978).

9. Judy PF, Swensson RG, and Szulc M. Lesion detection and signal-to-noise ratio in CT images. Med. Phys. 8, 13 (1981).

10. Hanson KM. Noise and contrast discrimination in computed tomography. [In] Technical Aspects of Computed Tomography, TH Newton DG Potts Eds., 3941 (CV Mosby, St. Louis 1981).

11. Burgess AE, Jennings RJ, and Wagner RF. Statistical efficiency: A measure of human visual signal-detection performance. J. Appl. Photog. Engr. 8, 76 (1982).

12. Burgess AE, Wagner RF, and Jennings RJ. Human signal detection performance for noisy medical images. [In] Proc. IEEE ComSoc Int. Workshop Med. Imag.,

Asilomar, CA, Mar. 1982.

13. Wagner RF, Brown DG, Burgess AE, and Hanson KM. The observer SNR penalty for reconstructions from projections. Mag. Res. in Med. 1, (1983).

14. Joseph PM, Hilal SK, Schulz RA, and Kelzc F. Clinical and experimental evaluation of a smoothed CT reconstruction algorithm. Radiology 134, 507 (1980).

15. Wagner RF, Smith SW, Sandrik JM, and Lopez H. Statistics of speckle in ultrasound B-scans. IEEE Trans. SU-30, 156 (1983).

16. Smith SW, Wagner RF, Sandrik JM, and Lopez H. Low contrast detectability and contrast/detail analysis in medical ultrasound. IEEE Trans. SU-30, 164 (1983).

17. Wagner RF, Brown DG, and Smith SW. Rician statistics and signal detectability in ultrasonic B-scans. Ultrasonic Imaging 5, 181 (1983).

18. Hanson KM. Detectability in computed tomographic images. Med. Phys. 6, 441 (1979).

19. Wagner RF and Jennings RJ. The bottom line in radiologic dose reduction. Proc. of the SPIE 206, 60 (1979).

20. Jafroudi H, Muntz EP, Bernstein H, and Jennings RJ. Multiparameter optimization of mammography. Proc. of the SPIE 347, 75 (1982).

LIST OF ADDRESSES

S.ANGHAIE
University of Florida
Nuclear Science Center
Gainesville, FL 32611
U.S.A.

C.R.APPLEDORN
Indiana University
School of Medicine
Dept. of Radiology
Divison Nuclear Medicine
926 West Michigan Street P-16
Indianapolis, IN 46223
U.S.A.

J.D.AUSTIN
University of North Carolina
107-A New West Hall 035A
Chapel Hill, NC 27514
U.S.A.

Stephen BACHARACH
National Institutes of Health
Building 10, Room 1C401
Bethesda, MD 20205
U.S.A.

David.C. BARBER
Dept. Medical Physics and Clinical Engineering
Royal Hallamshire Hospital
Glossop Road
Sheffield S10 2JT
U.K.

H.B.BARBER
Optical Sciences Center
University of Arizona
Tucson, AZ 85721
U.S.A.

Harrison H. BARRETT
Optical Sciences Center
University of Arizona
Tucson, AZ 85721
U.S.A.

J.P.BASSARD
Laboratoire d'Optique
Faculté des Sciences
Route de Gray
F-25030 Besançon Cedex
FRANCE

M.BAUD
Laboratoire d'Optique
Faculté des Sciences
Route de Gray
F-25030 Besançon Cedex
FRANCE

Brent BAXTER
University of Utah
Medical Center
Salt Lake City , Utah 84132
U.S.A.

Jean Pierre BAZIN
INSERM
IGR - rue Camille Desmoulins
F-94805   Villejuif Cedex
FRANCE

G.W.BENNETT
Brookhaven National Laboratory
Medical Department
Upton, New York 11973
U.S.A.

P.BERTHOUT
Laboratoire d'Optique
Faculté des Sciences
Route de Gray
F-25030 Besançon Cedex
FRANCE

R.BIDET
Laboratoire d'Optique
Faculté des Sciences
Route de Gray
F-25030 Besançon Cedex
FRANCE

Yves BIZAIS, M.D.
Brookhaven National Laboratory
Medical Department
Upton, New York 11973
U.S.A.

C.BLACKBURN
University of Utah
Medical Center
Salt Lake City , Utah 84132
U.S.A.

S.H.BLOOMBERG
University of North Carolina
207-A New West Hall 035A
Chapel Hill, NC 27514
U.S.A.

R. BOLLEN
Agfa Gevaert
Systems Research
Septestraat 27
2510 Mortsel
BELGIUM

R.O.BONOW
National Institutes of Health
Bethesda, MD 20205
U.S.A.

Axel BOSSUYT
Dept. Radioisotopes
A.Z.-V.U.B.
Laarbeeklaan 101
1090 Brussels
BELGIUM

E.BOTVINICK
University of California
San Francisco, CA 94143
U.S.A.

Annick BOUILLER
Tivoli - Centre Hospitalier
Avenue Max Buset 34
7100   La Louvière
BELGIUM

L.BOXT
Harvard Medical School
Brigham Women's Hospital
Radiology
44 Binney Street
Boston, MA 02115
U.S.A.

P.BRIANDET
Section of Nuclear Medicine
University of Illinois, Medical Center
1740 West Taylor street
Chicago, Illinois 60612
U.S.A.

A.Bertrand BRILL, M.D., Ph.D.
Brookhaven National Laboratory
Medical Department
Upton, New York 11973
U.S.A.

B.H.BROWN
Dept. Medical Physics and Clinical Engineering
Royal Hallamshire Hospital
Glossop Road
Sheffield S10 2JT
U.K.

D.G.BROWN
National Center for Devices and Radiological Health
5600 Fishers Lane - HFX-250
Rockville MD 20857
U.S.A.

Nicholas BROWN
The Institute of Nuclear Medicine
The Middlesex Hospital Medical School
Mortimer Street
London W1N8AA
U.K.

D.D.BUSS
University of Florida
J.H.M. Health Center
Gainesville, FL 32610
U.S.A.

Jean-Claude CARDOT
Centre Hospitalier Régional
2 Place St Jacques
Besançon
FRANCE

E.L.CHANEY
University of North Carolina
107-A New West Hall 035A
Chapel Hill, NC 27514
U.S.A.

G.CLARKE
Dept. Medical Physics
University College London
Gower Street
London WC1
U.K.

Sharon K. CLAYTON
Orlando Regional Medical Center
50 West Sturtevant
Orlando FL 32806
U.S.A.

J.H.CLORIUS
Deutsche Krebsforschungszentrum
Institut für Nuklearmedzin
Im Neuenheimer Feld 180
D-6900   Heidelberg
GERMANY

C.R.CONTI
University of Florida
J.H.M. Health Center
Gainesville, FL 32610
U.S.A.

L.E.CROOKS
University of California
400 Grandview Drive
South San Francisco, CA 94080
U.S.A.

Janos CSIRIK
Department of Computer Science
6720 Szeged
Somogyi u. 7.
HUNGARY

Maurits DE BELDER
Agfa-Gevaert N.V.
Septestraat 27
2510   Mortsel
BELGIUM

Cornelis N. DE GRAAF
Institute of Nuclear Medicine
Catharijnesingel 101
3511   GV   Utrecht
THE NETHERLANDS

Michel DEFRISE
Vrije Universiteit Brussel
TENA
Pleinlaan 2
1050   Brussel
BELGIUM

C.DE MOL
Vrije Universiteit Brussel
TENA
Pleinlaan 2
1050   Brussel
BELGIUM

Marie-Paule DERDE
Farmaceutisch Instituut
ANSB
Laarbeeklaan 103
1090   Brussel
BELGIUM

Robert DI PAOLA
INSERM
Institut Gustave-Roussy
39 rue Camille Desmoulins
F-94805 Villejuif
FRANCE

André DOBBELEER
Polderstraat 147
2760 Kruibeke
BELGIUM

M.A.DOUGLAS
National Institutes of Health
Bethesda, MD 20205
U.S.A.

J.DUVERNOY
Laboratoire d'Optique
Faculté des Sciences
Route de Gray
F-25030 Besançon Cedex
FRANCE

Elscint Benelux
Diegemstraat 31
1930 Zaventem
BELGIUM

P.A.ERVIN
Optical Sciences Center
University of Arizona
Tucson, AZ 85721
U.S.A.

R.FAIVRE
Laboratoire d'Optique
Faculté des Sciences
Route de Gray
F-25030 Besançon Cedex
FRANCE

D.FAULKNER
University of California
San Francisco, CA 94143
U.S.A.

William D. FLATMAN
St Bartholomew's Hospital
Dept. of Nuclear Medicine
West Smithfield
London EC1
U.K.

M.A.FLOWER
Institute of Cancer Research
Dept. of Physics
Royal Marsden Hospital
Downs Road
Sutton, Surrey SM2 5PT
U.K.

I.L.FREESTON
Dept. Medical Physics and Clinical Engineering
Royal Hallamshire Hospital
Glossop Road
Sheffield S10 2JT
U.K.

G.FRIJA
Hôpital Cochin
Service des Radioisotopes
27 rue du Fb. St Jacques
F-75014 Paris
FRANCE

K.FU
University of Florida
J.H.M. Health Center
Gainesville, FL 32610
U.S.A.

Henry FUCHS
Computer Science Department
University of North Carolina
New West Hall (035A), UNC,
Chapel Hill, NC 27514
U.S.A.

Edward A. GEISER, M.D.
University of Florida
Box J-227
J.H.M. Health Center
Gainesville, FL 32610
U.S.A.

C.J. GIBSON
Regional Medical Physics Department
Dryburn Hospital
Durham DM1 5TW
U.K.

Maria Carla GILARDI
CNR Centro Studi di Fisiologia del Lavoro Muscolare
CSFLM Ospedale S. Raffaele
V. Olgettina 60
I-20132   Milano
ITALY

J.L.GOLMARD
Hôpital Cochin
Service des Radioisotopes
27 rue du Fb. St Jacques
F-75014 Paris
FRANCE

E.GORDON
Stanford University
School of Medicine
Stanford, CA 94305
U.S.A.

Michael L. GORIS, M.D., Ph.D.
Stanford University
School of Medicine
Stanford, CA 94305
U.S.A.

M.V.GREEN
National Institutes of Health
Bethesda, MD 20205
U.S.A.

Jean-Baptiste GUILHEM
Centre Hospitalier Régional D'Orléans
Service de Médecine Nucléaire
F:45100   Orléans
FRANCE

Hamphrey R. HAM
Free University of Brussels
Dept. Radioisotopes
St Pieters Hospital
Rue Haute 322
1000   Brussels
BELGIUM

D.P.HARRINGTON
Harvard Medical School
Brigham Women's Hospital
Radiology
44 Binney Street
Boston, MA 02115
U.S.A.

R.S.HATTNER
University of California
San Francisco, CA 94143
U.S.A.

E.R.HEINZ
University of North Carolina
107-A New West Hall 035A
Chapel Hill, NC 27514
U.S.A.

Dieter HELLWIG
University of Ulm
Inuversitätsklinik Ulm
Radiologie III (Nuklearmedizin)
SteinhoevelsraBe 9
D-7900   ULM
GERMANY

Alexander Stewart HOUSTON
Dept. Nuclear Medicine
Royal Naval Hospital, Haslar
Gosport, Hants P12 ZAA
U.K.

N.M.HYTTON
University of California
400 Grandview Drive
South San Francisco, CA 94080
U.S.A.

A.M.JACOBS
University of Florida
Nuclear Science Center
Gainesville, FL 32611
U.S.A.

P.H.JARRITT
The Institute of Nuclear Medicine
The Middlesex Hospital Medical School
Mortimer Street
London W1N8AA
U.K.

A.E.JONES
National Institutes of Health
Bethesda, MD 20205
U.S.A.

R.H.JONES
Duke University
Medical Center
Department of Surgery
Box 2986
Durham, NC 27710
U.S.A.

F.H.M.JONGSMA
University of Limburg
P.O.Box 616
N-6200 MD Maastricht
THE NETHERLANDS

Michel JOSSA
Université de Liège
5 Place St Barthelémy
4000 Liège
BELGIUM

Edmond KAHN
INSERM
IGR - rue Camille Desmoulins
F-94805 Villejuif
FRANCE

L.KAUFMAN
University of California
400 Grandview Drive
South San Francisco, CA 94080
U.S.A.

J.J.KOENDERINK
Physics Laboratories
Dept. Medical and Physiological Physics
State University Utrecht
Princetonplein 5
N-3584 CC Utrecht
THE NETHERLANDS

George KONSTANTINOW
Duke University
Medical Center
Department of Surgery
Box 2986
Durham, NC 27710
U.S.A.

H.B.KRONMAN
University of Chicago
Dept. of Radiology
950 East Fifty-Ninth Street
Chicago, Ill. 60637
U.S.A.

P.J.LAMING
The Institute of Nuclear Medicine
The Middlesex Hospital Medical School
Mortimer Street
London W1N8AA
U.K.

Daniel LAMOTTE
Université de Liège
Centre de Recherche du Cyclotron
Sart-Tilman
4000   Liège
BELGIUM

Martin LEACH
Institute of Cancer Research
Dept. of Physics
Royal Marsden Hospital
Downs Road
Sutton, Surrey SM2 5PT
U.K.

J.F.LEBRUCHEC
Hôpital Cochin
Service des Radioisotopes
27 rue du Fb. St Jacques
F-75014 Paris
FRANCE

Margaret H. LEWIS
University of Texas
Health Science Center at Dallas
Radiology, 15.270/UTHSCD/5323 Harry Hines
Dallas, TX 75235
U.S.A.

J.C.LIEHN
Institut Jean Godinot
1 Rue du Général Koenig
B.P. 171
F-51056   Reims
FRANCE

R.LUYPAERT
Dept. Radiology
A.Z.-V.U.B.
Laarbeeklaan 101
1090   Brussel
BELGIUM

M.A.MACLEOD
Dept. Nuclear Medicine
Royal Naval Hospital, Haslar
Gosport, Hants P12 ZAA
U.K.

E.T.MACHARDY
University of North Carolina
107-A New West Hall 035A
Chapel Hill, NC 27514
U.S.A.

R.MARSH
Dept. Medical Physics
University College London
Gower Street
London WC1
U.K.

J.P.MAURAT
Laboratoire d'Optique
Faculté des Sciences
Route de Gray
F-25030   Besançon Cedex
FRANCE

Charles E.METZ
University of Chicago
Dept. of Radiology / Box 225
950 East Fifty-Ninth Street
Chicago, Ill. 60637
U.S.A.

P.H.MILLS
University of North Carolina
107-A New West Hall 035A
Chapel Hill, NC 27514
U.S.A.

K.J.MYERS
Optical Sciences Center
University of Arizona
Tucson, AZ 85721
U.S.A.

K.S. NIJRAN
Dept. Medical Physics and Clinical Engineering
Royal Hallamshire Hospital
Glossop Road
Sheffield S10 2JT
U.K.

R.NORMANN
University of Utah
Medical Center
Salt Lake City , Utah 84132
U.S.A.

W.O'CONNELL
University of California
San Francisco, CA 94143
U.S.A.

C.R.OLIVER
University of Florida
J.H.M. Health Center
Gainesville, FL 32610
U.S.A.

Bernard E. OPPENHEIM, M.D.
Indiana University
School of Medicine
Dept. of Radiology
Divison Nuclear Medicine
926 West Michigan Street P-16
Indianapolis, IN 46223
U.S.A.

Douglas A. ORTENDAHL
University of California
400 Grandview Drive
South San Francisco, CA 94080
U.S.A.

R.J.OTT
Institute of Cancer Research
Dept. of Physics
Royal Marsden Hospital
Downs Road
Sutton, Surrey SM2 5PT
U.K.

Dan G. PAVEL, M.D.
Section of Nuclear Medicine
University of Illinois, Medical Center
1740 West Taylor street
Chicago, Illinois 60612
U.S.A.

R.G.PAXMAN
Optical Sciences Center
University of Arizona
Tucson, AZ 85721
U.S.A.

Amy PIEPSZ
Free University Brussels
Dept. Radioisotopes
St Pieters Hospital
Rue Haute 322
1000 Brussels
BELGIUM

Stephen M. PIZER, Ph.D
University of North Carolina
107-A New West Hall 035A
Chapel Hill, NC 27514
U.S.A.

L.PRONZATO
Hôpital Cochin
Service des Radioisotopes
27 rue du Fb. St Jacques
F-75014 Paris
FRANCE

ROBERTS
Bioengineering Department
Adac Laboratories
255 San Geronimo Way
Sunnyvale, CA 94086
U.S.A.

Dominique ROMARY
Hôpital St Anne
Service de Médecine Nuclèaire
6 rue Cabanis
F-75014 Paris
FRANCE

J.G.ROSENMAN
University of North Carolina
107-A New West Hall 035A
Chapel Hill, NC 27514
U.S.A.

J.C.ROUCAYROL
Hôpital Cochin
Service des Radioisotopes
27 rue du Fb. St Jacques
F-75014 Paris
FRANCE

R.W.ROWE
Brookhaven National Laboratory
Medical Department
Upton, New York 11973
U.S.A.

Biagia SAITTA
Nuclear Medicine Service
General Hospital Castelfranco
Via Zermanese 157/C
Treviso
ITALY

Tamas SANDOR
Harvard Medical School
Brigham Women's Hospital
Radiology
44 Binney Street
Boston, MA 02115
U.S.A.

Peter SCHMIDLIN
Deutsche Krebsforschungszentrum
Institut für Nuklearmedzin
Im Neuenheimer Feld 180
D-6900   Heidelberg
GERMANY

M.A.SEIFALIAN
The Institute of Nuclear Medicine
The Middlesex Hospital Medical School
Mortimer Street
London W1N8AA
U.K.

W.E.SMITH
Optical Sciences Center
University of Arizona
Tucson, AZ 85721
U.S.A.

J.C. SOMER
University of Limburg
P.O.Box 616
N-6200 MD Maastricht
THE NETHERLANDS

C. SOUSSANA
Hôpital de Saint-Germain-En-Laye
Square Leon-Blum 10
F-92800   Puteaux
FRANCE

E.V.STAAB
University of North Carolina
107-A New West Hall 035A
Chapel Hill, NC 27514
U.S.A.

O.STEENHAUT
Vrije Universiteit Brussel
Pleinlaan 2
1050   Brussel
BELGIUM

D.C.STRICKLAND
University of North Carolina
107-A New West Hall 035A
Chapel Hill, NC 27514
U.S.A.

Jerry J. SYCHRA, Ph.D.
University of Illinois Hospital
Section of Nuclear Medicine
1740 W.Taylor Street, Room 2500
Chicago, Ill. 60612
U.S.A.

Eiichi TANAKA, Ph.D.
National Institute of Radiological Sciences
9-1, 4-Chome, Anagawa 4
Chiba-shi 260
JAPAN

Andrew TODD-POKROPEK
Dept. Medical Physics
University College London
Gower Street
London WC1
U.K.

Alex TOET
Physics Laboratories
Dept. Medical and Physiological Physics
State University Utrecht
Princetonplein 5
N-3584 CC Utrecht
THE NETHERLANDS

H.TOYAMA
Tokyo Metropolitan Geriatric Hospital
Sakae-cho, Itabashi-ku
Tokyo
JAPAN

S.R.UNDERWOOD
The Institute of Nuclear Medicine
The Middlesex Hospital Medical School
Mortimer Street
London W1N8AA
U.K.

John W. VAN GIESSEN
Onderafdeling der Wiskunde en Informatica
Delft University of Technology
Julianalaan 132
N-2628 BL Delft
THE NETHERLANDS

Peter P.VANRIJK
Physics Laboratories
Dept. Medical and Physiological Physics
State University Utrecht
Princetonplein 5
N-3584 CC Utrecht
THE NETHERLANDS

W.VAN SPEYBROECK
Sonotron N.V.
Onderwijsstraat 58
1930   Zaventem
BELGIUM

Alain VENOT
Hôpital Cochin
Service des Radioisotopes
27 rue du Fb. St Jacques
F-75014 Paris
FRANCE

Josette VERDENET
Centre Hospitalier Régional
2 Place St Jacques
Besançon
FRANCE

Franklin L. VERMEULEN
Rijksuniversiteit Gent
Electronics Laboratory
St Pietersnieuwstraat 41
9000   Gent
BELGIUM

Dino VITALE
Cattedra di Gerariatria e Gerontologia
University of Naples
Via Morghen 187
I-80129   Napoli
ITALY

Robert F. WAGNER
National Center for Devices and Radiological Health
5600 Fishers Lane - HFX-250
Rockville MD 20857
U.S.A.

E.WALTER
Hôpital Cochin
Service des Radioisotopes
27 rue du Fb. St Jacques
F-75014 Paris
FRANCE

S.WALTON
The Institute of Nuclear Medicine
The Middlesex Hospital Medical School
Mortimer Street
London W1N8AA
U.K.

P.WANG
University of Chicago
Dept. of Radiology
950 East Fifty-Ninth Street
Chicago, Ill. 60637
U.S.A.

Steve WEBB
Institute of Cancer Research
Dept. of Physics
Royal Marsden Hospital
Downs Road
Sutton, Surrey SM2 5PT
U.K.

G.WHITE
National Institutes of Health
Bethesda, MD 20205
U.S.A.

W.J.WILD
Optical Sciences Center
University of Arizona
Tucson, AZ 85721
U.S.A.

J.M.WOOLFENDEN
Optical Sciences Center
University of Arizona
Tucson, AZ 85721
U.S.A.

Y.XIA
Laboratoire d'Optique
Faculté des Sciences
Route de Gray
F-25030 Besançon Cedex
FRANCE

L.ZHANG
University of Florida
J.H.M. Health Center
Gainesville, FL 32610
U.S.A.

I.G.ZUBAL
Brookhaven National Laboratory
Medical Department
Upton, New York 11973
U.S.A.

P.ZUIDEMA
Physics Laboratories
Dept. Medical and Physiological Physics
State University Utrecht
Princetonplein 5
N-3584 CC Utrecht
THE NETHERLANDS

PROCEEDINGS OF PREVIOUS IPMI CONFERENCES.

INFORMATION PROCESSING IN SCINTIGRAPHY, Proceedings of the
3rd conference, Cambridge, Mass., 1973. Document number
CONF-730687, USERDA Technical Information Center, Oak
Ridge, Tennessee, 1975. Contact: National Technical
Information Service, U.S. Department of Commerce,
Springfield, Virginia 22161, U.S.A.

INFORMATION PROCESSING IN SCINTIGRAPHY, Proceedings of the
4th conference, Orsay, 1975. C.Raynaud and A.Todd-Pokropek,
Ed.. C.E.A., Service Hospitalier F.Joliot, 91406, Orsay,
France.

INFORMATION PROCESSING IN MEDICAL IMAGING, Proceedings of
the 5th conference, Nashville, Tennessee, 1977. A.B.Brill
and R.Price, Ed.. Document number ORNL/BCTIC-2. Contact
National Technical Information Service, U.S. Department of
Commerce, Springfield, Virginia 22161, U.S.A.

INFORMATION PROCESSING IN MEDICAL IMAGING, Proceedings of
the 6th conference, Paris, 1979. R. Di Paola and E. Kahn,
Ed.. Editions INSERM, Paris, France.

MEDICAL IMAGE PROCESSING, Proceedings of the 7th
International Meeting on Information Processing in Medical
Imaging, Stanford, California, 1981. M.L.Goris, Ed.,
Division of Nuclear Medicine, Stanford University,
Stanford, U.S.A.